A COMPREHENSIVE GUIDE TO

Budgeting

FOR HEALTH CARE MANAGERS

Thomas K. Ross, PhD

Associate Professor of Healthcare Management
Appalachian State University
Boone, North Carolina

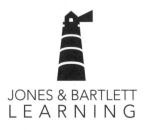

JONES & BARTLETT
LEARNING

World Headquarters
Jones & Bartlett Learning
5 Wall Street
Burlington, MA 01803
978-443-5000
info@jblearning.com
www.jblearning.com

Jones & Bartlett Learning books and products are available through most bookstores and online booksellers. To contact Jones & Bartlett Learning directly, call 800-832-0034, fax 978-443-8000, or visit our website, www.jblearning.com.

Substantial discounts on bulk quantities of Jones & Bartlett Learning publications are available to corporations, professional associations, and other qualified organizations. For details and specific discount information, contact the special sales department at Jones & Bartlett Learning via the above contact information or send an email to specialsales@jblearning.com.

Production Credits

VP, Product Management: David D. Cella
Director of Product Management: Michael Brown
Product Specialist: Danielle Bessette
Production Manager: Carolyn Rogers Pershouse
Director of Vendor Management: Amy Rose
Vendor Manager: Juna Abrams
Senior Marketing Manager: Sophie Fleck Teague
Manufacturing and Inventory Control Supervisor: Amy Bacus
Composition: codeMantra U.S. LLC

Project Management: codeMantra U.S. LLC
Cover Design: Kristin E. Parker
Director of Rights & Media: Joanna Gallant
Rights & Media Specialist: Robert Boder
Media Development Editor: Shannon Sheehan
Cover Image (Title Page, Part Opener, Chapter Opener):
 © 10255185_880/iStock/Getty
Printing and Binding: Edwards Brothers Malloy
Cover Printing: Edwards Brothers Malloy

Library of Congress Cataloging-in-Publication Data
Names: Ross, Thomas K., author.
Title: A comprehensive guide to budgeting for health care managers / Thomas. K. Ross.
Description: First edition. | Burlington, Massachusetts: Jones & Bartlett
Learning, [2019] | Includes bibliographical references and index.
Identifiers: LCCN 2017038329 | ISBN 9781284143546 (pbk.: alk. paper)
Subjects: | MESH: Health Services Administration—economics | Budgets
Classification: LCC RA971.3 | NLM W 84.1 | DDC 362.1068/1—dc23
LC record available at https://lccn.loc.gov/2017038329

6048

Printed in the United States of America
22 21 20 19 18   10 9 8 7 6 5 4 3 2 1

This book is dedicated to my family; past, current, and future students; teachers; and colleagues without whom this book would have never been conceived, let alone completed. I am grateful to the staff of Jones & Bartlett Learning—Michael Brown, Danielle Bessette, Juna Abrams, Robert Boder, and Shannon Sheehan—and to the reviewers for their comments and efforts. The debt I owe all of you can neither be calculated nor be repaid; thank you all. All errors are solely the responsibility of the author.

Contents

About the Author

Thomas K. Ross is a member of the faculty at Appalachian State University, Boone, NC, USA, in the Department of Nutrition and Healthcare Management, where he teaches courses in healthcare finance and healthcare budgeting. He received his PhD in economics from St. Louis University, and an MBA in finance and accounting and a BBA in accounting and management from the University of Cincinnati. His first book, *Health Care Quality Management: Tools and Applications*, was published in 2014, and he is working on a text on applying Lean Six Sigma in health care. He previously taught at East Carolina University, King's College (PA), and Indiana University South Bend. Dr. Ross has worked in hospitals as director of patient accounts and financial analyst, and in healthcare information technology companies supporting budgeting and cost reimbursement systems.

Reviewers

Jan Boller, PhD, RN
Associate Professor
Western University of Health Sciences
Pomona, California

Nancy G. Cameron, DNP, RN, NEA-BC, COI
Associate Professor
East Tennessee State University
Johnson City, Tennessee

Yolanda S. Garcia, MS, MLS(ASCP)CMSBB
Assistant Professor and Laboratory Manager
Rush University Medical Center
Chicago, Illinois

Ellen K. Hamilton, DNP, RN, MSN, FACHE
Assistant Professor
Georgia Southern University
Statesboro, Georgia

Denise Hancock, PhD, RN, LCCE
Undergraduate Academic Director &
    Associate Professor
William Carey University
Biloxi, Mississippi

Nalin Johri, PhD, MPH
Assistant Professor
Seton Hall University
South Orange, New Jersey

Carl Kirton, DNP, RN, MBA
Adjunct Professor
St. Peter's University
Jersey City, New Jersey
Adjunct Professor
New York University
New York, New York
Chief Nursing Officer
University Hospital
Newark, New Jersey

Preface

The principal problem with financial education is that finance does not prepare students for the work they need to perform in their professional and personal lives. Universities do a questionable job of preparing students to select a profession, make major purchases, or file their income taxes. The burden of debt, $90,336 per household, as well as student loans, $48,172 for households with this type of debt, are often-discussed issues, but little guidance is provided to be cautious in acquiring debt or minimizing the cost of debt (Frankel, 2016). On the other hand, it often seems that financial aid offices and federal policies encourage reckless use of debt. The $20 trillion of national debt provides yet another example of irresponsible debt use for citizens. A 1.0% increase in interest rates will translate into an additional $200 billion annual outflow of funds, reducing what can be spent on health care, education, defense, highways, or any other government-provided good or service.

Corporate finance likewise fails to prepare current and future managers for the primary financial tasks they are called upon to perform. Multiple chapters in other finance books are devoted to understanding the capital structure, setting prices, allocating overhead, and securing working capital but operating managers rarely need this information. Managers will need to work with budgets on a monthly, if not daily, basis and budgeting is not a topic that finance books devote significant attention to. The primary goal of this text is to rectify this situation by demonstrating how to construct and interpret budgets and highlighting the cost of using resources. The first goal is to remedy a problem I find in most books and articles on budgeting; that is, their inability to impart the "why it should be done," "what can be done," and "how to do it" to the reader. U.S. universities seem to relish in providing courses such as "Fairy Tales," "The Philosophy of Harry Potter," and "Witchcraft in the 16th Century." This author values competency-based education—teaching learners concrete skills that will be applied, rather than abstract and/or outdated ideas. Readers should feel comfortable that when called upon, they will be able to construct a budget required to accomplish a task. Similarly, at the end of a budget period, they will be capable of analyzing performance: why were more or less resources consumed than budgeted?

Even if you are never called upon to produce a budget, you will live and work under a budget, so you should be able to contribute to budget discussions by asking fundamental questions: what is the goal, what methods or alternatives are available to achieve this goal, and which path should be taken? What production method produces the best result, which method can be performed at the lowest cost, and which should be selected if there is a trade-off between the best outcome and the lowest cost? A naive approach—the best outcome and damn the cost—is not acceptable. Decisions must be made recognizing the alternatives foregone. Is the best result worth giving up other things, or are we willing to accept less than the best to enjoy other goods and services? Understanding the larger picture is the second goal: how our choices affect every part of our lives, the lives of those around us, and the lives of people we do not even know.

My students were uncomfortable with textbook discussions of budgeting that lacked detail and failed to impart essential budget skills. Finance texts devote a large amount of time to who, what, and when, and less time to how and why: who must send the budget to whom, who approves the budget, what procedures are followed, what are budget timetables, etc. Books contained procedural minutiae, and rather than building an understanding of budgeting goals, they covered dry facts and procedures and ignored ideas. As Confucius noted, "I'm told and I forget. I see and I remember. I do and I understand." The traditional approach to budgeting leads to forgetting.

To understand the how and why, my students prepare budgets using different methodologies and evaluate how the different systems and assumptions affect resource estimates. In budgeting, it is essential to understand goals and see the entire process in action, whether you are the CEO or CFO responsible for overall organizational performance or an operating manager running a single department. Budget building often entails simply increasing the amounts previously expended by a department or organization for expected future work—little insight is gained from this exercise. Budgeting should highlight how departments and organizations operate: how goods and services are produced and the resources required to produce output. Seeing the interrelationships between the desired end, the committed resources, and their cost is the essence of budgeting, expands one's understanding of operations, and is the foundation to make organizations more effective and efficient.

The primary question is whether the organization is doing the best it can. Are employees maximizing the value of the organization? Secondary questions include whether we want to produce this output, in this quantity, with

these resources, in these quantities, at these prices. The budget should guarantee that value is maximized, but the pertinent question is *value in whose eyes?* In for-profit organizations, shareholders want maximum profits, employees want higher salaries, and consumers want high-quality and low-price goods. Budgeting is a means to recognize and balance competing interests. Managers should understand the roles of their departments or divisions vis-à-vis the organization, the role of the budget vis-à-vis the organization's operation and mission, and the relationships between stakeholders. Budgets are *information systems*, and goals and resource allocations define an organization's priorities and plans.

This book is not a bureaucratic exercise to show readers how to fill in budget forms. Readers should be as comfortable scratching out a budget on the back on an envelope as they are creating a budget in Microsoft Excel. It is more important to accurately estimate resource requirements on an envelope than to have a spectacular slide presentation with tables and charts that misstate resource needs. The quality of information is the most important attribute, not its presentation. The primary objective of budgeting is to understand the relationship between inputs, outputs, and outcomes, and financial training should impart the skills necessary so that managers can accurately estimate the cost of running an operation. The budget presentation is secondary; a monkey in a silk suit reading presentation slides is still a monkey.

Budget procedures per se—who sits on the budget committee, when budgets must be submitted, who reviews and approves the budget, etc.—are briefly discussed. Managers will find these issues dictated within the confines of their particular organizations, and they will have to deal with the specified guidelines and employees. The procedures established within an organization are more important than any set of general guidelines that could be provided, so little time is spent on these issues.

This text introduces the reader to the logic of budgeting and the types of budgets. When properly constructed, budgets are systems of cause and effect. Resources, labor, supplies, machinery, and buildings are purchased to produce a result. Managers should understand why expenditures are made, what higher budget allocations add to output, and whether the expenditures increase the value of the organization.

Budgeting tools are introduced and connected to their practical uses and theoretical foundations. The first question that should be answered before undertaking budgeting is why the organization exists. An organization's survival may depend upon its employees' understanding of "the big picture" and their ability to build and analyze budgets that advance organizational goals. To impart these skills, budgeting structures and relationships are presented in forms, flowcharts, examples, and tree structures. The multifaceted presentation is designed to impart an organic understanding of what is taking place, what questions are being asked, why it is occurring, and how the questions are answered.

The primary budget question is, how much will it cost to conduct activities and produce results in the following year? The typical response is what it cost last year with an increase to accommodate rising resource prices. This answer is unfortunate and all too common; it assumes what the organization did last year is worth continuing and there is no reason to delve deeper and evaluate performance—life on automatic pilot. Economists assume individuals are always comparing the benefits and costs of their actions and changing their behavior when opportunities arise to increase their satisfaction. Budgets should be the vehicle to produce this same dynamic within organizations.

A budget is a simplified model of a system constructed to achieve a purpose—it describes a production process in dollars and cents. A budget specifies what is to be accomplished, the resources planned to be consumed in achieving this end, and the expected cost of those resources. The power of budgeting comes from this simplified understanding of reality; it provides a lever on the world, where one can ask and evaluate the question, is a change likely to produce a better outcome? Will different inputs or production methods produce a better or lower-priced good or service, lower the quantity or cost of resources consumed, and/or increase consumer satisfaction?

A second departure from traditional approaches to budgeting is the emphasis on economics. The optimal budget provides just enough resources to accomplish the tasks set forth. A tight or efficient budget is the ultimate goal. More resources should not be expended to produce a good or service, because it is wasteful. People are better off when goods and services are produced efficiently and resources are allocated to their best uses. Reaching efficiency, however, creates winners and losers; lower-cost outputs benefit consumers, but employees required to increase their productivity may believe themselves to be worse off.

Adam Smith noted that one of the wondrous elements of market systems is that when people work to obtain the greatest benefits for themselves, they often produce the greatest benefit for everyone else. Striving for higher profits and incomes leads people to produce better products and lower costs to overcome their competitors, and these efforts benefit consumers. Markets work automatically; an inability to produce goods consumers want at prices they are willing to pay generally results in business failure. Competition for resources takes resources away from inefficient or ineffective organizations and reallocates them to uses where they produce higher value.

Resource allocation decisions within organizations are not automatic. Budgets should fulfill the same role in organizations as markets perform between producers and consumers. Budgets should identify and encourage value-adding activities and reduce low-value activities. The ultimate goal is maximizing effectiveness and efficiency; however, the reader will see that incentives matter and managers frequently strive to maximize the size of their budgets. Budget maximization is seldom compatible with producing the best product at the lowest price. Readers will become familiar with strategies to maximize a budget and mechanisms to prevent inappropriate, excessive use of resources.

One of my biggest regrets as an economist is that economics is often seen as irrelevant. Basic and uncontroversial ideas about the role of prices and markets are often lost in the minutiae and controversy of macroeconomic intervention and government policies. My students report economic concepts are infrequently used in their classes. This book synthesizes the practical topic of budgeting with economic concepts. None of the concepts will be out of the reach of a reader who has yet to take an economics course, but if the reader has never taken a class in economics, I hope he or she might be encouraged to seek further economics training. For readers who have taken prior economics courses, I hope they gain a greater appreciation of the information they learned and see how economic ideas pervade all aspects of life.

Economics is the foundation of finance, and the goal of financial management is to ensure an organization has sufficient resources to carry on operations indefinitely. Cash inflows must equal or exceed cash outflows, and the primary mechanism to reach this result is creating a budget that balances revenue and expenses and operating according to the budget. The text provides you with the two critical finance skills that all managers should master: constructing a budget and evaluating budget variances.

You may think that budgeting is more important in your professional lives since many of us are paid to prepare and execute organizational plans, but intelligently allocating scarce resources is probably more important in our personal lives. In our private lives, we control *all* major decisions: how much we earn and spend; in our professional lives, we may be told what to do and how to do it. Budgeting is the same for everyone: what do we want, what do we have to spend, and what should we buy? To paraphrase one of Charles Dickens's characters: the difference between hell and heaven is spending one dollar more or less than we earn; having a plan of what we earn and what we spend is the first step toward heaven.

▶ Reference

Frankel, M. (2016). *The average American household owes $90,336: How do you compare?* Retrieved from https://www.fool.com/retirement/general/2016/05/08/the-average-american-household-owes-90336-how-do-y.aspx

PART 1

The Foundation and Practice of Budgeting and Financial Management

A budget is an organization's operating plan expressed in monetary terms. A budget defines goals, outlines how operations are expected to be conducted, and sets performance standards. Actions are random without a plan or budget. A random action could be possible with unlimited resources, but in the face of limited resources and competitors seeking to steal customers, it is a prescription for failure. Budgets provide a framework to set and pursue goals and evaluate performance.

Budgeting encourages people to think about what they will spend before they actually spend their funds. The difference between budgeting and spending is as stark as the difference between being proactive and reactive. Budgeting requires individuals to determine where they want to be, how they expect to get there, and whether they can reach their goals with the resources at their command. Spending requires little more than reacting to events as they arise, and may be a viable strategy if one had unlimited funds. No individual, organization, or country has unlimited resources, so budgeting is needed to increase the probability of achieving goals.

Budgeting and financial management are often overlooked (or actively avoided) skills in the pantheon of management abilities; that is, they are often viewed as a technical activity best left to specialists. The chapter "Financial Planning and Management" introduces readers to the primary budgeting and financial management functions. The specialist view undercuts those who hold it, managers responsible for planning, organizing, leading, and controlling cannot fully complete their duties without financial competency. Financial competence is having the knowledge, skill, and ability to respond to issues and challenges to improve the economic performance of an organization. The managers' primary responsibilities are assuring effectiveness and efficiency, which cannot be achieved without financial information.

While we would hope that the people creating a budget have a thorough understanding of the systems they are working in, managers are often thrust into positions of authority without a clear knowledge of inputs, throughputs, outputs, and feedback mechanisms used in production. Budgeting provides the means to acquire this knowledge. Once managers have this knowledge, they can then assess what type of budget would provide the greatest support for the activities of their departments. Readers are introduced to five types of operations (cost, expense, revenue, profit, and investment centers) and five types of budgets (incremental, flexible, zero-base, program, and activity-based budgets). There is no one-size-fits-all approach that maximizes value; incentives matter, and managers should use the budgeting system that provides the greatest encouragement to the desired behavior.

The chapter "Accounting and Economics" discusses the obstacles (uncertainty, bounded rationality, and opportunism) to maximizing the value of an organization from a set of resources. Assigning resources to their optimal use is impeded by uncertainty. We often do not know what the best use of a resource is, and even if we know the answer today, it may not be the same tomorrow. While uncertainty recognizes that the future cannot be known, bounded rationality acknowledges that we may be less than clear on the best use of resources today. Individuals must work within their knowledge and experience, and their understanding of customer desires and production methods may be incomplete. Finally, opportunism recognizes that even with certainty and unbounded rationality, the inherent drive to improve one's self-interest often results in the pursuit of personal goals at the expense of others. The choice of a budgeting system should be made on the basis of its ability to minimize and control the conflicting goals of individuals, organizations, and society.

Accounting provides the essential foundation to measure success. The question of viability, that is, whether operations can be continued, is answered by the income statement, that is, whether total revenue is greater than or less than total costs. Solvency, that is, whether total assets are greater than or less than total liabilities, is assessed by the balance sheet. Understanding each is essential to determining how profitability and equity can be increased. Economics supplies the idea of opportunity cost, the recognition that everything we do or spend precludes other activities or purchases and maximizing value from resources requires that they be allocated to their best uses. Similarly, the idea of marginal decision-making recognizes that the return from resources devoted to an activity will decrease as the resources are increased. An understanding of accounting and economics is required to understand cost behavior and reach efficiency.

Organizational architecture and evaluation of department performance are key elements in this text. Managers should be accountable for only the things they control. Readers should understand that a cost center manager should be held accountable for the resources used and what they produce, while an expense center manager may be responsible for only the mix of resources used, given the lack of a clear output measure to assess efficiency. Accountability should also be different for managers charged with selling products (revenue centers); divisional directors who control product mix, output prices, and input mix (profit centers); and the C-suite, which sets goals and investment policy (investment centers). Budgeting should provide metrics that clearly and equitably measure the performance of different managers.

The chapter "Budget Incentives and Strategies" begins by recognizing the balancing of interests in market transactions that encourages efficiency among producers and discourages overconsumption among consumers. The chapter explores the incentives toward overproduction, inefficiency, and overpaying for resources in nonmarket systems, where the recipients of goods and services and the providers of resources are not the same. The chapter also talks about who participates in the budgeting process, what roles they normally fill, and what their behavior is. First, a typical budget cycle, or calendar, is provided to demonstrate when each participant enters and exits the process. Next, budget strategies are reviewed. The chapter focuses on activities and outcomes rewarded in the budget. Readers should recognize that individuals will attempt to optimize their well-being under any system, so the budgeting process and system need to be carefully designed and implemented to ensure individual interests are not pursued to the detriment of organizational objectives.

The chapter concludes by reviewing what a budget is and what it is not. A budget is a means to understand an organization, its goals and priorities, its operations, and its incentive structures. A budget is not an end in itself; the goal is not to create a financial plan but rather to facilitate the achievement of organizational goals. Budgeting seeks to obtain the greatest amount of output from a set of resources and can only reach its potential when all participants in the process understand what a budget is and how it can improve their performance as managers.

CHAPTER 1

Financial Planning and Management

▶ Introduction

There are two types of managers, financial managers and nonfinancial, operating managers. Although the number of operating managers greatly exceeds the number of people working in finance, finance has a disproportionate hold on organizations. Operating managers oversee the primary activities in the value chain (e.g., inbound logistics, operations, outbound logistics, sales, and service) and are entrusted with ensuring the organization satisfies its customers. Finance is a support function that should facilitate the primary activities by providing employees interacting with customers with the resources and information they need to succeed.

The primary functions of management are planning, organizing, leading, and controlling (Robbins & Coulter, 1999, p. 11). Planning sets the big picture: what are the goals, strategy, and plans of a department or organization? Organizing defines the tasks to be completed: who performs each task; how, when, and where tasks should be performed; and who makes decisions? Leading is where plans and the organization are tested; managers should direct and motivate employees toward desired ends and resolve conflict. Controlling is the day-to-day monitoring and evaluation of results and the implementation of correction, when needed. Some managers believe that planning, organizing, leading, and controlling can be completed without reference to finance; however, no function can be conducted without financial information. A firm understanding of cost and revenue is essential to setting goals, an understanding of costs is vital to designing efficient work processes and allocating resources, and leading and control cannot occur without knowledge of whether the organization is on track to meet its goals.

The prominence of finance in organizations lies in the fact that all managers, whether trained in finance or holding a financial position, are responsible for how resources are employed. At the end of the day, bills must be paid, and everything operating managers do has economic implications, from the purchase and use of labor, supplies, and equipment to changing inputs, processes, and products. While managers may have intuitive reasons for proposing or implementing change, finance requires that managers explicitly define how systems will change, and quantify in dollars the degree of improvement expected. Finance provides systematized thinking about means and ends and a method of ordering information. Structured thinking is always preferable to undisciplined thought and rash action but can be intimidating to those unversed in its practice. Operating managers are often challenged by the financial method of organizing information because of their lack of training in accounting, economics, and finance.

If your job is to attend to patients in a nursing unit, run and report lab tests, clean rooms, or monitor government healthcare policy, you need to navigate financial waters. When planning change, it is insufficient to simply claim it will increase output, improve quality, or reduce costs. A financial case should be made that quantifies the cost of the change and the increase in output (or revenue) expected, the degree of improvement expected in quality, or

the reduction in costs anticipated. Accounting not only establishes the rules of the game, it also *is* the language of business and all managers should be fluent. The text is designed to elevate your financial vocabulary and skills, increase your managerial effectiveness, and enhance your ability to understand and interact with finance professionals.

What is financial management? This question can be answered from two related but different perspectives. The first perspective is the specialist view encompassing people trained in and/or working in finance. Financial activities from the specialist perspective include planning and budgeting, financial reporting, capital investment decisions, financing decisions, working capital management, contract management, and financial risk management (Gapenski, 2012). Weston and Brigham (1978) define finance functions as raising and allocating funds and managing the use of funds, including ensuring the availability of cash to meet commitments.

The second perspective is that of operating managers, whose primary responsibilities are not finance per se but rather completing tasks under monetary constraints. The perspective pursued in this text is that of an operating manager with minimal financial training. The work of financial and nonfinancial managers overlaps in budgeting; therefore, operating managers must produce acceptable goods or services and remain within their budget to reach organizational goals and secure favorable performance reviews. The challenge facing operating managers is that although they are knowledgeable in their primary area of responsibility, they are often greenhorns in financial management.

It matters little whether a person is managing a pathology department, an auto assembly plant, a school, or a church; the person's expertise is probably not finance. Yet, each is responsible for economic performance. Likewise, most college graduates are often less than fully competent in financial management unless they majored in finance or accounting, and most never take a finance course. Yet, once they assume a managerial position, their performance will be determined by their **financial competence**. Financial competence is having the knowledge, skills, and ability to respond to issues and challenges to improve the economic performance of an organization. Managers are entrusted with resources that determine the cost of producing goods and services and/or the ability to generate revenue that shape customer satisfaction and the financial success of the organization.

The problem is that many managers do not understand how they contribute to the success of the organization. This confusion is the direct result of how students outside of finance and accounting are educated. Introductory healthcare finance courses cover the gamut of finance activities, that is, the seven functions noted by Gapenski (2012). This approach provides a 40,000-foot view of the financial topography but fails to bring students to a level of competency in *any* area of finance. Managers thus trained, and the untrained, face a rude awakening when they assume command of a department. Once in the trenches and responsible for running their area according to a budget, they begin to understand what they do not know about finance.

▶ Perceptions on Budgeting and Budgeting Perspectives

The budget most managers inherit is simply a record of past expenditure. Managers are given a budget, but many have little knowledge of how the amounts allocated to various expenses were determined, and are expected to complete their work, while keeping expenses at or below budget. The starting point for the examination and mastery of financial management is budgeting. No part of finance looms larger

in the day-to-day responsibilities of managers than creating a budget and responding to budget variances. A **budget** is a department's or organization's operating plan expressed in monetary terms. Budgeting is often a source of discontent among operating managers because of their lack of financial training and the impact of the budget on who gets what resources.

Budgeting competency requires that managers be able to (1) define the production system (the area where they are knowledgeable), (2) quantify expected operations in dollars (building a budget, the area where they are less knowledgeable), and (3) analyze actual results in light of the budget to determine where things went better or worse than expected (the area where they have the least knowledge). Budget construction and variance analysis are the two finance functions operating managers regularly work with, while opportunities to participate in capital investment decisions are rare, and financing and working capital management issues may never arise. In light of this reality, the text focuses on building a budget and comparing actual results with expected performance, so managers can more effectively complete their duties when they assume responsibility for a department, division, or organization.

The text covers all traditional financial topics, such as pricing, breakeven analysis, capital structure, and cost of capital, but does so from the standpoint of building budgets and managing operations. Budget construction and variance analysis, often covered in one or two chapters in finance textbooks, are comprehensively developed with data from actual organizations and the healthcare industry. The use of actual financial statements and industry statistics builds insight into the complexity of healthcare operations and points readers toward useful sources of data from which they can build their budgets and compare performance. (Chapter 15 provides an overview of the more rarefied topics, such as financial reporting, working capital management, contract and financial risk management, and capital structure and financial leverage, to complete the picture of financial management.)

Managers of cardiology programs, physician practices, clinical labs, and human resource departments face different budget situations. The manager of a cardiology program or physician practice may select what services will be provided, set the prices of those services, and determine the resources used to create those services. A lab manager may supply lab tests (a known quantity and quality), where he or she may have no control over prices or the quantity of tests preformed but is evaluated on their ability to stay within the budget. A human resources manager, unlike the lab manager, does not produce discrete outputs or outputs whose quality can be readily assessed. These differences argue against a one-size-fits-all budgeting approach. The goal of the text is to connect what a department does (and what a manager should control) with a budgeting system that facilitates management by providing insight and facilitating comparisons. Roles are clarified, conflict is minimized, and budget management is simplified when budgets are built that operating managers *and* their supervisors agree accurately estimate and fund the work expected to be done.

Budgets are often simply a bureaucratic exercise carried out by untrained and hostile managers to meet a directive set by some executive or accountant. A budget is constructed with little enthusiasm when it is seen as a bureaucratic exercise, another irrelevant task that delays the more pressing and important management of day-to-day operations. Managers put little effort into preparing their budgets when they believe their revenue and expense calculations will be ignored and their budgets may ultimately be set by accountants who have little knowledge of their departments and their operations.

Budgeting is often a contentious process in organizations, a contest for resources, where political power plays a large role in determining funding levels. Years ago, Moore and Jaedicke (1976, p. 555) attributed the negative attitudes toward budgeting to the fact that it is designed to be a restraint on action and spending and that few people welcome limits imposed on them by others. More recently, Libby and Lindsay (2010) reported the four main criticisms of budgeting: it consumes a lot of managerial time and the cost may exceed its benefit, it inhibits change, it is often disconnected from strategy, and it encourages budget gaming. These criticisms are legitimate, but they speak to how budgeting is used rather than what inherent flaws there are in budgeting.

Senior management, which has the most to gain from an effective budgeting process, is frequently hostile and dismissive of budgeting. Hostility arises from the nonfinancial members of the executive staff, who are intimidated by the accounting and budgeting processes and perceive the budget as an attempt by finance to increase its control over the organization. Among operating managers, the budgeting process is frequently seen as violating the **unity of command**: managers feel they must report to their direct supervisors for operational matters *and* to finance for budget issues.

Finance is partially responsible for cultivating the perception that it lords over other departments. Budget procedures are seen as arbitrary and obtuse and the finance staff aloof and unhelpful. The budgeting process is further undermined when senior management abdicates responsibility for accounting and budget matters and leaves subordinates to "work things out with finance." The "hands-off" approach makes it clear to subordinates that budget work is unimportant to their bosses and is performed solely to pacify finance. Managers in this situation effectively report to more than one superior and accordingly feel little commitment to the budgeting process. The resulting budget is designed to minimize conflict and contains trivial, if any, differences from prior budgets, and expenses are increased enough to cover expected price increases for resources, allowing operations to continue more or less as they have in the past.

Once finalized, the budget is put on the shelf—one more task accomplished. On-the-shelf budgets are not integral to the work of employees and are not used to control, evaluate, or improve operations. This is the inevitable result of budgeting where few employees understand the role and functions of a budget: the budget is simply an aggregation of numbers. This all-too-common and unfortunate result can be avoided if senior management demands more from budgeting and is willing to supply the resources necessary so that all managers can fully contribute to the budgeting process.

Budget Perspectives

Budgets are designed and should be used with three time periods in mind: the future, the present, and the past. The future (or prospective) stage is where the primary concern lies and often produces a dysfunctional budgeting process that spends disproportionate time predicting future output and prices and too little time analyzing what actually occurs. Hours are spent determining the amount of funding needed (what resources are required) to carry on operations in the upcoming year, but once the budget is finalized and the fiscal year begins, it has little impact on day-to-day activities. Using a budget primarily to predict future revenues and expenses ignores and negates its true function—a tool to guide and control operations. It is the responsibility of senior management, finance, and operating managers to ensure budgets are not a yearly exercise in foretelling the future to be prepared and forgotten.

The tendency toward dysfunction is encouraged by the budgeting system employed: many organizations use **incremental budgets**, which encourage overestimation of output and the resources needed to complete work. Incremental budgets are constructed by adjusting historical expenditures for inflation to create

future budgets. Other budgeting systems lessen the dysfunctional tendency of incremental budgets, but many people do not realize how systems' performance may be predetermined before the budgeting process begins. *Every system is perfectly designed to achieve the results it produces*—the choice of a budgeting system may have more impact on employee performance and production costs than any other factor. Does your budget encourage effort, economy, and innovation, or does it produce shirking, waste, and the status quo?

The value of a budget is maximized when the present, past, and future are simultaneously considered. The operating results of prior years and the current performance should inform the budget but not dictate future expenses. Present operations should be evaluated in terms of past performance and future needs: what will customers want tomorrow, next month, and next year? Budgets should enable managers to understand where they have been and how they are performing and guide them to where they want to go; "things have always been done this way" does not mean future operations should follow the past.

The budget is an organization's map to the future. Once a budget is completed and the operating year begins, the budget should serve as a management guide (the concurrent budget role). **FIGURE 1.1** highlights the three budgeting perspectives prospectively; the budget asks what resources should be consumed to produce a given quantity of goods or services? After the fiscal year starts, managers should use the budget to determine whether the expected amount of resources is being consumed. Is the plan being realized? The answer should dictate whether present practices are continued (when on target) or whether investigation is needed to determine why things are not going according to plan (when over- or underbudget). Analysis should determine when corrective action is required and what actions are required to obtain the maximum value from resources. The link between the budget and operations is frequently missed.

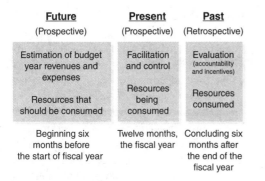

Future	**Present**	**Past**
(Prospective)	(Prospective)	(Retrospective)
Estimation of budget year revenues and expenses	Facilitation and control	Evaluation (accountability and incentives)
Resources that should be consumed	Resources being consumed	Resources consumed
Beginning six months before the start of fiscal year	Twelve months, the fiscal year	Concluding six months after the end of the fiscal year

FIGURE 1.1 Budget Perspectives

Managers often do not see how budgets can facilitate day-to-day control, but rather see them as a burden to struggle against, that is, "I get work done despite my budget."

After the close of the fiscal year, the budgeting process should retrospectively examine performance to determine whether operations could have been completed more effectively or efficiently. **Effectiveness** measures whether the organization met its goals. Were the goods or services produced willingly purchased by consumers? Were the consumers satisfied with the goods or services after purchase? **Efficiency** measures the amount of resources consumed in creating a product. Was the minimum amount of resources employed, or did the organization use more or pay more for labor, materials, equipment, and/or buildings than was necessary to produce its output? In the long run, organizations must be effective, producing satisfied consumers, and as efficient as their competitors. Inefficient producers may produce desirable products, but if their costs are too high, they will find themselves driven out of business by nimbler competitors.

Retrospective analysis assists managers in designing better systems that encourage employees to strive for the organization's goals. It is vital to see budgets as more than prospective exercises in estimating future revenues and expenses. The whole is greater than the sum of its parts; organizations lose most of the benefits budgets can provide when the concurrent or retrospective elements do not establish accountability or incentives.

Budgets can be outstanding tools that reflect and communicate the goals of an organization; increase understanding of the organization and its operations, products, and customers; and identify areas where improvements can be achieved, while providing incentives for employees to improve. Properly used budgets are the essence of management, defining goals (planning), directing resources and processes (organizing), influencing employees and customers (leading), and identifying when change is needed (controlling).

How does a tool that offers so much become an annoyance to those who use it? Part of the answer is that managers and employees do not come to budgeting naturally but are forced to construct budgets and respond to monthly variances as part of their job. Annoyance often results when knowledge regarding the use of a tool is lacking. Notice the number of people who damn technology because they have not learned how to use it. Personal computers, cell phones, and programmable thermostats offer a multitude of benefits if one takes the time to understand their uses and operations, but too many people believe they are too busy to read the instruction manual, and fail to obtain the benefits of the technology and waste time attempting to use it.

Like technology, the key to budgeting is an understanding of its uses and processes. Education is the answer, but operating managers often have little understanding of why budgets are created or how they should be used. People trained in medicine, engineering, theology, etc., cannot be expected to understand the complexities of finance, but these are exactly the people called upon to prepare and execute budgets. Increasing the understanding of the financially uninitiated on the fundamentals of accounting, economics, and budgeting will make them more effective managers.

▶ Strategic Planning, Operations, and Budgeting

Reinforcing budget frustration is the misperception of senior management, which is trained to think about the organization as a whole, and financial professionals, who focus on resource constraints but often fail to recognize the complexities and demands facing operating managers. Senior managers see themselves as planners or futurists, while accounting and budgeting personnel find themselves delegated to be the financial watchdogs of the organization. Senior management is responsible for ensuring the current and future success of the organization. Senior executives must see "the big picture" and provide the vision of where the organization will be in 5 years or more. Finance is responsible for determining whether the organization has sufficient money to continue operations and meet future needs, while operating managers want enough resources to complete their daily tasks.

Frustration is inevitable when senior management and finance attempt to dictate output levels *and* costs to operating managers. A prime benefit of budgeting is to reconcile the department or process view of operating managers with the broader goals and vision of senior management and the constraints and trade-offs of finance. Each group understands a different aspect of the organization, and all views are necessary for success. Operating managers should not be allowed to determine their expenses without reference to the larger organizational goals and constraints, nor should senior management or finance, who may not understand production processes, dictate costs. A useful budget synthesizes the forward-looking, functional, and financial perspectives and provides greater understanding to senior management, operating managers, and finance of the other perspectives.

As seen in **FIGURE 1.2**, all three groups should focus on where their responsibilities overlap (i.e., the core). The core is where goals are connected to resources (whether goals can be achieved within the organizational constraints) and an action plan (how the goals will be achieved, and what processes will be used). Organizations generally do not provide adequate training to help operating managers understand the goals, structure, and processes of budgeting. Organizations commonly provide managers with only enough information to prepare a rudimentary budget and provide trifling responses to budget variances. Operating managers frequently have neither the time nor the information to see the big picture, the constraints on the organization, how their operations fit into the organization's goals and vision, and whether their budget and performance are treated equitably relative to other departments. However, managers quickly learn how to work budgeting systems to secure their personal goals. It is easy to see that when people perceive constrained spending, unrealistic performance expectations, and resources given to others, they harbor resentment against the people and processes that nurture these perceptions and manipulate the system for their own benefit.

Education and openness are key to a productive budgeting process. Operating managers

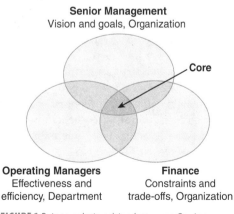

Senior Management
Vision and goals, Organization

Core

Operating Managers
Effectiveness and
efficiency, Department

Finance
Constraints and
trade-offs, Organization

FIGURE 1.2 Interrelationships between Senior Management, Operating Managers, and Finance

should see themselves, their departments, and their budgets as integral components to the success of the organization. They should understand the organization's mission, its chosen means to achieve the mission, the resources committed to those means, the tools used to monitor performance, and the incentives designed to ensure follow-through, a rapid response to problems, and process improvement. Problem solving and process improvement require timely information to understand and control operations.

Timely and accurate information is necessary but insufficient to ensure managers and workers pursue goals in the best interest of their employers; they also require motivation. The satisfaction of doing a job well is seldom enough to encourage high performance when managers and workers are aware that nonperformers receive similar compensation. There must be some added incentive (praise, advancement, salary, etc.) to encourage employees to excel; the budget should provide the basis for recognizing those who perform above and below par. Timely and effective action on financial information is essential to achieve organizational objectives and establish the credibility of management and the budgeting process.

Budgets should identify potential (what an organization should be able to produce with a given set of resources), define accountability (who is responsible for meeting goals), and provide appropriate incentives to individuals to strive toward this end. The continuing demands for government subsidies for Amtrak provide a case in point of lack of accountability. In 1997, Congress passed a law requiring Amtrak to cover its operating expenses by December 2002; operating losses in 2002 were $1.18 billion. In 2002, Amtrak officials said the 1997 breakeven dictate was impossible, and they knew it when they accepted the goal. What does this say about the credibility of Amtrak's oversight? It indicates Amtrak's management never expected to be held accountable and explains why

Amtrak has never covered its expenses since its formation in 1971. Amtrak's operating loss in 2016 was $1.080 billion, and proceeds from federal paid-in capital were $1.530 billion (Amtrak, 2016). The larger issue is what control society has over operations whose managers expect ongoing public subsidies.

Accountability is a bad word to those who believe they are subject to unrealistic demands or who have had the luxury of being unaccountable. Everyone would like to be given a task without a resource constraint; that is, we would like jobs where we could consume as many resources as we want. If everyone acted without economic restraint, it is easy to see resources would be squandered, less goods and services would be produced, and the world would be poorer. Proper oversight of resources requires a standard of appropriate use and incentives to conserve resources.

A properly constructed budget is the antidote to the empty and often mindless calls for reduced spending; it should tell managers whether it is possible to produce a specified level of output, given the allotted resources, before production begins. Budgets more often than not make too generous resource allocations rather than too low or efficient resource allocations. Accountability makes sense only when an efficient amount of resources is provided. Managers who find it too easy to meet their budgets and those who find it impossible have little respect for the process or those involved in it.

Budgeting quantifies in dollars where managers intend to go (goals), how they plan to get there (an operations guide), and how much it should cost to get there (resource constraints). Budgeting should serve planning and operations by informing goal setting and providing standards against which operations can be evaluated and managed.

Who Does What?

Senior management sets short-term goals and provides the long-term vision for the organization, operating managers run day-to-day operations, and finance provides accounting reports and ensures access to resources. Senior management and operating managers direct and motivate employees, and budgeting is essential to setting goals (are they feasible?), assessing performance (is the organization on-track?), and establishing a climate where employees strive to achieve organizational goals (are incentives in place to encourage employees to produce the best product at the lowest cost?). Operating managers and accounting provide the day-to-day structure to assess and control performance. Does output meet the targets set in the operating plan? Is the product selling as expected? Are defects at or below targeted levels? Is production on schedule? Are final products delivered to end users at the time promised? Have costs been minimized? Are customers happy? The intersection of senior management, operations, and finance is a budget that provides quantitative targets to assess these questions and serves as a guide for adjusting performance; it is the essence of organization, leadership, and action.

Senior management should provide the mission, vision, and goals for the organization before a budget is constructed. The budget is the organization's map to its desired destination, the success of which requires managers find and follow the limited number of routes that make the most of the opportunities available. The failure to plan, like randomly selecting a road to arrive at a desired destination, is unlikely to carry an organization to success. Budgets do not ensure success, but the failure to specify where you want to go and how you intend to get there increases the likelihood of failure.

Senior management's role is strategic decision-making, while operating managers are tasked with making tactical decisions. **Strategic decision-making** determines what an organization should be, where it is heading, and how it should get there. **Tactical decision-making and action** is the day-to-day work required to keep the organization on track, achieve its goals, and use resources as planned. Strategic management broadly describes what the organization

hopes to accomplish; tactical management assembles and coordinates resources to achieve the mission.

After an organization's strategies and goals are formulated, the role of budgeting is to determine whether the goals are feasible, given its resources, and assist managers in identifying the best means to achieve those goals. Some people believe that the role of finance is simply to provide funds for operations and that finance should not impose its view on the organization that revenues must cover costs. This view is strong among nonprofit and public employees, who believe they pursue noble ends and should be exempt from financial constraints. This view is as wrong as it is strongly held; every organization must cover its expenses to survive. Organizations must generate sufficient revenues to cover their costs by selling goods and services or recoup any deficiency through voluntary (donations, gifts, loans, etc.) or involuntary (taxes and subsidies) sources of funds, or they cease to exist.

Employees often become upset when lack of funds kills a favored project or requires expenses to be lowered and interpret this as an unwarranted financial intrusion into operations. These people are either unable or unwilling to see the burden money-losing programs place on other departments and the organization's viability. Given limited resources, everyone should understand the need to be efficient and work within resource constraints. Plans and operations must be adjusted to the resources the organization can draw upon. Finance would be negligent if it allowed managers to start down a path they cannot complete because of insufficient resources. Unfortunately, the bearer of financial limits, like the bearer of bad news, seldom gets an enthusiastic reception.

When sufficient funds are available to fulfill a strategy, budgets should guide the management of resources on an ongoing basis (facilitate operations) and evaluation of performance (management, use of resources, and achievement of goals). **FIGURE 1.3** demonstrates

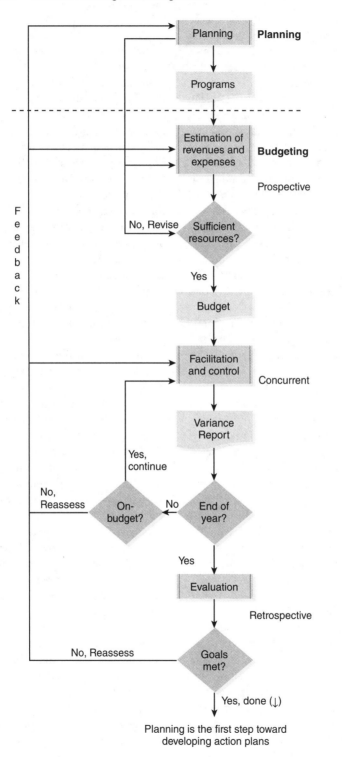

FIGURE 1.3 A Budgeting Flowchart

Cleverley, W. O., & Cleverley, J. O. (2018). *Essentials of Health Care Finance* (8th ed.). Burlington, MA: Jones & Bartlett Learning

the relationship between the planning process and the budget stages and the need for feedback to ensure each part of the process communicates with and improves earlier functions when deficiencies are identified. To operate effectively, each stage in the budgeting process requires different perspectives, skills, and information.

Planning and determining organizational goals is the responsibility of senior management and precedes the formal budgeting process. Planning defines what programs will be pursued, what work should be done, how much output is expected, and when it will be produced. Budgeting, being subordinate to planning, communicates back to the planners whether the organization has sufficient resources to carry out the plan. If sufficient resources are not available, plans should be altered so that they can be accomplished with the resources available to the organization. If a plan can be achieved with the organization's resources, the budget communicates to the operating managers responsible for carrying out the plan what is expected of them and what resources they will have to fulfill their tasks.

Like a thermostat, a budget evaluates whether an organization is "too cold" (spending too much for the output produced) or "too hot" (producing too much output, given its resources) and signals the "heating and air-conditioning system" to provide cooling or heat. Organizations running cold should reduce input use, and those running hot should commit more resources to maintain the quantity and quality of output. When the temperature falls within an acceptable range, the heating and air-conditioning system turns off. Unlike a thermostat, however, a budget monitors multiple criteria and should provide managers with detailed information on a range of outcomes to allow them to adjust operations as needed. The goal of planning and budgeting (estimation of revenues and expenses, facilitation and control, and evaluation) is to improve the effectiveness and efficiency of production systems.

Organizations exist to serve the desires and needs of owners, customers, employees, and the communities in which they are located. In for-profit organizations, the main goal is to maximize the wealth of the owners, whether they are mom-and-pop operations or large multinational enterprises with millions of shareholders. While maximizing owners' wealth is the goal, the means to greater wealth require these organizations to provide goods and services at prices that attract and retain customers. The result, as Adam Smith noted, is that individuals pursuing their own interests serve the public more effectively than if they had consciously set out to assist others (1977, p. 477).

Planning is the first step in developing action plans that maximize the value of the organization. In sole proprietorships, mom and pop are the strategic planners; they not only are employees but also determine the direction of their business goes. If mom and pop select the right goals and follow an effective action plan, they reap the benefits of their foresight and ability to carry out the plan. If they choose the wrong goal or cannot manage the plan, they lose money and may end up bankrupt.

In large, for-profit corporations, ownership and management are divided. Mom and pop may own 10,000 shares of Google, but they are not going to be directly involved in setting Google's goals or strategies. These decisions are delegated to professional managers, who are responsible for protecting the interests of shareholders and may be accountable if operating results fall short of expectations. The performance of for-profit corporations is judged by the equity and debt markets. Organizational goals, plans, and performance are followed by fund managers and bankers, and organizations that cannot attract and retain customers, manage resources, or grow as rapidly as they led their investors to believe find themselves with falling stock prices and limited ability to borrow money. These organizations may cease to exist unless improvements are made.

The concept of ownership is clouded in nonprofit organizations and public enterprises. Who exactly owns these organizations? Who should benefit from their operations? How is managerial performance evaluated and controlled? While ownership and control in nonprofit and public organizations may be unclear, the planning process and the goal of maximizing organizational value are the same as for-profits. Nonprofit and public organizations are owned by the community and should be run for the benefit of the community (versus private inurement of individuals). Managerial performance should be judged on how well the managers meet the organizational mission; while this is harder to evaluate than the simple objective of maximizing profits, performance is still evaluated by the people who provide funds. In the case of nonprofits, these will be philanthropists and/or lenders, and in the public sector, the executive and legislative branches of the government, taxpayers, and bond markets.

Regardless of ownership, managers must determine why the organization exists, what they hope to accomplish, and how they are going to accomplish their goals. Strategic planning should be a continuous process of decision-making (versus an episodic goal designation process) based on how well managers achieve current goals, given changes in the operating environment and control over resources. The budget should report whether goals are achieved and whether output, revenue, and expense projections are realized. Deviations from the operating plan require investigation: What internal or external factors changed to prevent actual expenses from meeting budget projections? Were budget deviations attributable to uncontrollable events, or were they due to the action or inaction of management? Budgets should assist in identifying uncontrollable factors and feeding information on performance and exogenous events into the planning, facilitation and control, and evaluation processes. Budgeting is a crucial link between an organization's achievement and its future.

The first step in strategic planning is defining the organization's **mission**. The mission provides the broadest and simplest answer to the question of why the organization exists. What is the organization's reason for being? The mission determines who will be served and what goods and services these customers or clients want. Understanding the needs and desires of potential consumers should guide senior management in determining what the organization should do: what goods and services to produce and how many of each to produce.

Looking inward, senior management must ask what owners want the organization to be. Should the organization strive to meet the demands of a broad market, or should it focus on a subsegment of a market? Hospitals sponsored by religious orders may choose not to provide services they believe conflict with their beliefs, despite a demand for those services. Senior management and owners of GE saw its future in high-tech products and elected to move out of financial services and home appliances to concentrate resources on an energy-centric strategy. An organization's mission should guide strategic and tactical decision-making and the behavior of its employees.

Unfortunately, the clarity of a mission is often lost when managers attempt to put these ideas into a mission statement. By attempting to be all things to all people, mission statements often degenerate into overly broad and generic statements that fail to define the organization or its goals. Too often, a mission statement is little more than an overly ambitious and ambiguous public relation statement: "We want to be number one in <name of field>," or "We want to make the world a better place by <providing a good or service>." Instead of inspiring or motivating employees, these statements appear as banal as answers delivered from memory by beauty pageant contestants.

A second problem arising from a primary appeal to external constituencies is that the mission statement may fail to provide guidance to internal constituencies. A mission statement that does not provide guidance is not taken seriously by anyone (if it is even known) in the organization. Effort expended crafting a meaningless mission statement that does not define goals or standards by which employees can measure and assess their performance undermines an organization rather than strengthening it. In extreme situations, the quest for a mission statement encourages dissension or indifference. Employees are divided between those seeking realistic and useful direction and those seeking an "all things to all people" missive that cannot guide decisions or actions.

Some people argue that asking for specificity from an instrument that must be broad misconstrues the role of mission statements. The practical problem is that mission statements are sold as essential to the organization's existence but employees frequently see them as irrelevant. An irrelevant mission statement undermines an organization's management, goals, and action plans. At a minimum, a mission statement should provide guidance when conflicts in goals and vision arise and resource limits are encountered. When all things are not possible, which alternatives should be pursued and what should be abandoned? Which of the available alternatives best fulfill the organization's mission and vision? It is not what the mission is but rather what the mission does that is important. The mission statement should unify the organization and guide operations; if it does not, it should be rewritten.

The next step requires senior management to translate the mission into goals. Goals define the operation: who will be served, what products and services will be produced, and what is success? Employees should know who they are expected to serve (types of customers), where operations will be provided (service areas: local, regional, national, or international), and what goods and services will be provided to customers and markets. Management should know whether customers can be provided with goods and services at prices they are willing and able to pay, while providing an adequate return to the people who supply the organization with resources. After goals are defined, concrete plans of what is expected must be developed (**TABLE 1.1**).

Programs are the third and final step in the planning process and the first step in creating a budget. The mission and goals are used

TABLE 1.1 Strategic Planning Examples		
	Nonprofit/Public	**For-Profit**
Mission	Serve the poor	Maximize shareholder value
Goal	Reduce infant mortality	Concentrate efforts on high-profit, high-growth markets
Program	Build and staff a 10-bed NICU. Establish community health clinics in areas A, B, and C	Expand personal electronics product line—international
		Expand consumer finance offerings—domestic

to create action plans that specify how objectives will be achieved. Programs specify what the organization will do: who will be served, how many customers will be served, how customers will be served (the resources needed to accomplish the desired tasks), what markets the organization will operate in, what types and quantity of output it will produce, and what scale of operations is needed to produce the specified output.

The planning process starts with the mission and ends with specific programs. The three steps in planning (setting the mission, goals, and programs) define what managers expect in the budget year. The role of budgeting is to determine whether plans are achievable: does the organization have sufficient resources to operate on the scale envisioned? Budgets do not set direction but assess the probable financial consequences of the directions considered; they do not veto higher-level decisions but, rather, attempt to ensure sufficient resources are available to pursue the chosen goals.

Sun Tzu, more than 2000 years ago, noted in *The Art of War* (c. 400 BCE) that success hinges on planning: "The general who wins a battle makes many calculations in his temple, here the battle is fought" (p. 26). To mount effective action, leaders must understand the resources needed, their cost, and where funds will be gathered—planning must be carried to the level of line item budgeting to ensure success. The following proverb describes the result of failing to pay attention to small but vital details:

For want of a nail the shoe was lost.

For want of a shoe the horse was lost.

For want of a horse the rider was lost.

For want of a rider the message was lost.

For want of a message the battle was lost.

For want of a battle the kingdom was lost.

And all for the want of a horseshoe nail.

The role of budgeting is to facilitate the achievement of chosen goals, and the first step in the budgeting process is to determine the resources an organization needs to meet its goals. Budgeting translates programs into dollars and cents. What types of resources are required? How many of each are needed to fulfill the programs expected? What will the resources cost, and does the organization have sufficient funds to purchase the resources? Planning supplies a set of programs to guide the estimation of revenues and expenses in the budget year.

▶ The Budgeting Process

The first job of a budget is to quantify the revenues and expenses expected from the projected programs, that is, estimate future cash inflows and outflows. The operating plan should quantify expected output: What does senior management expect to produce and in what volume? What production methods will be used, and how much revenue is expected from the sale of output? With information on expected outputs and volume, managers can determine the types and amount of resources they need to produce the output and, given expected input prices, estimate the total cost of those inputs in the budget year. The key question is, will the organization have sufficient revenues (inflows) to cover its costs (outflows)?

Economics poses three fundamental questions: (1) what will be produced, (2) how will it be produced, and (3) who will receive the output? Budgeting is managers' answers to these questions. The first two questions are answered by planning and operations. The third speaks to customers and clients and sources of revenue. Where will money come from to pay employees, purchase supplies, and use equipment and facilities? Will funds come from market transactions (i.e., customer payments, donations, and/or government grants)? When donations and grants are available, will goods and services be offered at a subsidized price or at no cost to clients? Budgeting is a systematic process tying revenues to expenses and the main tool managers use to determine whether the organization can survive, given its revenues and production costs.

Operating managers often only see their own expenses, and their departments may not produce revenue. It is the job of the budget office to summarize departmental budgets into a **master budget** that reports total budgeted expenses and revenues to determine whether the operating plan is financially feasible. If the organization has insufficient resources to cover its projected expenses, the revenue shortfall must become feedback to planners to decide whether to reduce the number or scale of programs in order to match the organization's ability. It bears repeating that the role of finance is not to decide what to produce or the number of units to produce but rather to assess whether the operating plan is feasible. It is the job of senior management to decide what will and will not be attempted when resources are limited. When financial infeasibility is not conveyed to planners or planners ignore resource constraints, the organization is set on a path that can only lead to failure—attempting to do too much with too little.

Estimation of Budget Year Revenues and Expenses

Economics holds that the primary problem facing humanity is unlimited needs and desires and limited resources to produce the goods and services we want. Limited resources and unlimited desires are analogous to the sources and uses of funds in organizations. Organizations must have sufficient revenues to cover operating costs. There are unlimited ways in which organizations can spend money to improve or expand their output, but are customers or others willing to pay for these activities? Organizations could expand to serve new markets, but are resource suppliers willing to

pay the cost necessary to produce additional goods? If existing customers, philanthropists, or taxpayers are unwilling to pay for expanding output or enhancing goods and services, then neither increased output nor improvements should be undertaken. The role of budgeting is to prospectively determine whether production costs can be recouped.

The estimation phase is integral to planning as it attempts to discern what an organization can and cannot do. The first step in the estimation process determines the relationship between revenues and costs: will a program be a net source of funds, generating more revenue than its costs, or a use of funds, with costs exceeding revenue? When costs are not covered, budgeting does not categorically reject the plan or programs but asks where funds will come from to ensure the long-run survival of the organization. Do some programs produce sufficient excess revenue over expenses to allow other programs to operate at a loss? Can other funds be raised to support programs where expenses exceed revenues? Organizations can survive with one or more money-losing programs if they have other sources of revenue, but no organization can survive over the long run if total expenses continually exceed total revenues.

The relationship between revenue and expenses is a question of value: is output perceived to be worth more than its production costs? Value is created when people are willing to pay more for a good or service than its production cost. Resources are squandered when people are unwilling to pay production costs and production occurs anyway. The resources used to produce low-valued output should be employed in areas where the inputs would produce more highly valued goods or services that people would willingly purchase. Agricultural surpluses and below-cost inventory reduction sales are two examples where the world would have been better off if the resources used to produce excessive amounts of milk, grain, and consumer products had been used to create goods and services for which there is insufficient supply.

A simple miscalculation is one reason products are created in greater abundance than desired. Management could overestimate the demand for a consumer good or service or underestimate production costs. In either case, customers may be unwilling to pay production costs. Another reason for overproduction is that some people benefit when the value of output produced is less than the cost of resources consumed. The first group is input suppliers, who receive their wages, interest, or rents, even if products go unsold or unused because no one is willing to pay a price that covers cost. The second group is clients, who receive free or subsidized goods and services and are unconcerned with total production costs. Employees and subsidized consumers ask, "Is what I'm receiving worth more or less than my cost?" Employees ask, "Is my salary greater than or less than the value of my time?" Clients ask, "Is the benefit I receive from a subsidized good worth what I have to pay for it?" Individuals typically do not ask, "Is the good or service worth at least as much as the cost of resources consumed to produce it?" but only ask, "Is it worth more than I have to pay for it?" Subsidies alter market transactions and benefit the workers and consumers of goods and services that are distributed free or below their production costs. Debates on sports arenas are a case in point. Team owners, players, and fans desire public-subsidized arenas. But do sporting facilities create value, and is the benefit to society, not just owners, players, and fans, worth the hundreds of millions or billions of dollars required for construction?

After determining total costs, budgeting asks the financial feasibility question: "Will revenues cover costs?" We want to know *before* resources are purchased and funds are committed whether costs can be covered. Programs specified in the planning phase are the primary input to estimates of resource needs and cost. The budget should determine whether an organization can afford the inputs required to produce the planned output and where funds will come from to purchase resources.

There are only three parts to a budget: output, revenue, and costs. The responsibility of planners and the budget office is to prepare an accurate output forecast, that is, the type and quantity of output expected, so that operating managers can construct accurate expense budgets. The task of estimating revenues may fall on the operating managers or the budget office. If the organization is divided into revenue and profit centers, operating managers may be responsible for revenue projections. But in many cases, revenue estimates are the responsibility of marketing or finance. Revenue estimates are built on projections of future sales and price increases. Sales, units sold, and the price at which output is sold are impacted by the degree of competition in the output market, consumer demand, and regulation. Other revenue streams, such as donations, grants, investment income, and loans, must also be estimated and incorporated into the budget to determine the total resource constraint.

Costs are typically estimated by department managers who understand both their production processes better than anyone else in the organization as well as the costs of resources needed to complete assigned tasks. The job of the budget office, after specifying the quantity of output expected, is to provide managers with guidance on cost increases, the predicted prices of inputs in the budget year, and specify budget procedures and deadlines.

The resulting budget is a specification of the type and number of goods and services expected to be produced, the revenues associated with the sale of these outputs plus other revenues, and the expense associated with acquiring inputs, if not the physical quantity of each input needed. The budget is the operating plan defining the cost of resources expected to be consumed and the way these expenses will be financed. There are two possibilities: revenues are greater than or equal to costs, or revenues are less than costs. If projected revenues are greater than or equal to costs, the estimation process may be complete. The completed budget can be sent to senior management and the board for approval, and if no changes are needed, the budget is complete.

If expenses exceed revenues (or a higher profit is desired), managers can continue to plan the same amount of activity and attempt to reduce cost (is there fat in the budget?), raise revenue (can higher prices be charged?), or revisit the planning process to reduce the scope of activities to be consistent with revenues. When revenue shortfalls constrain operations, budgeting is an essential tool to refine (not direct) the operating plan by providing timely and relevant information to senior management to affirm the organization's core objectives and focus efforts. The budget should define the extent of the revenue shortfall and provide options so that senior management understands the trade-offs faced. A third option may be to run an operating deficit, identify where additional funds to cover the costs (such as selling assets or soliciting loans or subsidies) will come from, and send the unbalanced budget for approval. Running a budget deficit is a short-term alternative and cannot be continued over the long run—no organization can survive if its costs continually exceed revenues.

Facilitation and Control

After the budget is approved and all parties agree that the plan is achievable and should be implemented, the second stage of budgeting is to operate according to the plan. The budget specifies where the organization will be if its projections of output, prices, and performance are accurate (the budget plan is met). If revenues just cover expenses, the organization will be no worse or better off than it was in the prior year. When revenues exceed costs, the organization's wealth increases and it will be more capable of achieving its mission. Organizations with increasing wealth can purchase more and/or better resources, expand output,

or pursue other endeavors. When costs exceed revenues, accumulated wealth is consumed, and if costs continue to outstrip revenues, the organization will have to reduce its scope of programs and may eventually be forced to terminate operations. Given the necessity of covering costs over the long run, it is essential that managers use the approved budget as an operations guide. Failure to keep costs below or on budget weakens the financial strength of organizations.

For a budget to be an operations guide, it must clearly define output targets and resource limits so that managers can determine whether they are efficiently accomplishing their tasks. If department functions are not met or are being inefficiently achieved, the budget should be the basis for determining why this is occurring and how to correct the situation. Performance information must be delivered timely to managers to enable them to adjust operations as needed. Typically, managers receive monthly variance reports comparing actual and expected costs of operation. Variance reports should provide sufficient information for managers to monitor input usage and output, pinpoint the causes of variance, and adjust input consumption to meet budget standards for those inputs they control and to explain the variance for costs that cannot be controlled.

The job of managers is to effectively and efficiently produce goods and services, but before this can happen, managers must design goods and services that meet the needs and desires of consumers. Second, these products must perform at the level desired by customers *and* be offered at attractive prices. The desire of customers for the best product at the lowest price demands efficiency. Efficiency requires that no more resources be used than absolutely necessary to produce a good or service and the output be of sufficient quality to satisfy consumer expectations, industry standards, and/or government regulations. Producing low-cost and low-quality goods or services that no one wants to purchase is neither effective nor efficient. In health care, restoring a patient

TABLE 1.2 Performance and Sustainability

	Effective	Ineffective
Efficient	Long-run sustainability	Unsustainable
Inefficient	Short-run sustainability	Unsustainable

to health is the goal; it is pointless to provide healthcare goods and services at minimum cost if they do not improve the health of the patient. On the other hand, restoring health, while consuming an inordinate amount of resources, is a path to failure. Successful organizations operate in cell 1 in **TABLE 1.2**; they are both effective and efficient.

Effectiveness and efficiency may or may not occur together; organizations may be efficient but ineffective (cell 2), that is, producing a good or service at the lowest-possible cost that no one wants or is willing to pay for. As customer dissatisfaction grows, securing continued patronage will be difficult. An effective but inefficient (cell 3) organization produces a good or service that fulfills people's needs or desires but consumes too many resources. People want the good or service but may be unwilling or unable to pay the price required to obtain it. The organization may succeed in the short term, but its customers may switch suppliers as soon as a competitor emerges that produces the same outcome at a lower price. Finally, an organization may be ineffective and inefficient (cell 4): it produces high-cost goods and services that no one wants. This is the worst of all worlds and threatens the short- and long-term viability of the organization. The only viable position for an organization is to be effective and efficient; the other possibilities do not meet customer demands and/or consume too many inputs in satisfying consumers. Long-term success in markets requires an organization to deliver the best product at the lowest price. When market forces are absent,

regulation is used to protect customers from price gouging and defective products.

Regardless of whether markets or regulation impose control on an organization, budgets are the primary internal mechanism managers use to allocate resources and evaluate their use. Monthly variance reports (Chapter 11) assess performance, but evaluation cannot be reduced to "Is a department or organization meeting its budget?" A major consideration in using variance reports is identifying controllable and uncontrollable costs. It makes no sense to hold managers accountable for costs beyond their control; effective budgeting systems concentrate the managers' attention on resources they can and should control.

If actual expenses are running ahead of the budget, what does this tell us about performance? It could be that the operating manager is not performing well, it could indicate problems in the budgeting or planning process, or it may be the result of unforeseeable and uncontrollable external factors. When the budget is met, planning, budgeting, and operations are congruent, that is, output, costs, and revenues correspond with projections. When operations are over- or underbudget, it signals the need for examination and feedback to the planning and budgeting processes. The problem may be ineffective management; that is, it was possible to achieve the tasks set forth in the budget with the amount budgeted, but resources were poorly used, resulting in cost overruns. When resources are poorly used, managers should examine why this is occurring. Does the manager have the skill and/or desire to control the resources he or she is entrusted with? A manager who has neither the skill nor the desire to steward the resources at his or her command should be replaced. However, competent and diligent managers also overrun their budgets. The question is, did the manager have access to timely and accurate information and the authority to alter resource use? When an organization's accounting systems do not provide detailed information on resources used and outputs produced, efficiency should not be expected.

Regardless of the efforts of managers, when planned programs cannot be achieved with the budgeted resources because of errors in the planning and estimation processes, operating managers should not be held responsible for the overruns. Managers finding themselves with insufficient resources are not without blame, as they should have made the underfunding clear during the expense estimation process. Underfunding of expenses could be due to unrealistic and overenthusiastic programming—the failure of senior management to recognize limits or the failure of budgeting to accurately determine resource needs and/or demonstrate to planners the financial impossibility of the scope of programs envisioned. Managers lose faith in a budgeting process that provides too little resources for the tasks required, despite the fact that the allocations may still bind them.

The integrity of the budgeting process also suffers when too many resources are budgeted and little managerial effort is required to meet targets. When costs are underbudget, planners and expense estimators need to know why: was it the result of a one-time saving, or is it an ongoing situation? When it is a recurring situation, planners need to identify where excess resources can be extracted and reallocated to increase the value of the organization. Budget personnel should also recognize why too many resources were allocated and how overestimation of resources requirements can be avoided in the future.

Upward feedback from operations to the planning and estimation processes is as essential to the budgeting process as the downward communication of goals and programs. Managers who use resources ineffectively and inefficiently need to be identified and trained. When the planning and financial feasibility processes systematically under- or overestimate resources requirements, this also needs to be identified and corrected. Regardless of where the problem lies, the budgeting process should provide the means to identify, inform, and correct prior inadequacies in planning, estimation, and management processes. The budget should serve as the basis for demonstrating to senior management the inability to carry forth programs, given available resources, and indicating to operating managers where costs are excessive. Effective budgeting requires four actions: (1) planners must produce a set of achievable programs, (2) operating managers must accurately determine costs of this set of programs, (3) budgeting must determine whether sufficient revenues are available to cover expected costs, and (4) all should be responsible for seeing that operations are effectively and efficiently carried out. Planners, operating managers, and finance share the responsibility for building a realizable budget to link programs to operations and fulfill the organization's mission and goals.

Evaluation

Guiding and assessing operations is the primary purpose of budgeting; it is where the "rubber hits the road." Variance reports are the tool managers should use to identify the way resources are being used, problems as they arise, and required remedial actions. Monthly variance reports should allow managers to modify their operations *before* cost variances grow to a size that jeopardizes organizational plans and/or are recognized by senior management. Retrospective, year-end evaluation enhances day-to-day management when it produces a greater understanding of the production process and the factors driving budget variances. Evaluation is the final phase of budgeting undertaken *after* the budget year is completed.

Retrospective, annual reviews may seem an unnecessary task, since monthly variance reports have been provided, resources have been expended, and history cannot be altered. This view fails to recognize that evaluation has a different objective than facilitation and control. Evaluation is a means to judge management performance and reward managers who met goals and institute remedial action for those who did not reach their objectives. Retrospective evaluation provides an opportunity to understand longer-term phenomena and improve future performance in a way month-to-month reports do not.

Managing performance using monthly variance reports is designed for rapid adjustment of operations during the budget year; year-end reports assess the managers' performance. Monthly variance reports are subject to month-to-month deviations; it is typical to see deviations from the budget on a period-to-period basis due to unforeseen events that make accomplishing tasks more (or less) difficult. Timing differences are also common, as expenses budgeted in 1 month may be paid in different months, creating a temporary surplus (if paid later than expected) or a deficit (if paid earlier than anticipated) during the budget year. Over a year, month-to-month positive and negative variations should offset, and thus the retrospective, annual assessment should provide a valid indicator of manager performance.

How should a manager's performance be evaluated if he or she meets the budget 1 out of 12 months or 8 out of 12 months? Obviously, this is a silly question, and month-to-month performance can be manipulated. What we want to know is, how did the manager perform over the entire year? Are total expenses less than the budget, and did the manager take effective action based on the monthly variance

reports? Being underbudget for more months than overbudget may provide little insight into the effectiveness of managers. Assume manager A's actual expenses exceed the budget by $500 over 11 months, and in the 12th month, the department is underbudget by $8000. Then, for the year, manager A would be underbudget by $2500 ($-$5500 (11 * $-$500) overbudget + $8000 underbudget). This performance is obviously superior to a manager who came in underbudget by $500 eight times and was overbudget by $1500 in the other 4 months, resulting in being $2000 overbudget for the year ($4000 (8 * $500) underbudget $-$ $6000 (4 * $-$1500) overbudget). All other things remaining constant, managers who come in underbudget for the year perform better than managers who are underbudget for more months than overbudget but are overbudget for the year.

Budgeting should provide an intelligent guess of what the future will bring, but with any prediction, it is likely that unforeseen events will produce an environment where projections are unachievable. Effective management in the face of positive and negative events uses monthly variance reports to alter operations to achieve the best-possible outcome. Poor management clings to the budget, as one clings to a life preserver after a ship sinks, and does not change operations despite environmental changes. The evaluation stage asks not only how the managers met their budgets but also how they performed when events did not match assumptions. Did the managers identify changes and appropriately alter resource consumption when output increased or decreased? The monthly variance reports provide the information necessary to facilitate operational change, given environmental changes. The year-end reports establish accountability and evaluate the managers' ability to adapt their operations when unforeseen events arise.

If actual expenses are consistently above the budget, it may indicate the assumptions used in the planning and cost estimation processes were unrealistic and nonachievable. If actual expenses are consistently lower than the budget, it may indicate planning is underestimating what the organization could achieve. Consistent surpluses (or year-end spend-downs) demonstrate that the budget underestimated the amount of output that could be produced, overestimated the cost of resources needed, or both. When costs are consistently lower than the budget, the goal should be to reallocate unneeded resources to other areas that can produce outputs of greater value to customers and the organization. The problem, as we will see, is that most managers spend unused funds on items of little or no value to prevent "their" resources from being reallocated.

The budget office is responsible for providing year-end reports comparing actual expenses to budget expenses that can be used to evaluate the managers' performance. Was the budget met? Were output volumes, input and output prices, and production processes different from those anticipated in the budget? If foreseen, would these changes have increased or decreased expected resource utilization? What factors caused these changes? Were these factors within the manager's control? Did the manager adapt to these changes and use resources wisely? Individuals who understand the budgeting process and participate in the prospective and concurrent phases should be able to move away from the simple question of whether the budget was met to a more complex understanding of what should have taken place. Budgets are built on estimates of what could happen; the evaluation phase should provide the information necessary to draw conclusions of what would have occurred if the future could have been perfectly predicted.

Use of year-end reports should not be limited to evaluating managers but should also assess the planning and estimation processes. How accurate were output and price projections? Were the projections significantly different from expected, and if so, why? To improve the planning and estimation processes, managers should take a multiyear view of operations and develop year-to-year comparisons to calculate growth rates in outputs, resource use, revenues, and costs and assess the accuracy of prior budget estimates. Is there a historic bias toward over- or understatement of these variables? If so, can this information be used to improve the accuracy of future forecasts? If forecasts can be improved, managers can rely more on planning for what will occur than reacting to budget variances. Information learned in the evaluation stage should be conveyed back to operating managers, the budget office, and planners to improve the efficacy of management, budgeting, and planning processes.

▶ Systems and Budgets

Every production process can be better understood through the lens of system theory. A **system** is a set of inputs and procedures for accomplishing a task or achieving a goal. All systems comprise four parts with a feedback mechanism; **FIGURE 1.4** presents a generic system. A system starts with inputs that are assembled and transformed into outputs to fulfill some human need or desire. There are three primary inputs: humans, buildings and equipment, and raw materials (i.e., labor, capital, and land). Entrepreneurship or management is frequently cited as a fourth input. Inputs come in different grades and capabilities. Inputs are easy to see and control as they are generally tangible. The job of a budget is to identify the types of inputs required, balance the cost of inputs against their capabilities, and determine how much of each input is required to produce a given level of output.

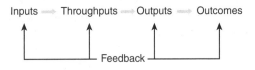

FIGURE 1.4 A Generic System

The second stage of a system transforms inputs into outputs. The throughput process encompasses everything required to coordinate the production process—policies, procedures, management, algorithms, recipes, etc. Throughputs are often intangible and difficult to conceptualize. Some throughput processes are "black boxes," as it is easy to see the inputs going into a black box and the outputs that emerge, but there remains some mystery as to what happens to transform the inputs to outputs. Management is a black box, what exactly is management? Management involves motivating others to accomplish tasks, but what motivates people? Motivational techniques vary by manager, and a manager may employ different techniques on different employees in different situations or the same employees in different situations. What happens within a black-box system is often nondeterministic, meaning neither performance nor output can be predicted with certainty.

In some industries, like automobile production, the throughput process is a "white box," that is, the amount and type of inputs are known and the production steps are well established. In white-box systems, it is easy to determine when excessive resource use occurs or when steps are missed, duplicated, performed poorly, or done out of sequence. In white-box systems, throughputs are easy to manage; in black-box systems, control often focuses on inputs or outputs as they are more easily quantified.

In most systems, it is easy to determine when the production process is completed and an output is produced. Products can be counted as they come off the assembly line and services when the interaction with the consumer ends (a physician visit begins when the patient appears at the office and ends when the patient leaves). Outputs are generally measurable: one sees the number of patients seen, students graduated, or widgets produced. It is natural to evaluate the input and throughput processes at this point since outputs are easy to count and evaluate. Complications arise with nontangible services, or services whose quality is difficult to define and measure. Effective control over the production process requires an output measure that captures the amount and quality of work performed and is accepted as valid by employees.

The effectiveness and efficiency of inputs, throughput processes, and outputs may be for naught if the organization is not producing a good or service that meets a real or perceived need. The essential measure of success for any organization is how well it meets a human need or desire, that is, what outcome is produced. Outcomes, like throughputs, are more difficult to measure than inputs or outputs. Outcomes for goods and services transacted in markets can be assessed by the ability to sell outputs at a price above cost. In voluntary market transactions, managers can ask whether customers were willing to pay the full cost of a product or whether customers believed the product was worth at least as much as they had to pay for it.

In health care, the number of patients seen or tests run is known, but do we know whether patients are better off? Did the health status or quality of life improve because of the care rendered? A better measure of healthcare success would determine whether patients were satisfied with the care they received and whether they perceived their life as better 1 year after receiving care. Ernest Codman recommended this standard in 1914, yet health care continues to evaluate patient satisfaction at the point of service (Codman, 1914). The ability to measure outcomes accurately and at the appropriate time is essential to enable managers to modify inputs, throughputs, or outputs to increase customer satisfaction.

Feedback loops are designed to keep systems coordinated and allow employees to improve outputs and outcomes by identifying problems and concerns so that corrections or enhancements can be made as early as possible in the production process. If the output does not produce the desired outcome, the feedback loop should focus the search for problems: Is the problem at the point of output (the wrong good or service is being produced), in the throughput process (production errors or problems are reducing the value of the output produced), or with inputs (improper or inadequate inputs are being employed, making it impossible to deliver a good product)?

The goal is to identify problems before substandard goods and services disappoint customers. Information on system performance should allow managers to pinpoint whether it is a problem with inputs, throughputs, or outputs that results in poor outcomes, customer dissatisfaction, low revenue, and/or high costs. Higher-than-expected usage of labor hours, supplies, machine time, etc., may indicate that substandard inputs are hampering the transformation process or the transformation process is operating suboptimally. Examining defective or deficient outputs allows employees to identify substandard performance, but discovery at this point does not allow corrective action before the production process is complete. Effective inspection of outputs can prevent the unknowing sale or delivery of substandard products to customers but requires duplicate efforts to correct defects. Properly constructed and used budgets allow managers to compare actual operating results with the expected standards and make timely system changes. As more information is typically better than less and as information is more valuable when received early in a process, managers should strive for prevention rather than detection of defects.

Management should facilitate production processes by ensuring the availability of inputs, the efficiency of the transformation process, and the quality of outputs and by ensuring that the output fulfills some need or desire. Feedback is essential to determine when system performance is substandard, identify the source of deficiency, and move the process to a level of performance that satisfies customers.

Three budget functions were identified: the first prospectively determines what it should cost to produce the types and quantity of goods and services set out by planning and whether the organization can generate sufficient revenue to purchase the resources necessary to produce the expected output. The operating plan, the approved budget, includes a set of inputs, production procedures, and total cost and establishes standards against which operations should be measured. The second, concurrent function of the budget facilitates day-to-day control over operations by providing information on actual performance and standards: is the process operating as expected? This question deals with the quantities and costs of inputs used, the outputs produced, and the outcomes achieved and should provide timely information to managers so that corrective action can be taken before resources are squandered. The last function is retrospective evaluation undertaken with a full year of data so that temporary fluctuations are minimized and performance can be fairly assessed. Were organizational goals achieved? Who, if anyone, is responsible for positive and negative deviations from the budget? What incentives are in place to tie organizational and employee goals together? System theory allows managers to move beyond analysis (what is happening) to synthesis (how thing work together toward a common goal).

Budgeting Systems

The primary focus of a budgeting system is typically on one point of a system or production process (**FIGURE 1.5**). Incremental budgeting (Chapter 6) focuses on the use of inputs. A major reason incremental budgets are used is that inputs are easy to measure and building a budget does not require comprehensive insight into production processes. The goal of incremental budgeting is to prevent the waste of inputs, or, more accurately, to ensure no more resources are used than budgeted. The job of a manager is to ensure all inputs purchased are employed in producing a good or service, that is, employees are working their scheduled hours, supplies have not been wasted or diverted to other uses, etc.

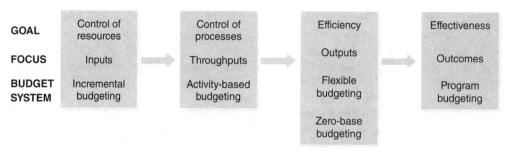

FIGURE 1.5 Budgeting Systems

The problem with incremental budgeting is that although employees may be at their appointed positions and resources may not be diverted, they may not be employed efficiently or effectively in the production process. The goal of flexible budgeting (Chapter 7) and zero-base budgeting (Chapter 8) is to ensure resources are used efficiently: not only should resources be in place, but no more should be employed than are necessary. This requires a greater understanding of the production process and the relationships between inputs and outputs. How many labor hours are required per output produced to ensure high-quality output? Flexible and zero-base budgets establish incentives for operating managers to minimize the cost per output produced.

Producing an output at the lowest-possible cost does not guarantee that anyone will want the output, so program budgeting (Chapter 9) shifts to a focus on outcomes. Program budgets are built around desired outcomes and attempt to quantify the impact of outputs on customers. Are customers satisfied, did they obtain the benefit they sought or expected, and will they continue to patronize the organization? Under program budgeting, managers are encouraged to maximize outcomes, including producing at the lowest-possible cost and possibly employing more resources when more or better outcomes can be produced at a low cost.

Activity-based budgeting (Chapter 10) adds realism to the budgeting process by recognizing that not all activities are created equal. A focus on outputs or outcomes ignores how they are produced, and activity-based budgeting identifies what employees do and for whom. In a hospital, the cost of providing inpatient care varies by patient, provider, and/or payer. For example, elderly patients may require a broader range of services, more services, and additional time to complete common services. Activity-based budgets recognize that changes in customers (the ratio of elderly to nonelderly patients) may have a profound effect on resource use, even if the number of admissions or patient days does not change. Activity-based budgeting focuses on throughputs and provides a basis for more effective management of resources and a differential pricing system that recognizes process and cost differences between customers.

The search for an effective way to monitor the totality of an organization's operations led to the development of **balanced scorecards** (Kaplan & Norton, 2000). Budgeting systems focus on one part of a system (inputs, throughputs, outputs, or outcomes) and the relationship between revenues and cost, whereas balanced scorecards examine the organization from four perspectives: financial, customer, internal or process, and learning and growth (**FIGURE 1.6**).

Balanced scorecards assess an organization's ability to pursue its goals. A balanced scorecard is a pyramid, with the pinnacle, or goal, of earning sufficient profits (or maximizing the value of the organization) to allow the organization to survive and thrive. The profit perspective asks the overarching question, is

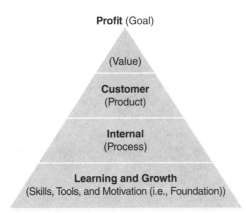

FIGURE 1.6 The Balanced Scorecard Pyramid

the organization meeting its goal? Are revenues greater than expenses, and is value being created? Sustained profit requires satisfied customers, so balanced scorecards identify, monitor, and encourage things that customers value (level 2). Measures of how well the organization delivers products that satisfy customers include satisfaction surveys, an expanding customer base (an increase in the number of customers), an increase in the percentage of repeat customers (do past customers return?), and a larger market share.

The profit and customer perspectives rest upon internal processes (level 3), or how the organization delivers products that satisfy customers. Customers seek effective and efficient internal processes, as evidenced by low prices based on cost minimization, timeliness, and high reliability. The learning and growth perspective (level 4) recognizes that the world is continually in a state of flux and organizations have to adapt to change or be left behind. Although profits and customer satisfaction may be high today, this does not guarantee future success. Changing consumer tastes and preferences, new technology, and the emergence of new competitors and products sink organizations that fail to recognize and respond to changes. The learning and growth perspective asks what an organization needs to ensure effective and efficient processes. Changing consumer preferences and technology require

organizations to have the ability to anticipate and react to change; develop capable employees through training, education, and high performance standards; and provide workers with the right tools (information, equipment, etc.) to maximize their performance.

Balanced scorecards identify the major areas that determine an organization's success, but at this point, they do not tie these factors to resource allocation. Most budgeting systems do not take the comprehensive view that balanced scorecards pursue, although activity-based budgeting comes closest to a holistic understanding of how organizations operate, while program budgeting emphasizes outcomes received by customers. A balanced scorecard is not a substitute for budgeting, but it is clear that its emphases (the cost of satisfying customers, effective and efficient processes, and learning) can improve planning, management, and budgeting.

▶ Evaluating Performance

The existence of for-profit organizations is based on their ability to generate adequate returns for their owners. Suppliers of inputs continually evaluate how their resources are employed, and economists utilize the concept of **opportunity cost**, the alternative foregone, to analyze resource allocation choices. This concept is helpful in understanding how individuals and organizations should approach budgeting decisions.

A mom-and-pop operation may choose to close its doors if the monetary return the business produces is less than what it can earn by employing their labor and capital in another type of business or working for someone else. As long as mom and pop earn more for the time and resources they invest in their business than they could earn by working for Google (or another employer) and putting their nonlabor resources into income-earning assets, they continue their business. At the point where they can earn more by working for Google, say, and lending their capital to others, they may alter the employment of their resources. Of course, there are intrinsic benefits from running your own business, and being your own boss can outweigh marginal income differences.

Large, publicly held corporations face the same constraints: do operating profits keep stockholders and lenders satisfied? If stockholders foresee that earnings may not be equal to comparable investments, they sell their stock (driving down its price) and reinvest in other companies (driving up the price of their stock). The continual re-evaluation and repricing of investments in equity markets produce comparable returns for comparable risks, and the only way to earn higher income is to invest in riskier ventures. Managers face the same trade-off when constructing budgets: which programs and processes add the most value to the organization, which should be funded, and how much funding should each receive?

Value matters. This is the bottom line of budgeting: what is the relationship between the benefits and cost of production? Are the benefits of production sufficient to justify the resources employed? In for-profit organizations, this rule can be reduced to whether the organization is earning an adequate profit for the risk assumed. If returns are inadequate, for-profits have two options: they can increase revenues and/or decrease expenses to improve operating results or go out of business. Organizations with inadequate returns on the resources employed who do not take effective action will see their resources involuntarily redeployed to uses that are more profitable. The marvel of markets is they operate automatically: well-managed organizations are rewarded with higher stock prices and lower interest rates, while poorly managed operations see stock prices decline and interest rates increase. The efficient allocation of resources does not require an expert or czar but functions because individuals desire the highest return for their resources and maximize their well-being by moving resources from low-yield to high-yield investments.

Profits are a simple means to understand the value of an organization and where resources should be increased and reduced. Resource decisions are less clear in nonprofits and public organizations, where profit signals are absent. The goal of maximizing value remains, but how does one measure the value of nonmarket transacted goods and services produced by nonprofit and public organizations? Overlooking this measurement issue, if a nonprofit is ineffective, inefficient, or both, it is in jeopardy of losing its customers to other organizations that can produce a higher-quality good or service at a lower price. Ineffective and/or inefficient nonprofits will have difficulty raising capital through donations or debt markets. Nonprofits cannot raise capital through equity markets and are regulated by the same mechanism as for-profits in debt markets. Lenders will analyze nonprofit operations to determine whether debt is likely to be repaid, and nonprofits that cannot cover their expenses will be unlikely to get loans. Similarly, philanthropists wanting to achieve a certain goal, for example, maximizing health or knowledge, will seek medical or education institutions that they think are best able to meet their desired outcome. Institutions that waste resources, that is, produce a small amount of goods and services for the resources employed, will see their donations redirected to more effective and efficient institutions.

The exception to this rule is public agencies. Government agencies do not have to operate effectively or efficiently, since they rely on public financing. Their revenues do not come from voluntary transactions with customers, investors, lenders, or philanthropists but from compulsory taxes, and inefficient performance is more likely to produce higher taxes than discontinuation of operations. Ineffective or non client-satisfying performance is also unlikely to lead to agency failure. The ballot box regulates public operations, but it is questionable how effective this mechanism is in minimizing production costs or maximizing client services. The main problem is that the interests of the two primary beneficiaries of free or subsidized government services, clients receiving the goods and services and public employees paid to produce the outputs, have an interest in continuing or expanding programs regardless of performance, since they receive large benefits and provide little, if any, of the resources required to fund operations.

▶ The Benefits of Budgeting

A well-structured and well-understood budget provides multiple benefits for its customers, owners, and employees. First, the budgeting process is a means to educate employees on how the organization operates. The process of allocating resources, managing to a budget, and evaluating year-end results should provide employees with a greater understanding of the organization's sources of revenue, inputs and input costs, operations, outputs, and outcomes (**BOX 1.1**).

The second benefit is securing the involvement and buy-in of employees. The involvement of operating managers is crucial to the

construction of realistic budgets, as they have the best understanding of their operations. Their involvement provides an opportunity to educate senior management and finance on their departments' processes. Senior management and finance operate at the organizational rather than the departmental level, focus on different matters, and often have a minimal understanding of operating department processes. This knowledge problem is often more severe in large and diversified organizations. The involvement of operating managers in the budgeting process is essential for cultivating their attachment to the plan and maximizing the usefulness of the budget.

Third, the budget is a means to communicate the organization's priorities to internal and external constituencies. The budget shows what the organization intends to accomplish, and budget allocations demonstrate management's commitment to goals. Managers committed to building a customer-friendly organization will devote resources and have a plan to cultivate and monitor the behaviors required to meet such a goal. A $4 million allocation toward achieving a goal demonstrates greater commitment to the activity than a budget of $1 million. An organization's mission statement may emphasize increasing employee wellness, but if the budget allocates only $500,000 to wellness programs out of a total budget of $100 million, one-half of 1%, is it really a priority? Budget allocations demonstrate management's commitment in dollars and provide the means by which the organization expects to achieve its goals.

The budget demonstrates what is important to managers and where they will focus their attention and efforts. The selection of a budgeting system tells employees what is going to be measured (i.e., inputs, outputs, outcomes, or activities) and how it will be measured, and may establish the metrics for employee performance evaluation. Incremental budgets create cost awareness, flexible and zero-base budgets emphasize productivity, program budgets focus on outcomes, and activity-based

---

BOX 1.1 The Benefits of Budgeting

- Educating employees on how the organization works
- Securing the employees' buy-in through their participation in budget construction
- Communicating organizational goals and priorities
- Establishing performance measures (what is important, and what will be monitored)
- Elevating the organizational view above department perspectives
- Establishing an operational plan
- Setting a standard for evaluation

budgets aim at controlling work processes. What is measured gets attention, and the budgeting system chosen can increase or reduce accountability. Accountability is essential to achieving the objectives of the organization and is diminished or lost when focus is placed on less relevant but more easily measured factors. Healthcare organizations should target improving health (an outcome) rather than increasing the number of admissions, patient days, surgeries, or office visits (outputs), while educational organizations should focus on increasing the knowledge and skills of students rather than graduation rates.

The master budget highlights the need to cover costs; unfortunately, managers in non-revenue-generating departments often do not see the necessity of balancing revenues and expenses and develop an incomplete and naive view of the organization and its constraints. Without profit, or excess revenue over expenses, organizations do not survive. The saying "no margin, no mission" neatly encapsulates this thought; organizations that cannot cover their expenses will be unable to serve their customers or clients, owners, or employees over the long run.

Budgets should make employees and others aware of the necessity of producing adequate returns on investment that allow capital to be replaced as it wears out. Revenues equal to expenses is not a sustainable position. Assume a building was constructed in 1988 and needs to be replaced in 2018. Its replacement cost will be substantially higher than its original construction cost because of an increase in the price of raw materials and wages, as well as more stringent building codes. Budgets should raise employee awareness of the constraints and trade-offs facing the organization. When an organization chooses to operate programs at a loss, the budget should indicate where funds will come from to pay the unmet expenses and replace capital. Understanding the totality of an organization's economic situation should encourage employees to take actions consistent with its long-term survival and emphasize the tie between their individual interests and behavior and the well-being of the organization.

The budget is an operational plan that plans, guides, sets expectations, minimizes surprises, avoids shortages and excesses, and moves the organization toward its desired future. Employees should continuously evaluate performance using variance reports to make timely alterations to input use, production processes, and output to meet internal standards and external demands.

Lastly, the budget provides the standard for evaluating performance: was the plan followed? Against this standard, managers should be able to identify what went according to plan, better than expected, and worse than expected. When better- or worse-than-expected results arise, managers should identify the causes of favorable and unfavorable changes to continue the former and avoid the later, when possible. Budgeting is a tool for establishing expectations and interpreting actual performance, improving future performance, and evaluating and compensating employees.

The introduction to financial planning and management began by describing the problems impeding the effective development and use of budgets, and it concludes with the advantages that accrue to organizations that fully utilize budgets. Budgeting is often reviled within organizations as a waste of time, if not counterproductive; this is not due to any lack of usefulness of budgeting but rather to the poor way budgets are used. Organizational life is simplified, and conflict reduced when employees understand the goals, processes, and reward mechanisms in budgets. When employees understand the purpose of a budget and utilize the benefits it provides, they may stop seeing budgeting as another bureaucratic task to endure and may instead see it as a tool to elevate their understanding and performance.

Summary

Budgeting comes in threes. There are three primary parties: senior management, operating managers, and finance. There are three budget functions: estimation of budget year revenues and expenses, facilitation and control, and evaluation. These functions occur in three distinct time periods: before, during, and after the budget year. Budgeting pursues three goals: controlling resources, ensuring efficiency, and guaranteeing effectiveness. Senior management and the budget office should ensure that employees with little or no financial training understand the goals of budgeting and serve as resources for managers to improve their ability to plan, manage, and evaluate operations. Finance professionals should strive to elevate nonfinancial managers' understanding of the budgeting process rather than simply providing them with the minimal tools needed to construct a budget.

The prospective role of budgeting translates senior management's goals into monetary terms and determines whether the organization has the resources needed to complete the work it has set for itself. Once achievable plans are established and approved, the budget should be used throughout the budget year to determine whether the plan is being met. Are revenues and expenses on budget? When goals are not achieved, monthly variance reports should facilitate the discovery of what is preventing success and what corrective actions should be taken. After the close of the budget year, the budget should be the basis for understanding operating results, establishing accountability, and motivating employees. The incentives managers follow and the results organizations achieve are determined by the budgeting system used. Budgeting systems can be constructed around inputs used, outputs produced, results achieved, or activities performed. What the budget focuses on, measures, and rewards will largely determine where employees invest their efforts.

Performance matters regardless of the ownership status of the organization. Budgets fulfill the same functions in for-profits, nonprofits, and public organizations: they exist to maximize the value of the organization by establishing standards and accountability. Budgeting may be more important to public and nonprofit organizations than for-profits, given the lesser control market forces play in determining the survival of these organizations. Managers who fully understand the budgeting process should see their role not only from the perspective of their departments but also as an integral part in the achievement of the larger goals and future of the organization.

Budgets not only establish the financial, operational, and evaluation standards, but when shared, they also are potent communication tools. They educate customers, employees, and other members of the public on the organization's operations and priorities. Management's willingness to share financial information and ensure employee understanding of financial issues will benefit the organization by focusing the employees' attention and increasing their commitment to its goals. Budgets are an opportunity to unify organizations and launch them on a path toward success, but this vision cannot be realized if managers and employees do not understand their roles and the functions of budgeting.

The remainder of the text takes you on a tour of financial management so that you understand the functions of finance and produce budgets to achieve desired objectives. Managers should not only be technically knowledgeable about their operations but also understand how accounting, economics, finance, strategic behavior/game theory, and program analysis concepts and tools can improve the performance of their area of responsibility. The text is not about accounting and how to fill in forms; rather, it is about how to improve operations by understanding the focus, goals, processes, and strengths and weaknesses of budgeting systems.

Key concepts include planning, management, accountability, revenue-driven costs, incentives, information, efficiency, effectiveness, and choice. Management needs a budgeting system that will work with it instead of against it to obtain the desired behaviors and outcomes that will benefit management and the organization. Knowing which budgeting system to use is the goal of this text.

Key Terms and Concepts

Balanced scorecard
Budget
Effectiveness
Efficiency
Financial competence

Incremental budget
Master budget
Mission
Opportunity cost
Strategic decision-making

System
Tactical decision-making
Unity of command

Discussion Questions

1. What is a budget, what is the goal of a budget, and what are the three functions of budgeting?
2. Explain the chief criticisms of budgets.
3. What are the roles and responsibilities of senior management, finance, and operating managers?
4. Why do departments and organizations spend more than what was budgeted?
5. Define effectiveness and efficiency and describe the relationship between them.
6. Why is profit (or excess revenue over expenses) necessary?
7. What is the difference in budgeting for for-profit, nonprofit, and public organizations?
8. Explain the five components of a system.
9. What is the goal of system thinking?
10. What are the benefits of budgeting?

References

Amtrak. (2016). *Consolidated financial statements.* Retrieved May 15, 2017, from https://www.amtrak.com/ccurl/736/320/Audited-Consolidated-Financial-Statements-FY2016.pdf

Cleverley, W. O., & Cleverley, J. O. (2018). *Essentials of health care finance* (8th ed.). Burlington, MA: Jones & Bartlett Learning.

Codman, E. (1914). *A study on hospital efficiency.* New York, NY: Classics of Medicine Library.

Gapenski, L. C. (2012). *Healthcare finance* (5th ed.). Chicago, IL: Health Administration Press.

Kaplan, R., & Norton, D. (2000, September/October). Having trouble with your strategy? Then map it. *Harvard Business Review, 78*(5), 167–176.

Libby, T., & Lindsay, R. M. (2010). Beyond budgeting or budgeting reconsidered? A survey of North-American budgeting practice. *Management Accounting Research, 21*(1), 56–75.

Moore, C. L., & Jaedicke, R. K. (1976). *Managerial accounting* (4th ed.). Cincinnati, OH: South-Western.

Robbins, S. P., & Coulter, M. (1999). *Management* (6th ed.). Upper Saddle River, NJ: Prentice Hall.

Smith, A. (1977). *An inquiry into the nature and causes of the wealth of nations.* Chicago, IL: University of Chicago Press.

Sun, T. (2002). *The art of war.* Boston, MA: Shambhala.

Weston, J. F., & Brigham, E. F. (1978). *Managerial finance* (6th ed.). Hinsdale, IL: Dryden Press.

CHAPTER 2

Accounting and Economics

CHAPTER OBJECTIVES

1. Explain the role of department budgets and organizational performance.
2. Explain the fundamental accounting equations and the purpose of financial statements.
3. Apply marginal decision-making.
4. Explain the different types of costs and how they impact product costs.
5. Calculate product cost based on output.

▶ Introduction

Budgeting should strive to ensure that the maximum value is received from a set of resources. The effort to obtain the maximum value faces three primary obstacles: uncertainty, bounded rationality, and opportunism. **Uncertainty** recognizes that budgeting attempts to foretell the future, a future that changes rapidly in often unpredictable ways. **Bounded rationality** deals with the inherent limitations of the human mind, compounded by incomplete information and limited time to make decisions. Not everything can be known, and decisions must often be made quickly within the limits of our understanding. **Opportunism** recognizes that people may take every chance they get to improve their well-being and that these efforts often come at the expense of others.

Humans desire maximum satisfaction with minimum effort, and this is true whether we view humans as individuals, in groups, or as a whole. The problem is that while individuals, groups, and society pursue the same maximizing goal, the efforts of each often prevent the realization of the goals of others. Individuals often want to maximize consumption, while minimizing their effort, that is, the maximum income from the smallest amount of work. Owners of organizations want to maximize their value by obtaining the largest-possible revenues and holding down costs or creating the greatest amount of output from their resources. The desire of individuals to minimize effort runs counter to the organizational goal of obtaining the maximum output from workers.

Societal goals add another layer of complexity to the maximizing goals of individuals and organizations. Society seeks the optimal production of goods and services and an adequate distribution of output across the population. The existence of **public goods, externalities,** and the desire for **income redistribution** complicates value calculations and does not use the value-determining mechanisms employed by individuals and organizations. Government provision of public goods and goods with positive externalities may be warranted because of **free riding,** that is, individuals receiving benefits may be unwilling to contribute to the cost of those goods, resulting in a less than optimal provision of the good. Goods with negative externalities, like pollution, may be overproduced and may force nonparticipants to bear part of the cost of their production—the opposite of free riding. Government action to restrict output or dictate production methods to reduce negative externalities is used to prevent or lessen shifting of costs to nonparticipants.

The extent of government-initiated income redistribution requires a value judgment; value in the public sector is determined in political markets, unlike private action that relies on economic markets. Resource transfers simultaneously discourage effort from higher-income groups by reducing after-tax earnings *and* lower-income groups by subsidizing their consumption. Society turns to the government to increase **social welfare** by remedying **market failures** and transferring income; government, however, is not known for either responsiveness or efficiency.

The behavior pursued by individuals in attempting to maximize their own interests may undermine both organizational and societal goals. Likewise, the actions employed by organizations can undermine the goals of society and vice versa, and the actions taken by organizations and society can undermine the goals of individuals. The tendency of individuals to minimize effort does not sit comfortably with the desire of organizations to obtain the maximum effort from employees or society's goals of economic growth and income disparity reduction.

It is sensible for individuals motivated by extrinsic rewards to reduce effort if it does not lower their income; however, shirking duties makes it impossible for organizations or society to obtain the highest-possible output from resources. On the other hand, some people believe that effort is its own reward and strive to do their best without the promise of an extrinsic reward or in the face of active opposition. Organizations attempting to maximize profit favor high-profit goods and services rather than a mix of products that some find more socially desirable (pop art versus high art or curative versus preventive care). The choice of profit-maximizing goods may lead to overproduction of goods accompanied by negative externalities and underproduction of goods with positive externalities, encouraging calls for government intervention to produce a more desirable output mix. Of course, government is itself a service, and there are questions of whether public services are over- or underprovided and whether society is receiving an adequate return on its investment in government. Should society expect more and better output from public workers?

Budgets are one way to navigate the inherent conflicts between individuals, organizations, and society and direct behavior to ensure that the maximum output (or as much as is practical) is produced from available resources. Budgets identify what can and should be produced and are a means to evaluate performance: are individuals putting in the expected effort, are for-profit and nonprofit organizations using their resources wisely, and are public agencies lessening market failures?

Budgeting has always been torn between two opposing goals. The idealistic or normative goal is to produce a budget that maximizes value, that is, obtain the maximum output from a set of resources. The opposing view is the pragmatic goals of individuals who do not want to be pushed to the extent of their capabilities and prefer budgets that pursue lower output and supply more resources. The pragmatic view of individuals impedes the realization of the idealistic goal. If budgets that provide high wages and require less effort from workers can be constructed, so much the better; however, consumers may decide that the limited product at high prices is not worth their patronage and spend their money elsewhere.

Budgeting in organizations encompasses both competition and cooperation. Competition arises between departments as managers try to increase the size of their budgets and share of an organization's resources. Cooperation is mandatory in every organization with more than one employee, as no person or department is individually capable of producing and delivering product. Budget building is always a contest between small, tight budgets and larger, easier-to-meet budgets. While managers may see budgeting as a zero-sum game within an organization, an increase in one department's allocation must come at a cost of smaller budgets for other departments; managers should recognize that their collective success depends on their joint ability to extract more resources from the external environment. Mutual interest explains why groups with seemingly opposing interests, such as unions and management, support the same competition-suppressing initiatives such as international trade regulations.

Readers should first recognize the magnitude of the budgeting task. Large organizations are multibillion-dollar enterprises operating in rapidly changing environments. Organizations challenged by rapid changes in customers' expectations, technology, competition, and regulations must formulate plans to carry themselves into the future. The smallest Fortune 500 company in 2016, Burlington Stores, had

$5.13 billion in revenue (Fortune 500, 2016). Understanding where and how $5.13 billion in sales is produced and assembling the resources to generate this revenue are monumental tasks. The ability of managers to accurately estimate revenues and expenses and manage within the budget may determine organizational and individual success or failure.

After recognizing the enormity of the budgeting challenge, the fundamental accounting equations and financial statements defining organizational performance and **net worth** are reviewed. Accounting provides the tools required to break the complex budgeting task into manageable parts. Organizational performance is the difference between revenue and expense, that is, profit or net income. The net worth of an organization, assets minus liabilities, at least in the short run, may *not* be determined by the inflow of revenues and the outflow of expenses. In the short run, the organization can have higher expenses than revenues and in extreme cases zero revenue. Such organizations, however, should have a long-range plan to not only recoup past losses but also generate substantial future profit. A start-up pharmaceutical company pursuing a patent may have zero sales revenue until the Food and Drug Administration (FDA) approves the drug for human use, a process that can take 7 years or more and $1 billion expenses. Only 0.3% of drugs become profitable (Swayne, Duncan, & Ginter, 2006, p. 438), but start-up companies can obtain funding, equity investments, and debt on the basis of their future earning prospects. These companies have long-range business plans demonstrating how they intend to build profit and net worth. Investors rely on business plans to determine whether an operation is worthy of their support and resources. For most organizations, additions and deductions from net worth are driven by the relationship between revenue and expenses.

After reviewing accounting, the discussion switches to economics to explore marginal decision-making, cost behavior, and economies of scale. **Marginalism** explains real-world processes and is the foundation for many budgeting systems. Understanding how costs change with output is synonymous with understanding how output is produced. It is not enough to understand total inputs used and output produced (measured in dollars); astute managers should also understand how output is affected by the amount and type of inputs used, the substitutability of one input for another (the marginal rate of substitution [MRS]), and whether the optimal mix of inputs is being used. Optimality asks the following questions: Is the revenue (or benefit) produced by the output greater than or equal to the cost of resources consumed, are resources fully employed, and can costs be lowered by employing a different mix of inputs? The best outcome from the organization or society perspective is that goods and services are produced at the lowest-possible costs, while satisfying customers or clients.

In the real world, cost minimization is rarely the goal or outcome of budgeting. Managers regularly pursue the goal of budget maximization as control over more resources makes managing easier and confers power, status, and income on department heads. Budgeting is a means to an end and, ideally, a means to direct resources to their highest-value uses and maximize the well-being of humanity. Ensuring that each department obtains the maximum benefit from its resources requires different metrics, given the varying control managers exercise over products sold and inputs consumed. Budget and performance evaluation systems should hold managers accountable for the things they should control and harmless for matters beyond their control. Managers who can set the prices at which products are sold or the prices paid for inputs should be evaluated differently than managers who cannot influence input or output prices. Budgets should be the basis for performance evaluation systems that maximize organizational value and judge each manager according to the control he or she should exercise over resources.

Budgets should clearly identify organizational objectives and define success regardless of whether the organization is for profit, nonprofit, or public. Budgets should stimulate discussion, resolve questions of whether the ends chosen are appropriate, and secure the buy-in and approval of interested parties. The approved budget should provide the financial plan to guide operations and incentives to ensure that organizational goals are diligently pursued.

▶ Budget Scope

The challenge facing management and budgeting is that organizations are large and complex social organisms, where thousands of people carry on a wide variety of activities and millions, if not billions, of dollars flow in and out. Given the scope and scale of operations, it is difficult to see the whole. No matter how hard anyone tries, it may be impossible for any single person to understand how the entire organization functions. Operating managers and specialists may only concern themselves with their areas of responsibility, but effective management requires the coordination of all parts. Many organizations suffer from **silo thinking**, the unwillingness to share information or coordinate work between departments, which reduces overall effectiveness and efficiency. Organizations should have a unified plan of operation and a system to coordinate activities, that is, a budget to maximize their chances of success.

To conceptualize the task that large, diversified organizations face in assembling a budget, one only needs to examine an organization chart. **FIGURES 2.1** and **2.2** provide examples of divisionally and functionally structured organizations, respectively. In **divisionally structured organizations,** activities are arranged by product line. Each product line controls all the essential activities required to design, produce, and deliver a product to a customer. Each division may be an autonomous business

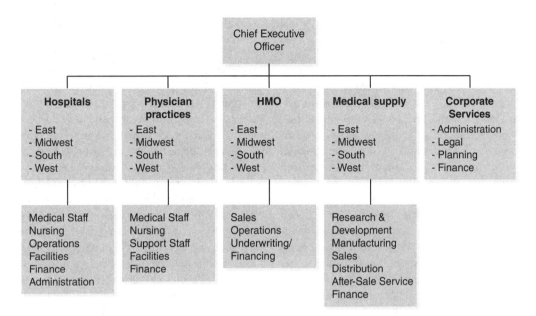

FIGURE 2.1 Divisional Organizational Structure

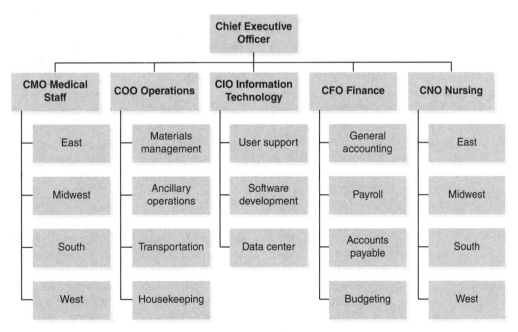

FIGURE 2.2 Functional Organization Structure

unit responsible for setting prices and generating sufficient revenues to cover its expenses plus the cost of corporate services.

The second major organizational form is a functional structure; organizations structured along functional lines consolidate all activities of a certain type within a single unit. **Functionally structured organizations** attempt to capitalize on specialization and **economies of scale** by limiting duplication of activities across units. Functional organizations have a single unit responsible for research and development (R&D), finance, marketing, etc., reporting to a single vice president (VP) who supports all product lines. In functionally structured organizations, changes must be coordinated through multiple authority lines. Divisionally structured organizations concentrate knowledge of a particular industry or product in a single authority center to allow decision-makers to respond swiftly to changes in customer desires or market direction without seeking and obtaining the cooperation of other units. As seen in Figure 2.2, many authority lines control only expense or cost centers and have no control over revenue-generating activities. In functional organizations, it is imperative that budgets provide focus and demonstrate the interdependencies between authority lines.

The difference in philosophy is clear. In the functional structure, the belief is that a single operation (or information technology, finance, etc.) group that can produce a wide range of products will be more effective and efficient than multiple units concentrating on a single product or customer. Functional organizations operate on the belief that one center of technical expertise for medical staff affairs, nursing, or finance is more effective and efficient than having multiple small, specialized staffs. Divisionally structured organizations work on the premise that specific customers require specific solutions and that it is better to build smaller staffs with specialized knowledge of specific industries, customers, and/or products. The trade-off that organizations must make is between technical expertise and knowledge of a particular product or group of consumers. The choice of which structure is best for a particular organization should be based on the size and scope of the organization,

the rate of environmental change, the degree of market competition, and other factors.

Regardless of structure, the reader can see that dozens of department budgets must be created to compile a comprehensive master budget for an organization. Each second-level (directly below the chief executive officer [CEO]) division or functional area will have dozens of departments divided by type of operation performed or customer served. In the divisional structure, it is clear that the hospital division that delivers inpatient and outpatient care may have a clear understanding of its revenues and cost but employees may be unaware of the performance of other operating units and have little understanding of the cost of corporate services and their departments' need to contribute toward defraying that cost. In the functional structure, the nursing division may not understand revenues, given that this function is handled in finance and finance may have a limited understanding of patient care processes and costs. A successful budgeting process elevates organizational interests over the parochial concerns of divisions and departments.

Organization charts demonstrate the difficulty in seeing the complete financial picture. In functionally structured organizatisons, most operating managers will see only the cost half of the picture (and a small part of that half). The medical staff and nursing units may understand their operations and expenses but may have little understanding of the costs of materials management, ancillary operations, and information technology. Similarly, support divisions and departments may have little comprehension of the costs and challenges faced by caregivers. Finance may understand revenues and input prices but be largely unaware of the complexities of medical treatment, that is, production costs. In divisionally structured organizations, each division has revenues and expenses and can be seen as a complete and distinct business unit, but division managers may not understand the allocation of corporate costs. While division managers may think that generating revenues that are 5% or 10% greater than their expenses is adequate, they may not understand that better performance is necessary to cover corporate expenses. It is doubtful whether even the CEO has extensive experience in more than one or two areas of the organization. Should the head of a hospital be a doctor or a nurse with medical experience or a business manager who can handle planning, finance, logistics, hotel and food service functions, etc.?

The master budget aggregates all the departments' revenues and expenses into a single statement to determine whether the total organizational revenues will be greater than costs in the budget year and whether the organization can sustain over the long run. Because of the different scope of authority they hold, the reader should see the inappropriateness of evaluating the CEO, division directors, and managers in the same manner. Managers of single departments, like nursing, respiratory therapy, and human resources, should not be evaluated in the same manner, given the different outputs their departments produce and the different levels of control they exercise over output, costs, and revenues. CEOs, VPs, and division directors should also be evaluated differently as their authority expands to cover multiple or all departments. This chapter explores the tools available to direct resources to their highest-value uses, that is, the uses that generate the greatest benefit for society. Chapter 3 explores the tools and strategies managers use to maximize the size of their budgets.

▶ The Accounting Foundation

Accounting plays the same role in the life of organizations as rules do in games. Accounting establishes the rules of the game: how performance is evaluated (how points are scored), and who is winning or losing during or at the end of a game. Budgeting, working within the confines of the system defined by accounting, sets the strategy and tactics managers plan to use in pursuing organizational objectives. Budgeting specifies which players will be fielded, what equipment they will play with, and what contributions each player is expected to provide to achieve victory. Accounting organizes data and facilitates performance evaluation. In conjunction with a budget and specific performance measures, accounting provides managers with the means to control and improve operations.

Winning in sports is simply a matter of scoring more points than your opponent scores against you. For example, in football, there are points for (PF) greater than points against (PA). In business, too, there are two primary and distinct processes to be managed, offense and defense. PF are revenue, or the value created by a team. In business, revenue (sales), or "offensive" production, requires managing labor, supplies, equipment, and facilities; in sports, the primary resource to be managed is the players. In non revenue-generating organizations, offensive production is defined as the amount of goods and services provided, such as the number of patients seen or vaccinations delivered.

PA signify what it costs the organization to produce its revenue or outputs. Production expenses, or the value consumed in production, is the "defense." The pertinent question is, are revenues greater than production costs or, for non revenue-generating organizations, is the benefit of the output produced greater than the expense incurred? Besides sales revenues and production costs, there are also the costs of special teams, including management, finance, and R&D. The question that must be answered is, is the value of the output greater than the cost of putting the team on the field? Are revenues greater than costs, that is, is value created greater than value consumed? A team that continually incurs more expenses than revenues must assess its performance: what areas of its team, offense, defense, or special teams, are underperforming? Is lower-than-desired performance a question of not having the right people, supplies, equipment, facilities, or some combination of each?

The two essential characteristics of successful organizations are **viability** and **solvency.** Viability assesses the relationship between revenue and expenses, and solvency examines the ratio of assets to liabilities. An organization with higher revenues than expenses is viable and should be able to carry on operations into the future. Solvency is the condition of having more assets than liabilities, or a positive net worth. Viability and solvency are the core accounting measures, as seen in the two fundamental accounting equations:

$$\text{Profit } (\pi) = \text{Total revenue (TR)} \\ - \text{Total cost (TC)} \quad (2.1)$$

$$\text{Equity} (E) = \text{Total assets (TA)} \\ - \text{Total liabilities (TL)} \quad (2.2)$$

Readers knowledgeable in accounting will recognize that these equations are the linchpins in the two major financial statements, the income statement and the balance sheet. The job of management is to largely control revenues and expenses. To paraphrase Charles Dickens (Mr. Micawber in *David Copperfield*), the difference between happiness and misery is simply making one dollar more or less than you spend. Organizations with more revenues than expenses, more money flowing in than

flowing out, build net worth and have unlimited horizons. Organizations whose outflows exceed their inflows erode their net worth and, if expenses continue to exceed revenues, are on the road to **bankruptcy.** The job of a budget is to ensure that an organization's inflows equal or exceed its outflows in the upcoming fiscal year, while strategic financial planning creates budgets to predict revenues and expenses over multiyear periods (**TABLE 2.1**).

Organizations are complex organisms requiring coordination to function at the highest level of effectiveness. Management's job is to ensure that desired outputs are produced and delivered to customers or clients at a reasonable cost to maximize sales revenues or secure other funding. While the managerial goal can be stated in three words, "revenues exceeding costs," coordinating large organizations requires managing dozens, if not thousands, of people, operating and maintaining buildings and equipment, paying employees and vendors, and tracking thousands of revenue and expense accounts.

Using the accounting equation, $\pi = \text{TR} - \text{TC}$, and examining the income statement, it is easy to assess the performance of an organization. **TABLE 2.2** shows the 2-year income statement of Oyam Hospital. The income statement is divided into revenues (the top half) and expenses (the bottom half). Revenues are divided into operating and nonoperating

TABLE 2.1 Revenues, Expenses, and Net Worth

Relationship Between Revenue and Expenses	Net Worth	Implication for the Future
Revenues (cash inflow) > Expenses (cash outflow)	Equity ↑	Growth
Revenues = Expenses	No change in equity	Stable
Revenues < Expenses	Equity ↓	Contraction

TABLE 2.2 Oyam Hospital Income Statement		
	2015	**2016**
Operating revenue	$766,473,000	$870,598,000
Nonoperating revenue	$6,535,000	$6,519,000
Total revenue	$773,008,000	$877,117,000
Salaries and wages	$311,710,000	$317,583,000
Fringe benefits	$66,007,000	$94,759,000
Supplies	$150,957,000	$160,468,000
Rent	$10,033,000	$10,353,000
Depreciation	$32,052,000	$32,247,000
Interest	$1,363,000	$819,000
Other	$150,963,000	$156,403,000
Total expenses	$723,085,000	$772,632,000
Profit	$49,923,000	$104,485,000

revenues. Operating revenue is derived from the sale of output, that is, the organization's primary line of business. Nonoperating revenue is derived from noncore activities such as investment income and rents, which are not the primary business of most healthcare organizations but arise due to the holding of financial assets (cash, marketable securities, etc.) or rental of unused space.

The bottom half, expenses, shows what the funds purchased and is known as the natural classification system. The primary expenses of an organization involve acquiring and using personnel (salaries and wages, fringe benefits), supplies, equipment and buildings (rent, depreciation), and money (interest), with an Other category for miscellaneous, lower-cost expenditures. A second reporting system, functional classification, reports expenses according to what they were used for, for example, administration, production, and sales.

In 2016, Oyam Hospital generated $877,117,000 in revenues and paid $772,632,000 in expenses for a profit of $104,485,000. The organization is viable and appears to be performing well, but we do not know how much it should earn, a topic to be covered in Chapter 12. A second way of assessing performance is to recognize that profits more than doubled from 2015, when $49,923,000 was earned. The jump in profit is attributable to management increasing revenue by 13.5%, while holding expenses to an increase of 6.8%. The job of budgeting is to determine whether future profits will increase, decrease, or stay relatively constant. Profit signifies the value created by an organization and is a primary measure of the performance of management, that is, is the value of the output worth more than the resources consumed in its production? Nonprofit and public organizations often avoid the use of the term "profit" in favor of net income, margin, excess revenue over expenses, additions to the fund balance, etc. The critical point is that regardless of the terminology used, the difference between revenue and expense is the primary measure of the value an organization creates.

The accounting equation, $\pi = \text{TR} - \text{TC}$, is the key to predicting future performance. The accounting equation can be disaggregated into the following equation:

$$\pi = (P * Q) - (\text{AVC} * Q) - \text{TFC} \quad (2.3)$$

Profit = Total revenue cost − Total variable cost − Total fixed cost

Equation 2.3 clarifies the roles of management and budgeting. Management must estimate revenue for the budget year on the basis of projections of prices (P) and output (Q). Projections of future revenue ($P * Q$) will be heavily influenced by past performance and anticipated events. Past performance provides a starting point for budget estimates, but forecasters should recognize that it does not guarantee future performance and that unforeseen events can substantially increase or decrease actual revenue. In organizations that do not generate revenue from the sale of goods and services, sources of funds and the amount of funds obtainable must be identified. In nonprofits, this may require estimating the proceeds of fund-raising or grants, while public organizations must forecast revenues expected from taxes on income, sales, property, etc., or deficit financing.

On the cost side, expenses must be estimated; management must determine whether an expense varies with output produced (average variable cost [AVC] $*$ Q) or is constant (total fixed costs [TFCs]). When expense varies with output, managers must determine the AVC per unit. Forecasts of variable costs, like revenues, are susceptible to two sources of variation: a manager may incorrectly estimate output (Q) or the cost per unit (AVC). TFCs, like management salaries, occupancy costs, and insurance, should be easy to forecast as they do not vary with output, although it is still important to employ the appropriate level of resources. For example, a hospital should avoid filling 50% or 110% of its beds. At 50% capacity, too much capital remains idle, and at 110%, patients may be housed in hallways because of insufficient investment. Current managers may not be accountable for prior investment decisions, but they are responsible for obtaining the maximum possible output from existing resources. The challenge managers face when excess capacity exists is to employ the resources, as intended, by increasing demand, reassigning resources to other tasks, or releasing assets.

The output of the budgeting process should be a set of **pro forma financial statements** establishing where the organization intends to be at the end of the budget period. The pro forma income statement projects revenues and expenses to determine whether the budget plan is feasible, that is, is TR > TC? Equation 2.3 demonstrates that there are four primary variables to be estimated and managed in the budget: the price of outputs (P), the number of units expected to be produced and sold (Q), the average cost to produce a unit of output (AVC), and the expenses needed to produce output that do not vary with the quantity of output produced (TFC).

The budget, returning to the sports analogy, establishes the game plan and details how managers expect to reach organizational goals. Will success arise from superior offense (sales), defense (production), special teams (management, R&D, etc.), or a balanced game? Accounting provides the game statistics, such as revenue per salesperson, cost per unit, and total profit, on a regular basis to inform managers of performance and allow them to change tactics, when necessary.

The second criterion for a healthy organization is solvency, having more assets than liabilities, a condition intimately related to the ability to generate higher revenues than expenses. When an organization's revenue exceeds its expenses, it earns a profit and builds wealth (or increases its equity). The balance sheet, **TABLE 2.3**, comprises three sections: assets (the resources the organization uses), liabilities (the resources in use not owned by the organization), and equity (the difference between assets and liabilities). The balance sheet lists assets and liabilities by **liquidity**, a measure of how quickly an asset can be converted to cash at full value.

Cash can be immediately used at full value and is listed first on the balance sheet. Other current assets such as accounts receivable are less liquid than cash as it may take 60 days or more to collect amounts customers owe to the organization or it can be sold at a discount from its current book value if immediate funds are needed. Fixed assets, including buildings and equipment, can be sold immediately, but the value received may be considerably less than their book value, so they are listed last, and the organization may be unable to recoup book value regardless of how long they are held.

Liabilities are also listed by how soon they should be paid. Current liabilities, accounts payable, should be satisfied in the short term, 90 days or less, while long-term debt such as bonds or mortgages may not come due for 30 years. The difference between assets and liabilities measures the net worth (equity) of the organization, while the difference divided by total assets reports the percentage of resources owned by the organization.

Table 2.3 shows that in 2016, Oyam Hospital controlled $638,184,000 in assets and $246,268,000 was owed to creditors, leaving a net worth of $391,916,000 (or 61.4% of the assets used by the organization were

TABLE 2.3 Oyam Hospital Balance Sheet		
	2015	**2016**
Cash	$25,435,000	$25,270,000
Other current assets	$162,936,000	$142,851,000
Fixed assets	$520,463,000	$470,063,000
Total assets	$708,834,000	$638,184,000
Current liabilities	$28,638,000	$32,344,000
Long-term debt	$192,874,000	$213,924,000
Total liabilities	$221,512,000	$246,268,000
Equity	$487,322,000	$391,916,000

owned by the organization). If no assets are transferred out of the organization (as dividends to stockholders, transfers to affiliated organizations, etc.), profit adds to the net worth of the organization. In 2015, Oyam earned $104,485,000, which should have increased the organization's net worth by an equal amount, but the balance sheet shows a decrease in net worth of $95,406,000 ($487,322,000 − 391,916,000). The decrease was due to a transfer of $199,891,000 to related organizations. Similar to the pro forma income statement, a pro forma balance sheet should be created when the budget is finalized so that managers will know the relationship between assets and liabilities anticipated if the budget is met.

TABLE 2.4 demonstrates the desired position of an organization is cell 1, earning profit, with assets exceeding liabilities. If both conditions are not capable, earning profit while liabilities exceed assets, cell 2, is the second best position. An organization earning profit can eventually accumulate assets that exceed its debts. The obstacle organizations in this situation face is that creditors may demand immediate payment, which cannot

be satisfied since total assets are lower than total liabilities. The third best position is cell 3, expenses exceed revenues but assets exceed liabilities. In this case, assets provide a temporary cushion to absorb current losses; the challenge for managers is to restructure their operations to establish profitability before the net worth is exhausted. The worst position is operating losses with liabilities exceeding assets, cell 4. In this situation, immediate shutdown may be the best option before operating losses widen the gap between assets and liabilities.

The problem in many organizations is that managers have difficulty in envisioning the total operation, given their focus on their departments and lack of knowledge of other functions and departments. The master budget is a means to incorporate managers into the larger organization by allowing them to see the entire financial plan for future years. The income statement and balance sheet, Tables 2.2 and 2.3, demonstrate that even with accounting tools, comprehending the magnitude of the dollars involved adds yet another level of complexity to management and budgeting processes.

TABLE 2.4 Viability and Solvency

	Balance Sheet		
		Assets ≥ Liabilities	**Assets ≥ Liabilities**
Income Statement	**Revenue ≥ Expenses**	Viable and solvent	Viable but insolvent (profit provides ability to achieve solvency in time)
	Revenue < Expenses	Non viable but solvent (accumulated wealth provides ability to absorb losses while working toward viability)	Non viable and insolvent

▶ Economics and Marginal Decision-Making

The goal of budgeting is to maximize the value of an organization by allocating resources to areas where they generate the greatest benefit. Maximizing value is an easy-to-state goal, but what does it mean and how is it done? When consumers shop, they attempt to maximize their satisfaction from spending a given amount of money. While many people do not see themselves as consciously evaluating the benefit of one good versus all the other goods and services that can be purchased, it is clear that some analysis, weighing of goods against one another, is carried on continuously to navigate the tens of thousands of potential purchases consumers could make.

Budgeting is an attempt to establish a conscious, forward-looking mechanism that produces the same result for an organization as the conscious and subconscious weighing processes individual consumers engage in daily. Organizations and their owners, employees, and customers want the greatest-possible enjoyment from a limited amount of resources, and there is a vast range of inputs (labor, land, and capital) an organization can purchase. The question is, how do managers get the most value from the resources they command?

Complicating resource allocation decisions is the fact that inputs have widely different prices and capabilities. When making a purchase, the consumer asks himself or herself, "Is the satisfaction I get from a good or service worth what I have to pay for it?" More precisely, the question is, can another good or service provide greater satisfaction per dollar expended than the one under consideration, that is, what is the opportunity cost of the purchase? Few people explicitly calculate the benefits received with the price paid for a good or service and then evaluate this ratio against the ratios of other goods and services, but the process occurs

nonetheless. We all have developed short-hand mechanisms for comparing goods that allows us to shop effectively—imagine how difficult shopping at Walmart would be if you had to compare all the items offered, when the average store stocks 120,000 items and a supercenter, 142,000 (Walmart, 2005).

Economics provides a procedure to compare one item against others and determine what must be given up to acquire a good or service to simplify purchasing decisions. An easy way to think of this weighing process is that if good X provides twice as much satisfaction as good Y, how much more should a consumer be willing to pay for good X? Without any calculation, it is easy to see that a consumer should be willing to pay twice as much for good X as for good Y. If good X is offered at a price less than twice the price of good Y, then X is the better buy. The consumer could buy one unit of good X, get as much satisfaction as two units of good Y, and have money left over for other purchases. Conversely, if good X is more than twice the price of good Y, the consumer could buy two units of good Y, get the same satisfaction as consuming one unit of good X, and have money left over. Few people go through the mathematics, but everyone, at some level, compares what he or she receives from an expenditure and what he or she could have received.

The weighing process managers face in the budgeting process is similar to consumers' purchasing decisions. The budget allocation process is, perhaps, simplest for for-profit organizations. For-profits exist to maximize profits, and their basis for a decision is whether the per dollar return generated by one investment exceeds the return of alternative investments. The value-maximizing decision rule does not mean that organizations allocate their money to investments that generate the highest dollar return. An organization will not necessarily invest in a machine or market that returns $1 million (investment A) over another that returns $500,000 (investment B). The critical factor is the relationship between the dollar return and the size of the investment. Assume investment A requires an outlay of $10 million and investment B $4 million. Investment A costs more than twice investment B does and its return is only two times higher, so investment B provides a larger return per dollar spent.

Another way of assessing value is to calculate **return on investment (ROI)** by dividing profit by the investment:

$$\text{Investment A} = \frac{\$1,000,000}{\$10,000,000} = 10.0\%$$

$$\text{Investment B} = \frac{\$500,000}{\$4,000,000} = 12.5\%$$

Changes in profit (the numerator) and/or the cost of either investment (the denominator) could change the decision. Assume the cost of investment B increases to $5,500,000 rather than $4,000,000. Investment B's ROI falls to 9.1% ($500,000/$5,500,000), and it is now less desirable than the 10.0% return achievable with investment A.

Of course, investments have different degrees of risk, and higher-risk projects must provide higher returns to attract investors, but we will assume away this complication. Assuming risk is the same for all projects, for-profits allocate their funds to alternatives with the highest ROI until their funds are exhausted or ROI is less than the cost of acquiring funds. Most people can conceptualize the organization's budgeting and investment process more easily than the purchasing decisions of individuals undertaken to maximize their satisfaction. Maximizing ROI appears simpler than maximizing satisfaction, because ROI can be quantified in dollars, a readily understood metric. Satisfaction, on the other hand, is an inscrutable idea—what is a unit of satisfaction, and how is it measured? The marginal decision-making sidebar provides an example of maximizing consumer satisfaction.

TABLE 2.5 shows the six projects an organization could invest in, and its **cost of capital,** the cost of using money, is 6.0%. Deciding which projects to undertake is determined by calculating the ROI for each project. After the ROI is calculated, the projects are sorted from the highest ROI to the lowest and graphed. The projects that will be invested in are determined by the availability of funds, the expected ROI, and the cost of capital.

TABLE 2.5 Calculating Return on Investment			
Project	**Investment**	**Profit**	**Return on Investment (%)**
A	$10,000,000	$1,000,000	10.00
B	$4,000,000	$500,000	12.50
C	$500,000	$80,000	16.00
D	$1,750,000	−$25,000	−1.43
E	$1,500,000	$135,000	9.00
F	$6,500,000	$350,000	5.38

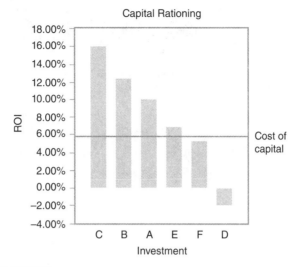

FIGURE 2.3 Ranking Investments

FIGURE 2.3 demonstrates that the first investment that should be undertaken is C, given that it has the highest ROI of 16.0%. If $16,250,000 in funding can be raised, projects C, B, A, and E should be undertaken ($500,000 + $4,000,000 + $10,000,000 + $1,500,000). Project F should *not* be invested in as its ROI, 5.38%, is less than the cost of acquiring money, 6.00%. Similarly, D should not be invested in, even if interest rates drop to zero, as it will not return the funds invested. While financial analysis rules projects F and D out of consideration, there may be extenuating circumstances, such as critical community need, that may impel organizations to undertake projects that will not return their investment.

While Table 2.5 and Figure 2.3 approached a project as a single cash outlay, budgeting operations require higher levels of granularity. A department or an investment does not comprise a single resource, so managers need to look at the contributions of individual inputs. Managers may have to decide between employing labor or equipment or between workers with different levels of skill and wage rates to accomplish work.

To construct a budget, managers should quantify the cost and productivity of the inputs that can be used to produce the desired output or fulfill the required tasks. Managers must make multiple choices between different types of labor, supplies, equipment, and facilities that have different capabilities, while recognizing the complementary nature of these inputs, that is, no input can complete a job alone. The first step toward employing an optimal set of inputs is to calculate the amount of output a set of inputs can produce.

TABLE 2.6 shows the maximum output that can be produced from different combinations of inputs with a budget of $1 million. It also shows the **marginal product (MP)**, the change in output attributable to increasing an input by one unit, while holding other inputs constant. Of course, some inputs require proportional increases in other inputs; it would be silly to increase labor if the additional workers had no supplies to work with. Adding labor may not require additional equipment or space if the present equipment and building are not fully utilized. Table 2.6 calculates the **marginal revenue product (MRP)**, the change in total revenue attributable to increasing one input by one unit, while holding all other inputs constant, that is, MP * Output price, $1000.

In Table 2.6, the manager must employ the minimum level of each resource to produce

SIDEBAR: Marginal Decision-Making

John Doe has a budget of $100, and the table given provides the total and (marginal) satisfaction he receives from consuming one unit of a good. What collection of goods should he purchase to obtain the highest-possible satisfaction with his $100 budget?

Quantity	Ribeyes $10/lb.	Apples $4/lb	Shoes $60/pair	Movies $10/ticket
1	32 (32)	8 (8)	270 (270)	40 (40)
2	60 (28)	15 (7)	390 (120)	70 (30)
3	82 (22)	21 (6)	470 (80)	88 (18)
4	96 (14)	26 (5)	500 (30)	93 (5)
5	100 (4)	30 (4)	500 (0)	90 (0)

Purchasing one pair of shoes and four pounds of ribeye provides 366 units of satisfaction (270 + 96) and costs $100. Purchasing a pair of shoes, one pound of ribeye, one movie ticket, and five pounds of apples produces 372 units of satisfaction (270 + 32 + 40 + 30), providing greater satisfaction than a pair of shoes and four pounds of ribeye for the same $100. Instead of willy-nilly adding up the satisfaction from various combinations of goods, economics offers a simple means to maximize satisfaction: purchase the goods that provide the highest satisfaction per dollar spent until the budget constraint is met. The following table reinterprets the first table by dividing marginal satisfaction by price.

Marginal Satisfaction per Price				
Quantity	Ribeyes $10/lb	Apples $4/lb	Shoes $60/pair	Movies $10/ticket
1	3.20[3]	2.00	4.50[1]	4.00[2]
2	2.80[5]	1.75	2.00	3.00[4]
3	2.20	1.50	1.33	1.80
4	1.40	1.25	0.50	0.50
5	0.40	1.00	0.00	0.00

Purchasing goods with the highest marginal satisfaction per dollar invested means that a pair of shoes is purchased first[1], followed by a movie ticket[2], one pound of ribeye[3], a second movie ticket[4], and, finally, a second pound of ribeye[5]. Total satisfaction is 400 units (270 + 40 + 32 + 30 + 28), selecting the highest-satisfaction goods per dollar spent ensures that no other combination of goods can produce greater satisfaction, given the budget constraint.

TABLE 2.6 Output, Marginal Product, Marginal Revenue Product, and Input Selection

Total Output

	Labor	Supplies	Equipment	Building	Land
Input price	$50,000	$50,000	$150,000	$200,000	$200,000
Input Quantity	/Worker	Each	Each	Each	/10 acres
1	100	100	300	400	400
2	250	200	570	400	400
3	350	300	810	400	400
4	425	400	1020	400	400
5	475	500	1200	700	700

Marginal product $\left(\text{Total output}_{n+1} - \text{Total output}_n\right)$, productivity of each additional input employed

	Labor	Supplies	Equipment	Building	Land
Input price	$50,000	$50,000	$150,000	$200,000	$200,000
Input Quantity	/Worker	Each	Each	Each	/10 acres
1	100 (100 − 0)	100	300	400	400
2	150 (250 − 100)	100	270	−	−
3	100 (350 − 250)	100	240	−	−
4	75 (425 − 350)	100	210	−	−
5	50 (475 − 425)	100	180	300 (2)	300 (2)

Marginal revenue product (MP $*$ P), revenue generated by each additional input employed

(continues)

TABLE 2.6 Output, Marginal Product, Marginal Revenue Product, and Input Selection   *(continued)*

Total Output

	Labor		Supplies	Equipment	Building	Land
Input price	$50,000		$50,000	$150,000	$200,000	$200,000
Input Quantity	**/Worker**		**Each**	**Each**	**Each**	**/10 acres**
1	$100,000 (100 * $1000)		$100,000	$300,000	$400,000	$400,000
2	$150,000 (150 * $1000)		$100,000	$270,000	–	–
3	$100,000 (100 * $1000)		$100,000	$240,000	–	–
4	$75,000 (75 * $1000)		$100,000	$210,000	–	–
5	$50,000 (50 * $1000)		$100,000	$180,000	$300,000	$300,000

Input selection (MRP/Input price), revenue generated per dollar invested in input

	Labor	Supplies	Equipment	Building	Land
Input price	$50,000	$50,000	$150,000	$200,000	$200,000
Input Quantity	**/Worker**	**Each**	**Each**	**Each**	**/10 acres**
1	$2.00 ($100,000/$50,000)	$2.00[a]	$2.00[a]	$2.00[a]	$2.00[a]
2	$3.00 ($150,000/$50,000)	$2.00[a]	$1.80[a]	–	–
3	$2.00 ($100,000/$50,000)	$2.00[a]	$1.60	–	–
4	$1.50 ($75,000/$50,000)	$2.00	$1.40	–	–
5	$1.00 ($50,000/$50,000)	$2.00	$1.20	$1.50	$1.50

[a]Input mix selection.

While the MRP identifies the increase in revenue due to adding inputs, it provides only half the information needed to determine whether inputs should be increased. The second factor is how much it costs to acquire an input. It is easy to see that inputs should not be employed that produce less revenue than their acquisition cost; however, in most cases, the choice managers must make is among inputs that produce more revenue than their input cost. To determine the most efficient input mix, managers should employ inputs that produce the highest revenue per dollar expended, that is, MRP divided by the input price until funds are exhausted or inputs generate less revenue than their acquisition cost.

output. If any of the five inputs is missing, no output can be produced. Organizations may have supplies, equipment, buildings, and land, but without labor, orders cannot be taken, machines cannot be set up, and, subsequently, output will be zero. The current building and land can support the production of 700 units of output and are fixed inputs as long as the total output is 700 units or less. After the minimum level of complementary inputs are in place (costing $650,000), the manager must decide which additional inputs to employ to expand output. Economics dictates that the greatest value will be created if the remaining $350,000 is allocated to inputs with the highest MRP per dollar invested in the input. The first input that should be increased is labor; the second unit of labor increased revenue by $150,000, costs $50,000, and has the highest MRP/input price. Given $300,000 remains to be spent, the manager should purchase additional labor (third increment, +$50,000), supplies (second and third increments, +$100,000), and equipment (second increment, $150,000). Should available funds decrease, the second increment of equipment should be foregone as its MRP/input price, $1.80, is less than the MRP/input price for the third increments of labor or supplies, $2.00. Selecting the inputs with the highest MRP per dollar invested ensures that resources produce the maximum-possible value.

Continuing operations as they are, that is, the status quo, is only acceptable if processes are effective and efficient. If effectiveness or efficiency has not been maximized, managers should explore ways to improve quality and/or reduce cost. Managers should focus on what could be rather than continue what is. Managers must understand what inputs produce, what inputs costs, and how much outputs sell for in order to build better systems. Only then can they ask whether a different mix of inputs will produce better output and greater value.

Cost Behavior

The size of a budget should depend on the relationship between outputs and inputs, that is, how revenue (or benefit) changes with changes in costs. The distribution of fixed and variable costs is essential to determining whether the price of output exceeds the AVC and justifies production. Fixed costs are expenses that do not change with output, that is, the same amount of an input is used and the same amount is paid regardless of the level of output. Variable costs are expenses that change with output, that is, as output increases, more inputs are used and higher costs are incurred. In the real world, costs are more complicated, so four types of cost will be discussed: fixed, variable, variable with a fixed component, and stepwise.

Fixed costs are expenses associated with employing resources that do not change with output: the same amount of a resource is used, and the same expense is incurred for a wide range of output. That is, more or less of the resource is not consumed as the quantity of output produced changes. Examples of fixed costs include senior management salaries, rent, interest expense, and/or depreciation on buildings and equipment. Only one CEO or chief financial officer (CFO) is required regardless of output. Likewise, buildings owned or rented will not change over a wide range of output in the short run. While the amount of fixed inputs should not change with output, the efficiency of operations will be determined by the level of output produced, and managers should strive to make the maximum use of fixed resources.

If the annual rent is $200,000 and 100 units of output are produced, the average fixed cost (AFC) per output is equal to $2000. The AFC falls to $500 per unit when 400 units are demanded and produced. The AFC graph in **FIGURE 2.4** demonstrates the impact of spreading fixed costs over different levels of output.

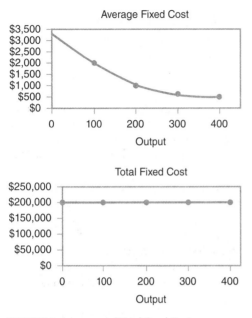

FIGURE 2.4 Average and Total Fixed Costs

is produced, and the quantity of resources consumed and their cost increase proportionately with increases in output. In a hospital, the costs of building and furnishing a nursing unit (depreciation) will be incurred even if the unit is empty, but the organization may not have to incur any labor costs or utility (lighting, heating, and cooling) expenses if it closes the unit.

There is often a one-to-one relationship between variable inputs and output. Assume it takes 12.5 hours of nursing time to treat an inpatient. If the average nursing wage is $40 per hour and staff are effectively employed, the cost per output will be a constant $500 per admission (**FIGURE 2.5**). When 100 inpatients are served, the total variable cost (TVC) will be $50,000, and if the number of inpatients increases to 400, the TVC will be $200,000,

When production involves a single fixed-cost resource, the average cost of output is minimized when the TFC is spread over the maximum output. Fixed costs (or resources) are not infinitely spreadable, that is, at some level of output, it becomes impossible for management to oversee operations, machinery to produce additional units of output, or the current space to contain operations, and additional fixed resources must be added.

From management's perspective, fixed costs are sunk costs and should only affect decision-making when reinvestment, renewal, or recommitment is an option; at all other times, these costs must be paid. While TFCs are noncontrollable in the short run, this does not mean that managers cannot influence the contribution these costs have on the total cost of output. When the quantity of output is variable, managers can determine how efficiently fixed resources are utilized.

Variable costs are expenses associated with inputs whose use changes with output. The quantity of variable resources used and their cost can be zero when no output

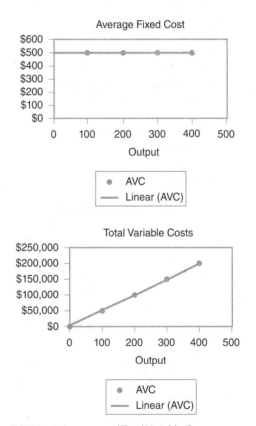

FIGURE 2.5 Average and Total Variable Costs

assuming no inputs are wasted. Examples of variable costs include production (piecework) salaries, sales commissions, and supplies. Blood products and pharmaceuticals are variable costs, where the total cost incurred should be determined by the number of inpatients served; of course, the total cost per patient will be higher than necessary if blood products or drugs beyond their expiration dates must be discarded or pharmaceuticals are diverted.

Variable costs with a minimum charge (**FIGURE 2.6**) are resources with a minimum cost component (licensing fee, connection charge) and a per unit consumed component (usage charge). Economics calls this pricing structure **two-part tariff**. Examples of two-part pricing structures include on-call pay, where nurses must be paid 10% of their hourly rate for being on call outside their regular hours and one and a half times their hourly wage when they work in excess of 40 hours a week; utilities, such as gas, water, and telephone, where

there is a monthly connect fee and use charge; and country club memberships, where there are initiation fees, annual dues, and monthly restaurant fees.

The average cost of a variable resource with a fixed component behaves similar to a fixed-cost resource in that managers have an incentive to spread the fixed component over a high volume to achieve a per unit cost that approaches the AVC for a purely variable resource. That is, the fixed component should be spread over the maximum number of units to push its per unit cost as close to zero as possible, leaving only the usage fee as the relevant expense. Another commonly incurred cost is overtime; overtime paid at the hourly wage rate plus 50% is incurred when hourly employees work more than 40 hours in a week. Assuming productivity is constant, outputs produced by a worker earning $40 an hour and producing two units per hour after they have completed their 40-hour workweek will increase the labor component to $30.00 per unit versus $20.00.

Step costs are "lumpy" resources that must be purchased in discrete quantities and may or may not have a minimum cost component. For example, an emergency room may be required to maintain a minimum staff around the clock regardless of whether there are any patients (zero output); a restaurant, on the other hand, could incur no salary expense at zero output by scheduling no staff and remaining closed. As soon as the restaurant decides to open its doors, it will require a minimum staffing level—hostess/host, server, cook, and dishwasher. Similarly, an organization may maintain a minimum four-hour pay rule for all employees called in to work. That is, once an employee comes to work, he or she will be paid for at least four hours, even if he or she is sent home because of lack of work before 4 hours are completed. Whether an organization requires minimum staffing or it doesn't, managers need to determine how many units of output the staff can handle (or produce) before more resources (labor,

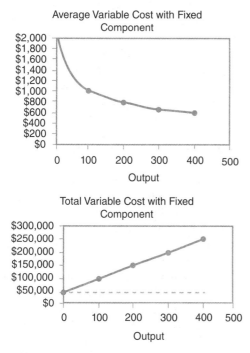

FIGURE 2.6 Average and Total Variable with Fixed Component

machinery, space) are required. **FIGURE 2.7** shows the average and total costs for the labor decision given in Table 2.6. The first worker can produce 100 units, two workers can produce 250, and so on.

If 101 (or 251) units of output were required, the cheapest method of producing one more unit would be by utilizing overtime. Managers must decide when is it cheaper (more efficient) to stretch existing labor by paying overtime (time and a half) or hiring additional workers (step costs). Often on-call staff or pool (registry) nurses have a minimum number of hours paid when they are called in. Managers

should be cognizant of the breakeven point, that is, when is it cheaper to pay overtime, and when should additional help be called in?

The question revolves around the number of hours of work to be done, the overtime pay differential, and the cost of on-call workers. Assume workers earn $15.00 per hour; therefore, overtime is paid at $22.50 per hour. On-call workers earn the same $15.00 per hour but will be paid for a minimum of 4 hours every time they are called in. The breakeven number of hours is as follows:

$$\text{Overtime wage} * \text{Required number of hours} = \text{On-call wage} * \text{Minimum guaranteed hours}$$

$$\$22.50 * x \text{ hours} = \$15.00 * 4 \text{ hours}$$

$$x = \frac{\$60}{\$22.50} = 2.67 \text{ hours, or 2 hours and 40 minutes}$$

If there is more than 2 hours and 40 minutes of work to be performed, it is cheaper to call in additional staff; when work can be completed in under 2 hours and 40 minutes, overtime should be paid. Examples of step costs include labor, equipment, and facilities.

Variable costs, variable costs with a fixed component, and step costs are marginal costs, that is, an increase in output generates additional expenses the organization must pay. The job of management should be to ensure that the marginal costs of producing output are less than or equal to the marginal revenue (or benefit) it creates.

No discussion of cost behavior is complete without relating input use and cost to output, more specifically how output changes when more inputs are used. Economists hold that most systems are characterized by **diminishing marginal returns**. Diminishing marginal returns occur when an additional unit of a variable input, such as labor, given a fixed factor, such as equipment or facilities, produces less output than prior units. That is, productivity falls as more and more units of the variable factor are employed in conjunction with a fixed factor.

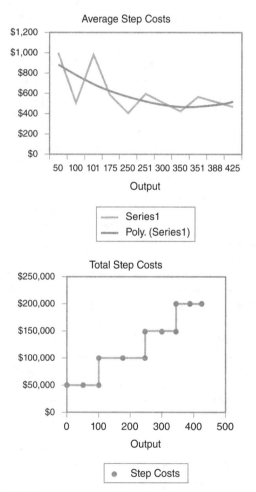

FIGURE 2.7 Average and Total Step Costs

FIGURE 2.8 demonstrates that diminishing marginal returns, initial expenditures for a variable input such as labor, increase the quantity of output produced more than later expenditures. As an individual or organization increases spending on an input, later expenditures produce less output because they have less fixed inputs to work with. Diminishing marginal returns are introduced because some people believe that spending additional money on an endeavor will produce returns comparable to earlier expenditures—this is not often true. In this example, diminishing returns occur because additional units of labor utilize a fixed amount of equipment and facilities, and as investment per worker declines (each worker has less equipment to work with), the output of the added labor declines. Beyond a given point, the curve flattens out, suggesting that additional input expenditures will produce little or no additional benefit. It is entirely possible that if additional resources are added, they will reduce rather than increase output—too many cooks in the kitchen.

Diminishing returns also occur in preventive health programs; early dollars should be spent on those in the high-risk groups most susceptible to the disease or condition. The first expenditures spent on those most likely to contract a disease or those who will experience the greatest reaction to a disease will produce the highest benefit by either preventing the disease or minimizing its consequence. Expansion of prevention programs leads to serving people who are less likely to contract a disease, may have less reaction to a disease, or

may be more difficult and expensive to identify and/or treat; thus, benefit declines as costs increase. The overuse of antibiotics and pain medications has given rise to negative returns due to increases in antibiotic-resistant bacteria and addiction. Diminishing marginal returns stand as a warning: spending more money does not ensure value is created.

Economies of Scale

Understanding how the cost of individual inputs changes is vital to determining the total cost and average total cost (ATC). Organizations have costs that increase proportionately with output, like supplies. Each additional unit produced requires a set amount of a resource and increases cost by a fixed amount, and fixed costs that do not change with output like facility costs. The relationship between labor costs and output is intricate, given how workers are employed and given the inability to store unused labor. Management must balance the incentive to produce the highest-possible output to spread fixed costs, since no additional cost is incurred against the potential jumps in variable costs due to overtime or step costs, to ensure that increases in output cover their production costs.

Employees are generally hired and paid for a 40-hour week, and when there is insufficient work to fill 40 hours, employees are idle and the labor cost per output increases. On the other hand, if more than 40 hours are needed to complete work, wages are paid at time and a half. **FIGURE 2.9** assumes that an employee is paid $20 per hour and produces one unit of output in 24 minutes (or 100 units per week). The average labor cost reaches a minimum of $8.00 per unit at 100 units per week where the employee is fully employed; any change in output increases the cost per output. If output falls to 90 units, the average labor cost increases to $8.89 ($800/90). If output increases to 110, the average labor cost increases to $8.36 ([$800 + $120]/110, or 4 hours of overtime at $30/hour). For a single employee, it is easy to see that efficiency requires having enough work

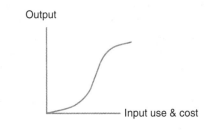

Output

Input use & cost

FIGURE 2.8 Diminishing Marginal Returns

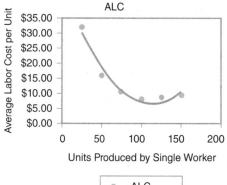

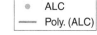

FIGURE 2.9 Average Labor Cost

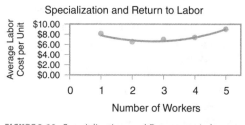

FIGURE 2.10 Specialization and Returns to Labor

to keep the employee busy and the per unit cost increases rapidly as idle time or overtime increases.

Not only is it important to keep individual employees fully employed to keep costs low, there is also an optimal number of employees needed to allocate duties efficiently. Adam Smith (1776, p. 13) noted that a pin factory could produce more output if the various tasks required to create pins were allocated to different employees. **Specialization** is the idea that an employee concentrating on a single or a small number of tasks will be more productive than if he or she has to shift between multiple activities. In Smith's example, a single employee performing every one of the 18 tasks required to produce a pin could make 20 pins per day. After the separate tasks of drawing wire, cutting, pointing, etc., were distributed among 10 employees, a single employee, as part of the team, could produce 4800 pins per day—employee productivity increased by 240-fold.

As seen in Table 2.6, a single worker can produce 100 units but two workers can produce 250 units—a gain due to specialization driving the labor component from $8.00 per unit to $6.40 (**FIGURE 2.10**). Past a certain point, employing additional workers leads to inefficiency as the capital per worker is reduced (too many employees using too little equipment) and management becomes more difficult.

These coordination problems lead to declining productivity: when two workers are employed, average productivity is 125 units per worker (250 units/2 workers), but when three workers are employed, average productivity falls to 116.67 (350/3) and labor cost increases to $6.86 per unit.

The example in Table 2.6 and Figure 2.10 demonstrate that to minimize cost per output, managers must employ the correct amount of a resource for the anticipated volume of output. The question is not what the appropriate level of use is for a single input but, rather, what the appropriate level of use is for all inputs, or what the cost-efficient scale of operations is. **Economies of scale** examine how average cost per unit changes with an increase in output. An economy of scale (or increasing returns to scale) reflects the situation in which a percentage increase in output results in a lower rate of increase in the ATC. Economies of scale exist if increasing output by 10% results in less than a 10% increase in the ATC.

FIGURE 2.11 demonstrates that the ATC declines with increases in output up to $Q^{optimal}$, which is the result of spreading fixed costs over a higher output. After $Q^{optimal}$, the cost per unit increases as additional variable inputs are needed to produce more output. The situation to the right of $Q^{optimal}$ is a diseconomy of scale (or decreasing return's to scale), where costs increase faster than output. The goal of managers should be to operate in the flat part of the curve, where costs are minimized and changes in output in either direction will have negligible effects on the ATC, that is, constant returns to scale.

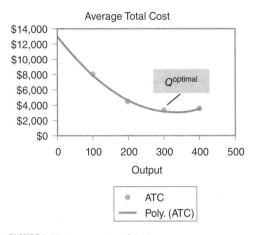

FIGURE 2.11 Economies of Scale

TABLE 2.7 Hospital Economies of Scale	
Bed Size	**Cost per Discharge**
<25	$11,568
25–99	$9,401
100–199	$9,239
200–299	$10,319
300–399	$11,286
>400	$12,851

Another way to envision increasing returns to scale is that the percentage change in output is higher than the percentage change in inputs used in production $\left(\%\Delta Q_{output} > \%\Delta Q_{all\,inputs}\right)$ because of gains from specialization (less non-productive task shifting and the ability to utilize techniques that were unavailable/nonoptimal at smaller output). At constant returns to scale, the change in output equals the change in inputs $\left(\%\Delta Q_{output} = \%\Delta Q_{all\,inputs}\right)$. In large organizations, coordination and accountability problems may drive decreasing returns to scale, that is, the inability to effectively manage resources may result in output growth that is less than the increase in input use $\left(\%\Delta Q_{output} < \%\Delta Q_{all\,inputs}\right)$.

The *2017 Almanac of Hospital Financial and Operating Indicators* provides a concrete example of economies of scale (Optum360°, 2016). TABLE 2.7 reports the average cost per discharge by bed size, which reaches a minimum for hospitals with 100–199 beds. FIGURE 2.12 demonstrates the U-shaped economy-of-scale curve showing that the smallest and largest hospitals have costs that are 25% to 39% higher than hospitals with 100–199 beds.

The challenge for management is to identify and manage the correct set of resources for the anticipated volume of output. Managers should (i) maintain full employment of resources (no idle time or waste) and (ii)

allocate resources to their best uses, that is, obtain the maximum contribution from each resource by assigning each to the task or tasks the resource is best suited for, while minimizing transitions. In any task, there is a problem of too small and too big; in small work groups, where employees perform a variety of tasks, costs may be higher than necessary because of the inability of the employees to do a single or a small number of tasks enough to maximize proficiency. Higher-than-necessary costs arise in large work groups from idle time, inflexibility, congestion, control, and transition problems.

▶ Organizational Architecture

Organizational architecture is a management system designed around decision rights (who has the authority to make decisions), compensation and reward systems (what employees receive for increasing the value of the organization), and performance reporting systems (which employee actions increase or decrease the value of the organization). Chapter 1 posed the question, does a budget

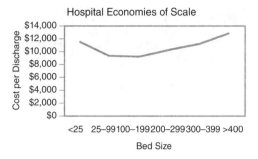

FIGURE 2.12 Hospital Economies of Scale

encourage effort, economy, and innovation or shirking, waste, and the status quo? Budgets can encourage either encourage effort, economy, and innovation or shirking, waste, and the status quo, so budgets and performance evaluation systems should be designed to recognize the factors managers can and should control, and establish incentives that advance the goals of the organization. The brief review of organization charts in Figures 2.1 and 2.2 demonstrates that different managers have different levels of authority over organizational resources—some only control inputs, while others decide what outputs will be produced, still others set the prices at which outputs are sold, and senior executives determine where future investments are made.

Budgets and performance evaluation systems should set goals that reward managers for effectively managing the resources at their command and explicitly recognize that different types of departments should be evaluated on the basis of the level of authority managers are given. Organizational architecture supplies the theoretical foundation for different types of budgeting systems. At the lower levels of an organization, managers typically control inputs and are responsible for producing goods and services that may or may not produce revenue. Lower-level departments are classified as cost, expense, or revenue centers on the basis of what they produce. Lower-level managers generally are not responsible for profitability. Questions of profit arise at the division level; while department managers may only produce

part of the final product, the division-level manager (or division director) is responsible for bringing the product to market and should be evaluated not only on production but also on sales—satisfying the consumer. Given the expanded responsibility of division managers, their operations are classified as profit centers. The responsibility of VPs extends beyond current operations to include what the organization will do in the future. Senior executives should be evaluated for investments that maximize the future value of the organization, and their areas of responsibility are labeled investment centers. The relationship between budgeting and performance evaluation systems and the five types of responsibility centers is discussed as follows.

Cost Centers

Cost center managers decide the mix of inputs (labor, supplies, equipment, etc.) employed to produce output and should be evaluated on efficiency, minimizing the cost per unit or maximizing output for a given budget. Output and quality must be measureable, that is, what the department produces must be easy to quantify (count) and it should be easy to distinguish acceptable from unacceptable output. A compensation system that rewards individuals for the number of units produced creates an incentive to maximize output. If quality is not measured, an output-based compensation system can encourage fast and flawed work. To maximize firm value, compensation and evaluation systems must ensure that output simultaneously satisfies consumers and minimizes costs. Cost center managers have no authority over sales, revenues, or profits, and hence, their budgets and performance should not be determined by fluctuation in these factors. Evaluating managers on the basis of efficiency should be used when managers can (i) measure quantity, understand cost functions, and set output levels and rewards, (ii) assess quality, and (iii) know the optimal input mix and have authority over input use (Brickley, Smith, &

Zimmerman, 1997, p. 324). Flexible and activity-based budgets may be most appropriate for cost center managers.

Expense Centers

Expense center managers decide the mix of inputs to be used to produce output, but output is subjective, for example, human resource functions, finance, and R&D. In human resources, the quality of new hires (or the screening and training processes) may only be apparent years down the line. Similarly, the quality of financial analysis or research may be known years in the future when the investment matures and its costs and benefits can be calculated. The problem with expense centers is that it is difficult to determine whether the right amount of inputs are being consumed relative to the output produced. In cost centers, where quantity and quality are measurable, charge-back systems are often used to establish control. Downstream departments that consume the goods and services "pay" their costs, and if these users can go and purchase inputs outside the organization when internal costs become too great, the upstream departments face market discipline and must maintain efficiency.

Unlike cost centers, the subjectivity of the quantity and quality of output in expense centers makes it difficult to establish charge-back systems for users that could discourage them from overusing the service. Departments that are not charged for use of services provided by other departments tend to overuse services. Brickley et al. (1997, p. 325) note that the costs of expense centers, typically overhead departments, have a tendency to grow faster than the organization as a whole, suggesting they may exploit the lack of a clear input/output relationship to increase their resource use and budgets. Evaluating performance and control often relies on benchmarking to similar-size organizations (is the human resource, finance, and/or R&D staff larger or smaller than similar-size organizations?) or

placing the department under the control of its largest user. The goal is to minimize cost for the level of service provided or maximize services for a fixed budget. Activity-based budgets may be most appropriate in this situation. One problem that arises when expense centers are placed under the control of its largest user is that the department may subsequently limit services to other departments to reduce cost.

Revenue Centers

Revenue center managers are tasked with selling a product or service (marketing, selling, and distribution) and may have limited authority to set prices. To maximize the value of the organization, managers should maximize revenue at a given price or quantity—the economic rule of equalizing marginal revenue and marginal cost. Revenue center managers control their input mix, that is, type of sales staff, amount spent on advertising, etc. Evaluating managers for equating marginal revenues and marginal costs should be used when the managers understand (i) the optimal price–quantity combination, (ii) the optimal product mix (does not allow sales staff to focus on high-revenue versus high-profit products), and (iii) the demand function of customers (Brickley et al., 1997, p. 326). Program budgeting and zero-base budgets may be most appropriate for revenue centers.

Profit Centers

Profit center managers decide the input mix, product mix, and prices and should be evaluated on the difference between actual and expected profits. A profit center is typically a set of cost, expense, and revenue centers. Complications, that is, profit shifting, can arise because of transfer pricing and allocation of overhead issues. In addition, there is the issue of interdependencies among business units and firm-wide profit. Program or zero-base budgets may provide the most effective monitor of managerial prowess.

Investment Centers

Investment center managers decide the input mix, product mix, output prices, and capital expenditures. An investment center is typically a set of profit centers, and the job of investment center managers, typically the C-suite, is to allocate funds to the most profitable profit centers. Investment center managers should be evaluated on the ROI and residual income (subtracting opportunity costs). Evaluation should also include assessment of risk assumed, that is, fluctuation in the ROI. Investment center managers are responsible for the profitability of the entire organization and should be evaluated on the master budget and realized profit. Program and zero-base budgets, again, provide the optimal structure to highlight and monitor decision-making effectiveness.

Whereas the managers of investment and profit centers should be evaluated on future and current profitability, managers of cost and revenue centers should be assessed on the cost per output produced or sold (throughput/output), while expense center managers should be evaluated on what is achieved compared to similarly funded departments (outcomes). Rational budgeting and performance evaluation systems must recognize the resources managers control, and establish incentives for managers to pursue organizational goals.

Summary

This chapter demonstrates that budgeting is a complex task encompassing a variety of operations and requiring the estimation of millions, if not billions, of dollars of revenue and expenses. Accounting provides a simple system to create budgets and determine how organizations are performing. Is the organization viable? Does the pro forma income statement show that revenues will exceed expenses if the budget is followed? If the budget is followed, will the organization be in a stronger position at the end of the fiscal year, and will the organization be solvent?

Marginal decision-making, cost behavior, and the way costs are combined are examined to explore operating expenses and identify how managers can minimize production costs. Spreading fixed costs over the highest amount of output minimizes the AFC, but only reduces the ATC if increases in variable costs do not offset the reduction in AFCs. Managers must understand how output changes with increases in variable inputs (MP), how cost increases with increases in inputs (cost behavior), and how the ATC changes with increases in output, given fixed resources (economies of scale) to determine whether consuming more resources benefits the organization.

Organizational architecture recognized the essential role played by incentives, decision rights, and monitoring systems in ensuring an organization's goals are pursued by its managers. Budgeting and performance evaluation systems should recognize the things a manager has authority over and build monitoring and compensation systems that track and reward senior and lower-level managers for maximizing the value of the organization.

Key Terms and Concepts

Balance sheet	Fixed costs	Marginal product
Bankruptcy	Free riding	Marginal revenue product
Bounded rationality	Functional organization	Net worth (equity)
Cost of capital	structure	Opportunism
Diminishing marginal returns	Income redistribution	Organizational architecture
Divisional organization	Income statement	Pro forma financial statements
structure	Liquidity	Public good
Economies of scale	Marginalism	Return on investment (ROI)
Externality	Market failure	Silo thinking

Social welfare	Step costs	Variable costs
Solvency	Two-part tariff	Viability
Specialization	Uncertainty	

Discussion Questions

1. Describe the goals of individuals, organizations, and society and how they interact.
2. What are the major challenges in preparing a budget for a large organization?
3. Explain the two accounting equations, including their purpose and relationship with the income statement and balance sheet.
4. Explain why the ATC tends to initially decrease as output increases and eventually increase.
5. Describe the differences between cost, expense, revenue, profit, and investment centers.

Problems

1. Calculate the ROI for each project and state which projects should be undertaken if the interest rate is 5%.

Project	Investment	Profit	ROI
A	$8,000,000	$1,000,000	_____
B	$5,000,000	$500,000	_____
C	$2,500,000	−$100,000	_____
D	$3,750,000	$250,000	_____
E	$4,000,000	$300,000	_____
F	$12,000,000	$1,250,000	_____
G	$6,500,000	$400,000	_____

2. Calculate the ROI for the following five projects. The total cost includes the initial investment. Which projects should be undertaken if the organization has a spending constraint of $7,000,000 and its cost of capital is 6%?

3. Assume you are the business manager for an outpatient surgical center that currently employs two surgeons. The table given provides the expected change in the annual surgical volume if additional surgeons are hired. If the salary for the to-be-hired surgeons is $200,000 and the practice earns $100

Project	Investment	Total revenue	Total cost	Profit	ROI
A	$3,000,000	$5,500,000	$5,000,000	_____	_____
B	$2,400,000	$4,000,000	$3,800,000	_____	_____
C	$1,350,000	$2,400,000	$2,300,000	_____	_____
D	$1,500,000	$3,200,000	$3,000,000	_____	_____
E	$2,000,000	$3,800,000	$3,700,000	_____	_____

per surgery after all other expenses (staffing, supplies, equipment/building costs, etc.) have been paid, how many additional surgeons should be added?

Surgeons	Total Surgeries
0	0
1	2,070
2	5,175
3	8,901
4	12,006
5	14,076
6	15,525

4. Given an output price of $500, the total output (in the body of the table), the quantity of each input (in rows), the price of inputs (in columns), and a budget of $1,200,000, calculate the MP and MRP for each input. Which resources in what quantities should be employed to maximize the value of the firm?

5. Assume the total cost for an appendicitis operation comprises supplies (AVC), the surgical team (step cost), and building and equipment (AFC). Calculate the ATC. What is the most efficient (minimum ATC) output quantity, given the costs in the table? What should be the cost to produce 900 operations?

Low Skill	High Skill	Low Capacity	High Capacity	Building and Land		
Labor	Labor	Supplies, Equipment	Equipment			
Input	$30,000	$50,000	$20,000	$100,000	$400,000	$500,000
1	64	120	50	250	1,000	1,350
2	130	220	98	475	–	–
3	200	300	144	675	–	–
4	266	360	186	850	–	–
5	330	400	228	1,000	–	–

Output	Average Variable Cost	Step Cost	Total Fixed Cost	Average Total Cost
0	$0	$50,000	$500,000	_____
150	$1,000	$100,000	$500,000	_____
300	$950	$100,000	$500,000	_____
450	$1,000	$100,000	$500,000	_____
600	$1,200	$200,000	$500,000	_____
750	$1,500	$200,000	$500,000	_____
900	$1,800	$300,000	$500,000	_____

References

Brickley, J. A., Smith, C. W., & Zimmerman, J. L. (1997). *Managerial economics and organizational architecture.* Chicago, IL: Irwin.

Fortune 500. (2017). Retrieved September 6, 2017, from http://beta.fortune.com/fortune500/list

Optum360°. (2016). *2017 Almanac of hospital financial and operating indicators.* Chicago, IL: Author.

Smith, A. (1776). *An inquiry into the nature and causes of the wealth of nations.* Chicago, IL: University of Chicago Press.

Swayne, L. E., Duncan, W. J., & Ginter, P. M. (2006). *Strategic management of health care organizations* (6th ed.). San Francisco, CA: Jossey Bass.

Walmart. (2005). Our Retail Divisions. Retrieved August 23, 2016, from http://corporate.walmart.com/_news_/news-archive/2005/01/07/our-retail-divisions

CHAPTER 3

Budget Incentives and Strategies

CHAPTER OBJECTIVES

1. Explain the difference in the flow of funds between market and nonmarket exchanges.
2. Explain the duties of senior management, finance, and operating managers in the budgeting process.
3. Describe the major strategies to increase, defend, or cut a budget.
4. Describe the major tasks needed to construct a budget.
5. Explain what a budget is and what it is not.

▶ Introduction

In the real world, we often observe egregious examples of waste. Given the tools at our command, why do we, as consumers, often think that we are not getting our money's worth? This belief regularly arises for goods and services not transacted in markets. Buyers do not purchase goods and services they think provide less benefit than other goods and services that could be purchased with the same money. When goods and services are free or heavily subsidized, the public often feels it is getting less than what it expects—shoddy products, poor service, and high costs.

Health care and education are two prime examples of heavily subsidized goods. Issues

with healthcare access, quality, and cost are routinely debated in public forums. Healthcare spending is high because the federal government or private health insurance pays for medical services and patients see little need to reduce their use of care. Patients demand more frequent visits and intensive care because additional consumption often costs them nothing. Providers recognizing that higher prices do not significantly lower the demand for healthcare services have little incentive to control costs. Primary education, a service for which local, state, and federal governments provide the bulk of the funding, is criticized for high cost and declining student performance. These two industries, and the nonprofit and public organizations that inhabit them, respond to a different set of constraints than organizations that sell their products to nonsubsidized customers.

This chapter explores how the flow of funds in input and output markets affects the demand for goods and services and organizational performance—employee desire to control costs.

After exploring the different external constraints on organizations, the roles of different personnel in the budgeting process are examined: Who in an organization looks out for the interests of society, customers or clients, resource providers (employees, stockholders, creditors, etc.), and/or taxpayers when market constraints are lacking? After defining budget roles, budget strategies are introduced and explored. Given that managers regularly seek to maximize their budgets, how do they present the best-possible case for more resources? Budgeting is a prime example of the old saying "Be careful what you wish for"; you get what you encourage, and it may not be what you want. Managers respond to the incentives budgets establish and take actions and pursue outcomes that enhance their salaries and status. The choice of budgeting systems, performance measures, and evaluation and control systems will direct employee attention to predictable ends. Senior management should ensure that the ends it desires are encouraged by the budgeting system employed.

After describing the flow of funds and incentives within input and output markets, the particulars of the budgeting process, and commonly employed budget strategies, Part 1 concludes with a discussion of what a budget is and is not.

▶ The Flow of Funds in Market and Nonmarket Exchanges

All organizations face similar constraints on success: they must satisfy customers or clients, resource owners (employees, stockholder/stakeholders, and creditors), and regulators. Satisfying these constituencies requires rational allocation of resources. Customers and clients want desirable goods and services delivered courteously and timely. Resource owners demand adequate returns on their investments, employees want high wages, providers of capital want high interest or dividends, and suppliers of buildings and land want high rents. Regulators seek to increase public safety, limit pollution, ensure propriety in financial dealings, etc. Managers must allocate resources to meet these often-conflicting goals and satisfy competing constituencies. High prices would please resource providers but would displease, if not drive off, customers. Government programs that distribute free or heavily subsidized services make clients and resource providers happy but upset the taxpayers who pay production costs.

Decisions must be made to determine what to produce and to what standard; how much to produce; how to produce it, including what resources to use; where production should occur; how to finance operations; and how to manage production processes. All of these actions must be taken within the constraints of the resources society is willing to pay to obtain the outputs of the production system. Organizations that cannot effectively manage their costs face the loss of customers or clients, restricted access to resources, and/or government scrutiny.

Increasing the value of for-profit organizations involves maximizing profits to build shareholder wealth. The first requirement for success and profitability in voluntary exchange markets is to produce goods and services people want at prices they are willing to pay. The second requirement is integral to the first: producing goods and services at the least possible cost to keep prices low, while maximizing the difference between price and cost. Maximum efficiency requires operating at the minimum average total cost or maximizing output from a set of inputs. Organizations that depend on voluntary transactions between them and nonsubsidized customers and compete with other producers for customers must be at least as efficient as their competitors. Managers and employees of for-profit organizations are driven by, evaluated on, and often compensated on profit; hence, personal interest and organizational goals are aligned in the pursuit of efficiency. Profits and value are maximized when the price of the last good or service sold equals its marginal cost of production ($P = MC$) (**FIGURE 3.1**).

Self-interest in voluntary exchange markets restricts the demand for goods and services and encourages efficiency. Customers, being simultaneously providers of resources (inputs), for which they are paid wages, interest, and rents, and consumers, who must pay for the goods and services they consume, have their conflicting interests balanced. As consumers, they want high-quality, low-cost products, low prices, and tight budgets; as resource providers, they want the highest-possible wages, interest, and rents that is, high costs and loose budgets. The conflict between low prices and high compensation for inputs within a

single group ensures that one group's interest cannot be sacrificed to another—since they are one and the same. In input markets, laborers do not sell their labor for less than what they think it is worth and employers do not purchase labor at prices that exceed its worth (i.e., the marginal revenue product [MRP]). Similarly, the sellers and buyers of land and capital transact these resources at mutually agreed prices.

In output markets, consumers do not purchase goods or services for more than they think they are worth. When organizations produce unwanted products or set prices too high, customers refuse to purchase and thus drive output and costs to acceptable levels. Resource providers may have to accept lower compensation or reallocate their resources to markets that are willing and able to pay more for labor, capital, and/or land. Opposing interests are balanced in voluntary exchange markets, and increasing the value of the organization requires producing goods and services at prices customers are willing to pay. The system results in mutually advantageous trade, customers believe the value of what they receive is greater than what they must pay, and producers/resource owners receive the best-possible return for their inputs to the production process. Customers and producers both must believe they benefit from the exchange, otherwise no transaction occurs.

Checks over demand and incentives toward efficiency are disrupted when the people who pay for inputs and the people who receive outputs are not the same. The separation of consumption of outputs from payment for inputs weakens, if not destroys, the equilibrium in market systems and encourages excessive and inefficient outputs. Unlike the two parties in voluntary exchange markets, **FIGURE 3.2** shows that there may be up to four distinct parties in involuntary or subsidized markets and the interests of resource providers, taxpayers, producers, and clients do not balance: gains of one group come at the expense of other groups.

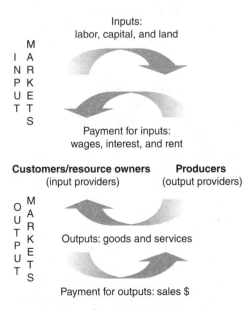

FIGURE 3.1 Flow of Funds: Market Exchange

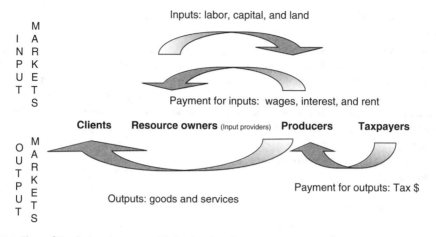

FIGURE 3.2 Flow of Funds: Involuntary and Subsidized Exchange

Major changes occur in the input and output markets, and self-regulation is weakened by divorcing payment for output from distribution of goods and services produced. The major change occurs in the output market, where clients may be able to obtain goods and services without contributing to their production costs and taxpayers may receive no benefit but are required to finance production. Medicaid recipients pay little if any taxes and have no incentive to reduce their consumption of healthcare services or concern for production costs. Medicare Part D provides a less extreme case, where patient payments accounted for 14.2% of program outlays in 2015 (Federal Hospital Insurance & Federal Supplementary Medical Insurance Trust Funds, 2016), but this contribution hardly encourages recipients to be conscientious in their use of pharmaceuticals. A subsidized client only asks, is a good or service worth what I have to pay to consume it? In the case of Medicare Part D, recipients obviously believe the $12.8 billion they pay for $89.8 billion in pharmaceuticals is worth it, but do taxpayers think it is worth the $77.0 billion they pay?

The second change is in input markets, where resource owners may or may not be taxpayers. If resource owners are taxpayers, they may be circumspect in how resources are used. But their interest as income recipients outweighs their role

as taxpayers, and hence, they seek higher remuneration for their resources. If resource owners do not pay taxes, they would have no reason to seek or demand fiscal restraint over input payments or output. Korte (2014) reported 318,462 federal employees owed the federal government $3.3 billion as of September 30, 2013.

The problem in the involuntary and subsidized exchange model is the small influence taxpayers have over the quantity of goods and services produced. Clients and resource owners have a direct interest in expanding the budget of subsidized operations: they are net beneficiaries (or winners) of expanding budgets. Resource owners want higher budgets because their incomes are directly tied to output: budget increases tied to higher wages, interest payments, or rents directly benefit resource owners. Expanding output also calls forth a need for more labor, capital, and land and may increase the prices of these inputs. The second group seeking expansion consists of subsidized clients. Expansion could occur by increasing the amount or quality of goods or services provided to current clients or increasing the number of people eligible for subsidized goods and services.

The opposing interest in involuntary exchange markets is the taxpayers who provide the funds to produce free or below-cost goods and services. Taxpayers, being net benefactors (or losers) in this exchange, have an interest in restricting the quantity of goods and services provided and want output produced as efficiently as possible. Opposition to expanding budgets, however, must be made through the political process and must abide by the majority rule. Federal taxpayers amounted to only 29.9% of the total population and 65.3% of employed persons in 2013. Unlike voluntary market exchanges, taxpayers in involuntary markets *cannot* choose not to withhold their resources.

Nonprofit and public organizations, like for-profits, should strive to maximize the value of their organizations; however, complications immediately arise over how to define and measure value. Nonprofit and public managers often claim that ideas of value maximization are foreign and perhaps inappropriate for their operations. This belief may stem from a simple misunderstanding: these organizations serve broad constituencies and produce goods or services that are provided free or at substantial subsidies to their clients, but the idea of value remains pertinent. The question of value revolves around the question of the worth of the output, and defenders of subsidized operations argue that the nonmonetary benefits produced exceed the monetary value of the resources consumed.

While it is true that not everything can be measured in dollars and cents, we are still left with the perplexing question of whether the value of a subsidized output is worth more than the resources consumed to produce it. The problem is that self-interest leads those who receive free or heavily subsidized services or whose livelihood depends on providing resources to nonprofit or public organizations to conclude that total benefit exceeds total cost. Clients receiving free goods or services, of course, think the outputs are worth more than what they pay. If subsidized clients pay 10% of the cost of a good or service, their calculation is simple: is the benefit received greater than or equal to the 10% they paid? Clients are generally unconcerned about where the other 90% is coming from to pay for the resources consumed by production. In tax-subsidized operations, there is an inherent incentive toward excessive and inefficient production. Expenditures on both Medicaid, an example of a free good, and Medicare, an example of a heavily subsidized good, have increased faster than the total healthcare spending or the U.S. economy.

People (as customers, clients, or taxpayers) desire the maximum benefit from invested resources, but the problem in subsidized markets is to determine whose benefit is to be maximized. Subsidized clients seeking the maximum benefit will demand more output as long as what they pay is less than the value they derive. Taxpayers who receive little from subsidized services may want to restrict output in order to reduce their taxes. Clients who do not pay the entire cost of the goods and services they consume and taxpayers who receive little or no benefit from subsidized services often cannot balance the cost and benefits of subsidized products, unlike customers in voluntary markets, who pay the entire cost of production and receive most, if not all, of the benefits of consuming a product. Failure to see both sides of production and consumption ensures non optimal resource decisions. It is easy to see that the total quantity of goods and services that could be distributed among the population is reduced when too many resources are used in production. But living standards are also reduced when too many (excessive consumption) or too few (insufficient output) goods and services are produced. Budgeting, by explicitly recognizing outputs, costs, and choices, should address the question of whether too many or too few subsidized goods are produced.

The conflict over output and efficiency can be illuminated by considering an example of two hospitals. It makes a significant difference to society if the cost to treat a patient (assuming similar medical problems and outcomes) is $10,000 in one hospital versus $8,000 in another hospital. A budget of $100 million allows 10,000 patients to be treated in the high-cost hospital and 12,500 patients to be treated in the low-cost hospital. Society is better off when more output is produced from a set of resources; however, in the high-cost hospital, employees may benefit from receiving higher wages (and possibly doing less work) and patients may enjoy more amenities and services. Inefficiency in any organization reduces output, but the problem is that organizations whose revenues come from compulsory taxes are likely to produce less output than possible and have excessive costs. The societal problem is that fewer subsidized goods and services are available to consumers, and ironically, too many high-cost, low-value goods and services are produced. Society could obtain greater value from another set of goods and services than what it receives from consuming subsidized products, or, in this case, overpaying for health care.

Evaluating the performance of nonprofits and government agencies is more complex than for-profits because it is more difficult to identify the components of value: what is the value of a subsidized good that is distributed free? Cost does *not* establish value: the value of a product may be higher, lower, or equal to the cost of resources used to create it. The lack of a profit mechanism, an easy-to-measure metric that indicates whether customers believe the value of a good or service exceeds its production cost, requires another mechanism to guide resource allocation. In the absence of prices and voluntary exchange, budgets should guarantee that the value of an output is greater than or at least equal to its production cost.

The differences between for-profit, nonprofit, and public organizations can now be highlighted. In for-profits, owners carry the risk of failure and enjoy the profits of success. The sources of funds in for-profits (ability to acquire labor, capital, and land and pay wages, interest, and rent) are equity, debt, and the sale of goods and services. The return on operations is total revenue less total cost. The demand for products comes from the ability of for-profits to produce goods and services that are desired by consumers at prices they are willing and able to pay. Failure to produce a desirable product at an acceptable price jeopardizes owners' investments since there is no requirement that their products be purchased at prices that cover the costs.

In contrast, the owners of a nonprofit hospital are the community. The hospital's sources of funds are the sale of goods and services, debt, grants, and donations. Returns to the community include net income, uncompensated care, and higher-than-market wages paid to employees. Demand, rather than being based on desire, may be based on the need for medical care, and the inability to pay does not preclude patients from obtaining services. Nonprofit hospitals are often committed to providing charity care, and hospitals participating in the Medicare program are required by the Emergency Medical Treatment and Labor Act (EMTALA) to provide emergency care. The desire and requirement to provide uncompensated care complicates the financial situation; hospitals must find other sources of funds to cover services for which they receive no payment. These funds must come from providing other profitable services, donations, or government grants.

In public organizations, like public health and police departments, all the owners are citizens. Unlike a nonprofit organization, where nonusers of services may not have to provide any financial support to the organization, in public organizations, all taxpayers must provide support. Public organizations also access the debt markets for funds and pay lower interest rates because of their ability to tap taxes to meet debt obligations and the tax preferences given to state and federal interest payments. The demand for the output of nonprofit and public organizations revolves around the necessity of their services and the potential inability of for-profits to supply goods and services in the desired or optimal quantities because of externalities or the public-good nature of the output or a desire for income redistribution. For these reasons, there does not have to be a direct link between consumption and financing, as cash inflows supported by compulsory taxes may be unrelated to the production of goods and services. The returns of public organizations are often stated in broad terms, such as improving

TABLE 3.1 Ownership Differences			
	For-profit	**Nonprofit**	**Public**
Owners	Stockholders	Community	All citizens
Sources of funds	Sale of output	Sale of output	Taxes
	Investment (equity)	Debt	Debt
	Debt	Donations, grants	Sale of output
Returns	Profit	Net income plus community need	Equity and stability
Demand	Ability to pay	Ability to pay plus community need	Voting

equity, maintaining order, and promoting stability. Controlling performance is difficult as the lack of a profit motive and mandatory tax support, in addition to being the sole provider of a good or service, undermines fiscal discipline (**TABLE 3.1**).

Organizations thrive by moving resources to the point where they generate the highest-possible value. This simple rule requires resources to be continually reallocated from low-value uses to those more highly valued by the public. The simple economic rule for profit maximization is that price (P) or marginal revenue (MR) should be equal to or greater than marginal cost (MC). This rule demands that the benefit of a good should exceed its production cost. While the benefit of consuming a good or a service does not have to be quantified in dollars to satisfy this rule, we still need to ask the question, is the value greater than, less than, or equal to the MC?

Consumers regularly purchase goods and services where the benefit or return cannot be quantifiable in dollars. We may not be comfortable saying that the value of hunger is $3.99, but we can definitely determine whether we are willing to spend $3.99 to purchase a Big Mac. Likewise, we all evaluate whether preventive health services are worth what we have to pay to receive them, even though it is commonly held that "you can't put a price on health." This belief implies we should be willing to pay any price for health care, which is clearly untrue. While "you can't put a price on health" may apply to efforts to stop a patient from bleeding out, it does not apply with equal force to preventive care. Flu vaccinations, for example, may not create substantial value, given the possibility that unvaccinated individuals may not contract the flu, vaccinated individuals may contract the flu, the cost of contracting the flu may be a miserable couple of days, and there may be rare but catastrophic adverse side effects of vaccination. Although the Centers for Disease Control and Prevention (CDC) reports tens of thousands deaths each year due to the flu, the *Statistical Abstract of the United States: 2012* documented only 411 deaths due to the flu in 2007.

Individuals spending their own money evaluate the value of health against all other goods to determine whether they want health care or food, clothes, and entertainment. Customers make purchasing decisions to maximize satisfaction and purchase goods and services that they believe will provide them with the greatest satisfaction for money expended, that is, products most urgently wanted, given the budget. The resource allocation decisions of nonprofits are similarly made using a mix of qualitative (value $\geq$ MC) and quantitative ($P \geq$ MC) measures, that is, they may choose a mix of a few profitable programs where revenues exceed expenses and a few unprofitable programs that meet a community need.

A nonprofit may consciously trade-off higher net income to provide needed but unprofitable community services. Organizations may choose to provide some essential, high-value services where costs cannot be recouped, and forego more profitable but less essential services. **TABLE 3.2** categorizes and prioritizes programs by profitability and community need; it is understood that programs that provide high profits and meet pressing community needs should be pursued first. Programs producing high profits are not urgently needed, and those with poor financial returns but meeting pressing community needs require greater consideration. Obviously, money-losing programs cannot be pursued if other sources of support are not available; hence, high-profit programs (whether urgently needed or not) must exist to support money-losing, high community

needs. In the end, no organization can survive if its operating expenses consistently exceed operating revenues, unless it can obtain other, non operating sources of revenue to cover the deficit. Unprofitable programs that do not serve pressing community needs should be avoided if other options can be funded.

Budgeting should assist in determining the mix between profitable and unprofitable services. Profitable services are essential to ensuring that unprofitable but needed services can continue and the organization can operate and replace its equipment and facilities over the long run. A for-profit hospital may have a better net income than a nonprofit hospital by providing fewer community services (emergency care, charity care, etc.), but this is a single, monetary measure of value. It may be that nonprofit and public hospitals create greater value when value is measured as an improvement in health per dollar consumed or a lower cost per patient served. Of course, the opposite could also be true: a for-profit hospital may have a higher net income and produce greater improvement in health per dollar expended than either nonprofit or public hospitals. A public health department providing free vaccinations may create more value per dollar expended than any hospital despite generating no revenue from the sale of its services.

The least fiscally constrained and flexible organizations are government agencies. Public organizations are least responsive to changing tastes and preferences, that is, once

TABLE 3.2 Program Mix, Profitability, and Need		
Profitability	**Community Need**	
	High	**Low**
High profit	Pursue	Pursue
Low profit/loss	Provide and offset	Avoid

started, government agencies are slow to adapt to a changing demand for their services. Often, government agencies provide a service for which there are no other suppliers and taxpayers supplying funds cannot withhold their support. The lion's share of funding for public organizations comes from involuntary taxes, thus insulating their production process from market forces. The public organizations' unresponsiveness to a changing demand arises from the small portion of their funds generated from usage fees. In public organizations, a declining demand for their goods and services may have little or no impact on their revenue, and they may not alter their processes or reduce output.

A second complication is that public organizations often operate as income redistribution vehicles, taking resources from one group to give to another. Politicians and public agency managers may see it as desirable to take a dollar from high-income groups and give 80¢ or 80¢ of service to a low-income group and maintain that society is better off as the loss to the first group is less than the gain to the second. That is, lawmakers may judge that 80¢ of medical service to a poor person is worth more than the $1.00 tax on a wealthy person. It is impossible to transfer resources from one group to another without costs due to the expense of collecting revenue and administering redistribution programs (i.e., Okun's "leaky bucket"). Transaction costs ensure that high-income groups pay more in taxes than other groups receive in goods or services. A final problem is that public agencies often judge their own performance: they decide how to measure their output and establish their own thresholds for success. All of these things, as well as political oversight, produce systems where efficiency is not a major goal.

A typical response to weakening demand in for-profit and nonprofit organizations is to cut back or eliminate services, but public agencies often do not respond this way. Public agencies often seem impervious to changing economic conditions because of the "iron triangle" (Rosen, 1988, p. 110). The iron triangle describes how the interactions of interested parties prevent resource reallocation and explains the difficulty encountered when people attempt to cut public budgets (**FIGURE 3.3**).

The reinforcing interests of each party in the iron triangle (decision-makers, producers, and consumers) make it desirable to cater to and work with the other two groups. In the iron triangle, each group controls items of value desired by the others. Politicians want to be elected or re-elected; hence, they work to secure votes. An easy way to obtain votes is to campaign for and support legislation for increased spending and fight attempts to reduce programs and public sector payrolls. Politicians expect that the returns from more government services to clients and more jobs and higher pay for public employees will be votes in their favor. Imagine a politician wanting to cut social security: the majority of senior citizens and social security administration (and federal) employees would vote against him or her.

Managers of public agencies desire higher budgets (to secure their position, increase their power, increase their salaries, etc.) and, for that, cultivate relationships with clients and politicians. Expanded programs provide more benefits to clients and secure the support of politicians. Public agency managers have the power to withhold resources from politicians and clients who do not support them. Hence,

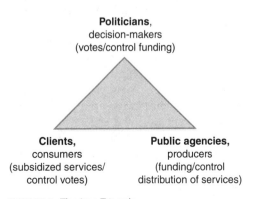

FIGURE 3.3 The Iron Triangle

an imaginary politician (one who supports reducing the size of government) may see poor service in his or her district, new government offices built in other districts, etc. Likewise, a client group that provides lukewarm support to an agency may see expansion of benefits for more supportive groups. Politicians and clients find it less risky and more advantageous to support an agency's expansion than oppose it.

Finally, clients want free or subsidized services, and politicians who do not cooperate in this pursuit lose votes and may be voted out of office, and uncooperative agency employees may face angry constituents, who might take their demands to their superiors, elected officials, and/or the media to press their case. The path of self-interest and least resistance leads public agencies to submit to, if not encourage, client and political demands in order to solidify political and public support for expanding public sector employment.

In the iron triangle, there is no countervailing power: the providers of resources, taxpayers, who stand to lose from the expansion of operations, lie outside the triangle. The question is, how much will taxpayers tolerate before demanding changes in public programs? The problem taxpayers face is concentrated benefits and diffused costs: those who receive direct and large direct benefits from public programs fight hard to maintain the status quo or increase the scale or scope of the programs. Taxpayers footing the bill may see the amount they pay as trivial and may be unwilling to devout significant time or energy into altering the current system. If 94.5 million individuals pay federal income tax and are concerned about an operation that costs the U.S. Treasury $3.7 billion, for example, sugar subsidies, the average cost per taxpayer is only $39.15—individual taxpayers will *not* see it as worth their time and energy to eliminate or reduce a program with a multibillion-dollar budget. The problem with sugar subsidies is that the majority of the cost does not come directly from the treasury but rather from higher retail prices, spreading the cost over

316 million people, a cost of $11.71 per citizen, while sugar producers receive, on average, $787,234 (Will, 2013).

Groups in the iron triangle pursue different goals, but all recognize that achieving their particular goal is based on the goodwill and cooperation of the other two groups. Each group controls and is controlled by the other two groups. Few, if any, individuals within the triangle have an interest in reducing the flow of resources. Missing in this system is the consideration of opportunity costs: can new or existing funds be more wisely spent on other things? Part of the problem in the public sector is the ease of seeing what could be lost (benefits, jobs, and votes) and the difficulty in seeing what could be gained (greater value and higher efficiency).

The outsiders, taxpayers, may not see what they will gain (and hence not lobby for resource reallocation), whereas the present beneficiaries see clearly what they will lose if their programs are reduced. There is also the simple problem of change; it is easier to look back than it is forward. Programs are routinely developed for a specific crisis. For example, sugar subsidies were a "temporary" program started during the depression of the 1930s, but the assumption of continuing need has not changed in the intervening years. The challenge for management and budgeting is to look ahead to determine what people will want in the future.

A second challenge is the inertia that afflicts most organizations; change agents fight uphill battles in attempting to alter systems in response to changes in the world. This is true in all organizations, but those that produce goods and services whose costs are not recovered by voluntary payments have the luxury of maintaining the status quo as the world changes around them. The World Bank (1995) held that in the absence of political desirability (a crisis and/or a change in leadership), political feasibility (the ability to purchase the support of opposition groups), and credibility (a reputation for keeping promises or restraints on reversing course), change would not occur in public organizations. Improvements in budgeting systems are needed to ensure that all organizations have incentives to minimize their costs similar to for-profits, whose revenues result from voluntary exchange with customers and battle with competitors to provide better and lower-priced goods and services.

▶ Budget Participants and Roles

Developing a budget involves three basic functions: budget preparation, review, and approval (**FIGURE 3.4**). These three functions, and the people performing them, find themselves variously in concert and at odds, depending on and competing against each other. The budget goal, maximizing value, is more effectively served if preparers, reviewers, and approvers share a common goal and utilize one another's strengths and knowledge.

Besides knowledge of the operation being budgeted, managers preparing their budgets should be familiar with efficiency, bargaining, and program evaluation (i.e., the assessment of the need, design, and impact of a program). Rather than being an accounting exercise, budgeting should be a dynamic, forward-looking process to realize organizational or social goals in the most efficient manner. A budget should serve the organization's reason for being, identify its objectives, define how those objectives will be pursued, and establish how performance will be evaluated. After the start of the fiscal year, the budget should provide a management guide (i.e., what is expected to be accomplished in the upcoming year), a tool to correct and improve operations, and a mechanism for measuring performance and establishing accountability.

Budget preparation, review, and approval require that budgets be constructed in concert with different members of the organization, where each member has a different set of knowledge and responsibilities. If any member's knowledge is omitted or a member shirks his or her responsibility, a non optimal plan will result. Each budget participant should supply accurate and relevant information and act in a manner that ensures what is best for the organization. This would be easy if goals were mutually reinforcing; however, budgeting processes must often navigate the conflict that arises when individual, department, and organizational goals are not the same.

Budget Preparation

Department managers are tasked with constructing the financial plan of operation for the following fiscal year. The financial plan may be as simple as specifying a given dollar amount (e.g., $2 million) and leaving the resources and what is to be done undefined. On the other hand, the plan may require identifying (1) what is to be accomplished, (2) what resources are needed for success, (3) how much the resources should cost and (4) providing a detailed plan that traces the dollar amount to a defined set of resources required to produce the quantified output.

An operating manager's primary concerns are departmental functions and customers or clients, whether they are the final consumers of a product or other members of the organization who use the department's output as an input in another production process. Managers are responsible for designing and managing how the operations of their departments are performed. Deming (1982, p. 315) holds that more than 90% of problems and the possibilities for improvement are due to the system and that system performance is management's responsibility. Managers should ensure their departments produce the output required by consumers and meet required quality standards. Managers should ensure consumers are happy with the output (what is produced) and the service they receive (how goods and services are delivered), while keeping expenses at or below the budget. Meeting all three

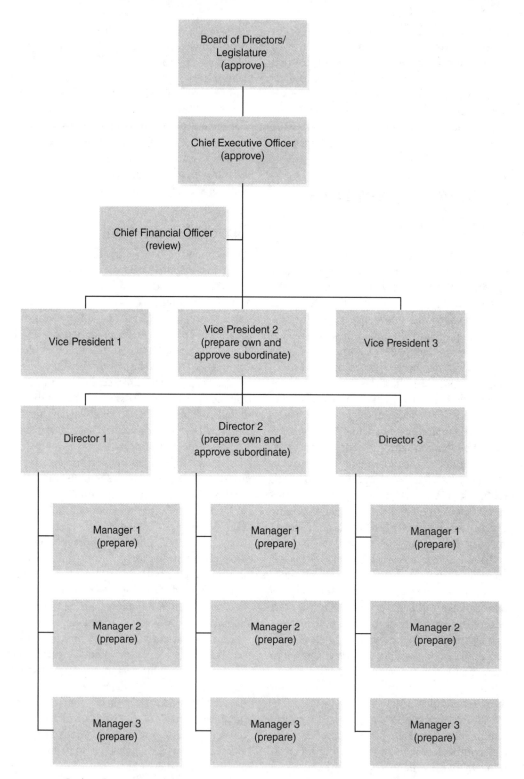

FIGURE 3.4 Budget Functions and the Organization Chart

objectives is easier with more resources, so the managers' primary objective in budget preparation is to obtain the highest-possible budget. The managers' performance is often assessed by whether they get the job done and whether they remain within the budget. Delivering consumer-pleasing products but overrunning the budget may be as unacceptable as not getting the job done but staying within the budget.

Maximizing the size of a budget produces a curious mix of optimistic and pessimistic (or best-case/worst-case) thinking in managers. Estimates of anticipated output are often overstated, while pessimism rules over the capability of resources employed to justify higher resources. Managers underestimate what resources can produce, including employee productivity, while they overstate unproductive time, the need for supplies, maintenance on existing equipment and facilities, and the need for new investments. Each appraisal is designed to maximize resources (or reserve capacity) to guarantee that unanticipated disruptions can be handled within the confines of the budget. Overstating of resource needs should be expected, as incomplete work is more noticeable than padded budgets.

Constructing an operating plan from scratch (see Chapter 5) is difficult because of all the variables that must be considered, and consequently, most budgets are built from past budgets or current performance. Budgets typically reflect where an organization has been rather than where it hopes to go. Future expenses are routinely based on past resource consumption and the anticipated prices for those resources in the following fiscal year (i.e., incremental budgets; see Chapter 6). Using past performance as a base for estimating future expenses simplifies budget calculations and plays into the mix of optimism and pessimism used in budget construction. To maximize budgets, managers assume few, if any, resources will be freed up or rendered unnecessary if output declines. This type of expense is a fixed cost, and given this assumption, the budget should be stable despite projections of falling output. On the other hand, when output is expected to increase, all expenses are classified as variable costs to obtain large budget increases.

While unwarranted budget maximization is wasteful, it is consistent with the managers' self-interest. A manager's job is to complete the tasks assigned, and the primary concern is not alternative resource uses. A manager's goal of maximizing the budget produces competition between departments and divisions, and it is the budget approvers' job to ensure that this competition allocates resources to their best uses. A manager's job should be to maximize the value of the organization, and managers should strive to increase output and reduce costs in order to demonstrate why budget increases should flow to their departments rather than other areas.

Should a manager maximize his or her budget or lower costs? Although these goals appear to be in conflict, they are not a contradiction; a budget should be maximized if, and only if, it provides greater benefits than alternative resource allocations. The role of the budget approvers is to evaluate alternatives and ensure resources are allocated to the best uses. On the other hand, a budget can be maximized without providing corresponding benefits, that is, one can simply increase costs without providing any service (i.e., featherbedding). The production of high-cost, low-benefit output should be a short-run phenomenon; it should only continue if the organization lacks competition and has a management team that does not or cannot weigh value and costs.

The review and approval processes should supply oversight to determine where resources produce their highest value.

Budget Review

Finance is charged with monitoring and controlling the financial health of the organization. The primary budget job of finance is to ensure that planned expenses are equal to or less than anticipated revenues, or can the operating plan be achieved with available resources? When budgeted expenses exceed revenues, finance must make senior management aware of monetary constraints and push them to develop a new plan with lower expenses, higher revenues, or both.

Managers often see a conflict between their goal of getting a job done and their view that finance simply wants to maximize profits by starving departments of resources. While this conflict may be real in some cases, it does not negate the fact that managers often seek budget increases that add little to the value of the organization. When unwarranted expenses are requested, the budget office has the unenviable duty to call the expenses into question. Finance is responsible for reviewing budget requests and asking tough and sometime impolite questions: Is this expenditure needed? Can the expense be reduced? Are existing resources used effectively (or can more output be produced from existing resources)?

Senior management and division directors are responsible for reviewing their subordinates' budget requests. A narrow view of this duty is to ensure that their areas of responsibility obtain all the resources they want. Reviewers at the division level should understand the broader issues facing the organization and be willing to forego resources if the funds could produce higher benefit in other areas. To encourage this broader view, senior management compensation should be partially based on the overall performance of the organization versus solely on the performance of the divisions.

Like operating managers, vice presidents (VPs) and division directors should be expected to be partial to their own areas and interests. While attempting to maximize their divisions' budgets, self-interest should lead the senior managers to ensure the best-possible allocation of resources within their areas of responsibility. VPs and division directors may be willing to see resources reallocated within their divisions or between their departments, but we should not expect them to eagerly accept resource shifts from their divisions to other divisions. In the contest for resources, senior managers generally can be expected to make the best case for own areas' budget requests and forcefully push back any attempts to reduce their budgets.

Budget Approval

At the budget approval stage, there should be a pronounced shift from a division or departmental perspective to the organizational view. Those approving the budget are responsible for the entire organization, and they should balance the conflicting, parochial interests of their subordinates.

The primary player in approving the budget is the chief executive officer (CEO) or president. CEOs are responsible for, and therefore should be evaluated on, the overall performance of the organization. A CEO should establish global priorities and direct resources to uses that produce the greatest benefit for the organization. When budgeted expenses exceed revenues and program cutbacks are required, we cannot expect VPs, division directors, or operating managers to scale back their operations; it is the job of the CEO to determine when cutbacks are needed, which programs receive funding, and which do not. This is an unenviable task, but it is the duty of the person sitting at the head of an organization. Likewise, when additional funds are available and multiple claims are made, it is the CEO's job to determine which of the emerging opportunities should be funded.

The final stop in the process is approval by the board of directors (or legislature for government agencies). The role of the board is typically thought to involve setting strategy, hiring, assessing, setting compensation, removing the CEO (when necessary), and approving budgets. On the other hand, many think that the board does not play an active role in management in for-profits and nonprofits. The text follows the "what the board should do" model versus "what boards actually do" and assumes that board members play an active role in planning and budgeting. The role of board members (or legislators) is to represent their constituents. In the private sector, board members typically include business leaders, members of the executive staff, employee representatives, and outside directors representing the larger community. In the public sector, the focus on particular constituencies is clear when we observe that a legislator takes a vastly different position on issues of spending and taxes according to who voted the legislator into office.

In the private sector, the role of the board parallels the role of the CEO; board members should focus on increasing the value of the organization regardless of whether this means maximizing profits or benefits to the community. Board members have a legal duty to protect the organization. For example, Worldcom and Enron directors had to pay $18 million and $13 million, respectively, out of their own funds to compensate investors for the frauds carried out at these institutions. The author doesn't expect directors to be sued as a result of constructing a poor budget. Worldcom and Enron are examples of the worst-possible misconduct by management, but they highlight the fact that directors should not shirk their responsibilities of assessing management and establishing the direction of organizations.

The usefulness of the budget is determined by how well each party fulfills its role. Operating managers, finance, and the CEO and the board must bring to the budgeting process their expertise on production processes, financial constraints, and goals and customers. The final budget should advance the best ends and find a proper balance between alternative resource uses. This requires determining what should be produced, how it should be produced, and who will receive the output. Answering these questions requires navigating the contentious issues of what should be funded and what will be foregone, what should be produced, and who should be served and making sure that enough, but no more than are needed, resources are committed to a production process.

▶ A Budget Construction Calendar and Overlapping Budget Cycles

Budget construction typically starts 6 months before the beginning of the following fiscal year (or 6 months prior to the end of the current fiscal year) to provide sufficient time to perform all the necessary budget-building tasks. Multiple months are needed to allow for budget preparation, review, and approval and to obtain participation from employees on the department floor to the C-suite. The process should begin with a set of programs detailing what senior management expects to accomplish in the upcoming year, including the type and quantities of output to be produced. Defining programs is the responsibility of senior management and/or planning. The budget office then develops a budget package, including instructions, forms, inflation forecasts, and output estimates, for distribution to department managers.

After receiving the budget package, managers may receive a month to complete and return their budgets. After managers submit their budgets, the budget office compiles the master budget by aggregating the department budgets to determine total expected revenues and expenses for the organization. If total expenses exceed total revenue, the department budgets may be returned to the managers for reducing expenses or to planners for reducing the scope of programs. The assessment of feasibility and the revision process may occur multiple times; hence, an early start is needed to ensure that the final budget can be completed before the start of the following fiscal year. Once the revenues and expenses are reconciled, the budget is sent to senior management and the board of directors for approval. **FIGURE 3.5** shows what budget work is needed, when it should occur, and which party is responsible for the task.

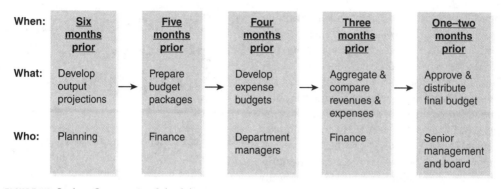

FIGURE 3.5 Budget Construction Schedule

Budget construction is the prospective phase of the process, and despite the fact that the concurrent and retrospective phases follow sequentially, organizations and operating managers have to operate in different budget phases at the same time. Managers may have to prepare the upcoming budget while executing the current budget and reviewing the results of operations of the previous fiscal year. A single budget cycle may require 24 months to complete from initial budget preparation through the final performance evaluation.

FIGURE 3.6 highlights the three budget functions and how they overlap in a single budget year. The *preparation* phase often begins 6 months prior to the start of a fiscal year and lays out the budgeting process, specifies resource needs, reconciles planned expenditures with expected revenues, and obtains necessary approvals. For example, in July 2016, the 2017 budget cycle begins with projections of programs and output from senior management, continues with the distribution of budgeting instructions and forms, and culminates with the approval of the final budget before the end of the year. The *facilitation and control* phase for 2017 spans from January to December 2017 and includes implementing the budget, managing the budget (modification of resource consumption according to output and/or environmental changes), and performing monthly analysis of variances. The final phase, *evaluation and accountability*, begins after the budget year is completed and accounting records

	2016		2017		2018	
	Jan–June	July–Dec	Jan–June	July–Dec	Jan–June	July–Dec
Budget year	Evaluate 2015					
2016	Execute 2016 →→→→→→→					
		Estimate 2017				
			Evaluate 2016			
2017			Execute 2017→→→→→→→			
				Estimate 2018		
					Evaluate 2017	
2018					Execute 2018 →→→→→→→	

FIGURE 3.6 Overlapping Budget Cycles

finalized. Finalizing the year-end income statement and balance sheet for 2017, for example, may take a month or more, and assessing performance, the retrospective phase, could continue through June 2018. The complete 2017 budget cycle, highlighted in Figure 3.6, may, thus, last from July 2016 through June 2018.

The overlap of evaluation of the prior budget and execution of the current budget in the first months of a fiscal year and the overlap of execution and estimation of the following year's budget in the final months of a fiscal year show that managers, senior management, and the budget office have to work in two budget cycles at the same time. If reviews of prior budgets require more than 6 months to complete or budget preparation begins more than 6 months before the start of a new fiscal year, managers may find themselves working in three budget years at the same time. Working on two budget years at the same time may be confusing, but it is easy to see that understanding the prior year's performance (e.g., fiscal year 2016) may provide insight into how current operations (fiscal year 2017) should be managed and that understanding performance in the prior and current years should inform the construction of the 2018 fiscal year budget. It is worth repeating that only when the budget is seen as a dynamic instrument to understand, control, and plan operations will organizations and managers reap the rewards of effective budgeting. If budgeting is treated as a one-time exercise to estimate expenses, where the results of one year are not utilized to improve current operations or plan future actions, the value of budgeting will be largely lost.

▶ Budget Strategy

Resources are valuable, and their control is always a source of conflict. Conflict is widely regarded as regrettable, if not outright undesirable, but many great thinkers believe that conflict can produce the best-possible outcomes. Conflict and competition are constructive and beneficial when they ensure that resources are employed in their most productive uses. In economics, competition manifests itself as rivalry between firms attempting to attract customers by producing better product or reducing the price below that of other firms. Competition among organizations benefits consumers. James Madison, in *The Federalist No. 51*, notes the necessity of competition in political systems and that "ambition must be made to counteract ambition." His vision was to divide the government and set the executive, legislative, and judicial branches of the government in competition with each other to ensure the rights of citizens. If one branch of the government should attempt to overstep its constitutional duties, it impinges on the authority of the other two branches. Madison expected that each branch would jealously protect its prerogatives and prevent transgressions by the other branches, while it itself is also held in check.

Budgeting is a similar, though smaller, version of a system of checks and balances. All organizations, whether for-profit, nonprofit, or public, have limited resources. Within organizations, managers are expected to strive for the maximum amount of the limited resources available, and resource grabs should be countered by those who will lose if another department or division obtains a large budget increase. The managers, directors, and VPs whose departments stand to lose resources should question why others need additional resources. They should ask what end the additional resources will serve, whether the end is more important than other things the organization is doing or could undertake, and whether present resources are being used effectively and efficiently. Every manager should be prepared to respond to these questions when his or her request for more resources is challenged. The role of the CEO and/or the board is to adjudicate conflicting resource claims and ensure resources flow to the areas that create the greatest value for the organization. The difficulty in expanding a budget "beachhead," grabbing a greater share of the organization's resources, will hopefully produce a system where only truly worthy undertakings survive the gauntlet.

Unfortunately, the idealist view espoused by marginal decision-making and competition for resources is regularly supplanted by the managers' desire to maximize their budgets. The choice of a budgeting system establishes incentives, and a poor choice leads directly to budget maximization rather than value maximization. Rosen (1988, p. 110) notes that the unwritten rule of the Congressional Ways and Means Committee was not to question the budget requests of other House members. In return for not questioning others' budget requests, the members do not question yours; this trade-off negates competition and leads to bloated, non value-maximizing budgets.

Brickley, Smith, and Zimmerman (1997, p. 27) recount how Soviet lighting manufacturers were compensated on the basis of the total weight of lamps produced. The use of a weight-based performance measurement system resulted in manufacturers producing the heaviest lighting fixtures possible because it was easier to meet production goals (measured in kilograms) by producing fewer and heavier fixtures than more lightweight lamps. In the end, chandeliers were produced, which were so heavy that they pulled down ceilings. Similarly, Moscow taxi drivers were compensated on the mileage driven, and to maximize mileage (and their pay), the drivers ran empty vehicles up and down the highways rather than transporting fares through busy Moscow streets. The mileage-based compensation system completely failed to achieve the desired results of transporting people, but mileage was maximized because higher speeds could be maintained and little time was wasted picking up or letting off passengers. Bureaucrats everywhere recognize that people need incentives, yet they fail to see that their evaluation measures and compensation systems lead directly to actions that reduce rather than increase value. Unintended negative consequences are obvious in retrospect, yet we do little to train people how to anticipate

predictable ill effects before systems are put in place.

Winning the Budget Game

The predictable consequence of implementing a budgeting system is that managers attempt to secure the greatest amount of resources they can and win the budget game. The obstacle to resource maximization is that this end must be pursued in a system where everyone else is pursuing the same goal and is inclined to see another's gain as his or her loss and vice versa. The author does *not* advocate the following actions but rather reports what happens versus what should happen. There are three simple rules for maximizing a budget:

Rule #1: Always request more resources than you need.

In the budget game, give-and-take is expected; managers should build excess resources into their initial expense estimates and plan to give back in the budget negotiations funds that were not needed. When budget requests are overstated, budget reductions can be achieved painlessly; that is, it is better to cut "fat" than "muscle," but if there is no fat in your budget, you may have no other choice than to cut muscle.

Rule #2: Be prepared and present the best-possible case for your budget request.

When requesting resources, managers should present the best-possible case to ensure favorable reception by reviewing and approving personnel. Know your audience; understand its goals; prepare a clear presentation, including graphs; highlight critical points or changes from the past; anticipate questions and provide support, as needed; and summarize key points in your conclusion. The last thing a manager wants is to have his or her competence questioned because of a poor budget presentation. Questions of competency give birth to increased scrutiny of budgets and performance. It is better to be prepared and project competence than to be forced to defend past and current performance and the necessity of future budget requests.

Rule #3: Always spend your entire budget.*

Once a budget is approved, it should be completely spent, as most budgeting systems unfortunately discourage cost reduction and thrift. If a manager does not spend all the money budgeted in a year, he or she will probably receive less funding in subsequent years. Senior management and finance assume that unspent monies prove that a department did not need the funding provided and that resources should be reallocated in future budgets.

Using the same thought process (see the footnote), if managers overspend, they "prove" that more money was needed and that their departments should receive higher funding in subsequent years. Many organizations employ this perverse incentive: managers receive fewer resources (are punished) for holding costs down and receive more resources (are rewarded) when costs go overbudget.

The primary objective of many managers is to maximize their budgets. The benefits flowing from a large budget include higher prestige, greater power over resources (the ability to hire, select suppliers, etc.), and potentially an increase in one's compensation. There is nothing inappropriate with large budgets unless they supply more resources than necessary to complete work.

Given the pecuniary advantages accruing to large budgets, managers have multiple reasons to seek the largest-possible amount of resources. The budget review and approval processes should prevent individual managers from undermining the larger goal of maximizing the value of the organization. Besides an increase in prestige, control, and income, managers also request more resources than they require because it is easier to manage with a cushion than when one has only enough and no more resources than are necessary to produce the expected outputs. Budget padding is a time-honored tradition. In some cases, excess resources are mandated to provide reserve capacity in emergencies, and more often than not, managers simply want the security that budget cushions provide.

Just-in-time inventory systems are similar to tight budgets in that both signal when resources are being used inappropriately. In just-in-time inventory systems, only enough supplies are held to complete a planned production run. As the production run approaches completion, additional material should be delivered by suppliers—the Kanban system. If supplies are misused, damaged, or stolen, the loss of resources will not allow the planned production run to be completed. The consumption of more resources than necessary alerts managers to the fact that the production system is not working as it should. This information motivates the managers to identify the problem and restore the system to optimal performance. A tight budget performs the same role: if the minimal level of resources is budgeted for a fixed amount of output and this output is produced but at a higher-than-expected cost, it indicates problems. The challenge of operating at maximum efficiency may be one that managers and employees would rather avoid.

Inefficient budgets also arise from managers' attempts to please employees, customers, or clients. It is important to recognize that one person's cost is another person's income and that a budget is an income and product distribution mechanism; employees want higher wages and lobby managers and the organization for higher compensation.

---

* If you can get away with it, spend more than you have been budgeted (to increase the base from which the following year's budget will be calculated).

Salary increases are one tool managers have to motivate and keep their employees happy (Herzberg categorizes money as a maintenance factor capable of making employees dissatisfied but ultimately unable to motivate them). Higher salaries for subordinates also provide a compelling reason for managers to seek raises for themselves.

On the consumption side, customers or clients want more and/or higher-quality outputs, especially when others pay the additional production costs. Managers could request more or better-skilled employees to improve output or increase timeliness, purchase higher-quality supplies, and/or provide more luxurious or customer-friendly facilities. The question that again arises is, at whose expense? In markets relying on voluntary transactions between buyers and sellers, the drive for more and better products or facilities is tempered by the realization that customers must pay for increases in quantity or quality. While some people are willing to pay the additional expense to shop at Macy's or other retailers providing more personal service, it is clear that more shoppers prefer the less luxurious facilities and lower-priced merchandise of Walmart. Clients receiving subsidized goods and services, however, will be more adamant in their demands, since the cost of expanding the output or service or improving facilities will be paid partially or entirely by others.

When goods and services are sold in voluntary exchange markets, increased costs arising from higher input prices, increased output, and/or higher quality (without higher productivity) must increase the price to the consumer. Demands by workers for higher wages or by consumers for more output or higher-quality output are moderated by the knowledge that these costs must be paid through higher prices. The problem that arises in nonprofit and public organizations is that the people receiving the benefit and those paying for the resources used in production may not be the same. Subsidized consumers will attempt to overconsume products when production costs are partially or fully paid by others (i.e., **moral hazard**).

Consumption of healthcare services among the elderly and the poor whose costs are primarily paid by workers is a prime example of the iron triangle and moral hazard. Politicians seek expansions in public financing of health care to capture votes of the elderly and the poor, healthcare workers see an expanded demand from these groups as a means to increase their incomes, and the elderly and the poor receive additional goods and services subsidized by others. All three groups benefit from expanding healthcare budgets, and taxpayers are left with lower disposable incomes. Public financing of health care succeeds because of concentrated benefits and diffused costs. The elderly, the poor, the healthcare industry, and politicians have a direct interest in expanding medical coverage and work for its realization. Taxpayers pay hundreds of billions of dollars a year to support Medicare and Medicaid, but this cost is diffused over tens of millions of workers. Taxpayers do not see it in their interest to actively oppose Medicare or Medicaid expansion, as the cost of opposing expansion is greater than the anticipated increase in taxes.

Further undermining opposition to the expansion of government programs is the use of debt financing. In an era of trillion-dollar federal deficits, taxpayers have less incentive to oppose expansion of government programs. Since the programs are funded by selling treasury bonds, they can be expanded, and taxes do not increase as costs are passed to future generations. The costs of federal programs today are not fully paid by the current generation; future generations, including those too young to vote and the unborn, have been co-signed to satisfy the debt.

The point is that budgeting in nonprofit and public organizations substitutes for the role of a market and should ensure that resources are used intelligently, that is, the value of what is created should be greater than or equal to the value of the resources consumed in the production process. Budgeting should equate the total costs and total benefits of an operation and be concerned with who pays. Economics seeks **Pareto improvements**, that is, reallocation of resources that make one or more persons better off without making anyone else worse off. At the point of **Pareto optimality**, no resource reallocation can occur without reducing another's well-being. Before any program is implemented, we should be certain that the benefit to one group (the consuming group) exceeds the cost imposed on another group (the payer group).

The next section reviews budget strategies recognizing that individuals' incentive to maximize their budgets and the organizational goals of maximizing output from a set of resources may not be in concert. Knowledge of the various strategies to increase or defend a budget can be used to protect value-adding activities or to prevent excess and unnecessary resources from being reallocated to better uses. Like all tools, budget strategies can be used for good or bad ends: they can support the efficient allocation of resources or be employed to maintain or expand nonproductive resources.

Economic Reasons for Budget Increases

Budgets should increase with changes in the environment that are beyond the control of managers and that increase the cost of producing the expected goods or services. Change is constant, and organizations simultaneously face factors that increase and decrease the cost of production. The discussion in this section assumes for the sake of simplicity that only one change arises at a time and there are no countervailing events. Managers attempting to maximize their budgets will make budget reviewers and approvers aware of changes driving costs higher, such as increases in input

prices, output, production technology, and product standards, while withholding information on cost-lowering changes.

Higher Input Prices

Budgets are typically constructed using current expenses increased for anticipated increases in resources prices (the change in the consumer price index, producer price index (PPI), or another measure of inflation). As input prices increase, budgets have to grow at the same pace to enable the organization to purchase the same set of resources and produce the same output. The problem (as well as a budget-padding opportunity) is that not all prices change at the same rate. Managers should be knowledgeable about specific price changes for the major inputs used and use this information to maximize their budgets. For example, the PPI in April 2017 (Bureau of Labor Statistics, 2017)) showed that all commodities increased in price by 5.3% from the previous year; however, fuel and related products increased by 17.6%, while healthcare services increased by only 1.7%. The use of the all-commodity increase would dramatically understate the rate of change in fuel and related products and their budget. On the other hand, the price increase for all commodities would overstate the increase in the price of healthcare services. If specific input prices are expected to increase faster than general inflation, managers should ensure that their budgets increase at the specific rate. On the flip side, if the prices of major inputs are less than general inflation, managers may want to accept the average price change and thus introduce an element of fat into the budget.

Increased Workload

Increases in the demand for the output produced, for example, a 5.0% increase in output, will require more inputs, and the budget should be augmented for the increased amount of inputs expected to be used, in addition to any anticipated increase in input prices. Expected increases in output provide another opportunity to pad the budget: a 5.0% increase in output should not produce a 5.0% increase in expenses, given the existence of fixed costs. Budget allocations should increase only to the extent that variable costs increase with higher output. On the other hand, when demand and output fall, managers do not voluntarily forego resources but wait to see whether others will identify and attempt to reduce their budgets. When others note that the falling output should translate into fewer resources, managers often argue that their costs are fixed and, thus, no reduction is appropriate.

Cost Increasing Change in Production Technology

Changes in production processes are often introduced to reduce costs. The classic case of cost-reducing technology is Henry Ford's introduction of the assembly line in 1913 (Ford, 1923). Before the assembly line was introduced, chassis assembly took 12 hours and 28 minutes; after its introduction, it took 1 hour and 33 minutes. Ford responded to this leap in productivity by increasing employee wages and reducing the price of the Model T.

Health care is a prime example of the introduction of cost-increasing technology. The decline of simple X-rays in favor of magnetic resonance imaging (MRI) increased costs for the same number of tests. MRIs produce higher-quality images, and hence, it may be argued that the output is better. But the point remains that health care, as opposed to other industries, often adopts cost-increasing technology. Changes in production technologies often lead to greater productivity and lower costs and again provide an opportunity for budget padding. A budget-maximizing manager would withhold information on cost-saving advances to appropriate those savings rather than letting them flow to the organization or its customers.

Pollution control regulations are a second example of cost-increasing technological change, Greenstone, List, and Syverson (2012) estimate that air quality regulations add roughly $21 billion annually to the manufacturing sector's costs.

Change in Output or Quality Improvements

Budgets should increase with changes in product features, such as improved appearance or expanded functionality and improvements in quality, that increase production time or require more qualified and higher-paid staff and/or better supplies and equipment. Again, changes may run in the opposite direction, and the substitution of cheaper components in a product or the acceptance of lower quality (less durable, etc.) would permit budget reductions that a budget-maximizing manager would ignore in his or her budget estimates.

Budgets should only increase when changes in the environment increase production costs. Legitimate or real reasons for higher budgets include higher production process, expanded output, cost-increasing technology change (often driven by regulation), and improvements to products. On the other hand, any of these factors moving in the opposite direction should translate directly into smaller budgets. Managers can be expected to identify factors that justify a higher budget and to ignore cost-reducing changes. The outcome will be higher budgets as budget approvers are at an information disadvantage in identifying cost-reducing factors.

Political Strategies to Increase or Defend a Budget

As opposed to legitimate reasons for higher budgets, there are a myriad of strategies employed to unnecessarily increase a budget or prevent budget reductions. The first set of strategies includes *all-purpose strategies* as their intent is to preclude budget scrutiny by cultivating defenders, developing the confidence of budget reviewers, and/or obfuscating department operations. The second set of strategies, *offensive strategies*, is employed to secure larger budgets, and these strategies are built on overstating the need for outputs and/or production costs. The last set, *defensive strategies*, is designed to prevent budget reductions during periods of austerity and include delay, responsibility shifting, and increase in the real or imagined costs of budget cuts.

All-Purpose Strategies

All-purpose strategies can be relied upon to seek additional funding or prevent budget cuts. All-purpose strategies are designed to lift a budget above scrutiny. Resources are valuable, and astute managers should never be complacent nor should they assume that current funding levels will persist. Dynamic and dramatic changes can affect the resources an organization or department will be able to call upon to fund its expenses and produce goods or services. Astute managers act to ensure that new funds flow their way, funding reductions are aimed at others' budgets, and demand (or need) for their goods and services grows.

Cultivate a Clientele and Advocates. This calls for increased funding or exemption from budget reductions. These requests coming from managers are seldom given complete consideration, since they originate from people with a stake in higher funding and represent a small number of people. Astute managers know that greater consideration is accorded to requests coming from external parties, typically consumers of the output produced, and the weight given to the request increases with the number of petitioners. Third-party demands for increased funding show a need (or at least a strong desire) for the good or service, a committed clientele that sees its interest as being tied to the funded program, department, or organization, and a large group, not simply employees, will be impacted. In 2013, the United States saw proposals to cut

back the postal service being actively opposed by the postal employees' union, who ran television commercials to whip up greater public opposition to the proposed cuts. The union successfully emphasized how the public and small businesses would be negatively impacted by ending Saturday mail service.

Cultivate Confidence. Cultivating confidence requires demonstrating the effectiveness and/or efficiency of your operation. The goal is to be respected and liked by those who review and approve your budget. When money is tight, the first targets for budget cuts are operations that are known to be ineffective or inefficient. One may not be ineffective or inefficient, but if the department has the appearance of either, it will rank high on the list of programs to reduce when budget cuts are needed. On the other hand, a department need not be either effective or efficient if it can maintain the appearance of each. To paraphrase Machiavelli, "Man lives by the eye rather than the mind"—all see, few understand.

Obfuscate. Obfuscation keeps operations a mystery. Mystery and indecipherability are often equated with complexity, skill, and value. Simplicity is often undervalued: if reviewers can understand an operation, they may think they can do the work better, cheaper, and faster. To avoid undesired contributions from direct supervisors, finance, senior management, and approving bodies, it is beneficial if these parties believe that the operation is beyond their comprehension and that they should defer to the operating manager's judgment. Obfuscation can use one or more of the following tactics:

- The voluminous data and numbers tactic inundates reviewers with details and makes it impossible for them to wade through data. Data is unorganized information, and managers should provide the maximum amount of data and a minimum amount of information. Data is difficult to deal with, organize, and summarize into information. The aim is to lead reviewers or approvers to the conclusion that data volume equates to complexity.

- You should provide half the picture. Describe the benefits created and ignore costs. Airbags are a perfect example: autosafety advocates reporting the number of lives saved, while ignoring the cost of installing hundreds of millions of airbags since 1989. According to Miller, Benjamin, and North (2001), in the first eight years when airbags were installed, 2600 lives were saved. However, 80 children were killed by exploding airbags in low-speed collisions, and 100 million airbags were installed in vehicles at a cost of $400 per airbag. The cost per life saved was $15,873,016 ($40,000,000,000/(2,600 − 80)). No one argues against saving 2,520 lives; however, many question the wisdom of spending $15,873,016 to save a single life and note that more lives could be saved at a lower cost through other interventions.

- You should *selectively use numbers and percentages*. When the output is large, report output increases as numbers, for example, demand increased by 10,000 units (if 1 million units are being produced, this amounts to a 1.0% increase). When 10,000 units are produced, an increase of 10,000 units should be trumpeted as a 100% increase.

- The policy or regulation trap tactic defends budget increases behind policy, regulation, and/or legislation changes and blocks budget cuts by asserting that reductions would violate existing edicts. In the latter case, managers only need to argue that existing expenditures must be continued because regulations demand it. The assertion may not be completely true, but budget reviewers and approvers will probably be outside their area of expertise and not challenge what must be done, why it needs to be done, how it should be done, and how much it should

cost. Similarly, how organizations respond to new or pending regulations will be determined by managers with an interest in responding quickly with a request for large increases in funding to meet the new or imagined requirements.

- Gold or chrome plating recommends that when you have nothing to say, say it well. Gold plating means adding expensive and unnecessary features to products and shifts the focus away from what is being spent to nurturing awe. Darrel Huff (1954) reported how a company that could not prove its cold remedy worked enhanced its appeal by changing the subject. The manufacturer demonstrated the nostrum killed germs, 31,108 in 11 seconds with only 1/2 oz. While this level of germ-killing ability seems impressive, it did not address the question of whether the germs killed caused colds. The goal of gold plating is to create in the minds of others the perception that the department's work is valuable, effective, and efficiently performed, often using visually appealing and sound-enhanced PowerPoint slides, strategically structured graphs, and irrelevant or biased statistics. In many situations, success is measured and reported as the use of inputs rather than higher output or better outcomes.

- Exclusive terminology resorts to the use of the proprietary language of the profession or field to obfuscate budget issues. Accountants, lawyers, doctors, and engineers resort to the arcane lexicon of their fields to perplex budget reviewers and approvers. The use of exclusive terminology is designed to suggest to noninsiders that they are unqualified to hold opinions regarding issues in consideration.

- A final tactic is to flatter and dissemble. Budget managers agree with the wisdom of those seeking budget reductions but act in a contrary yet nonconfrontational manner. Managers provide vigorous verbal support for an objective or directive, such as budget cutting and efficiency, but continue current operations as before or seek more resources. The goal of flattery and dissembling is to ingratiate one's self to reviewers and approvers, while actively opposing change.

All-purpose strategies recognize that budgeting is a political process. Managers must not only be able to provide legitimate reasons for increases in resources but also be capable of using political maneuvers to protect and enlarge the resources at their command.

Budget Increasing or Offensive Strategies

The primary purpose of budget-increasing strategies is to maximize funding. Legitimate reasons cover the increased cost of providing a good or a service, expansion, or quality improvement. Offensive strategies are predominantly illegitimate attempts to obtain more resources than needed and build an empire. These strategies are invoked when work does not require additional resources to be competently performed but resources may be available and managers want to pad their budgets.

Over Estimate Resource Needs

Estimate larger-than-expected increases in output. For example, a 10.0% increase in output is projected (although it may not be expected); therefore, the budget should be increased by 10.0% above inflation. Does the budgeting process, current or retrospective evaluation, recognize when anticipated increases are not realized? Overestimation is only effective when organizations use an incremental budgeting system and do not retroactively adjust the budget on the basis of actual production as flexible budgeting does. The reader should recall that requesting a 10.0% funding increase due to a 10.0% growth in output erroneously assumes that all costs are variable.

Round up

Rounding up is the systematic process of requesting slightly more resources than necessary. For example, instead of requesting the amount of resources needed, managers may round up budget requests to the nearest thousand, ten thousand, or hundred thousand dollars to increase their budgets. Less aggressive budget maximizers may round up an expenditure of \$65,500–\$66,000; managers who are more aggressive may request \$70,000 or \$100,000. The advantage of rounding up every expense line to the nearest thousand dollars is that it may achieve the same effect as rounding up a single line item from \$65,500 to \$100,000 and be more difficult for budget reviewers or approvers to detect.

Sprinkle

Sprinkling adds small amounts, \$100 or \$1,000, to every expense line. The logic, similar to rounding up, is that small amounts spread across multiple expense lines will be impossible for budget reviewers and approvers to detect. In the last example, rounding up from \$65,500 to \$70,000 (\$4,500) in a single line item may be easy to detect (in this case, it would be 6.9% over what is required [\$4,500/\$65,500]), but if \$100 is added to 45 line items, it would be next to impossible to detect. The impact on the budget is the same, but the budget padding is not as obvious.

Backlogs and Customer Complaints

The backlog and complaint strategy uses existing production problems to argue that the budget must be too low to support required operations. This *could* be a legitimate reason if the department has been underfunded and cannot keep up with the demand, or it could be the result of poor management. If backlogs and complaints are the basis for budget increases, incentives are established for managers to fall behind on production or deliveries to gain larger budget allocations—inefficiency and ineffectiveness would be rewarded in this system. The first question that needs to be asked is, should the function be backlogged, given its present resources? Similarly, are customer complaints due to underfunding or poor management of operations?

Crisis

The crisis strategy uses real or imagined crises as an opportunity for budget increases to prevent or minimize adverse outcomes. A fortunate or unfortunate point of emergency funding is that departments are seldom asked to relinquish funds after the conclusion of the crisis. Does a plane crash indicate that the Federal Aviation Administration (FAA) is underfunded or that it is poorly managed? The story the FAA will tell is one of previous understaffing, inadequate wages, and/or antiquated equipment and thus the need for budget increases. As seen by the Department of Defense and the Federal Emergency Management Agency (FEMA), federal departments seldom return to their prior size after a war or natural disaster.

New Programs

This strategy argues that the implementation of previously unperformed activities requires additional funding. If these activities or programs are valuable, then the overarching questions that should be asked are why they aren't presently funded and whether there is higher value in the existing or new services. Tactics for securing new programs include the following:

■ Old wine in a new bottle—repackaging existing programs to appear as new work to secure higher funding. Organizations often set aside funds for new initiatives to encourage efforts to provide better goods and services. A key weakness is that managers relabel existing programs to obtain new funding, and new initiatives are not undertaken.

■ The foot-in-the-door or camel-nose-under-the tent tactic knowingly starts programs with inadequate funds, builds a constituency, and then demands more funds to continue the work. Rejecting an expensive program is more likely before a constituency is created; after the constituency is built, it may be irrelevant that the original expense estimates were purposely understated. More funding is now needed to continue the program and ensure that the prior investment is not lost. The question that should be asked is will additional funding throw good money after bad? The initial request understated resource needs, oversold potential benefits, or did both, so what is the guarantee that the supplemental request does not have the same flaws?

■ The pays-for-itself tactic proposes new investments that are projected to produce revenues in excess of capital and operating costs. Fortunately, for managers using this tactic, postinvestment reviews (were the additional revenues realized?) are unlikely to take place. When undertaken, they often do not consider the impact of the project on other areas: if revenue increased, did it cannibalize another revenue stream? For example, do franchise food service operations in hospitals drain resources from the cafeteria, or do outpatient surgery centers reduce inpatient surgeries? Proposals that subsequently fail to deliver their promised results generally do not see funding cuts.

■ Use of the spend to save tactic promises funding increases will allow greater reductions in current expenses (labor, supplies, utilities, etc.). Thanks to short attention spans, additional resources are often invested and the expected cost savings are seldom followed up. For example, do electronic medical record (EMR) systems reduce documentation costs (or improve quality of care)? Like the pays for itself tactic, funding cuts are unlikely, even if the expected reductions in expenses do not occur and are recognized as failing to reach their targeted savings.

- Mislabeling is an appealing tactic that deliberately misstates the purpose of an expenditure to increase the probability of its acceptance. Mikesell (1995) gave a classic example of mislabeling pertaining to blast suppression areas around military bases and ammunition dumps. Blast suppression areas are designed to protect civilian populations from injury due to unintended denotation of munitions—an appropriate use of funds. Blast suppression areas, open green spaces, often end up as golf courses; if the Department of Defense asked Congress to fund recreation areas, it would receive a more severe review than in the case of seeking funds to improve safety.

- Requests for higher funding in anticipation of third-party actions argue that additional funding is needed to meet anticipated competitive threats or customer needs. The additional resources may be squandered if competitors' actions do not materialize or customers do not demand more output or seek improvements in products or services, but this cannot be known at the time of the request. Managers are incented to be proactive and overstate needs to capture additional resources, but postexpenditure reviews are essential to determine whether managers are crying wolf—how often do contingencies fail to be realized?

- Overreaction to third-party actions are requests for higher funding after a change has occurred, where managers select the most expensive means to meet the competitor actions or expand services to a growing customer population. Why budget for an ounce when a pound can be had? The question that should be asked is, are there other less expensive means to meet the challenge?

- Finally, the bandwagon tactic argues for higher funding to implement programs because everyone else is doing it. Following the bandwagon is a response to competition and the fear of being left behind. While this is a persuasive argument, it is also susceptible to the "if everyone jumps off a bridge" rejoinder—caution, patience, and skepticism are often underappreciated.

Even though the discussion of legitimate and illegitimate budget increases is drawn clearly, in the real world, things are rarely black or white. Legitimate increases are anything that requires a larger budget to complete the organization or department's goals, that is, price increases, higher output, changes in production processes, and service or product changes. Unfortunately, all of these factors can be gamed. Illegitimate tactics may be based on real or anticipated needs; however, these factors must be considered illegitimate if they do not result in changes in input prices, output, production processes, or services or products or if inappropriate (excessively costly) approaches are pursued.

Legitimate reasons for budget increases can also be leveraged to obtain higher-than-needed budget augmentations, including selective use of price changes, workload increases, and production process or product changes. The line between warranted and unwarranted budget increases is often blurred, reinforcing the need for all parties to be knowledgeable of what is being produced, how it is being produced, and how it could be produced. The lines between justifiable budget increases, prudent contingency planning (i.e., budget cushions), and outright budget padding are seldom clear.

The other important point is factors that increase the demand for resources are always highlighted in the budgeting process. When these factors move in the opposite directions, suggesting the need for fewer resources, they are ignored or withheld. Over time, budgets necessarily grow beyond the efficient point;

resources are added when output grows and seldom removed when output falls. Unnecessary resources may or may not be idle, and managers may find good uses, frivolous uses, or leave a resource unused. The question is whether the present use of a resource is the best use. Does the current allocation of resources serve the manager's goal, the organization's goals, or both?

Managers want budget cushions; they make work and life easier. Assume you only budget enough gas to take your car on anticipated trips. More likely than not, you will find yourself out of gas because of myriad events that could impact the number of miles actually driven versus the anticipated number of miles and your fuel economy (the miles per gallon your vehicle produces). Lack of maintenance (improper tire inflation, neglected tune-ups, etc.) will reduce fuel economy and highlight the lack of proper attention. Similarly, seeking more comfort (higher use of air-conditioning) or reducing the time traveled by driving at a higher speed reduces mileage and again raises questions. Third, you may take more trips than anticipated because of a higher demand or poor foresight (taking two trips when one properly planned trip would suffice). In each case, budgeting higher amounts for gas than you expect to use makes life simpler and does not raise questions about your ability to forecast resource needs or manage resources. Everyone notices when you run out of gas, but few notice how much gas remains in the tank after your travels are complete.

Preventing-Budget-Cut or Defensive Strategies

The goal of defensive strategies is to prevent reductions or termination of operations. During financial crises, departments are often asked to tighten their belts, that is, reduce their expenses. Reducing expenses is unpleasant or worse as it means foregoing something that one previously had. Given that the majority of operational healthcare costs are labor related, budget reductions may entail cutting staff or reducing employees' benefits (making employees contribute more to health insurance or retirement since salary reductions are seldom on the table). Budget cutting upsets employees and often produces employee turnover, creating additional problems. Managers avoid or minimize budget reductions by utilizing the following tactics.

Propose a Study

Proposing a study seeks to delay cuts and, hopefully, prolong action until budget reductions are no longer necessary or desirable. If cuts in funding can be delayed until after an impact study is completed, identifying the study team, collecting data, compiling findings, and distributing reports will require months and possibly years. By the time the "final" report is distributed, the need for reductions may pass. For physicians and hospitals, a cut in reimbursement rates may require cuts in expenses to hit the desired net income, but over time, increases in patient volume may replace the lost revenue—the organization may simply miss its financial targets in the short run. Similarly, city and state governments may see a drop in sales, income, or property taxes (due to job losses or declining property values) that create budget deficits, but if expenditure reductions can be delayed for 12–18 months, employment and property values may rebound, eliminating the need for cuts.

Cut High Visibility, Popular Programs

Proposing cuts or reductions in heavily utilized programs is designed to generate a public outcry. Managers typically avoid cutting the unseen, disliked, or low-value programs with limited public support. This strategy has been called the Washington Monument Ploy. In the 1996 budget "crisis," the National Park Service (NPS) closed the Washington Monument and the Grand Canyon (how do you close the Grand Canyon?) because it knew that closing these attractions would generate public support to stop the cuts. The NPS obviously did not want to suggest cutting the number of NPS personnel working in offices in Washington, D.C., or elsewhere, as this would not produce a public outcry.

Predict Dire Consequences

Forecasting significant negative outcomes as the inevitable result of budget reductions is another means to whip up public resistance to budget cuts. While neither the FAA nor the Food and Drug Administration (FDA) are "popular" programs, it was clear that the Obama administration thought sequestration (2013) could be stopped by threatening long delays for airline passengers and suggesting food safety would be endangered if the FAA and FDA budgets were reduced. Similarly, suggestions for cuts in the defense budget result in claims that wars will be more likely and the possibility of defeat will be greater, cuts in police or court budgets will set off a wave of crime, a cut in public health funds will lead to rampant epidemics, etc.

All or Nothing

The all-or-nothing strategy claims that any budget reduction is tantamount to shuttering the entire operation. This strategy attempts to overlook differential value. Most organizations conduct a variety of high- and low-value activities. Budget cuts should be concentrated in low-value areas or low-production employees. The fallaciousness of the all-or-nothing strategy can be seen by using the analogy of a newspaper. Would cutting one section of the newspaper, say, the horoscope, in response to tighter revenue destroy the entire value of the newspaper? Similarly, cutting the least productive salesperson does not drive revenue to zero. In the case of cutting low-value programs or low-productivity employees, it is clear that the potential loss is less than the average (total department activity, outputs, or outcomes/total inputs) and the overwhelming majority of output and value created by the department will continue.

You Pick

The you-pick strategy attempts to shift the choice (and responsibility) of what programs or expenses to cut to others, typically those seeking budget reductions. The intent of this strategy is to hope that any anticipated ill-will and the desire to be not held responsible for it will deter others from suggesting reductions or, should they persist, saddle them with the ire of customers and/or employees. This strategy follows Machiavelli's advice that unpleasant tasks should always be delegated to others.

We Are the Experts

This strategy directly challenges the understanding of those seeking budget cuts. It suggests that those seeking budget reductions do not understand the operations, so they should trust the managers running the programs when they conclude that no reduction is possible. This strategy parallels the all-purpose strategies of cultivating confidence and obfuscating operations by emphasizing the greater knowledge of department personnel to convince those seeking reductions that the operation is too complex and sensitive to sustain a cut and continue its mission.

Budget-Cutting Strategies

Like budget-supporting strategies, budget-cutting strategies can be classified as appropriate (legitimate) and inappropriate (illegitimate). The interesting result of budget review and budget cutting is that it encourages the strategic behavior it tries to prevent. The expectation of budget cuts leads managers to build fat into their budgets. The question is, do review and approval processes identify and remove more fat than they encourage?

Budgets should be cut for three reasons. The first is a revenue constraint. Revenues of the organization do not cover costs or provide an adequate return to the suppliers of resources, and expenses must be cut to provide an adequate return. Second, the organization changes its priorities and/or the demand for its output falls, so resources should be shifted to other uses. Third, the level of funding is too high compared to the output produced; operations can be continued at the same level of output and quality with fewer resources. The goal of budget cutting is to reduce fat and spare muscle, but in practice, this requires knowledge, and knowledge frequently resides with operating managers rather than budget cutters.

An inappropriate reason for cutting the budget is that the manager or department has fallen out of favor. Maximizing the value of the organization requires allocating resources to the functions that produce the greatest value, allocating resources according to the "politics" wastes resources. Given the potential conflict between individual goals and organizational goals, cutting a budget because of disfavor is inappropriate, yet it happens. Budget cutters use the following methods when expense cuts are desired or needed.

Make Across-the-Board Reductions

Across-the-board cuts require equal reductions in allocations from all departments, that is, shared pain. These cuts are the most commonly used method to reduce expenses, because it is indiscriminatory and easy. Across-the-board reductions may minimize employee dissatisfaction, since no favorites are played, but it encourages defensive actions by managers, that is, the building of fat into the budget in anticipation of cuts. The injustice of this approach is that it inflicts real pain on efficient departments and minimal pain where budget cushions are in place. The use of across-the-board cuts highlights a lack of knowledge of high- and low-value activities or

an unwillingness to target underperforming areas for reductions.

Cut New Programs

Cutting funding for new programs assumes that everything done in the past is valuable and should be continued and that new initiatives, categorically, have lower value. This budget-reducing method has the advantage of minimizing conflict: few people fight for what they never had, while developed constituencies, managers, employees, and customers/clients vigorously fight cuts in existing programs. While existing programs may be targeted toward higher needs, the automatic cutting of new initiatives ignores questions of how current programs are performing, what they are achieving, and whether a new program can achieve better results. The bias toward continuing funding of existing programs reduces the incentives for these programs to improve.

Cut Expansions in Existing Programs

Cutting funding for program expansions assumes that if the products or consumers did not have to be served in the past, they do not need to be served now. If the current program or output targets the highest-profit customers or the highest-need clients, expansion will provide less value, that is, diminishing marginal returns. This budget-cutting method again minimizes conflict, as new positions, supplies, and equipment are eliminated but existing operations are left untouched.

Cut Items Deleted from Prior Budgets

Cutting items that were removed from prior budgets relies on the logic that if it was not needed in the past, it still is not necessary. Managers often insert previously cut items into budget requests every year; they have a rationale for why it was needed previously, and the reason can be recycled. Managers have two avenues to success: one is that the request could slip through the review and approval process undetected, and the other is that revenue increases may permit higher spending. Inserting a budget request that is cut every year is better than missing an opportunity to expand the budget. When budget cuts are needed, budget reviewers look for things they have previously cut; they had a reason for cutting it before, so the reason may still make sense. The chief problem with cutting previously deleted items is that method is rooted in the past and may ignore emerging opportunities and needs.

Cut "Luxury" Items

Cutting luxury items targets expenditures deemed extravagant. In many organizations, luxury cuts are aimed at small and trivial items. For example, they often target food items (coffee and donuts at staff meetings) and travel. These are highly visibility items, which many see as expendable, but the problem is, how much is saved? Cutting or eliminating food and travel, which generally account for a small percentage of the total budget, has a limited impact compared to the cost of underutilized (or idle) personnel, yet in many cases, personnel cuts are sacrosanct. Another consideration is whether the trivial gains from cutting coffee and donuts are worth the employee dissatisfaction it arouses?

Seek Outside Assistance

Seeking outside assistance bring in consultants to suggest and take responsibility for cuts and is similar to the you-pick strategy of operating managers. This strategy attempts to shift blame to outsiders and keep relationships between people who will have to work together in the future cordial. Employing paid consultants, however, arouses employee animosity, as workers will ask why money is being spent on consultants when costs must be cut.

Reduce Budgets of Poorly Performing Managers

This strategy operates on identifying managers who appear to be ineffective and/or inefficient to concentrate cuts. The idea is that departments obtaining the most from their resources should be spared, and cutting the budgets of poor performers will have the smallest negative impact on the overall organization. This strategy has two problems: first, the department may be a potentially high-benefit department with poor management, and second, budget cuts may be targeted toward out-of-favor departments and managers rather than poor performers.

Cut Low-value Budget Items

Cutting low-value budget items reduces or eliminates funding for programs, processes, or expenditures whose costs exceed the benefits created—the goal of budget cutting. Indiscriminate cuts premised on the prior strategies are not needed; they fail to identify high- and low-value activities. Resources should be cut from low-value activities and given to programs that produce greater benefits. This may include expanding existing programs or developing new programs. Critically evaluating budget requests is, by far, the most difficult and worthwhile way to reduce expenses; it requires a clear understanding of what produces value and requires discriminating cuts. This approach to budget cutting generates fierce opposition from low-yield programs and calls of "unfairness," but it is the only way to ensure maximum benefit is obtained from an organization's resources.

The Budget Process

Budget building is a three-step and three-party process involving operating managers, finance, and senior management (Figure 3.4). The following discussion provides an overview of the primary functions of each party. Step-by-step procedures for preparing output forecasts and revenue budgets, generally the responsibility of finance and senior management, are covered in Chapter 4, while the responsibilities of managers to prepare expense budgets and the steps in creating them are the subject of the following six chapters.

Budget Preparation

The primary responsibility of operating managers is the assembly of the budget request, including a narrative, a statement of resources needs, and supporting data. The narrative should inform finance and approving bodies of each department's current situation: what it does; how it supports the larger organizational goals; what its strengths, weaknesses, opportunities, and threats are; and, possibly, what the prioritization of its needs is.

Following the narrative, detailed schedules identify the type and cost of resources required in the budget year. Operating revenue schedules identifying revenue sources and the amount expected should also be included if these projections are the responsibility of operating managers. The construction of expense budgets is covered in Chapters 5–10. Typically, the completed expense budget is presented side by side with current-year actual (or projected actual) expenses to highlight significant increases or decreases in spending. Budget preparers should recognize that reviewers often focus on and expect explanations for significant increases in requested expenses over prior-year expenses (or projected actual), so they should be ready to provide persuasive reasons to defend large expense increases. The final (and optional) component of the budget request is supplemental data. Supplemental data highlighting changes in the quantity of work performed, how work is performed, or what inputs cost is designed to support the budget request and reduce reviewer questions.

Financial Review

Finance fulfills three roles in the budgeting process. The first begins prior to the budget request. Finance often estimates budget-year output and expected input price increases. After the budget requests are completed and submitted, finance reviews the requests for compliance to organizational objectives and budgeting instructions, as well as simple arithmetic accuracy. **BOX 3.1** provides a list of items that finance reviews, and operating managers should double-check each prior to submitting their requests.

The last duty of finance is to assemble the master budget by adding together all individual department requests. After total projected revenues and expenses are compiled for the organization, the question is, is the plan feasible? Do revenues exceed expenses, and are net income and return on investment acceptable? If the plan is not feasible, budget requests may have to be redone by one, some, or all departments. The revision of budget requests may include respecification of expected output. For example, if expected output is lowered by 2.0%, by how much can expenses be reduced? When an acceptable master budget is reached, it is forwarded to senior management and the board of directors for approval.

BOX 3.1 Review of Budget Requests by Finance

1. Compliance with the mission: Are the requested resources consistent with the goals of the organization?
2. Compliance with budget instructions: Did managers use appropriate budget bases, inflation factors, and forms?
3. Logical connection between narrative and detail: Are the purpose and function of the department reflected in the resources requested?
4. Arithmetic accuracy: Are sums and products correct?
5. Completeness: Are complimentary resources included? For example, if motor vehicles are budgeted, are insurance, maintenance, gas, etc., included as well?

Budget Approval

The goal of the CEO's and the board's approval of the budget is to demonstrate that the financial plan is accepted and endorsed by top decision-makers. Top decision-makers review the budget to ensure it pursues desired objectives and the bottom line is acceptable. Approval by the CEO and the board should be a formality by the time the master budget is assembled and an acceptable bottom line is projected. Despite this expectation, it is imperative that sufficient time be allowed for approval. It is the author's opinion that there should be at least 1 month (or one board meeting) between the review by the last required approving body (typically the board) and the start of the budget year to provide sufficient time to revise the budget if it is rejected and approve the revision before the start of the budget year.

In the event the master budget projects that expenses will exceed revenues, more time should be planned. First, the projected loss may require finance to identify alternative means to fund the deficit, such as drawing down accumulated equity, selling assets, or assuming additional debt. Second, budgets projecting a loss will generally be more highly scrutinized by the CEO as well as the board. Philosophically, some executives and board members may find it unacceptable to project an operating loss and may withhold support for the budget. The budget will have to be revised if the executives or board members philosophically opposed to operating at a loss or with other objections have sufficient influence.

The approved budget is first a statement of priorities and how managers expect to achieve goals. Second, the budget is a communication mechanism to inform and coordinate internal and external parties. One of the prime problems in organizations is silo thinking; the master budget should allow each manager to see the big picture and increase his or her commitment to the organizational goals. Third, the budget provides the operations and financial guide for work and should be used to manage processes during the budget year. Variance reports contrasting the budget to actual operating results should allow managers to recognize whether operations are on track and when the plan is not being realized to identify whether internal and/or environmental factors are driving the differences and whether performance can be improved.

▶ What a Budget Is and What It Is Not

A budget is a means to understand an organization and its priorities, operations, and incentive structures. Budgets explain how organizations are expected to work in monetary terms. Monetary quantification of performance is an efficient means to organize information, facilitate decision-making, and gauge the effectiveness of actions. Managerial decisions should not be based on vague performance descriptors, such as over- or underbudget, but should be based on how far actual results differ from the target. If actual expenses exceed the budget, required actions will depend upon how far over expenses are as well as changes in output and revenues. Ultimately, budgets are a means to manage and safeguard resources.

A budget is not an end in itself; it is a means to achieve the larger mission and goals of an organization. The goal is not to create a financial plan but rather to create an operating plan that can achieve organizational goals. Unfortunately, the way many budgets are used, employees believe that creating a budget is the end. The primary purpose of a budget is lost if the completed budget is placed on the shelf and more time is spent estimating expenses rather than controlling processes. Budgets are not straitjackets; they neither demand nor justify continuing to do things as they were done in the past. A budget should be a means to identify better ways of doing things and react to contemporaneous changes: are new production methods better and/or cheaper than current methods? A budget should facilitate comparison of current costs with expected costs under new production methods and identify when production processes should change. A budget should also allow managers to quickly identify environmental or internal changes that do not allow the budget to be met and the size of their financial impact. Negative and positive impacts need to be communicated up the organization to determine whether departmental or organizational changes are needed. A budget is an information system, and if variations in plans are not recognized, communicated, and acted upon, a budget loses most, if not all, of its usefulness.

Budgeting is a tool, and it is only valuable if the information it provides is worth its cost; a complex, time-consuming (or destroying), and uninformative budget is not worth the effort. Budgeting is not and should not be equated to mindless cost control; it should ensure effectiveness and efficiency by providing just enough resources to complete a task at the level of performance expected—no more and no less. Budgeting can degenerate into all the things it should not be because of a lack of understanding of budgeting methods and goals, the inability or failure to use budgeting information to enhance operations, inappropriate use that is detrimental to operations, and assembling budgets primarily to satisfy external parties. Customers, owners, and employees benefit when managers at all levels understand budgeting goals and practices and incorporate budgeting information into daily decision-making and action.

Summary

This chapter describes how goods and services transacted in voluntary exchange markets are regulated by the opposing interests of producers and customers. In voluntary exchange markets, excessive output or pricing is prevented by the ability of customers to refuse to purchase (thus putting downward pressure on production, costs, and prices). When goods and services are transacted in subsidized markets, typically by nonprofit or public organizations, excessive demand can be unleashed. While budgets are important to all organizations to control resource use, budgets often substitute for the spontaneous order provided by market processes for nonprofit and public organizations.

This chapter also discusses the roles budget preparers, reviewers, and approvers play in the budgeting process and the various strategies used to increase, defend, or cut allocations. Legitimate reasons for budget increases are input price increases, higher output, quality increases, and shifts to cost-increasing production methods. One of the primary difficulties in constructing tight budgets that supply only needed resources is that legitimate reasons can be manipulated to maximize budgets. In addition, there is a host of political strategies developed to ensure that inefficient budgets are approved year after year. Some people think that discussing strategies and tactics to unnecessarily increase funding is tantamount to encouraging waste, but exposing the ways budget information is manipulated is the only way to improve budgeting and reduce waste.

The major parties and tasks in the budget-building process are described to pave the transition to the budget construction chapters. Part 1 concludes by recognizing what a budget is and what it is not. The goal of budgeting is to obtain the maximum value from available resources, but its ability to achieve this end is determined by the type of budgeting system chosen, the manager's understanding of budget practice, and the way individual interest is managed. Part 2 explores the focus of different budgeting systems and details how each type of budget is created and what its strengths and weaknesses are.

Key Terms and Concepts

Iron triangle   Pareto improvement   Pareto optimality
Moral hazard

Discussion Questions

1. Discuss how opposing interests are balanced in the market exchange model and how the introduction of subsidies and taxes impact the balance between producers and consumers.
2. Compare budgeting processes across for-profit, nonprofit, and public organizations.
3. Identify the parties in the iron triangle and their objectives.
4. Describe the major steps required to create a budget, who is responsible, and when they should be completed.
5. What are the three rules for winning the budget game?
6. What are legitimate reasons for budget increases?
7. Describe the differences between all-purpose budget strategies and budget-increasing strategies.
8. What are the best and the worst ways to cut budgets?
9. Discuss the differences between budgets as operating and financial plans. What is the proper role of a budget?
10. What are the major reasons budgeting often fails to reach it potential?

References

Brickley, J. A., Smith, C. W., & Zimmerman, J. L. (1997). *Managerial economics and organizational architecture*. Chicago, IL: McGraw-Hill.

Bureau of Labor Statistics. (2017). *Table 9. Producer price indexes*, Retrieved May 16, 2017, from https://www.bls.gov/web/ppi/ppitable09.pdf

Deming, W. E. (1982). *Out of the crisis*. Cambridge, MA: Massachusetts Institute of Technology, Center for Advanced Educational Services.

Federal Hospital Insurance & Federal Supplementary Medical Insurance Trust Funds. (2016). *2016 annual report of the boards of trustees of the Federal Hospital Insurance and Federal Supplementary Medical Insurance Trust Funds*. Retrieved November 17, 2016, from https://www.cms.gov/Research-Statistics-Data-and-Systems/Statistics-Trends-and-Reports/ReportsTrustFunds/downloads/tr2016.pdf

Ford, H. (1923). *My life and work*. Garden City, NY: Doubleday, Page.

Greenstone, M., List, J. A., & Syverson, C. (2012). The effects of environmental regulation on the competitiveness of U.S. manufacturing, NBER Working Paper No. 18392, Cambridge, MA.

Korte, G. (2014, May 22). Federal employees owe $3.3B in back taxes. *USA Today*. Retrieved September 7, 2019, from https://www.usatoday.com/story/news/politics/2014/05/22/congress-irs-tax-delinquencies/9442749/

Huff, D. (1954). *How to lie with statistics*. New York, NY: W. W. Norton.

Mikesell, J. (1995). *Fiscal administration* (4th ed.). Belmont, CA: Wadsworth.

Miller, R. L., Benjamin, D. K., & North, D. C. (2001). *The economics of public issues* (12th ed.). Boston, MA: Addison Wesley.

Rosen, H. (1988). *Public finance* (2nd ed.). Homewood IL: Irwin.

Will, G. F. (2013, June 7). George F. Will: Sugar subsidies are immune to even modest reforms. *The Washington Post*. Retrieved October 27, 2016, from https://www.washingtonpost.com/opinions/george-f-will-sugar-subsidies-are-immune-to-even-modest-reforms/2013/06/07/3c5318fe-cedd-11e2-8f6b-67f40e176f03_story.html?tid=a_inl&utm_term=.d75774117654

World Bank. (1995). *Bureaucrats in business*. New York, NY: Oxford University Press.

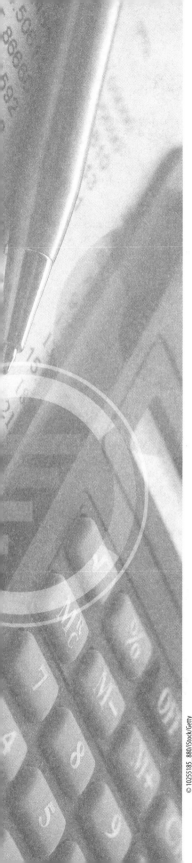

PART 2

Budgeting Construction

Part 2 emphasizes the mechanics of how budgets are constructed. The key to creating a budget is estimating how many units of a good or service will be produced in the upcoming fiscal year. The expected quantity of output should determine the amount of resources required and the way these resources will be financed. The chapter "Output Forecasts and Revenue Budgets" notes that six variables must be estimated to complete a budget: expected output, output prices, quantity of variable inputs, prices of variable inputs, quantity of fixed inputs, and prices of fixed inputs.

Output can be forecasted using quantitative methods based on historical data, qualitative methods relying on expert opinion, or a combination of both. Regardless of how estimates are derived, improving the accuracy of forecasts requires the forecasts to be critiqued at the end of the budget period. Was the forecast accurate? Should present practices be continued, or if the forecasts are under- or overpredicting demand, can future forecasts be improved? If the forecasts are consistently under- or overpredicting, should future forecasts be adjusted to increase their accuracy or should new forecasting methods be employed?

After output is forecasted, the next step is to estimate revenue: how much money will the organization receive from the output it produces? The composition of the industry and price elasticity should be considered to determine the latitude the organization has in setting prices, that is, will sales decline in response to a price increase? Healthcare reimbursement systems must also be considered, as price increases will not produce any additional revenue for patients covered by Medicare, Medicaid, and managed care payers with fixed payment systems such as per case, cost, or capitation reimbursement. Price setting is demonstrated to maximize revenue from charge-based patients despite the fact that additional revenue may not be forthcoming from the majority of patients.

The chapter "Scratch Budgeting" develops a scratch budget for a start-up. The chapter starts by exploring a generic chart of accounts to highlight common expense items and the way they are categorized by accounting systems. The goal of budgeting is to ensure that revenues equal or exceed expenses. When initial estimates indicate that this should not be expected, managers should consider all actions that could be taken to increase revenues and reduce expenses. The chapter also explores the essentials of business plans and breakeven analysis.

The chapters "Incremental Budgeting" and "Flexible Budgeting" explore the two most commonly used budgeting methods. Each of these systems estimates expenses by line item: how much will be spent on a particular resource? Incremental budgeting inflates base period expenses for expected price increases to produce fixed budget allocations. Flexible budgeting develops a cost standard per output per line item, increases the cost standard for expected price increases, and multiplies the product by forecasted output to develop a preliminary budget. The preliminary budget should be used to guide management, but the final budget is developed after the close of the budget period, when the inflated cost standard is multiplied by actual output. The benefit of flexible budgeting is that the budget increases and decreases with actual output, and meeting the budget does not get easier when output falls nor more difficult when output increases.

The chapters "Zero-Base Budgeting" and "Program Budgeting" shift to a planning focus (what should be produced) versus expense estimation (what resources are required). Zero-base budgeting and program budgeting are more appropriate for senior managers attempting to set the overall direction of the organization. Zero-base budgeting moves away from the idea that things should be continued simply because they were done in the past. Zero-base budgeting asks the question, should output continue at current levels, or should it be increased, reduced, or eliminated? This question is answered by comparing different uses of resources: can organizational value be increased by moving resources from one department or division to another? Program budgeting focuses the resource allocation question on what uses produce the best outcomes. This approach moves performance evaluation from inside an organization to the impact expenditures produce on customers. Can more people be served, or can existing customers be served better by reprioritizing the outcomes the organization pursues?

The chapter "Activity-Based Budgeting" provides the greatest insight into how an organization operates by basing resource decisions on the work performed. The number and type of activities performed should determine expenses. An activity-based budget supplies managers with the information they need to determine why actual operations deviate from the budget. Deviations can arise not only from increased output (considered in flexible budgeting) but also from changes in productivity and the number of activities needed to produce outputs. Activity-based budgeting facilitates identification of the eight wastes: budgets may be missed due to overproduction, overprocessing, excessive motion, excess transport of resources, defects, excessive inventories, idle resources, or underutilized talents. No other budgeting system provides the details managers need to facilitate and control production processes.

Budgeting systems determine incentives and performance, so managers should be careful in selecting a system that best advances their desired goals. If the goal is to reconsider how the organization uses its resources, zero-base and program budgets should be used as they require managers to consider alternative resource uses and the impact their operations have on external parties. If the goal is to estimate resource needs, incremental and flexible budgets produce concise line item budgets. In choosing between incremental and flexible budgets, managers should consider the fluctuation of output. Incremental budgets are easy to produce but require stable and forecastable output. If output is unstable or difficult to estimate, flexible budgets should be used to provide the necessary resources managers and employees need to complete work, that is, the budget should add resources when more work is done and reduce resources when output falls. While improving planning and resource estimation are primary budgeting goals, the main goal of budgeting is to improve operations, and activity-based budgeting does this best. Activity-based budgeting, built on tasks, supplies the necessary information to control what is done and how it is done. Managers with this information can make informed decisions and take the necessary actions to increase customer satisfaction and maximize the organization's value.

CHAPTER 4

Output Forecasts and Revenue Budgets

CHAPTER OBJECTIVES

1. Explain how output is forecasted using quantitative and qualitative methods.
2. Prepare output forecasts.
3. Explain the relationship between expected output and revenues and expenses estimates.
4. Explain how market organization and price elasticity impact an organization's ability to control prices and output.
5. Prepare a revenue budget.

▶ Introduction

The key to establishing an effective budget and operating plan is determining output: what goods or services will be produced in what quantities? Developing an operation plan shifts the job of a manager from reacting to events to anticipating and preparing. Managers should search for opportunities to redesign processes to reduce the eight Lean wastes: overproduction, idleness, excessive transport, overprocessing, excess inventory, excessive motion, defects, and underutilized talent. Managers should use the operating plan to ensure that the right type and amount of labor, supplies, and equipment are available at appropriate times and locations—prepositioning of resources. Without planning and prepositioning, an organization may run short of resources and have to acquire labor, supplies, and equipment quickly at premium prices, and it will lose time waiting for resources to continue production. Overinvestment in resources can be equally disruptive to production and generate unnecessary costs.

Budgeting is the monetary interpretation of the operation plan, defining expected output in the upcoming fiscal year and assessing total cash inflows and outflows. The accounting equation, *profit = total revenue − total costs*, succinctly states the budget goal. While few members of a large and diverse organization can envision the totality of the financial situation, managers provide pieces to budget: what revenues will their departments contribute, and what is the cost of the resources they will consume? The answers to these questions are tied to the goals of the organization. Is output expected to remain constant, increase, or decrease, and will the organization expand, contract, or remain the same size? Even in the simplest case, when the size of the organization is expected to remain constant, internal rearrangement of resources may be required if one department sees an increased demand for its output, while others have a lower demand; the attributes of goods and services change; and/or new production methods are introduced.

Output forecasts document the quantity of goods and services senior managers expect to produce in the budget year and are intimately tied to the organization's revenue and expense budgets. When more than one product is produced, the output forecast identifies the types of products expected to be produced and the quantity of each. Estimating output is the primary source of uncertainty in budget construction. Regardless of the type of organization, the demand for goods and services is shaped by an untold number of social, economic, political/regulatory, and technological factors. In the 1990s, health maintenance organizations (HMOs) were buffeted by changes that led many to seek protection in bankruptcy. Today, changing economic factors that disadvantage small providers continue to push small hospitals toward bankruptcy and propel their absorption into hospital chains. While the future cannot be known, it is vital that managers do their best to identify changes in demand so that they can allocate resources to meet shifting customer or client preferences.

Forecasted output is the key to the budget as it determines what it should cost to produce the targeted quantity of goods and services and when the goods and services are sold to customers—the budget constraint. The cash inflows from the sale of goods and services in most organizations provide the primary source of money to fund operations. To accurately estimate expenses, managers should have a clear understanding of what they will be called upon to produce in the budget year. The output forecast provides the foundation for estimating expenses—what type of resources are needed, and how many units of each are required for production?

The second role of the output forecast is to drive the revenue budget—the constraint on total expenses. There are two options: The first is that revenue increases with increases in output, that is, increases in output generate higher sales that wholly or partially cover the resources required to produce them. This is the case for organizations that sell their output to consumers, for example, hospitals and physician practices, Ford Motor Company, and Amtrak. The other option is that revenue is independent of output, that is, an organization receives a fixed amount of money to provide services for a given period, for example, public health organizations, Canadian hospitals, schools, and government agencies. When revenue is independent of output, the output is not sold in markets, and changes in output may not generate proportionate changes in revenue. Increases in the demand for nonmarketed outputs may put pressure on organizations by requiring more work from a fixed set of resources, and managers may need to lobby for budget supplements when output is expected to increase. When fixed budgets are employed, decreases in output make life easier: less work is required from a set of resources that could produce more. As discussed in Chapter 3, managers generally do not request smaller budget appropriations when output is expected to fall.

All employees of an organization should understand the relationship between output, revenue, and expenses, even if their departments produce no revenue or changes in output have no impact on revenues. All employees should understand how their work and departments affect the organization and, conversely, how revenue constraints impact the resources they can receive.

Output forecasts and revenue budgets are examined in this chapter since revenue is often intimately related to output. The first half of the chapter addresses output forecasts, but output and sales are often determined by the price charged for a good or service. The **law of demand** holds that people purchase more of a good or service at lower prices, so quantity and price should be simultaneously considered in markets where output is determined by voluntary transactions between buyers and sellers. Other factors that should be considered when estimating the demand for goods and services include the number of consumers (population), number of competitors, availability of substitutes, and environmental factors (weather, disease, etc.).

There are two primary approaches to forecasting output, top down and bottom up. Output forecasts are frequently developed at the top of the organization and transmitted down to operating managers. The top-down method is regularly used in functional organizational structures, where senior managers have a better understanding of customers and markets than lower-level managers, whose skills and responsibilities lie in a particular area or process. Senior managers can draw on their broader areas of responsibilities to construct the "best" forecast. Once the output forecast is developed by senior managers, it is handed down to operating managers, who use the expected outputs to construct their expense budgets.

The bottom-up approach is used in divisionally structured organizations (or where revenue centers are used), where output estimates are produced at the lower levels of the organization and transmitted up the organization for approval. This method is used when expertise of local information (in a particular geographic market or product line) is more important than centralized information. A prime example is a multistate hospital chain,

where differences in population growth and demography will significantly alter output forecasts. While the chain as a whole may see a rate of growth in admissions that is comparable to the nation, hospitals in states with increasing populations and a higher-than-average percentage of elderly patients may see admissions increase by two or three times the national rate, and hospitals in areas with declining populations may see admissions fall. A third factor that should be considered is the competitive situation in each market: are new hospitals entering or leaving an area, and/or are existing competitors adding or reducing beds? Under these conditions, the corporate staff may delegate the development of output forecasts to local hospital personnel, who have the best understanding of patients, referring physicians, and market conditions.

▶ Estimating Output

Projecting the demand or need for output is a challenging task, and predictions are seldom completely accurate. Yet, an idea of how many patients will be seen and what services they will need is essential to estimating revenues and expenses. Issues that should be addressed in output forecasts are trends, seasonality (not discussed here; since output in this chapter is estimated for an entire year, month-to-month revenue and expense budgets should recognize and incorporate seasonal fluctuations of output), and new initiatives. **FIGURE 4.1** highlights the six variables needed to construct a budget: quantity of output and price (Q and P), quantity and price of variable inputs (Q_{var} and P_{var}), and quantity and price of fixed inputs (Q_{fixed} and P_{fixed}).

Total expense (or cost) is the sum of variable and fixed costs; the reader can see that output is a direct factor in the calculation of total variable costs, but at one time output projections also determined an organization's investment in equipment and facilities. A hospital's investment in plant and equipment

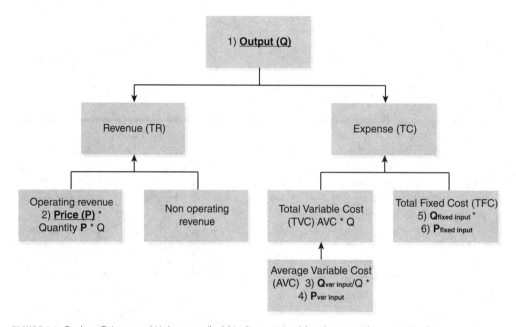

FIGURE 4.1 Budget Drivers and Unknowns (bold indicates variables that must be estimated)

was based on an estimate of the number of patients to be served and the facility size that would best accommodate them. Historical investments are **sunk costs**—a cost of previously committed resources that cannot be controlled by current managers in the short run but can impact profitability. Although the cost of previously committed resources cannot be changed, how effectively these assets are used, that is, how fixed costs are spread over output, affects the average total cost (ATC) and profitability.

Two variables, in addition to output, must be estimated to determine total variable costs. The first is the average variable cost (AVC), the product of the quantity of variable inputs needed (number of employees, doses, kilowatt-hours, etc.) to produce one unit of output and the price at which variable inputs can be obtained. Figure 4.1 divides the total quantity of a variable input by output (total variable inputs/total output) to determine average variable input use. For a hospital, the calculation of average nursing hours per admission would be total nursing

hours divided by total admissions. Multiplying average input use by its average price produces the AVC ($Q_{var} * P_{var}$), for example, *average nursing hours per admission * average nursing wage*. There may be an absolute minimum on the quantity of variable inputs required to produce a good or service, such as staff hours, that define the minimum achievable cost. Water is an example of fixed proportions: water (output) = H_2 + O (inputs). Actual variable costs will be greater than the minimum achievable cost when resources are ineffectively or inefficiently used.

The second unknown is the price at which variable inputs will be purchased. Input prices for variable expenses may or may not change during the budget year. Salaries may be set on an annual basis or by contract and should not change dramatically during the budget year, while the price of energy and other raw materials may fluctuate on a daily basis and produce large differences between budgeted and expected costs over the course of the fiscal year. The total variable cost is the product of the AVC and expected output.

The total fixed cost (TFC = $Q_{fixed} * P_{fixed}$) should be easy to estimate as the amount and price of these inputs should be known. In the absence of expansion, managers know the amount of property, plant, and equipment on hand and the prices at which the assets were purchased. Estimates for future occupancy and equipment costs should also be accurate since the quantity and price of new assets should be known. The job of management is to ensure that variable and fixed inputs are used effectively, not wasted or allowed to remain idle, and acquired at minimum cost. Constructing expense budgets is explored in Chapters 5–10.

Historical Trends in Output

The primary challenge in budgeting is estimating the demand for goods and services, and some products are more difficult to predict than others. Economic statistics demonstrates the dramatic swings in the demand for personal consumption expenditures. The three major categories of personal consumption expenditures are durable goods, nondurable goods, and services. A **durable good** is a product with an expected life span of more than 3 years, such as automobiles and furniture. **Nondurable goods** are expected to be used for less than 3 years, that is, they are rapidly worn out or used up. Clothing, food, and gasoline are examples of nondurable goods. **Services** signify nonphysical products such as health care, legal assistance, education, auto repair, entertainment, and haircuts. Forecasting the demand for services and nondurables is easier than for durable goods because services and nondurable goods are regularly repurchased.

Like personal consumption expenditures, some types of medical services are more predictable than others. Medical services can be classified into curative, chronic, and preventive care, with similar variability in demand as other goods. Curative care, like services, is stable in that patients are generally unwilling to go without treatment. Chronic care parallels nondurable goods, where patients may be tempted to postpone care by increasing the time between visits or dividing medication. Preventive care does not address a current health need and is the most volatile type of medical services since, like durable good purchases, it is largely at the discretion of the patient.

TABLE 4.1 shows that from 2003 through 2009, national health expenditures rose every year; however, these statistics do not help us determine whether the quantity of care demanded increased every year. Expenditures are the product of price and quantity, and increases in prices mask the change in the demand for medical services. When the number of services provided is studied, it shows that inpatient discharges, physician visits, and cosmetic surgery were not immune from an economic downturn. Like the overall economy, the demand for medical services declined in some years. Inpatient discharges, typically nondiscretionary care, showed the least variability, with a 3.9% growth in 2008 and a 1.4% decline in 2007. Cosmetic surgery, often discretionary care, saw large positive and negative swings in demand, increasing by 43.7% in 2004 and declining by 12.3% in 2008.

Table 4.1 documents the volatility in the healthcare industry that affects output forecasts. But budget builders have to decompose these larger, national trends into their specific services and markets. What type of goods or services do they provide, where do they sell or provide their products, and what has been the volatility of demand in their organization? Orthopods may not have to worry about the demand for their services as the overwhelming majority of patients will not forego bone setting, but cosmetic surgeons have discovered that the demand for cosmetic treatments is unpredictable and are actively promoting their services to less traditional groups, such as men, to stimulate demand.

While volatility resulting from changes in total economic activity (gross domestic

TABLE 4.1 Annual Changes in Health Expenditures, 2003–2009	Max. (%)	Min. (%)	Range (%)
National health expenditures	6.9	4.0	2.9
Inpatient discharges	3.9	−1.4	5.3
Physician visits	10.2	−6.4	16.6
Cosmetic surgery	43.7	−12.3	56.0
Gross domestic product	3.6	−2.6	6.2
Personal consumption expenditures	3.5	−1.2	4.7
Durable goods	7.7	−5.2	12.9
Nondurable goods	3.7	−1.2	4.9
Services	3.0	−0.8	3.8

product [GDP]) is one factor to consider in forecasting output, a second factor is **price elasticity**. Price elasticity measures how the quantity demanded of a good or service is impacted by a change in its price. While the mathematics of elasticity is discussed when creating a revenue budget, it is appropriate at this point to recognize that increases in anticipated demand will be lower if an organization raises prices, especially if its price increases exceed those of competitors.

One-Year-Ahead Forecasts

Predicting the future is a hazardous task rife with pitfalls that may subject the forecaster to harsh criticism. The more a forecast differs from what actually occurs, the more other employees attack the forecast and/or forecaster as the primary reason the organization failed to meet its goals. If the forecast underestimates demand, operating managers may be unprepared to produce the quantity necessary to meet actual demand and may have to overpay for resources (paying overtime versus regular pay, purchasing temporary help, etc.). If the forecast overstates demand, managers may have excess capacity and higher-than-needed costs.

Forecasting output for the budget year requires more than one calculation, given that predicting demand in the budget year must occur before the end of the current fiscal year. The first calculation estimates what total output in the current fiscal year will be, since less than 12 months of data are available. The second calculation requires extrapolating from the estimate of the current year's output to the budget year.

Before any calculation can be made, managers must decide what level of granularity is needed. At what level should output be estimated, and what information is available from accounting, marketing, and/or information systems? At the highest level of aggregation, an organization may simply specify its total output in dollars, a macromeasure. The dollar volume of sales provides little insight into what is being produced, so hospital managers may estimate expected admissions (a set of resources required to restore a patient to health) or patient days (a set of resources consumed by a patient on a single day), while physicians may specify their output as the number of patient visits or procedures they expect to provide.

At one time, admissions or patient days were good enough to build a budget on because if either increased, the hospital would receive higher revenue under charge- (fee-for-service) or cost-based reimbursement. Similarly, if the expected resources per admission or patient day exceeded the budget (due to higher intensity or lower efficiency), the hospital would receive higher revenue under the cost-based reimbursement system used by Medicare and Medicaid and could raise prices for charge-based patients. The shift to fixed reimbursement, including diagnosis-related groups (DRGs), requires hospital managers to understand and manage the set of resources required to deliver effective care. Hospital managers today need to understand patient volume by major diagnostic category (MDC), DRG, and payer to accurately project revenue and expenses.

MDCs break the 667 different DRGs into major body systems. **TABLE 4.2** shows the

TABLE 4.2 Major Diagnostic Categories, 2013			
MDC	**Name**	**Weights**	**Arithmetic Mean LOS**
PRE	Ungroupable	6.3640	12.5799
1	Nervous system	1.9867	4.3820
2	Eye	1.0524	3.0405
3	Ear, nose, and throat	1.2122	3.0879
4	Respiratory system	1.5149	4.5267
5	Circulatory system	2.9247	4.7412
6	Digestive system	1.7970	4.9200
7	Hepatobiliary system	1.9800	5.2758
8	Musculoskeletal system	2.2514	4.4476
9	Skin, subcutaneous tissue, and breast	1.4722	4.2819
10	Endocrine, nutritional, and metabolic systems	1.7198	4.2803
11	Kidney and urinary tract	1.7033	4.2978

(continues)

TABLE 4.2 Major Diagnostic Categories, 2013 *(continued)*

MDC	Name	Weights	Arithmetic Mean LOS
12	Male reproductive system	1.2365	3.2013
13	Female reproductive system	1.5067	3.7088
14	Pregnancy and childbirth	0.8028	2.4737
15	Newborn and other neonates	2.3952	7.5429
16	Blood, blood-forming organs, and immunological disorders	1.8006	4.4130
17	Myeloproliferative diseases and disorders	2.3737	5.8818
18	Infectious diseases and disorders	2.1707	5.7546
19	Mental diseases and disorders	1.0721	4.0964
20	Alcohol/drug use or induced mental disorders	0.9325	4.8167
21	Injuries, poison, and toxic effects of drugs	1.5398	3.9311
22	Burns	4.7773	8.1329
23	Factors influencing health status	1.2470	4.0566
24	Multiple significant trauma	3.4054	6.2656
25	Human immunodeficiency virus infection	2.3244	5.9830

LOS, length of stay

average weight for the DRGs that constitute each MDC and the mean length of stay (LOS) for hospital patients. Each DRG has a unique weight, so the table highlights the different reimbursement a hospital receives for treating a patient (weights) and how much care may be required (mean LOS). MDC 14, pregnancy, has the lowest average weight and LOS, while MDC 5, circulatory treatment, has a weight 3.64 times higher than that of pregnancy care and an average LOS that is almost double

(4.74 versus 2.47 days). The budgeting implications are clear: managers should forecast admissions by MDC because of the variability in payment and resource utilization. **TABLE 4.3** shows that forecasting output at the MDC level may also distort revenue and expense projections because of variability within each MDC.

Table 4.3 examines MDC 5 in detail, dividing the associated DRGs into surgical and medical cases. Circulatory patients treated surgically

TABLE 4.3 Variability Within MDCs

MDC	DRGs	Name	Average Weight	Geometric Mean LOS
5	216–316	All circulatory system DRGs	2.9247	4.7412
	216–265	Surgical DRGs	4.2771	5.8771
	266–316	Medical DRGs	1.0607	3.1754

DRG	Surg./Med.	Name	Weights	Geometric Mean LOS
216	Surg.	Cardiac valve with card. cath. with major CC	9.5190	13.7792
217	Surg.	Cardiac valve with card. cath. with CC	6.3495	8.9960
218	Surg.	Cardiac valve with card. cath. without CC	5.3429	6.5470
...				
280	Med.	AMI, discharged alive with major CC	1.7999	4.9497
281	Med.	AMI, discharged alive with CC	1.0961	3.2442
282	Med.	AMI, discharged alive without CC	0.7736	2.1318

card. cath., cardiac catheterization; CC, complications and comorbidities

have an average weight and LOS of 4.28 and 5.88 days, respectively, significantly higher than the values for patients treated medically, 1.06 and 3.18 days. The reimbursement for surgical cases is more than four times higher than that for medical cases, and surgical patients remain hospitalized 85% longer than medical patients. Given the differences in payment and inpatient utilization, accurate revenue and expense forecasts demand that patient volume be divided by the type of care expected to be delivered.

Table 4.3 also demonstrates the revenue and expense variability within surgical and medical care on the basis of whether the patient presents with complications. Reimbursement for DRG 216, cardiac valve with cardiac catheterization, for a patient with major complications and comorbidities is 1.78 higher than the same treatment for a patient without complications and comorbidities. Managers should also expect patients with major complications and comorbidities to be hospitalized more than twice as long as uncomplicated cases. Similar increases in reimbursement weights and LOS are seen for acute myocardial infarction (AMI) patients treated medically; major complications and comorbidities increase reimbursement and expected LOS by 2.32 times over uncomplicated cases. Managers would be remiss if output projections were based solely on total admissions, as the type of case (body system, type of treatment, and presence of complications and comorbidities) has a significant impact on the flow of funds the hospital receives and the resources it needs to treat patients.

Fixed reimbursement requires hospital managers to determine what resources should be consumed and whether current resource use is appropriate. Managers must know what type of patients are expected (DRG = 667) in order to determine the set of resources they need. Consumption of resources also varies on the basis of patient age, as older patients typically consume more resources for similar medical problems than younger patients. Head nurses need to understand the number of days different types of patients will be hospitalized, while the laboratory, radiology, and pharmacy managers should know the approximate number of lab tests, X-rays, and pharmaceutical orders they should expect in the budget year to appropriately schedule staff and order supplies. Differences in patients on

the basis of revenue and cost require more than a simple forecast of total admissions. Managers should understand prior volume and the distribution between relevant subgroups and determine whether changes in patient mix should be incorporated into forecasts.

FIGURE 4.2 shows the change in health consumption expenditures from 2000 through 2014. The story it tells is that total expenditures as well as hospital and physician expenditures have steadily increased over time. This type of knowledge may be useful for projecting revenue (the compound growth rate ranges from 5.4% per year for physician services to 6.3% for hospital care), but it is less useful for projecting expenses. Expenditures (revenues of healthcare providers) are the product of quantity and price, but estimating provider expenses requires understanding the expected quantity of output. **FIGURE 4.3** demonstrates that the quantity of inpatient care and cosmetic surgery (physician care) demanded annually is less stable than health expenditures.

FIGURE 4.3A illustrates the challenge of forecasting. From 1993 through 2013, hospital discharges increased in 12 years and decreased in 8 years. While hospital

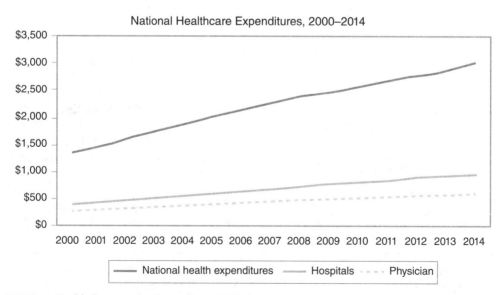

FIGURE 4.2 Health Consumption Expenditures, 2000–2014

discharges increased more times than they decreased over the past 17 years, 60.0% versus 40.0%, managers need to know how to flex their operations in order to deal with higher or lower workloads. In the 12 years when discharges increased, 5 of those years experienced increases exceeding 1.50%. In the 8 years with decreases, more years saw a decline over 1.25%. The largest decline in

discharges occurred between 2012 and 2013, when discharges decreased by 2.43%; conversely, the largest increase came in 2000, when discharges increased by 2.50% over 1999. The average length of stay (ALOS) throughout this period showed a steady and predictable decline.

The fluctuation in the demand for cosmetic procedures, **FIGURE 4.3B** overwhelms

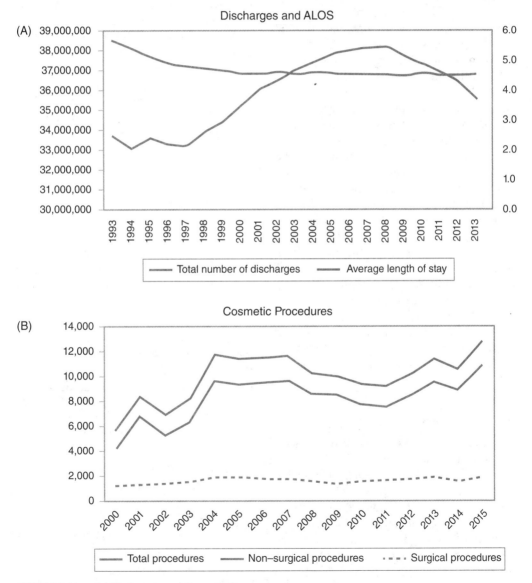

FIGURE 4.3 Hospital Discharges and Cosmetic Surgery

the variability seen in hospital discharges. The challenge for managers is to ensure that operations continue efficiently when demand is falling and sufficient resources are ready to handle higher volumes. A manager of a cosmetic and plastic surgery practice would be hard-pressed to adapt to the major changes in the demand for surgical and nonsurgical procedures. The total cosmetic procedures hit a new peak in 2015 and increased by 122.8% from 2000 but were lower than their previous high mark in 2007 for the previous 8 years. Providers had to adapt to not only this rapid increase but also a 21.4% decline in procedures between 2007 and 2011.

Historical data provides budget preparers with a wealth of information to use: what resources were consumed for the quantity of output produced in the past, and how has the composition of output changed over time? Budgeting is an art and a science; statistics and mathematics can be used to understand how things were in the past as well as project trends into the future, but the future often does not follow the past. While nature does not leap, it evolves, so detecting when a trend begins and ends or when growth accelerates or slows is more art than science. Will constrained government revenue alter healthcare policy and reduce healthcare utilization, or will the Affordable Care Act continue to exist, and if so, will it increase the demand for care?

Quantitative Forecasts

Quantitative forecasts use historical data to estimate future demand for goods and services and set output targets. The major assumption of quantitative forecasts is that the future can be determined from the past. Four types of quantitative forecasts are reviewed: compound growth rates, moving averages, exponential smoothing, and regression.

Compound Growth Rates

The simplest way to project the demand for future output is to calculate past rates of growth. The assumption underlying compound growth rates is that previously observed rates of growth provide an accurate estimator of future growth. Two formulas are needed to calculate the compound growth rate and estimate the need for future output. Equation 4.1 divides current output by base year output and raises the quotient to the power $1/n$, where n is the number of periods between the current and base periods, to determine the compound growth rate. Over short periods, compound growth rates are comparable to simple growth rates (((current output − base output)/base output)/n), but over long periods, simple growth rates overstate real growth.

$$r = (X/Y)^{(1/n)} - 1, \qquad (4.1)$$

where r is the compound growth rate; X is the current value; Y is the historical value, the base; and n is the number of periods between X and Y.

Equation 4.2 uses the compound growth rate calculated using Equation 4.1 to project demand n periods into the future.

$$Y \text{ (future estimate)} = X * (1+r)^n \qquad (4.2)$$

Estimating inpatient discharge growth in the United States using past history (Chapter04.xlsx) over the past 9 and 19 years produces different estimates of the rate of increase:

$$r_{(2005-2014)} = (\text{Discharges in 2014} / \\ \text{Discharges in 2005})^{(1/2014-2005)} - 1$$

$$r_{(2005-2014)} = (35{,}358{,}818/37{,}843{,}039)^{(1/9)} - 1 \\ = -0.0075, \text{or} -0.75\%$$

$$r'_{(1995-2014)} = (\text{Discharges in 2014} / \\ \text{Discharges in 1995})^{(1/2014-1995)} - 1$$

$$r'_{(1995-2014)} = (35{,}358{,}818/33{,}647{,}121)^{(1/19)} - 1 \\ = 0.0026, \text{or} 0.26\%$$

The use of different base years (2005 and 1995) provides dramatically different reports of how fast the demand for inpatient hospital care is growing or shrinking. The 9-year growth rate shows a contraction of 0.75% per year, while the 19-year rate indicates a 0.26% growth. The challenge for forecasters is to determine which base year should be used. Will demand for inpatient care return to the level it achieved from 1995 through 2014, or will discharges continue to decline as they have since 2005? To complicate matters, a third option may be more likely: history may not provide a valid estimator of the future because of the emergence of new phenomena that may drive growth above or below either rate.

As 2015 would be in process and the total number of discharges is not known, using the compound growth rates calculated in order to forecast the total U.S. discharges of 2016 on the basis of output in 2014 requires the following calculations:

$$Y_{2016} = \text{Discharges in } 2014 *$$
$$(1.0000 + r_{(2014-2005)})^{(2016-2014)}$$

$$Y_{2016} = 35,358,818_{(2014)} * (1.0000 - 0.0075)^2$$
$$= 34,829,304 \text{ discharges}$$

$$Y'_{2016} = \text{Discharges in } 2014 *$$
$$(1.0000 + r_{(2014-1995)})^{(2016-2014)}$$

$$Y'_{2016} = 35,358,818_{(2014)} * (1.0000 - 0.0026)^2$$
$$= 35,543,987 \text{ discharges}$$

The difference in discharges between these two estimates is 2.1%, or 714,683 discharges. A difference of 2.1% will have a substantial impact on national health expenditures as well as the organization's operations (employment, expenses, and revenues). Whether an individual provider has the capability to economically expand or contract production by 2.1% in the course of a year is the question. Hospitals are built with excess capacity, so while they should be quite capable of altering production by ±2.1%, the question is, will resources be fully utilized if demand falls short, or will adequate

care be provided if demand increases? For reference, a 2.1% change in patient volume for a hospital with $1.0 billion in revenue could increase or decrease its revenue and expenses by approximately $21 million.

National statistics frequently are at least 2 years old, complicating the forecasting problem. Projecting the demand for inpatient care or other care for an individual hospital should be relatively straightforward. If year-to-date current discharges in 2018 are known, the forecast for the following year, 2019, simply requires annualizing the current output and accounting for 1 year of growth (or contraction). If 17,243 patients are discharged in the first 6 months of 2018 and the historical compound growth rate is 1.0%, the 2019 forecast would be 34,831 (17,243 discharges * 12 months/6 months * 1.01). Alternatively, if current year statistics are not available, the forecaster could use 2017 statistics, 33,892, and the compound growth to extrapolate 2 years into 2019 (as done for national discharges). The 2019 forecast would be $33,892 * (1.01)^2 = 34,573$.

Historical growth rates simply examine how output has changed over some specified period and assume that the rate of growth will continue in the future. As demonstrated, selection of different base years provides different growth rates and estimates of the future demand for output. The forecaster should be able to explain why he or she believes that one time frame provides a better estimate of the future. A forecaster estimating discharges may believe that the drop in inpatient care starting in 2008 will not continue because of demographic trends, so the 1995–2014 growth rate should be more representative of future demand. On the other hand, another forecaster may believe that the shift of care to outpatient services will continue, and he or she may elect to use the 2005–2014 growth rate.

Organizations whose growth is based on acquiring other organizations can only expect to continue past growth rates if the acquisitions continue. For example, Wal-mart's and

McDonald's growth in total sales may be primarily due to opening of more outlets, and a budget preparer at any particular store or restaurant should be more concerned with growth in per store sales.

Moving Average

One of the simplest ways to construct a forecast is by averaging past history. A moving average forecast simply averages a specified number of historical periods to estimate future demand, that is, a 3-year moving average adds the totals for the 3 years prior to the forecast period and divides the sum by three. Similar to using compound growth rates, the current year needs to be annualized (X_{t-1}/Months $*$ 12) before being used in Equation 4.3. An estimate for 2015 discharges would add the total discharges from 2012 through 2014 and divide the sum by 3. Moving averages can be superior to growth rates when a series has no discernible trend.

$$Y_t = (X_{t-1} + X_{t-2} + X_{t-3})/3 \qquad (4.3)$$

$$Y_{2015} = (\text{Discharges in 2014} + \text{Discharges in 2013} \\ + \text{Discharges in 2012})/3\,\text{years}$$

$$Y_{2015} = (35,358,818_{(2014)} + 35,597,792_{(2013)} \\ + 36,484,846_{(2012)})/3 \\ = 35,813,819\,\text{discharges}$$

Microsoft Excel provides a moving average function. Under the **DATA** tab, select **Data Analysis** (an add-in available under **File** and **Options**), select **Moving Average** from the pop-up menu, and click **OK**. On the resulting data entry screen, enter the **Input Range** to use, specify the **Interval** (the number of periods to be averaged), and designate the **Output Range** where the forecast should be displayed. Click **OK**.

Like compound growth rates, the number of periods to include in the moving average depends on how volatile the output has been and should be rigorously examined. Forecasters should calculate moving average forecasts using different intervals (number of former

periods), analyze how well each model predicts output by calculating the forecast error (square root of $\sum (\text{predicted} - \text{actual})^2$), and select the number of periods that minimizes forecast error. Excel provides two options, **Chart Output** and **Standard Errors**, to compare forecasts generated using different numbers of former periods.

Exponential Smoothing

Exponential smoothing estimates future demand on the basis of current output and the prediction of current output. The key decision forecasters make is the value of the smoothing coefficient to be used. The smoothing coefficient, α, can range from 0.0 to 1.0 and determines the relative weight placed on actual and predicted output. When $\alpha = 1.0$, the output forecast depends entirely on current output; when $\alpha = 0.0$, the forecast is driven solely by the previous year's prediction of output; and when $\alpha = 0.50$, the forecast is the average of actual and predicted output. Exponential smoothing should be used when there is no predictable upward or downward trend in output.

$$Y_{2015} = \alpha * X_{2014} + (1 - \alpha) * Y_{2014}, \qquad (4.4)$$

where X is the current output (or an annualized estimate of current output), Y is the beginning of the year output forecast, and α is the weight between 0.00 and 1.00.

Excel provides an exponential smoothing function. Under the **DATA** tab, select **Data Analysis**, select **Exponential Smoothing**, and specify the **Input Range** to employ, specify the **Damping Factor** ($1 - \alpha$, the smoothing coefficient), and designate an **Output Range** where the forecast should be displayed.

Given 2014 is the last year of national discharges available, the exponential smoothing estimate for 2015 discharges using $\alpha = 0.90$ is

$$Y_{2015} = 0.90 * 35,358,818_{(2014\,\text{actual})} \\ + (1 - 0.9) * 36,691,107_{(2014\,\text{forecast})} \\ = 35,392,107\,\text{discharges}.$$

Assume the 2018 output forecast for a hospital was 34,869 cases and exponential smoothing is used to predict 2019 discharges. The fiscal year 2018 is halfway complete, and 17,243 inpatients have been treated. Assuming an equal number of patients will be seen in the second half of the year, the projected actual discharges for 2018 will be 34,486 (17,243 * 12/6). This estimate combined with the 2018 forecast produces a 2019 forecast of

$$Y_{2019} = 0.90 * 34,486_{(2018\,projected\,actual)}$$
$$+ (1 - 0.90) * 34,869_{(2018\,forecast)}$$
$$= 34,524\,discharges.$$

The smoothing coefficient determines the weight placed on actual and forecasted output, that is, in the past, did the current output or the forecast provide a better estimator of output in the budget year? The weight assigned to α can be determined by using various estimates of α, calculating the forecast error from each value (the retrospective difference between estimated and realized output) and selecting the smoothing coefficient with the smallest error for future forecasting. Estimates of $\alpha = 0.10$, 0.20,…, 0.90 were reviewed, and 0.90 produced the smallest forecasting error. Excel again provides two options within the exponential smoothing function, **C**hart Output and **S**tandard Errors, to assess the accuracy of forecasts generated using different damping factors.

Regression

Unlike the previous forecasting methods that focused solely on determining future output from past history, regression attempts to identify relationships between the output to be estimated and other, causal variables that may be easier to estimate. Estimates of inpatient discharges (the **dependent variable**) should change with changes in the size, income, and age of the population (the **independent variables**). A forecast for discharges in 2014 could be predicted on the basis of estimates of population size, average income, average

population age, and other independent variables. The regression formula is

$$Y = A + b_1 X_1 + b_2 X_2 \cdots b_n X_n, \qquad (4.5)$$

where Y is the forecast, A is the **intercept** (the expected value of Y when all Xs are zero), b_i is the slope (change in Y expected from a one unit change in X_i), and X_i is the independent variable (the variable expected to predict change in Y).

Unlike compound growth rates, regression assumes that output is the result of a demand or need based on other factors. The demand for inpatient care (discharges) should decrease with increases in price and increase with the size and age of the population, higher income, and more comprehensive insurance coverage. Other factors such as race/ethnicity and number of competitors could also be added.

$$Y_{Discharges} = f \quad (price, \quad population, \quad age,)$$
$$(-) \qquad (+) \qquad (+)$$
$$(income, \quad insurance, \quad …)$$
$$(+) \qquad (+) \qquad (+)$$

Regression complicates prediction and increases the number of variables that must be predicted, but it may provide a more accurate model of the demand for future output. **TABLE 4.4** displays the historical values for discharges (000), median age of the U.S. population, per capita GDP, and total population (000). $Y_{Discharges} = f(age(+), income(+), population(+))$.

Excel provides a regression function. Under the **DATA** tab, select **Data Analysis** and select **Regression**. Next, specify the **Input Y Range** (the dependent variable), specify the **Input X Range** (one or more independent variables), and designate the **O**utput Range where the results should be displayed. **FIGURE 4.4** shows the regression output for.

$$Y_{Discharges} = f(median\,age, per\,capita\,income[GDP],$$
$$population[number\,of\,citizens]).$$

TABLE 4.4 Discharges, Median Age, Per Capita Income, and Population

Year	Discharges	Median Age	GDP (per Capita)	(000) Population
1993	33,735,002	33.7	$36,631	259,919
1994	33,148,180	34.1	$37,645	263,126
1995	33,644,908	34.4	$38,211	266,278
1996	33,384,374	34.7	$39,203	269,394
1997	33,230,554	34.9	$40,473	272,647
1998	33,923,632	35.2	$41,783	275,854
1999	34,440,994	35.5	$43,241	279,040
2000	35,300,425	35.4	$44,511	282,172
2001	36,093,550	35.5	$44,486	285,082
2002	36,523,831	35.7	$44,853	287,804
2003	37,074,605	35.9	$45,711	290,326
2004	37,496,978	36.0	$47,001	293,046
2005	37,843,039	36.2	$48,129	295,753
2006	38,076,556	36.3	$48,942	298,593
2007	38,155,908	36.5	$49,319	301,580
2008	38,210,889	36.7	$48,724	304,375
2009	37,734,584	37.0	$46,965	307,007
2010	37,352,013	37.2	$47,793	309,330
2011	36,962,415	37.3	$48,207	311,583
2012	36,484,846	37.5	$48,920	313,874
2013	35,597,792	37.6	$49,386	316,126
Compound Growth				
Rate		0.55%	1.51%	0.98%
2014 forecast		37.8	$50,129	319,236

SUMMARY OUTPUT: Discharges					

Regression Statistics	
Multiple *R*	0.9440
R²	0.8911
Adjusted *R²*	0.8719
Standard Error	657,690.17
Observations	21

ANOVA					
	df	*SS*	*MS*	*F*	*Significance F*
Regression	3	6.01625E+13	2.00542E+13	46.3620	2.13086E−08
Residual	17	7.35346E+12	4.32556E+11		
Total	20	6.7516E+13			

	Coefficients	*Standard Error*	*t Stat*	*P-value*	*Lower 95%*	*Upper 95%*
Intercept	91,308,904.60	20,072,330.88	4.55	0.0003	48,959,988.24	133,657,820.97
Median Age	−4,007,484.85	1,167,210.75	−3.43	0.0032	−6,470,084.28	−1,544,885.43
GDPpc	476.97	112.49	4.24	0.0006	239.63	714.31
Population (000)	231.36	84.18	2.75	0.0137	53.75	408.98

FIGURE 4.4 Regression Output

The **adjusted *R²* (the coefficient of determination)** in the regression output shows that 87.2% of the change in discharges is explained by changes in median age, per capita income, and total population. The intercept states that discharges would be 91,308,904 if age, income, and population were 0. Discharges are expected to decrease by 4,007,485 for every 1-year increase in the median population age, and the result is significant, that is, its ***p*-value**, or the probability of obtaining the calculated coefficient when the independent variable is unrelated to the dependent variable, is 0.03%. Statistical significance requires the *p*-value to be 5.0% or less. For every one-dollar increase in per capita GDP, discharges are expected to increase by 476.97; this result was significant as the *p*-value is less than 5.0%. For every 1000-person increase in population, discharges are expected to increase by 231.36, which is significant. The formula for predicting discharges in 2014 is

$$\text{Discharges}_{2014} = (91,308,905 - 4,007,485 \\ * \text{Median age}) \\ + (476.97 * \text{per capita GDP}) \\ + (231.36 * \text{Population})$$

Using a regression equation to forecast discharges requires the forecaster to predict the median age, per capita income, and population for 2014 versus predicting only discharges when using compound growth rates, moving averages, or exponential smoothing. The advantage of regression is that median age, income, and population are more stable than discharges and hence easier to estimate. The compound growth rate for median age is 0.55% per year; per capita income, 1.51%; and population, 0.98% per year. The forecast for median age in 2014 would be 37.8 years; per capita income, $50,129; and total population (in thousands), 319,236. The predicted 2014 discharges are

$$\text{Discharges}_{2014} = (91,308,905 - 4,007,485 * 37.8) \\ + (476.97 * \$50,129) \\ + (231.36 * 319,236) \\ = 37,569,168$$

The power of regression analysis is that forecast errors can be tracked to specific elements. In this example, if the discharge forecast varies from the actual number, is it due to a higher-than-expected increase in median age, or did median age plateau or fall? Likewise, the forecast error could be the result of higher or lower growth in per capita income or population or a changing relationship between the dependent and independent variables. While increases in population age were expected to lead to higher use, it predicted fewer discharges. This could be the result of more aggressive channeling of older patients to outpatient settings or improved health status due to higher economic status. Increases in per capita income and population were correlated with higher admissions (more people with more money should seek more care), but forecasters must recognize that prior relationships, including their direction and magnitude, may not continue into the future.

Composite Forecasts

The last three forecasting methods provided different estimates for total discharges in 2014, so some forecasters use a combination of different methods to reduce the probability of large errors. The moving average method predicted 36,348,351 discharges for 2014, while exponential smoothing and regression predicted 35,691,706 and 37,569,168 discharges, respectively. A composite forecast giving equal weight to each estimate produces a simple average:

$$
\begin{aligned}
Y_{2014} = &(0.3333 \times \text{Moving average}) \\
&+ (0.3333 \times \text{Exponential smoothing}) \\
&+ (0.3333 \times \text{Regression discharges}) \\
&\rightarrow \text{Discharges}
\end{aligned}
$$

$$
\begin{aligned}
Y_{2014} = &(0.3333 * 36,348,351) \\
&+ (0.3333 * 35,691,706) \\
&+ (0.3333 * 37,569,168) \\
= &36,532,755 \text{ discharges}
\end{aligned}
$$

Composite forecasts do not allow extreme predictions to prevail as the forecast is a combination of multiple estimates. Different weights can be placed on each forecast to reflect which method has been the most accurate over time.

Similar to retrospective analysis of moving average and exponential smoothing models, different weights should be tested using historical data to determine the weights that minimize forecast error.

Composite forecasts, like the forecasts of Hurricane Irma shown in **FIGURE 4.5**, recognize different models reach different conclusions, and average the projections to arrive at the most likely results. Figure 4.5 shows the path predictions based on the location of Irma on September 6, 2017, of where it could make landfall, Central Florida at it most western point and the Outer Banks of North Carolina, on the eastern side. The extreme predictions allow affected parties to prepare for the worst-possible outcomes, while recognizing their low probability of occurrence. In this case, the western path was correct: Irma rapidly lost strength as it moved through Central Florida on September 10, 2017.

The preceding forecasts were demonstrated using national discharge statistics; readers should see the applicability of these forecasting methods to smaller data sets (their own data). Caution: what is past is not prologue. None of the forecasting methods can guarantee an accurate estimate of the future. Forecasting methods that rely entirely on history, compound growth rates, moving averages, and exponential smoothing assume that what came before will accurately predict what will happen in the future. Regression, utilizing a more sophisticated approach based on relationships between variables, also assumes that past relationships continue into the future. Neither assumption can be relied upon; things change in unpredictable ways. Forecasting was not introduced to provide "the answer" but to emphasize that forecasters who understand the demand for their products stand a better chance of guessing the future than individuals who produce forecasts out of thin air. Familiarity with where the demand for output arises and how output has fluctuated in the past provides

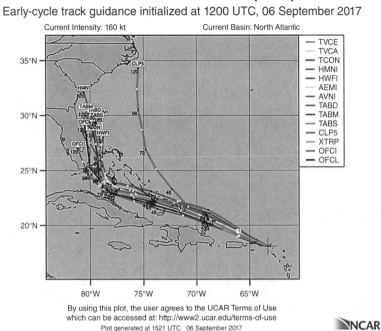

MAJOR HURRICANE IRMA (AL11)
Early-cycle track guidance initialized at 1200 UTC, 06 September 2017

Current Intensity: 160 kt   Current Basin: North Atlantic

By using this plot, the user agrees to the UCAR Terms of Use
which can be accessed at: http://www2.ucar.edu/terms-of-use
Plot generated at 1521 UTC   06 September 2017

NCAR

FIGURE 4.5 Projected Paths of Hurricane Irma, 2017
© 2017, University Corporation for Atmospheric Research.

a good foundation for estimating the need for future output and effectively managing operations.

Qualitative Forecasts

Quantitative forecasts assume that what has come before will continue and are weak in identifying turning points; on the other hand, qualitative forecasts substitute human judgment for data. Expert judgment relies on the insight of one or more individuals to predict future output. A qualitative forecast may be as simple as one person's intuition or may be an aggregation of the opinions of multiple individuals. Qualitative forecasts are used when historical data is missing or history is unlikely to provide an accurate estimate of the future. For example, history can provide little guidance on when an organization will

introduce a new product or start a new business. Qualitative estimates can be produced using the product life cycle model or the Delphi technique.

In the **product life cycle** model, sales (revenues) change systematically over four periods of a product's life: introduction, growth, maturity, and decline. When a new product is launched, the introduction phase, sales are low as customer recognition and acceptance are built. In the growth phase, sales grow rapidly as more customers become aware of and demand the product. Growth leads to maturity: as more and more people purchase the product, the market becomes saturated and sales level off. Decline comes when another product replaces the present product (e.g., ambulatory surgery displaces inpatient surgery) or the product loses its novelty and sales fall (e.g., compact disc sales have fallen by 82.9% since 2000,

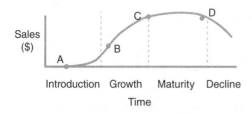

FIGURE 4.6 Product Life Cycle

Statisticbrain, 2016). **FIGURE 4.6** displays the product life cycle.

The judgment aspect of the qualitative forecast comes from where the experts position a product or organization. Points A through D in Figure 4.6 show where a good or service may lie on the product life cycle; the assumption of where the product *does* lie has a substantial impact on forecasts of future sales. Assuming a product is in introduction, A, or is moving toward maturity, C, implies sales may grow slowly. If the product is believed to be entering its growth stage, B, sales may increase exponentially. At maturity, C, the total industry sales may not change, and the only way for the organization to increase its revenue is by taking customers away from competitors. In decline, D, industry sales fall, and it may no longer be possible to increase sales by increasing market share; when this is the case, output forecasts should be reduced. The implications of misinterpreting the product life stage will have a profound impact on the revenue forecast: If the product is in its introduction and growth phases, A and B, revenues will increase; at maturity, C, little change should be expected; and when in decline, D, large revenue reductions may occur.

A second qualitative method is the **Delphi method**, where a panel of experts is physically separated and each person responds individually to a series of questions (what sales will be in the following year, what factors will drive sales in the following year, etc.). Physical separation prevents panel members from being unduly influenced by other members. After the initial responses are received, they are summarized and distributed to each panel member so that each can respond to the opinions of others and reassess his or her own answers. After a few rounds of response and review, a consensus of opinion is obtained and output forecasted.

The advantages of qualitative forecasts are that they rely on the judgment and experience of personnel and can be produced quickly and at little cost. The disadvantages are that forecasters may place too much emphasis on recent events and ignore data that does not support their own views.

It is essential to evaluate the accuracy of prior forecasts, whether using a quantitative or a qualitative forecasting method. The retrospective, or evaluation, phase of the budgeting process should include an assessment of the planning and forecasting processes. How close were the forecasts to the actual output demanded? If the forecasts were off, how can forecasters learn from their mistakes? Are forecasts under- or overpredicting demand, and if so, why? Can future forecasts be adjusted to achieve greater accuracy? If the forecasts are consistently under- or overpredicting, future forecasts should be adjusted up or down to increase their accuracy. Forecasters should examine their estimating techniques and explore new methods when there is a pattern to the forecast error.

The goal of forecasting is to accurately project future variables; for data series that show steady and stable trends (like expenditures), compound growth rates may be the best. Forecasting of outputs (discharges, patient days, procedures, and patient visits) that increase and decrease without pattern may require using moving averages, exponential smoothing, or regression to capture the dynamic nature of demand. Revenue and expense budgets are heavily dependent upon the output forecast; good forecasts provide the foundation for good budgets, and it is unlikely that an accurate budget can arise from a poor forecast—garbage in, garbage out.

Revenue Budgets

Revenue is typically determined as the product of price and quantity ($P * Q$) of the good or service expected to be sold. The question is, how much influence does an organization have over price and quantity? Does the organization control its destiny? Can it raise prices and/or increase the quantity of output sold to increase revenue? Not all organizations have the ability to set their own prices; in some cases, purchasers dictate prices, leaving organizations with only the option of increasing quantity to increase revenue. In public organizations, departments may have no control over either the price charged (the good or service may be provided at no charge) or the quantity of output they produce, and higher levels of output may not increase funding. Budgeting is straightforward when price and output are fixed; quantities and prices are multiplied to establish the revenue budget, and managers attempt to keep expenses under the total revenue. Rarely are prices and output fixed, so this section examines how revenue is determined on the basis of an organization's ability to influence output prices and the demand for output.

In economics, the idea of *market organization* holds that the type of industry an organization operates in determines its actions. The **structure–conduct–performance paradigm** holds that the industry structure (number of producers and type of product) determines conduct (organizational action such as pricing, marketing, and innovation) and that structure and conduct determine performance (profit). In **perfect competition**, many sellers offer homogeneous products, that is, the product of one producer cannot be distinguished from the competitors'. Individual organizations in perfectly competitive industries have no control over price and can sell as much output as they can produce at the market price. Competition and innovation are limited as neither price nor sales can be increased by marketing or research and development (R&D) activities. For example, farmers can produce as much grain or other agricultural product as they are capable of and sell it at the prevailing market price. In perfectly competitive markets, the only way to increase revenue is by expanding output.

In **monopolistic competition**, there are many sellers but products are differentiated. Buyers do not see the products of competing organizations as identical and may be willing to pay higher prices for the products they think are superior. Product differentiation provides organizations with limited control over prices. Competition may also arise through advertising, product innovation, and distribution to convince purchasers that the organization produces the best products in the market, provides superior service, and/or affords more convenient access. An organization's control over price is limited as consumers may select less desirable products or less convenient access if the price differential becomes too great, for example, restaurants. A fast-food aficionado may think a McDonald's hamburger is superior to the offerings of Burger King, Hardees, etc., but if McDonald's charges $0.50 more for comparable burgers, the consumer may be unwilling to pay this difference and patronize Burger King or other restaurants despite his or her preference for McDonald's hamburgers. Providers in monopolistically competitive markets can increase their revenues by expanding output or by limited price increases (**TABLE 4.5**).

Oligopoly describes a market characterized by a small number of producers who exercise significant control over price due to limited competition and their ability to differentiate their goods or services from competitors. Oligopolists, like automakers or airlines, engage in strategic behavior, as one organization knows its competitors and attempts to determine how to counter their actions. Will a price increase or decrease be followed, will improvements in products or services be copied, will an advertising campaign be countered, and/or will expansion of distribution outlets lead to similar expansion by competitors? Oligopolists consider how their competitors may respond to their actions when plotting strategy. If competitors generally follow price increases, managers can raise prices without the fear of losing market share. On the other hand, if competitors will not or cannot follow price reductions, lowering prices may be beneficial if the additional sales captured from higher-priced competitors more than offset price reductions. Oligopolists can increase their revenues by increasing prices (if competitors follow price increases) or reducing prices

TABLE 4.5 Market Organization

	Control over Price	Number of Sellers/ Producers	Type of Products	Example
Perfect competition	None	Many	Homogeneous	Farmers
Monopolistic competition	Limited	Many	Differentiated	Restaurants
Oligopoly	Extensive	Few	Both	Automobiles
Monopoly	Complete	One	Unique	Utilities

and expanding sales (if competitors cannot follow price reductions).

A **monopoly** has complete control over prices since it is the sole source for a product. Monopolists have no competition, and consumers have no close substitutes for their products. If you want natural gas, electricity, or water, you have to deal with the local utility company; if you want a diamond, you deal with DeBeers. Customers must pay the price a monopolist charges or go without the good or service. The only constraints on price increases for a monopolist come from consumers, who can refuse to purchase if prices go too high, or price-setting regulations.

The reader should see that any particular hospital or physician might be viewed by patients as a perfect or monopolistic competitor. One hospital stay or physician visit may be viewed as indistinguishable from another, or strong loyalties (that supersede pricing) may arise between patients and providers. Market organization predicts that a provider's control over price will increase as the number of comparable suppliers decrease. For example, the ability of a hospital or physician to raise prices will depend on whether the hospital or physician is one of many, one of few, or the sole provider in the market.

Output is the major determinant of revenues and costs, yet revenue often has a major impact on organizational expenditures. Parkinson's law states that expenditures expand to consume available income and organizations with excess revenues find uses for these funds, including expanding their work force, increasing the compensation of workers, purchasing higher-quality supplies and equipment, and building larger and more ornate facilities. On the other hand, revenue-constrained organizations find ways to cut costs by reducing or eliminating low-value activities, demanding more from employees, and making due with smaller, more basic facilities. Knowledge of revenue constraints, or the lack thereof, is a primary determinant of how large the expense budget can be versus how large it need be.

Monopolists and oligopolists with the ability to set prices and quantities have the greatest latitude to determine their revenues, but even these organizations must recognize limits on customers' willingness to pay for their output. Revenue budgets are often backed into in industries or geographic areas where an organization has no close competitors. That is, expected expenses are estimated for the budget year and divided by expected output to determine the minimum price needed to cover costs and provide an adequate return on investment (ROI). Setting the revenue budget to cover total expected expenses assumes that prices can be set independent of sales; in the real world, revenues often fall when prices are raised.

Market organization examines industry-level factors that affect prices and demand, and price elasticity focuses on the characteristics of individual goods and services to determine how sales respond to price changes. The law of demand holds that the number of units of a good or service purchased falls with an increase in price, but the key issue is, by how much will sales fall if prices are increased? Will an increase in price more than offset a drop in sales and increase revenue, or will the reduction in sales be greater than the increase in price and produce lower revenues? Point elasticity, Equation 4.6, measures the percentage change in quantity sold that accompanies a percentage change in price (subscript 1 indicates the quantity sold and price before a price change and subscript 2 after the price change).

$$P_e = \frac{(Q_2 - Q_1)/Q_1}{(P_2 - P_1)/P_1} \qquad (4.6)$$

Price increases only produce higher revenues when the percentage decrease in sales is less than the percentage increase in price, that is, demand is **inelastic**. Price elasticity (P_e) is categorized as **elastic** when the percentage change in price results in a greater percentage change in quantity sold in the opposite direction and **unitary elastic** when the percentage change in price results in an equal percentage change in quantity sold in the opposite direction. The degree of elasticity recommends different approaches to price setting. Price elasticity determines whether it is in the best interest of an organization to increase, decrease, or leave prices unchanged.

Raising prices only generates higher revenues when price elasticity is inelastic, that is, $P_e < -1.0$. In the extreme case, if $P_e = 0.0$, sellers can raise prices without losing any sales, so every percentage point increase in price increases the total revenue by the same percentage. When quantity demanded is inelastic, every 1.0% increase in price reduces sales by less than 1.0% and total revenue increases. The expected change in revenue is determined by multiplying the percentage change in price by $1 - P_e$. If price is raised by 10.0% and $P_e = -0.5$, the expected change in revenue is 5.0% (10.0% * (1 − 0.5)).

TABLE 4.6 shows the revenue calculation for an organization selling a single good at a single price, given different degrees of price elasticity. If price is raised by 10.0% and demand is perfectly inelastic, that is, $P_e = 0.0$, the seller sees no change in quantity sold and the total revenue increases by 10.0%. When price elasticity increases to −0.5, the 10.0% increase in price reduces the quantity sold by 5.0% and the total revenue increases by 4.5%. When $P_e = -1.0$, unitary elasticity, the 10.0% price increase is offset by a 10.0% reduction in quantity sold and the total revenue remains relatively constant. Producers facing unitary elasticity have no incentive to increase or decrease price. If $P_e = -1.5$, a 10.0% price increase reduces quantity sold by 15.0% and the total revenue falls. Producers facing elastic demand, $P_e > -1.0$, should reduce prices to increase the total revenue.

The price elasticity of a product is determined by the consumer's desire or need for the product. The demand for a good or service and the consumer's willingness to pay for it are impacted by whether the product is a luxury or a necessity: the percentage of the consumer's budget spent on the item, the length of time purchasers have to adjust to price changes, and the existence of close substitutes. Goods and services that are believed to be necessities have lower price elasticity. For example, medicine and food are items that people will purchase at about the same levels even if prices are increased. Luxury items, such as entertainment, jewelry, designer clothing, and yachts, are more price elastic. As prices of luxuries increase, buyers recognize that these things are not needed but are merely wanted, and demand may fall precipitously.

TABLE 4.6 Price Elasticity and Total Revenue

| Quantity | | | % Change in | |
Price Elasticity	Sold	Price	Revenue	Total Revenue
Current revenue	200,000	$50	$10,000,000	Baseline
After Price Increase				
0.0 (inelastic)	200,000	$55	$11,000,000	+10.0%
−0.5 (inelastic)	190,000	$55	$10,450,000	+4.5%
−1.0 (unitary elastic)	180,000	$55	$9,900,000	−1.0%
−1.5 (elastic)	170,000	$55	$9,350,000	−6.5%

The second factor, the percentage of budget spent on an item, speaks to the ability of the consumer to cope with price increases. A 10.0% or 20.0% increase in the price of a 15 oz. can of baked beans from $1.32 to $1.45 or $1.58 ($15.79 for 12 cans @ Amazon.com on November 4, 2016) may not be noticed or, if noticed, may not change the consumer's buying behavior. A rent increase of 10.0% (from $800 to $880 per month) may put such a crimp into a person's budget that he or she may seek another place to live. The point is, what behavioral change does a price increase impose on the consumer's other purchases? Change is easily accommodated when a price increase amounts to a small percentage of a person's budget; changes amounting to 5.0% or more of a consumer's disposable income may require undesired reductions in other purchases and reduce the demand for the item increasing in price.

The third factor is the length of time a consumer has to adjust to a price increase. In the short run, consumers may be forced to pay higher prices, but given time, they can locate alternatives for items that increase in price. Gasoline is a prime example; if the price of gas increases by $1.00 per gallon tomorrow, drivers will still have to get to work and run essential trips—their demand for gas may be undiminished. Drivers may consider other alternatives, such as carpooling or public transportation, and more extreme measures, including purchasing a more energy-efficient vehicle or moving closer to work if gas prices remain high. Price elasticity increases as consumers have more time to adjust their spending to higher prices.

The final consideration is whether close substitutes exist for the good or service. Items with close substitutes are more price elastic as consumers can easily switch from higher-priced goods or services to other items that fulfill the same need or desire at a lower price. An increase in the price of beef may be met with an increase in the demand for pork, chicken, and seafood if their prices do not increase at the same rate, that is, consumers will switch to other meats (or foods) as the relative price of beef increases. An increase in the price of insulin will not reduce demand significantly, given the lack of a substitute. NBC News reported that the price of insulin has increased between 380% and 400% since 2004 (Popken,

2016). A lack of close substitutes explains why monopolists have so much control over their prices—their consumers cannot purchase other goods and services to meet their need or desire, for example, utilities.

Feldstein (2005) reviewed multiple studies and reported that price elasticities for hospital admissions ranged from -0.14 to -0.20. Using the midpoint of this range would conclude that a 10.0% increase in the price of a hospital admission would reduce admissions by 1.7%. Hospitals face an inelastic demand for care and can increase revenue by raising prices; the increase in revenue, however, will be constrained by the number of patients reimbursed under fixed payment arrangements. Feldstein also reported that the price elasticity for physician visits ranged from -0.09 to -0.35 and nursing home services from -0.73 to -2.40. Research suggests that nursing homes face an elastic demand curve and could increase revenue by lowering prices; at the high elasticity estimate, a 10.0% reduction in price would raise demand by 24.0%.

How managers perceive other suppliers of a good or service will respond to a price change has a significant impact on price setting. If other providers are expected to follow price increases, managers do not have to fear losing sales to competitors and thus face less elastic demand. If all hospitals or physicians raise prices by 3.0%, their relative positions are unchanged and none should fear losing customers to competitors; however, total admissions or office visits could be lost if consumers opt to purchase other goods and services in lieu of healthcare services. If price increases are not followed, a provider increasing its prices should expect to lose patients to competitors that do not raise prices. Strategic behavior based on the recognition of conflicting interests and interdependency should dictate when prices are increased, decreased, or held constant.

Assume a nursing home sells one item, assisted living services, for $8000 per month, and every resident pays the same price. Sales have increased over the past 10 years at a compound growth rate of 2.0%. **TABLE 4.7** demonstrates what the future revenue will be, given different degrees of price elasticity, if the nursing home currently sells 4500 months of care annually and is considering raising prices by 5.0%.

TABLE 4.7 Calculating Total Revenue

	Price Elasticity	Units Sold		Price	Total % Change in Revenue	Total Revenue
Current revenue		4,500		$8,000	$36,000,000	Baseline
Budget, $P_e =$	0.00	4,590	4,590 * (1 + (5% * 0.00))	$8,400	$38,556,000	+7.1%
	−0.73	4,422	4,590 * (1 + (5% * −0.73))	$8,400	$37,144,800	+3.2%
	−1.56	4,232	4,590 * (1 + (5% * −1.56))	$8,400	$35,548,800	−1.3%
	−2.40	4,039	4,590 * (1 + (5% * −2.40))	$8,400	$33,927,600	−5.8%

Table 4.7 highlights the potential impact of price elasticity on the revenue budget from $+7.1\%$ to -5.8%; as long as $P_e <= -1.0$, price increases lead to higher revenue, but the expected change in revenue decreases as P_e approaches -1.0. When $P_e > -1.0$, any increase in price reduces the total revenue; however, this impact is masked by the 2.0% annual growth in units sold. Price increases reduce the total revenue even after factoring in the 2.0% growth if $P_e >= -1.32$. If the nursing home is at the midpoint or upper limit of the previous identified range of price elasticity (-0.73 to -2.40), managers should consider reducing prices.

Calculating the revenue budget is less complicated for organizations that cannot set their prices. Hospitals or physicians whose patients are covered by Medicare, like agricultural producers who sell their output at the prices set by commodity markets, have to determine the price they will be paid for their output and the quantity of output they want to produce. Healthcare providers can sell as much care as they like, assuming it is medically necessary at the current reimbursement level, but their ability to increase revenue by raising prices is extremely limited. Before the advent of DRG reimbursement, hospitals could simply determine their costs that would be paid for Medicare patients under cost reimbursement, and set prices for charge-based patients to generate the required revenue to cover costs (including uncompensated care) plus profit. After DRGs were introduced, there was no guarantee that costs for Medicare patients would be covered, so all losses had to be recouped by increased prices for charge-based patients.

As Medicare shifted to fixed reimbursement, other healthcare insurers implemented their own fixed payment systems to minimize cost shifting. Healthcare providers now face the situation of other organizations: can treatment be provided within the constraint of what third-party payers are willing to pay? DRG reimbursement provides an opportunity to hospitals to increase revenue by increasing the number of cases treated. However, capitated reimbursement, where an organization is paid a flat fee per member covered (divorced from the number of cases treated or the level of treatment provided), shifts hospitals from a system where revenue can be controlled by adjusting the number of cases handled to a system where reimbursement is fixed and where increasing the volume of services provided will not increase revenue.

Capitation establishes a fixed revenue budget, where an organization may have no control over price or the quantity of output. This arrangement is common in public organizations. For example, the Department of Defense (DOD) received $696.3 billion in 2010, but with combat operations simultaneously occurring in Iraq and Afghanistan, the DOD found it could not meet all its expected duties and sought supplemental appropriations. Many organizations, like public health departments, are allocated a budget at the start of the year and see no additional revenue if output expands. These organizations find themselves managing (i.e., limiting) output, when possible, or reducing quality (cutting the cost per output) to stay within their budgets. Examples of organizations with fixed revenue budgets include public sector agencies, Canadian hospitals operating under global budgets, or U.S. healthcare providers with capitation contracts. In each case, managers know at the start of the budget year the total revenue they will receive and cannot raise prices or increase output to increase revenue.

In accordance with Parkinson's law, managers find themselves looking for ways of using their available funds when revenues increase and excess funds are expended on "nice to have if you can afford it" items. Organizations flush with funds can lose focus; they can afford to be extravagant, be inefficient, or provide money-losing services. In the golden years of healthcare financing, 1966–1983, massive increases in salaries, the number of workers employed, services provided, and investments in plant and equipment occurred. The legacy of easy money continues to haunt health care. The shift to fixed reimbursement is difficult;

it requires organizations to get a better handle on their operations and to cut "fat" as well as the expectations of their stakeholders. Hospital employees no longer expect annual salary increases above the rate of inflation, physicians recognize that investment in technology is constrained, and all should recognize the limits on providing uncompensated care.

Healthcare organizations now face rigid spending limits, that is, what revenue can be brought in through patient services? Non operating revenues can ease the limits placed on healthcare providers from revenues generated from patient services. The income statement in Figure 2.3, Chapter 2, shows $6,518,282 in non operating revenues that accounted for only 0.75% of the total revenue but obviously provided the organization with expanded investment opportunities. Revenue constraints place additional emphasis on accurate budgeting; the failure to provide goods and services within the limit set by the revenue budget means that the organization will lose money and possibly cease to exist.

Budgeting Revenue

There are two primary approaches to determining the revenue budget: the revenue budget may be calculated prior to or after the expense budget is compiled. In organizations that exert significant control over prices, the revenue budget may be the last piece of the master budget. The budget preparer takes the output forecast, collects expense estimates from operating managers, and compiles the total expense budget. After all department expenses are compiled, the total expense is divided by the forecasted output to determine the price that must be set to cover expenses. The ability to set prices allows the organization to cover its expenses and enjoy whatever net income it desires.

Organizations that are price takers often calculate their revenue budget prior to their expense budget and use the revenue forecast to inform the expense budget. The budget in a price-taking organization again starts with forecasted output but then switches to determining the price it will receive for its output. Expected output and price are multiplied to establish the revenue budget. The year-to-year change in the revenue budget should guide the subsequent construction of the expense budget. If total revenue is expected to increase by 3.0%, the budget directions given to managers may specify an acceptable rate of increase in their expenses as something less than 3.0%. The final step reconciles the total expense budget to the fixed revenue budget, that is, are total expenses less than total revenue?

Output forecasts to this point assumed a single homogenous good; in the real world, however, organizations produce a variety of distinct outputs. Whether an organization is a hospital, a physician practice, or an automobile manufacturer, the budget should identify as closely as possible what is intended to be produced and who will purchase it. As suggested by the earlier discussion of DRGs and MDCs, two hospitals may admit 10,000 patients per year, but they can have dramatically different revenues and expenses, depending on the type of patients admitted. Medicare provides higher reimbursement for surgical care and cases with complications and comorbidities, so hospitals providing a higher percentage of surgical services and treating sicker patients will have higher revenues and expenses than providers serving uncomplicated medical patients. Revenue projections in Table 4.7 are based on a single product sold at a single price. Two additional systems will be demonstrated. The first is for a physician practice that provides different levels of patient visits at different prices, but each type of visit is reimbursed at the same rate. The second is for a hospital providing inpatient care and receiving different reimbursement for the same type of admission.

Assume a physician practice provides 10 services, new and established visits, and all patients are under Medicare or all payers pay the same rate for each type of visit. The physician or office manager needs to construct reasonably accurate estimates of the type of patients that will be seen (new or established patients) and the level of care they will need (brief to comprehensive visits). Medicare reimburses physicians for treatment on the basis of the expected treatment time, training and training costs, and practice expenses under the resource-based relative value system (RBRVS). **TABLE 4.8** provides the healthcare common procedure coding system (HCPCS) codes for the 10 types of visits rendered, the number of each type expected in the budget year, the relative value units (RVU), and the reimbursement rate. The revenue budget is determined by multiplying price by quantity.

The type of patient seen and the level of care provided must be accurately forecasted to produce an accurate revenue budget. A shift of patients from one type of service to another will have a substantial impact on revenue: If 200 new patients (99203) are replaced in the patient mix by 200 established patients (99213), revenue will fall by $16,012 ($-2.4$%). A shift of 200 established patients from limited (99212) to extended (99214) visits would increase revenue by $16,720. Changes in the type of patient seen or the level of care provided also impact the time needed to treat patients and the expense budget.

TABLE 4.8 Calculating the Revenue Budget for a Physician Practice					
Output	**HCPCS**	**RVU**	**Price**	**Quantity**	**Revenue**
New Patient					
Level I, Brief	99201	0.95	$67.31	112	$7,538.72
Level II, Limited	99202	1.70	$120.45	165	$19,874.25
Level III, Moderate	99203	2.52	$178.54	402	$71,773.08
Level IV, Extended	99204	3.59	$254.35	109	$27,724.15
Level V, Comprehensive	99205	4.58	$324.49	52	$16,873.48
Established Patient					
Level I, Brief	99211	0.56	$39.68	269	$10,673.92
Level II, Limited	99212	0.99	$70.14	541	$37,945.74
Level III, Moderate	99213	1.39	$98.48	3,269	$321,931.12
Level IV, Extended	99214	2.17	$153.74	632	$97,163.68
Level V, Comprehensive	99215	3.18	$225.30	309	$69,617.70
Total				**5,860**	**$681,115.84**

It is well known that third-party payers reimburse healthcare providers at different rates for similar services, so the following example demonstrates the impact of changes in the patient (or payer) mix on hospital revenues. To simplify the presentation, the assumption is that a hospital provides one output—inpatient admission. The patient mix must be defined since reimbursement depends on whether the admission is reimbursed by Medicare under a per case (DRG) system, a commercial insurer paying charges, a managed care paying a capitated rate, or a charity case (no pay). In this case, shifts in patients treated (rather than shifts in the type of care provided) have a substantial impact on the total revenue and on whether the hospital meets its budget.

Determining the revenue forecast for a hospital involves estimating inpatient revenue on the basis of the number of inpatient admissions and the average reimbursement per case. Hospitals are largely price takers; reimbursement is set by third-party payers on the basis of the cases admitted (DRG), cost, inpatient days (per diem), and capitation, and charge-reimbursed patients make up a small percentage of the total patients.

Under charge reimbursement, a hospital establishes its price and the patients or their third-party payers pay billed charges. Under a percentage-of-charge system, third-party payers negotiate a discount and pay billed charges less the discount. If a third-party payer negotiates a 20.0% discount, it pays 80.0% of the billed charges and the remaining balance is written off as a contractual discount. In the following example, $15,000 is billed, $12,000 is paid, and $3000 is written off as a contractual discount. In cost-based reimbursement, allowable costs are identified and the total allowable cost is divided by the total charges to establish a cost-to-charge ratio that is used to reimburse cases. In the example, the total cost is $58,000,000, the total revenue is $90,000,000, and the ratio of cost to charge is 64.44% ($58,000,000/$90,000,000). Given that $15,000 is billed per case, a third party reimbursing the hospital on cost would pay $9667 per case ($15,000 * 64.44%). The difference between the billed charges per case and the cost per case, $5333, is written off.

Per case (DRG) reimbursement establishes a flat rate per admission on the basis of the type of admission, the body system involved, the type of care rendered (surgical or medical), and the presence of complications or comorbidities. Under DRG reimbursement, hospitals have an incentive to increase efficiency and discharge patients as soon as medically appropriate in order to keep costs low and maximize the difference between cost and the per case payment. In this example, the case payment is $10,300 and $4,700 is the contractual discount. Per diem reimbursement pays hospitals on the basis of the number of days a patient is hospitalized: $1900 per day is paid, and charges above $1900 are written off. Capitation pays a flat rate per member per month (PMPM) for all required services, and revenue is independent of charges. Charges in excess of the monthly capitated payment, *covered members * PMPM*, are written off. The challenge facing a hospital is that patients may be reimbursed under each of these systems, in addition to any charity care the hospital provides.

TABLE 4.9 assumes that a hospital admits 6000 patients per year (Q) and the ALOS is 5 days. The average billed charges per admission equal $15,000, the AVC is $1,350/day, and the total fixed cost (TFC) is $17,500,000. Patients whose charges are paid in full account for 6.0% of admissions, with an additional 10.0% reimbursed at 80% of the billed charge. Cost reimbursement covers 15.0% of admissions, and DRG reimbursement covers 55.0% of patients at $10,300 per admission. A managed care payer has negotiated a per diem arrangement paying $1900 per day that covers 5.0% of patients. Another managed care payer has negotiated a capitation arrangement that pays the hospital $90 PMPM and covers 52,000 members. These 52,000 members account for 6.0% of the total admissions. Charity care and bad debt (no pay) constitute the remaining 3.0% of admissions.

TABLE 4.9 Calculating the Revenue Budget for a Hospital

			Reimbursement			Patient Mix
Quantity (Q)	6000		Charge 100%			6%
Price/day	$3,000	($15,000/5 days)	Charge 80%	Discount	20%	10%
Price (P)	$15,000		Cost	Per Diem	$1,900	15%
Average length of stay	5.00		Per Case	Per (DRG) Case	$10,300	55%
Total fixed cost	$17,500,000		Per Diem	Capitation rate	$1,080	5%
Variable cost/day	$1,350	($6750/5 days)	Capitation	Covered lives	52,000	6%
			No pay			3%

	B	C	D	E	F	G	H
	Charge	80% Charge	Cost	Per Diem	Per Case	Capitation	Composite
Total revenue	$90,000,000	$90,000,000	$90,000,000	$90,000,000	$90,000,000	$90,000,000	$90,000,000
Contractual discount	0	$18,000,000	$32,000,000	$33,000,000	$28,200,000	$33,840,000	$30,890,400
Net revenue	$90,000,000	$72,000,000	$58,000,000	$57,000,000	$61,800,000	$56,160,000	$59,109,600
Expenses							
Total fixed cost	$17,500,000	$17,500,000	$17,500,000	$17,500,000	$17,500,000	$17,500,000	$17,500,000
Total variable cost	$40,500,000	$40,500,000	$40,500,000	$40,500,000	$40,500,000	$40,500,000	$40,500,000
Total	$58,000,000	$58,000,000	$58,000,000	$58,000,000	$58,000,000	$58,000,000	$58,000,000
Net income	$32,000,000	$14,000,000	$0	-$1,000,000	$3,800,000	-$1,840,000	$1,109,600

Table 4.9 and the accompanying spreadsheet, BudgetCh04.xlsx, allow the reader to evaluate the impact of different scenarios, changes in the payer mix, prices, costs, and utilization on the net revenue and profitability. Columns B through G demonstrate the impact of price, reimbursement rates, cost, and utilization changes on how much the hospital would earn if *all* admissions were paid under that reimbursement system. The composite column, H, estimates the total net revenue for the hospital by incorporating the mix of patients served under each reimbursement system.

The most advantageous reimbursement system is a charge-based system (column B), where the hospital has complete control over its revenue, that is, it can increase price and quantity. If all cases were paid at 100% of charges, the hospital would earn a profit of $32,000,000. A percentage of the charge reimbursement system is almost as advantageous as 100% of charges, assuming the hospital can raise prices at its discretion. Column C demonstrates that the impact of a 20%, or $18,000,000 ($90,000,000 * 20%), contractual discount is a dollar-for-dollar reduction in net income. If all cases were reimbursed at 80% of billed charges, the hospital would earn $14,000,000. The good news for a provider is that any discount given to third-party payers can be negated by price increases. Assume a third-party payer negotiates a higher discount, increasing the discount from 20% to 25%; the negative impact on net revenue can be eliminated by increasing prices by 6.67%. The hospital currently receives 80% of $15,000, or $12,000, per case; if the third-party payer negotiates a 25% discount, the average charge per case only needs to be increased to $16,000 to continue to net $12,000 per case ($16,000 * 75%).

The high profits achievable under charge-based reimbursement led third-party payers to establish greater control over their medical outlays through cost-based or fixed reimbursement. Under cost-based reimbursement, third-party payers reimburse providers for the cost of services delivered and do not cover profit,

so gross revenue less cost determines the contractual discount. Providers may not be able to generate a profit under this system, but they benefit from the guarantee that their costs will be covered. The hospital in this example would recoup its $1350 per day variable cost and its $17,500,000 fixed cost, or reimbursement equals the hospital's average total cost of $9666.67 per case. Cost reimbursement encourages providers to increase costs by employing more and higher-priced resources. Under cost reimbursement, employees, suppliers, and patients may benefit from higher employment and wages, greater use of supplies and reduced incentive to negotiate better prices, and more medical care.

Medicare eventually learned that cost-based reimbursement rather than restraining outlays led to a rapid increase in cost and payments to providers and began the shift to fixed case-based payment in 1983. Initially, Medicare specified 372 different DRGs with different payments rates; as of 2015, the number of DRGs stands at 667. The incentive under per case reimbursement is toward higher efficiency (lower costs) and increased number of cases. Medicare recognized the incentive to increase admissions and limited reimbursement to medically necessary care. Admission of non-medically necessary cases would not be paid by Medicare and could not be billed to patients. While per case reimbursement reduced the ability of hospitals to increase their revenues, it provided a clear objective for management: the total cost of medical care had to be kept below the case payment rate. The Medicare per case (DRG) reimbursement of $10,300 is desirable as long as the hospital can hold its average cost per case below this amount. Currently, the average cost is $9666.67, and if all patients are covered by Medicare, the hospital would earn a profit of $3,800,000 (or $633.33 per case).

After Medicare introduced case-based payment, other third-party payers recognized that costs could be shifted to them if they continued to reimburse hospitals on charges, and so they introduced reimbursement based on the number of days hospitalized (per diem) or the number of people covered (capitation). The per diem rate of $1900 per day in this case does not cover the total cost of providing daily care of $1933.33 ($58,000,000/6,000 cases/5 days), and the hospital would lose $1,000,000 if all patients are paid under this system. Per diem reimbursement gives an incentive to providers to reduce costs, increase admissions, and keep patients longer. Third-party payers using per diem reimbursement recognized these incentives and, like Medicare, limited payment to medically necessary cases and days.

Given a capitation rate of $90 PMPM ($1080 per member per year), total expenses would be greater than their reimbursement, creating a loss of $1,840,000. Capitation is the most radical departure from charge-based reimbursement as it does not reimburse hospitals on the care provided but, rather, on the number of patients the hospitals contract to provide care for. Under capitated reimbursement, hospitals must understand utilization rates and production costs as they accept a fixed PMPM payment and assume responsibility to provide all needed care. If a hospital can keep patients healthy and out of the hospital, it keeps any excess revenue; if the cost of treating exceeds the total PMPM payments, the hospital loses money. Capitation changes the traditional incentive in health care from treatment after a patient becomes ill to prevention and keeping patients healthy.

The reader should note that charity or bad debt (no pay) does not produce any revenue, and all costs associated with treating these cases must be recouped from other payers, or the organization will lose money. Given the posited patient mix, this hospital earns a profit of $1,109,600 and the charge- and case-based patients subsidize the losses incurred on the per diem, capitation, and charity cases.

Pricing

If a hospital is a price setter, prices for outputs should be based on costs. In Table 4.9, variable costs are $1350 per day (or $6750

per case) and the TFC is $17,500,000 per year (or $2916.67 per case when 6000 cases are treated). These two costs provide the basis for a brief discussion of pricing. There are two types of pricing, full **cost** and marginal cost pricing. **Full cost pricing** establishes the minimum prices to cover all costs; it requires recovering at least $9666.67 per case, the $6750 (5 days ∗ $1350/day) variable cost and the $2916.67 fixed cost per case. Any reimbursement above this breakeven point increases profit.

Marginal cost pricing aims at recouping the costs that arise from increasing output by one unit (treating one more inpatient) and ignores fixed costs. Fixed costs must be paid regardless of output, so these costs can be ignored when setting prices. Under marginal cost pricing, as long as a payer pays more than the variable cost ($6750 per case), it is in the interest of the hospital to provide care. Any reimbursement over $6750 will defray some of the hospital's fixed expenses. In Table 4.9, the per diem and capitated patients are desirable because they contribute toward paying down fixed expenses; the average capitated payment per admission is $9360, or $2610 over its variable cost of $6750. The payment received from the per diem payer, $1900 per day, exceeds the $1350 AVC per day and thus provides $550 per day toward meeting fixed costs. In total, the per diem payments contribute $825,000 ($550/day ∗ 5 days ∗ 300 patients) toward fixed costs, and although this does not fully recoup the fixed cost of $875,000 ($2916.67 ∗ 300 patients), the hospital is better off with these patients than without them.

Similarly, the average capitated payment per admission is $9,360 ($56,160,000/6000 patients), or $2610 over the variable cost. If the capitated patients do not utilize the hospital and no other patients take their place, the hospital would lose an additional $940,000 ($2,610 ∗ 360 patients). If any payer should seek to pay less than $6750 per case, the hospital's total loss will increase as the payment will fail to cover not only the its fixed costs but also the additional variable costs incurred to deliver care, so the hospital should reject the offer. Any reimbursement above the marginal cost will increase profit if fixed costs are met by other payers or reduce losses if fixed costs have not been fully satisfied.

Marginal cost pricing is a short-term option appropriate for organizations that are price takers. Organizations cannot offer marginal cost pricing to all payers, as fixed costs must be recouped (through sales, donations, and/or tax-supported funding), or the organizations will not be able to carry operations into the future.

Accurate revenue budgets require that managers understand their patient population, the services they provide, and the different reimbursement rates they receive for providing services. Output should be specified by type of care and payer when reimbursement rates are based on these factors. The reader should understand that *none* of the examples provided in the chapter meets the realities of healthcare markets. The multiple-Q/single-P model (Table 4.8) ignores the fact that different payers reimburse physicians differently for physician services, while the single-Q/multiple-P model used for the hospital (Table 4.9) ignores the 667 different DRGs used by Medicare to pay inpatient stays. These complications are often circumvented by calculating average (historical) reimbursement per physician visit or admission, but when these shortcuts are used, the budget preparer should understand that any significant change in output or patient mix could dramatically increase or reduce actual revenue and expenses.

Preparation of output forecasts and revenue budgets may be done by senior management, with the planning and finance departments providing the lion's share of information. On the other hand, output and pricing projections may emanate from medical service lines that have the best understanding of their patient populations and may be conveyed up the organizational structure.

Regardless of the direction that output and pricing information travels, senior and operating managers should have a firm grasp of the total need for care, how the need will be satisfied, and how treatment will be reimbursed in order to determine the level of resources they will be able to command during the budget year.

Summary

Predicting output and revenues may not be required from operating managers overseeing cost or expense centers, yet they should know how it is done and what its impact is on expense budgets in order to understand the total budgeting process. The key to revenue and expense budgeting is output; it is the predominant factor in determining the flow of funds into the organization and the amount of resources needed, that is, the outflow of funds. While many managers have no control over output or prices, each manager controls a set of resources and should understand how his or her resource allocations are affected by changes in output and total revenue. On the other hand, managers of revenue, profit, and investment centers need to estimate output, revenue, and expenses.

Output forecasts can be derived from quantitative or qualitative methods. Quantitative methods attempt to forecast output on the basis of history (how output has grown in the past, or what the average of past years is) or identify relationships between output and other variables. Qualitative forecasts have the advantage of being easy to prepare since they rely on the judgment and experience of the forecaster and must be used in the absence of historical data. Astute budget preparers evaluate forecasts to determine which have provided the most accurate estimates of demand, and adapt their techniques to improve future forecasts.

Revenue projections require an understanding of how revenue is generated: does the organization control price, and is revenue tied to output? If an organization can set prices, the prices set will be determined by the structure of the industry and the characteristics of the goods or services provided. Managers attempting to maximize revenues should consider how their customers and competitors might respond to price and output changes. Healthcare providers have the added challenge that prices do not often determine net revenue, so output must be projected by type of care and payer, since the same treatment is reimbursed at different rates by different third-party payers.

Knowing the expected demand for output in the budget year should enable managers to make better projections of expenses, and understanding revenue should inform and discipline their use of resources. Managers who recognize revenue constraints (and the relationship between prices and consumer purchases) should be more likely to internalize the goals of the organization and its customers and exert more control over their expenses compared to managers who disregard spending limits and believe they should be provided with more resources.

Key Terms and Concepts

Adjusted R^2 (coefficient of determination)	Independent variable	Price elasticity
Compound growth rate	Inelastic	Product life cycle
Damping factor	Intercept	Qualitative forecast
Delphi method	Law of demand	Quantitative forecast
Dependent variable	Marginal cost pricing	Regression
Durable goods, nondurable goods, and services	Monopolistic competition	Slope
Elastic	Monopoly	Structure–conduct–performance paradigm
Exponential smoothing	Moving average	Sunk cost
Full cost pricing	Oligopoly	Unitary elastic
	p-value	
	Perfect competition	

Discussion Questions

1. Explain why the output forecast is integral to the preparation of a budget.
2. What are the strengths and weakness of quantitative forecasting methods?
3. Describe the four phases of the product life cycle and their implications on output forecasts.
4. Explain the differences between an organization operating in a perfectly competitive industry and a monopolist.
5. Explain the factors that increase the price elasticity of a product.
6. Explain how charge, cost, per case, per diem, and capitation reimbursement affect a hospital's ability to control revenue.

Problems

1. Forecast the demand for dental services (data in Chapter04.xlsx, under the Figure 4.2 tab, line 33) for 2015 using (a) historical growth rates using 2000 as the base year, (b) exponential smoothing with α = 0.50, (c) a three-year moving average, and (d) an unweighted composite using (a)–(c).

2. Forecast the demand for hospital admissions (data in Chapter04.xlsx, under the Figure 4.3a tab) for 2015 using (a) historical growth rates using 2000 as the base year, (b) exponential smoothing with α = 0.20, (c) a three-year moving average, and (d) an unweighted composite using (a)–(c).

3. Use regression to determine how physician visits have changed with changes in population size, population age, and income between 1997 and 2011 (Chapter04.xls, under the problem 4.3 tab) and forecast physician visits for 2012 if population size, population age, and income are estimated to increase by 0.48%, 1.26%, and 0.96%, respectively, annually.

4. Calculate the revenue budget for the physician practice (Chapter04.xls, under the Table 4.8 tab) if the total patients seen is expected to increase by 5% and the intensity of care delivered to established patients is expected to increase, that is, shift by 100 from 99211 to 99214 and by 100 from 99212 to 99215.

5. A hospital admits 500 patients per month, who stay for an average of five (5.0) days per admission. It charges $12,000 per admission and incurs $7000 in costs ($4000 fixed and $3000 variable) per patient. First, assuming all patients are reimbursed under the same reimbursement method, complete the table and calculate net income for the hospital under each reimbursement method. Second, in the **Composite** column, calculate the hospital's expected net income, given the payer mix specified below (% of admissions). Assuming the per diem payer is offering a contract for the upcoming fiscal year that will pay $1200 per day, should the contract be accepted? Explain your answer.

80% of charges, 35% of admissions

Cost, 5% of admissions

Per diem, $1500 per day, 10% of admissions

Per case, use DRG payment calculated in #2.45% of admissions

PMPM, $200 capitation for 15,000 covered lives, 5% of admissions

6. Calculate the profit for a hospital (Chapter04.xls, under the Table 4.9 tab) if prices are increased by 5%, the AVC increases to $1450 per day, the average discount given to a percentage of charge-reimbursed payers increases to 25% and case-reimbursed patients increases to 57% of the patient mix, and cost-based patients fall to 13%.

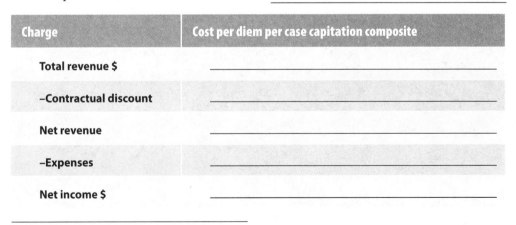

Charge	Cost	per diem	per case	capitation	composite
Total revenue $					
−Contractual discount					
Net revenue					
−Expenses					
Net income $					

References

Feldstein, P. J. (2005). *Health care economics* (6th ed.). Clifton Park, NY: Thomson Delmar Learning.

Popken, B. (2016). Is insulin the new EpiPen? Families facing sticker shock over 400 percent price hike. Retrieved November 4, 2016, from http://www.nbcnews.com/business/consumer/insulin-new-epipen-families-facing-sticker-shock-over-400-percent-n667536

Statisticbrain. (2016). Retrieved November 4, 2016, from http://www.statisticbrain.com/music-albums-sales-statistics

CHAPTER 5

Scratch Budgeting

CHAPTER OBJECTIVES

1. Explain the steps in assembling an expense budget.
2. Explain the structure and purpose of the chart of accounts.
3. Prepare an expense budget.
4. Assemble a master budget.
5. Discuss the actions that can be taken to increase net income.
6. Calculate the breakeven volume.

▶ Introduction

Businesses fail for many reasons. Two of the primary reasons are insufficient planning and insufficient capital. People starting a business often do not understand the amount of resources required to run a venture or the cost of resources. Statistics on business failures show that 36% of businesses fail before they are 2 years old and 50% fail within 4 years. Success is easier for healthcare and educational organizations, where 56% survive for more than 4 years (versus the average of 50% for all businesses), while information technology (IT) start-ups have the lowest survival rates, with only 37% surviving past 4 years (Statistic Brain, 2017). Planning and determining whether an organization has sufficient capital to survive are two of the primary goals of budgeting.

This chapter examines how expense budgets are constructed for a new enterprise. The chapter "Output Forecasts and Revenue Budgets" explored two important elements in the construction of the expense budget: output (what is to be produced) and revenue (a constraint on how much can be spent in producing the specified output). This chapter focuses on estimating what it should cost to produce a defined amount of output.

Starting a new endeavor presents numerous challenges; the budget preparer should account for all costs, but it is difficult to foresee everything needed in new ventures. Think of any activity you performed for the first time; once begun, it becomes generally apparent that you could have prepared and equipped yourself better for the task. In hindsight, we often catch ourselves saying, "I should have thought of that," but in fairness, not everything can be foreseen, for example, how much output will be demanded.

A start-up budget is simply a tool to reduce the margin of error, that is, establish a framework where major and minor expenses will be harder to overlook. Capital budgeting (Chapter 14), dealing with major investments to replace equipment or buildings or expand operations, faces the same challenge: what will be the total increase in expenses, and can these costs be recovered? The uncertainty facing a start-up is many times greater than that facing replacement or expansion decisions, as managers assessing these investments have prior information and knowledge to rely on. People starting new enterprises rarely have complete information, and many only have vague ideas of what resources are needed, how many of each are needed, and what they cost. This lack of knowledge and preparation contributes to low business survival rates.

Given the enormity of the challenge facing start-ups, it is useful to research similar operations, when available, to understand how they operate: how are they structured, what resources are consumed, and what results do they produce? There is a profound difference between scratch budgeting and the more common incremental budgeting (Chapter 6). In incremental budgeting, the budget preparer has historical information about the cost of resources consumed and the benefit of seeing how expenses and output have changed over time. For a new endeavor, the budget preparer is often given a blank sheet of paper and the task of estimating likely output, the type of and amount of resources needed to produce that output, and input prices. The goal is to budget just enough resources to accomplish the assigned job. Given the uncertain nature of demand and the production process to be employed, it is likely that the scratch budget will deviate from actual resource use and over- or understate expenses.

The goal of reviewing scratch budgeting is to demonstrate the fundamental relationships between inputs consumed and outputs produced:

how much output is expected, how will goods and services be produced, what resources will be needed, what quantities are need, and how much should they cost? These relationships are implicitly embedded or explicitly used in all budgeting systems, but nowhere is the incentive to be efficient greater than in a start-up budget. Given the unknowns facing a start-up, the budget preparer seeks to determine whether the venture is worth undertaking: will revenue exceed expenses? People starting new businesses have an incentive to not budget for unnecessary or nice-to-have items, because these costs may not be recoverable. Similarly, when new goods or services are planned, managers enter a realm paralleling scratch budgeting, where they cannot rely on past financial data and must identify cause-and-effect relationships and work with new resources.

Few managers will be called upon to construct an expense budget from scratch, so Chapter 6 focuses on the more common task of incremental budgeting. Incremental budgeting is simply the process of identifying what has been spent, augmenting those expenditures for expected increases in input prices, and adjusting them for any anticipated changes in output. Incremental budgets provide an incentive for featherbedding or nice-to-have items if revenues are sufficient to cover their expense. Even so, understanding scratch budgeting practices will illuminate the underlying relationships in existing budgets and provide a launching point for readers who may be asked to create a business plan for a new business line.

▶ Assembling an Expense Budget: Manufacturing Table Lamps

Assume you want to open a business producing high-quality wooden table lamps. You may be a master woodworker, but you probably lack extensive training in finance and budgeting, so you have two choices. The first is to simply start producing and selling table lamps, pay expenses as they arise, make sales when possible, and see what happens. The second is to build a budget outlining what you think will be needed in terms of resources and the sales you anticipate to cover your expenses. The prudent approach builds a financial plan before commitments are made, as blindly plunging in is risky and undesirable. A five-step budget process (**BOX 5.1**) is recommended in order to enhance your financial acumen and odds of success.

The first task in budget building is to decide what will be produced, that is, the type of goods or services needed or desired by customers or clients. What to produce is related to the type of customers the business wants to serve and the geographic area it plans to cover. Output should be defined in terms of the type of goods and services to be produced, including their attributes (size, appearance, functionality, quality, etc.). The more precisely output is specified, the more accurate the estimates of revenues and expenses, given the different prices the products may command in the marketplace and their different demands for inputs. After defining the type of outputs expected to be produced, the quantity of output expected in the budget period must be estimated (see Chapter 4). Assume your business will initially produce one output, wooden table lamps, and 5000 units can be sold in the next year.

The second task defines how each product will be produced, that is, how will the table lamps be constructed? What mix of inputs, labor, supplies, utilities, and capital is required to produce the specified products, and how much of each input is needed? Economics defines the relationship between inputs and output as a **production function**, i.e., output $(Y) = f$ (labor, supplies, energy, etc.). Products and services can be produced in a variety of ways, depending on the volume of output to be produced (individual, batch, mass, or

---

BOX 5.1 Steps to Construct an Expense Budget

1. Identify the type and quantity of expected output.
2. Select a production method and identify inputs needed.
3. Calculate the quantity of inputs needed to produce the desired output.
4. Identify input prices.
5. Multiply input quantities and their prices for each input and total for all inputs.

---

continuous), use of resources (capital versus labor-intensive production methods), and percentage of product produced versus purchased (self-contained start to finish or partial assembly). Will table lamps be produced individually, will components be produced in bulk and table lamps assembled later, or will an assembly line be utilized?

Capital-intensive production systems substitute machines for workers. The trade-off is that machinery is expensive and long lasting but may lower the average variable cost (AVC) versus labor, which is divisible, amendable, and assignable to other tasks and can be released as demand falls. In labor-intensive processes, managers may have to decide between employing higher-skilled and paid workers or lower productivity and paid workers. Products can be built from a variety of materials (metal, wood, or plastic), which will affect the product, production method, and cost. Consumer expectations and their willingness to pay will determine which materials are used. The Hershey Company provides an excellent example of input substitutability and production flexibility. The ingredient label on a Hershey's Milk Chocolate with Almonds bar specifies cocoa butter and/or sunflower oil to allow Hershey to shift ingredients as input prices change. If the price of cocoa butter increases or that of sunflower oil falls, the company can substitute sunflower oil to either prevent costs from rising or reduce costs and vice versa.

An example of a function that can be satisfied in different ways and at different costs is getting the product to the customer, that is, freight. Will the producer use air, water, rail, or road transport? Managers must weigh consumer expectations (how quickly buyers want a product) against the cost (how much more consumers are willing to pay to obtain a good or service a day earlier). Amazon.com pushes this decision to its customers by allowing them to select their shipping method and balance earlier delivery against a higher shipping cost. Two keys to success are flexibility to allow the production process to switch to the lowest-cost production method and incentives for those in the system, whether workers or customers, to use the highest-value methods.

The question of what inputs should be employed requires the budget preparer to specify what is needed (a task or a function) and how the resource will fulfill the task, that is, what role will each resource play in producing and delivering a product? Every organization needs various types of labor, including management, production, housekeeping, and maintenance. In small organizations, a single person can perform two or more functions, while in larger organizations, each function

may be specialized, and in mass production, every production task may be subspecialized. Organizations also need a variety of supplies to achieve their objectives, including office supplies to record transactions, pay invoices, pay salaries, and bill customers; production supplies to build the product; and housekeeping and maintenance supplies for the repair and cleaning of equipment and facilities. Additional expenses include the costs of acquiring, operating, and insuring facilities and equipment, such as rent, interest, utilities, and insurance.

The last paragraph hints at the enormity of the task facing the budget preparer: How will the budget preparer identify the various resources required to run a business? Once the expenses are identified, how will the budget preparer know whether too many resources are being consumed? Accounting assists with this task through the **chart of accounts**, a list of all items that result in the inflow or outflow of money. The chart of accounts (**TABLE 5.1**) provides detailed tracking of revenues and expenses as well as assets and liabilities.

The reader can see that a range of account numbers are assigned to various financial transactions, for example, 1000–1999 record transactions that increase or reduce assets. Total assets can be increased by revenue, account numbers 4000–4999 and acquiring liabilities, 2000–2999, and are reduced by

TABLE 5.1 Chart of Accounts

Account Numbers	Description
1000–1999	Assets
2000–2999	Liabilities
3000–3999	Equity
4000–4999	Expense
5000–5999	Revenue

expenses, 4000–4999 and paying down liabilities. Under double entry accounting, every transaction undertaken by an organization changes two accounts, sales increase cash or accounts receivable (debit) and equity (credit), the payment of employee salaries reduces cash (credit) and equity (debit). Double entry accounting balances debits and credits, recognizes transactions that increase and decrease the value of the organization, and facilitates the production of accurate accounting statements. **TABLE 5.2** provides further details; the chart of accounts provides the details necessary to build income statements and balance sheets examined in Chapter 2.

The purpose of the chart of accounts is to break financial transactions into homogenous categories for tracking and control. The accounting structure allows managers and employees to track expenses by line item to determine whether excess resources are being consumed. It does not matter whether the organization is a healthcare provider or an automobile manufacturer; managers should know whether labor costs are out of line with similar producers. If labor costs are excessive, is it because of too many managers or production personnel, too much overtime, and/or the use of temporary workers? Other costs should also be monitored. For example, hospitals should determine whether pharmaceutical use is excessive relative to the number of patients treated, while automakers want to know whether their use of steel is excessive relative to the number of cars produced. The chart of accounts allows managers to better understand their costs by tracing the costs to their source and purpose. **FIGURE 5.1**, a chart of accounts tree, provides a visualization.

Controlling costs requires managers to know the amount of each input needed to produce a product, that is, managers should be able to identify when excess resources are consumed and initiate action to reduce waste. Cost behavior and economies of scale were explored in Chapter 2 to illuminate the potential relationships between input use and expected output. When use of an input increases, should an

TABLE 5.2 Detailed Chart of Accounts			
Assets	Current assets	1010	Cash
		1020	Inventory
		1030	Accounts receivable
		1040	Prepaid expense
	Long-term assets	1200	Land
		1300	Equipment
		1350	Accumulated depreciation, equipment
		1400	Building
		1450	Accumulated depreciation, buildings

(continues)

TABLE 5.2 Detailed Chart of Accounts			*(continued)*
	Other assets	1800	Other
Liabilities	Current liabilities	2010	Accounts payable
		2020	Notes payable
		2030	Accrued wages
		2385	Current portion of long-term debt
	Long-term liabilities	2510	Long-term debt
Equity		3000	Owner's equity/fund balance
Expense accounts (check)		4010	Management (physician) salaries
		4015	Staff salaries
		4110	FICA
		4120	Health insurance
		4130	Retirement
		4140	Unemployment
		4150	Other fringe benefits
		4210	Clinical supplies
		4250	Office supplies
		4310	Rent
		4350	Repair and maintenance
		4410	Electricity
		4420	Gas
		4430	Water and sewage
		4440	Telephone

		4510	Insurance (malpractice, casualty, automobile, etc.)
		4610	Depreciation
		4710	Interest expense
		4810	Shipping and freight
		4910	Marketing expenses
		4920	Uniforms and laundry
		4930	Housekeeping
		4940	Travel, lodging, and meals
		4950	Education and training (CME)
		4960	Other expenses
Revenues		5010	Operating revenue
		5210	Non operating revenue

FICA, Federal Insurance Contributions Act; CME, continuing medical education

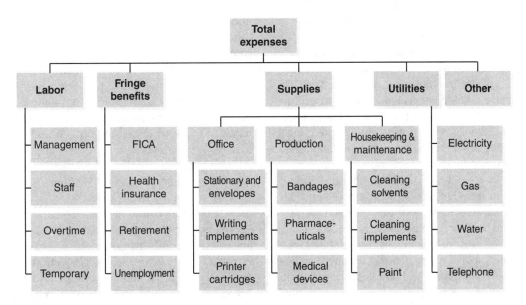

FIGURE 5.1 Chart of Accounts Tree

increase in output be expected, and if so, by how much should output rise?

For example, after basic managerial functions are met, increases in management staff should have no positive effect on output; of course, too many managers could have an adverse effect on production through excessive paperwork, slow decision-making and action, etc. Staff salaries should clearly be related to the amount of output produced: a productivity standard should be set that defines the amount of output expected when workers are properly utilized. A productivity standard requires defining how many minutes of labor are needed to produce one unit of output. After the standard is defined, managers can determine how many units of output can be produced by one worker and how many workers are required to produce the anticipated output. A wooden table lamp requires one and a half hours of labor (not including unnecessary work or idle time) to prepare wood, turn the base on a lathe (half hour—more later), finish the base, assemble the table lamp, wire it, and pack it for shipping. The total worker compensation is the sum of wages and fringe benefits, and fringe benefits depend on the number of employees (health insurance) or total salaries (social security taxes, retirement, and/or unemployment insurance).

Like labor, supply expenses should be determined by identifying the minimum number of resources required per unit of output. The budget should not plan for misuse, waste, obsolescence, or losses to theft. If you plan for waste, you probably will not be disappointed; waste will meet, if not, exceed your expectations. The planned table lamp will have a wooden base, $5'' \times 5'' \times 19.5''$, before turning, that is, each table lamp requires 7.9 board feet of lumber. In addition, a lighting kit (socket, electrical cord, and harp) and a lampshade are needed.

The third major input decision (after labor and supply requirements are defined) is, how much equipment and how big a space (square footage) are required to house the operation?

Equipment and facility costs should be determined by the expected output and be fixed in the short run. Managers should balance the ability to expand output if demand rises with the need to minimize under- or unused resources. Purchasing or leasing more space and equipment than are immediately needed makes it easy to expand output if demand should increase. On the other hand, if demand does not increase or falls below expectations, the organization may be saddled with significant expenses for unused resources for many years. When acquiring fixed resources, managers should consider the incremental costs of acquiring excess capacity now, the ability and cost of incrementally adding capacity in the future (is it cheaper to lease 20,000 square feet today or add on to buildings as the need arises?), and how quickly can demand be expected to grow (how long will excess capacity remain unused?).

Equipment and facility decisions determine the last major set of expenses: how much will utilities cost? Gas and electric costs will be determined by the need to heat and air-condition a fixed space, as well as the energy consumption of equipment. Water, sewage, and telephone expenses will be determined by the size of the facility, the type of production performed, and the number of employees.

The third task defines the total amount of variable inputs required: total labor hours and total supplies (inputs/output * total output) plus fixed resources. If each table lamp requires 1.5 labor hours and 5000 units are desired, 7500 productive hours are needed. Assuming each employee works 52 weeks per year, 40 hours per week, or 2080 hours, 3.61 workers will be needed. Given that few people actually work 8 hours a day, 5 days a week, 52 weeks per year, consideration must be made for nonproductive time due to breaks, vacation, and sick time. Productive effort in a normal 8-hour day should be no more than 7.5 hours after subtracting two 15-minute breaks; in addition, 4 weeks of productive time will be lost annually because of vacation and sick leave.

After adjusting for nonproductive hours, the maximum amount of productive effort in a year may be 1800 hours per worker; the organization will need 4.17 workers (7500/1800) instead of the 3.61 originally calculated. The 0.17 worker requirement can be met by hiring a fifth full-time employee, hiring a part-time employee, or paying overtime. A lighting kit and lampshade are required for each table lamp, so 5000 of each are necessary. The entrepreneur has located a 1600-square-foot building to house operations, and rent and utilities are based primarily on square footage. Equipment and tools will be needed, which will entail **depreciation**, rent, and repair and maintenance. Telephone and Internet service are needed to support communication, insurance to cover casualty losses, and an Others category for unforeseen expenses.

The fourth task is to determine input prices for each resource. What is the wage for each type of labor required? The entrepreneur budgets a salary of $50,000 and assumes that the production workers required all have similar skills. The prevailing wage rate is $30,000 per year per worker. If a part-time worker can be employed at the prevailing wage rate, the wage cost would be $125,000 (4.17 * $30,000). If overtime is used, the wage cost would increase to $127,650 ([4 * $30,000] + [0.17 * 1.5 * $30,000]), and if five full-time workers are hired, the wage cost would be $150,000 (5 * $30,000).

While wages are expected to be $175,000 ($50,000 management + $125,000 production), the **total compensation** will be higher because of fringe benefits. Budgeting for mandatory payroll expenses, such as social security and Medicare taxes (FICA, 7.65% of payroll) and unemployment insurance (1.1%), and optional expenditures for health insurance ($5,000 per employee) and retirement plans (5.0%) adds 28.3% to labor costs. The

"true" cost of employing production workers is $39,135 per year rather than $30,000.

A lighting kit can be purchased for $5.39 and lampshades for $14.40 at wholesale prices. The cost of the base will be determined by the wood used: if red oak is used, the cost is $2.50 a square foot versus $7.50 for mahogany. While the acquisition cost for supplies is straightforward, the price paid, one always needs to be cognizant of complementary costs, including transportation costs and storage costs. Many suppliers give volume discounts for bulk purchases, which could reduce acquisition costs but increase storage expenses, and thus the trade-off should be considered. In addition to production expenses, office supplies to support administration, billing, human resources, etc., add an additional $1.00 per unit.

For equipment and facilities, besides their acquisition costs, repairs, maintenance contracts, insurance, etc., must also be budgeted. If the buildings and equipment are purchased, the budget preparer must decide how they will be depreciated (straight line or accelerated). For example, if the building is purchased for $600,000, with an expected life of 20 years, straight-line depreciation allows $30,000 ($600,000/20 years) to be deducted from income to recognize the annual cost of using the resources. If the entrepreneur does not have $600,000 to invest, a second option would be to rent a furnished 1600-square-foot facility for $26 per square foot per year, that is, an annual rental cost of $41,600.

Equipment is purchased for $40,000 and depreciated over a 10-year life, resulting in an annual depreciation expense of $4000 per year. Repairs and maintenance are estimated at $1500, while utilities, telephone and Internet, and insurance are paid monthly. The last expense, Others, is for unforeseen events and is calculated as 2.5% of the total nonlabor expenses.

The final task is to calculate the total line item expense: multiply input quantities and input prices plus related costs. Actual expenses are generally higher than expected because of non obvious factors that increase the amount and price of resources needed, for example, nonproductive time and payroll taxes, which increase the total cost of hiring productive workers from $108,300 (3.61 workers at $30,000 per year) to $163,193 (4.17 workers at $39,135).

Methods of Estimating Expenses

There are four primary ways of estimating expenses: fixed, variable with output, variable with other inputs, and arbitrary (Mikesell, 1995, p. 115). Method 1, fixed expenses based on current market prices, involves costs that do not change with increases in output (or other inputs used); they are truly fixed costs. Market prices will vary, but once purchased, neither the price nor the amount of resources required should change. Examples include management salaries, rent, and insurance premiums.

Method 2, variable expense with output (or sales), involves costs that change directly with changes in output. These are resources like labor and supplies, where there is a one-to-one relationship with output. For example, when one more table lamp is produced, 1.50 hours of labor, 7.9 board feet of lumber, a lighting kit, and a lampshade are required. Of course, no additional labor may be required if the present complement of labor is not fully utilized, that is, full-time employees work for less than 7.5 hours per day. Bad debt or sales commissions are expenses that change with gross revenue; when 1.0% of sales is expected to be uncollectible, bad debt increases as the number of units sold or the price of output increases.

Method 3, variable expense with other inputs, is based on a constant relationship between inputs; it is a cost driven by the use of other inputs rather than by output. For example, FICA, retirement, and unemployment insurance expenses have a one-to-one relationship with payroll. For every additional dollar of salary paid, the organization owes 7.65 cents to the Social Security Administration. Similarly, organizations frequently contribute to employee retirement accounts as a percentage of their salary, and state unemployment taxes are calculated as a percentage of the total payroll. Payroll taxes and fringe benefits will be unaffected by changes in output if the current labor complement is not fully employed and total hours do not change. Administrative costs such as general management, human resources, and payroll expenses may be determined by the number of people employed rather than by output—the expenses of these functions are likely to be step costs. For example, an organization may assume that for every six or eight employees, one supervisor will be employed.

Arbitrary estimates are used when an expense cannot be related to other variables. Method 4 boils down to "pick a reasonable number," for example, equipment repairs may not be predictable, but something should be set aside for the contingency. An appropriate starting point is to research what similar organizations spend or budget for unpredictable expenses. In some instances, insurance may be available to deal with contingencies and, hence, convert a low-probability and high-cost outlay to a smaller, predictable periodic payment. In other cases, insurance may not be available or may be too expensive and managers may choose to self-insure. In businesses with a history, the arbitrary method may involve averaging past expenditures, but in new operations, there is no experience to rely on, although prudence dictates that a contingency fund be created. A fifth method is introduced and used in Chapter 6, which is based on past history; the budget estimate is calculated by adjusting the prior year's expenses for expected price increases. This method cannot be used in a new business that has no prior history or experience; a scratch budget will be based on the first four methods (**BOX 5.2**).

TABLE 5.3 shows the completed budget. The entrepreneur can now determine whether to set prices high enough to cover the costs. The scratch budget demonstrates that to recoup the estimated costs, table lamps must sell for at least $101.10 each if red oak is used. If table lamps are made of mahogany, the minimum price to break even goes up to $141.59. The entrepreneur should also factor into the output price the minimum rate of return expected for putting the resources at risk as well as inflation; a 10% mark-up is included in the table. Imagine if the entrepreneur thinks table lamps can be produced with $175,000 (after factoring in nonproductive time) allocated to productive labor and later realizes that $49,000 for fringe benefits was not factored in. Will the prices be high enough to pay the bills? Will the business survive?

An important point in the scratch budget is that it often records the minimum amount of resources needed, that is, the budget preparer expects one-to-one relationships between inputs and outputs. The assumption is that only one lighting assembly, one lampshade, and so on would be needed per table lamp. People starting a business typically do not plan for excessive amounts of waste. Crosby (1979, p. 38) estimated the cost of quality failures to be equal to 20% of sales in some organizations. According to the Institute of Medicine (IOM), in health care, it is common to hear that 30% of expenditures are due to waste (2013).

While some loss is unavoidable, it is inconceivable that an entrepreneur opening a business would plan for 20% waste; for example, our table lamp manufacturer would not expect to purchase 6000 lampshades to build 5000 table lamps. If inputs are consumed at a higher rate than expected, managers should investigate to determine the cause. Is output higher than

BOX 5.2 Building a Budget to Produce 5000 Table Lamps

1. Establish a target output: 5000 units.
2. Define budget standards (how to produce the output, what mix of inputs to use, etc.): Variable inputs are 1.5 labor hours, 1.0 table lamp hardware (socket, harp, and cord), 1.0 lampshade, and 7.9 board feet of wood per unit. Fixed resources, used in combination with the variable resources, are building, equipment, and utilities.
3. Calculate the total quantity of variable inputs required: Total person-hours (1.5 labor hours per unit * 5000 units/1800 productive hours per worker per year = 4.17 workers), 5000 hardware setups and lampshades, and 39,500 (7.9 * 5000) board feet of wood. Calculate the total amount of fixed inputs required: building (minimum square footage), the type and number of machines, the amount of insurance coverage, etc.
4. Determine the prices for each input: Variable inputs include $30,000 wages per year, and fringe benefits include 7.65% social security, health insurance ($5000) per worker, 5.0% retirement, and 1.1% unemployment compensation. Supplies include $5.39 for the lighting kit, $14.40 for lampshades, and $2.50, $4.50, or $7.50 per square foot for red oak, walnut, or mahogany, respectively. Fixed inputs are $26 per square foot for occupancy and 10% annual depreciation on machinery; occupancy and machinery costs depend on whether the building and equipment are purchased (depreciation) or rented (lease payments), plus repairs, maintenance contracts, etc.
5. Calculate total expenditures (input quantity × input prices). Staff salaries are 4.17 full-time employees * $30,000 = $125,000, while total compensation is 28.3% higher for fringe benefits. Total expenses = (Quantities of variable inputs × Prices of variable inputs) + Fixed expenses.

TABLE 5.3 Budget for 5000 Table Lamps

| Object Code | Step 2 | | | Step 3 | Step 4 | Step 5 |
	Type of Input	Productivity (Budget) Standard		Quantity	Input Price	Budget
4010	Management and clerical staff	1	per year	1.00	$50,000	$50,000
4020	Staff salaries and wages	1.5	Hours/ unit	4.17	$30,000	$125,000
4110	FICA	1	Salaries	$175,000	7.65%	$13,338
4120	Health insurance	1	per employee	5.17	$5,000	$25,833
4130	Retirement	1	Salaries	$175,000	5.00%	$8,750
4140	Unemployment	1	Salaries	$175,000	1.10%	$1,925
4210	Supplies					
4214	Socket, harp, and cord	1	per unit	5000	$5.39	$26,950
4216	Shade	1	per unit	5000	$14.40	$72,000
4222	Red oak	7.9	Board feet/unit	5000	$2.50	$98,750
4224	Walnut	7.9	Board feet/unit	0	$4.50	$0
4226	Mahogany	7.9	Board feet/unit	0	$7.50	$0
4250	Office supplies	1	per unit	5000	$1.00	$5,000
4310	Rent	1	Square feet/year	1600	$26	$41,600
4350	Repairs and maintenance	1	per year	1	$1,500	$1,500

4410	Electricity	1	per month	12	$180	$2,160
4420	Gas	1	per month	12	$150	$1,800
4430	Water and sewage	1	per month	12	$100	$1,200
4440	Telephone	2	per line/ month	24	$75	$1,800
4510	Insurance	1	per month	12	$200	$2,400
4610	Depreciation	1	per year	1	$4,000	$4,000
4810	Freight	1	per dozen units	417	$25	$10,417
4960	Other expenses (glue, stain, etc.)	1	Nonlabor expenses	$259,160	2.5%	$6,479
						$500,602

Step 1

Output	**Statistics**		5,000
	Cost per table lamp		$100.12
	Price (10% mark-up)		$110.13

expected, was the original budget (input quantities or prices) underestimated, or are resources being used inappropriately? Time will reveal actual losses, but managers should ensure that losses are kept to a minimum by acting in a timely manner when input use appears excessive. While the budget to produce 5000 table lamps demonstrated general concepts and processes, the next section moves on to a more practical healthcare application.

▶ **Estimating Expenses for a New Physician Practice**

Assume you have your medical license, have just completed your residency, and want to open your own practice. Where do you start? Throughout your residency, you were responsible for your patients' health, but you drew a paycheck every week. Now you are responsible for your patients' health as well as the livelihood of you, your family, and your employees. Running a business was not a class in medical school or in your undergraduate program, yet it is obvious that you need to generate sufficient patient revenues to cover your practice expenses, generate sufficient income to cover your living expenses, and save money for future large expenditures like purchasing a home, having children and sending them to college, and eventually retiring. In medical practice, the difference between practice revenues and expenses is the doctor's income. An independent physician is not guaranteed a salary but receives a residual income from his or her practice. Revenues above expenses increase the physician's income, while any shortfall reduces the income dollar for dollar.

When a new business is opened, the owners want to know whether the operation can be carried on profitably or whether revenues will cover costs. A physician could plunge in, open a practice without any planning, and hope for the best, but this would be imprudent. Healthcare businesses are the least likely to fail in their first 4 years, but a physician who commits himself or herself to high fixed costs for potentially underused building and equipment would increase the odds of failure.

In many cases, the "blindly plunging in" approach is not possible; the physician may require capital, and few people are willing to extent credit without a business plan (see the sidebar). A business plan and a budget are required to answer the question of whether a business can sustain itself. A budget is a monetary plan for a proposed business, defining the inflow and outflow of resources, how money will be raised and spent, and whether the business can be self-sustaining. Will the proposed venture generate sufficient revenue to cover expenditures? No organization can continue if its inflow is habitually less than its outflow. When expenses exceed revenue, an organization faces three options: increase inflow, reduce outflow, or cease to exist.

To avoid cutting costs or failing, the physician wants to know, before funds are committed (and potentially unrecoverable), whether the practice can generate sufficient revenues. A budget specifying what will be produced and sold and what the anticipated operating expenses are is required. Budgeting is a means to quantify and control risk—planning before committing resources and undertaking action.

The physician is targeting 90 patients per week. The average number of patients per week per physician is 107, so the physician sets the sights slightly lower (15.9%) to allow for gradual practice growth. The first and largest expense to estimate is wages and benefits. Our physician (the entrepreneur) may first set a desired target income. In 2016, the average salary for a physician in family medicine was $207,000 (Medscape, 2016), so the physician salary expense is set as $175,000—a fixed price (method 1), but in reality, it is a residual, the difference between practice revenues and expenses.

In addition to the physician, additional staff is needed; given 90 patients per week, the physician believes that all required medical support can be provided by a single resident nurse (RN) and office functions by a single receptionist/billing clerk. RN salaries average $58,240 ($28 per hour), and a receptionist earns $35,360 ($17 per hour), for a total of $93,600. These salaries are based on current market wages and are a fixed expense. Regardless of how many patients are seen, both individuals will work 40 hours per week and be paid for 52 weeks (Table 5.4).

While the salary expense is approaching $300,000, there are additional expenses directly related to payroll. The five major employment-related fringe benefits are FICA, health insurance, retirement, unemployment insurance, and tuition assistance.

While creating a scratch budget is rare, managers starting a new business line or students entering into consulting may be called on to create a business plan. A business plan is a detailed description of how managers expect the organization or program will meet its goals. A business plan is generally required in order to obtain funding and recruit talent. It provides goals, strategies, and resources and should be used to translate goals into actions, for example, how much sales by what date. Here are the typical elements included in a business plan:

Executive summary: A concise summary of what will be sold, where the organization has been and where managers expect it to go, how it will succeed, when mileposts will be reached, and what resources will be required to reach goals.

Company description: A history and position of the organization to date, including the business purpose and aims, products and services offered, management, and proprietary rights (Barrow, Barrow, & Brown, 2008, p. 2).

Market analysis: Specification of the current and expected market size, including expected units to be sold, prices, revenues, and market share. The market analysis should discuss obstacles to achieving sale projections, including expected responses of competitors.

Organization structure and management: A focus on who all are employed and what their roles, skills, and prior accomplishments are. The organizational structure should clarify who makes decisions and how quickly decisions can be made and implemented.

Service or product line: A definition of the product or service to be produced: what does it do for whom, why do customers purchase it, can it be used immediately, and does it require training and/or alteration in how the customer does things (Brooks & Stevens, 1987, p. 17)? Emphasis should be on distinguishing the organization's product(s) from the competitors'. For a product in development, the product stage should be identified: conceptual, conceptual testing, general design, detailed design, prototype, limited production, test marketing, or entering full production (Brooks & Stevens, 1987, p. 28). The discussion should also fully define the product(s) to be sold and, when multiple products are offered, the total sales expected from each line.

Marketing and sales: Specification of how the organization will reach and satisfy customers and a discussion of how competitors are expected to react.

Funding: A discussion of where existing funds were raised, how much additional funding is needed, and where it will be obtained.

Financial projections: Historical and pro-forma income statements, balance sheets, and cash flow statements, past and expected capital expenditures, and ratio analyses.

Business plans, like budgets, are a means to assess and control risk. As seen, the elements of finance and budgeting contribute two parts of the larger plan of how managers expect to succeed. The business plan should clarify in the minds of the writer(s) and readers of the plan that the organization has employees who are knowledgeable about the customers' desires, production processes, and potential competitors and who have the ability, drive, and resources to successfully produce and sell a product. People who understand the components of a business plan and can produce accordingly have a highly valued skill.

Estimation of these expenses is based on their relationship to other inputs (method 3). FICA is assessed against the employer and the employee; each party pays 6.2% of the first $113,700 in wages for retirement payments and 1.45% for Medicare applied to every dollar earned—no income limit (mandatory). The inclusion of this tax increases employee compensation by $16,704 (roughly half of what the practice will pay to employ the receptionist/billing clerk). The second mandatory tax is unemployment insurance levied by the state; in the state where the physician will be practicing, the tax is 1.1% of payroll—an additional $2955.

The remaining employee benefits, health insurance, retirement, and tuition assistance, are voluntary. Health insurance is market-priced (method 1) and varies with the type of plan, individual ($3000) or family ($6000), and the coverage (copayments and deductibles). Budgeting for family coverage for all three employees adds $18,000 to the budget. Retirement benefits are also voluntary, and the physician elects to contribute 5.0% of each employee's pay to a 401(k) plan (method 3). Retirement contributions provide employees with an opportunity to receive nontaxed, more appropriately delayed taxed, compensation, this compensation will be taxed when withdrawn after retirement. Finally, additional monies, $1500, will be allotted for tuition assistance; the physician wants to encourage lifelong learning but recognizes that free goods are overconsumed, another example of a moral hazard, and so intends to cover 75% of tuition assistance costs. The physician does not know whether either of the to-be-hired employees will be interested in continuing their education, so the budget amount is arbitrary (method 4). Next year, the physician will have a better idea of whether this amount was too little or too much when actual expenditures are reviewed.

The total benefits add up to $53,059, or 19.75% of wages. A common error of new businesses is to fail to consider the impact of fringe benefits; similarly, employees often fail to consider how fringe benefits increase their total compensation. It is easy to see what is in your paycheck, gross and net pay, but the necessity of paying FICA taxes as well as providing health insurance and retirement adds substantially to the cost of employing a worker; the failure to include the expense of fringe benefits will severely understate cash outflows during the budget year.

The second set of expenses, supplies, is directly related to output (method 2). The number of patients seen will determine both clinical and office supply use. Each patient may result in the use of gloves, tongue depressors, examination gowns, etc., for an average cost of $5.50 per patient for medical supplies. Similarly, medical records must be compiled and bills prepared and sent for services performed. Creating files, billing, and postage are estimated to cost $2.00 per patient visit. These two line items add $23,760 and $8640 to expenses—a variable cost. In addition to the variable cost associated with documenting treatment and billing, $600 a month is needed for electronic medical record (EMR)/billing software (subsumed in 4310).

The third set of expenses, rent (or occupancy), is market-priced (method 1). Rent is variable and is based on the size of the space rented and the amenities offered. Rent depends on location, square footage rented, amenities provided (lobby, parking, landscaping, etc.), and the age of the building. Our physician has located a medical office building renting suites for $1500 per month, a fixed cost. While the rent seems high, the building is part of a medical campus with convenient access to a hospital and an opportunity to expand the practice without moving. Rent covers external repairs but does not cover internal renovations, so the physician decides to set aside $4000 just in case (method 4).

Utilities are not covered in rent, so additional monies must be allocated for electricity, gas, water, and telephone. Electricity and gas expenses are related to the size of the space to be lit, heated, and cooled; the desired illumination or temperature; and the duration the space will be lit or heated (office hours?). On the basis of the size of the office, and assuming lighting and heating/cooling will be active from 8:00 A.M. through 6:00 P.M., Monday through Friday, the physician expects to spend $200 per month for each, a fixed cost (method 3). Water for washing hands after each patient, drinking, housekeeping, and toilet functions is estimated at $100 per month. Telephone, paging, and off-hour answering are determined by features desired and are market-priced (method 1). The physician expects the monthly telephone bill to run to about $80 per month and has received a 2-year quote for answering and paging services at $100 per month.

Malpractice insurance varies by specialty and region; the physician receives a quote for 1 year at $8000, with a $2 million coverage per event and $25,000 deductible. The physician estimates having to purchase $40,000 in medical equipment and office furnishings; the Internal Revenue Service (IRS) allows a business to write off a portion of the investment as expense each year. Using straight-line depreciation and assuming a 10-year life, the physician can deduct $4000 per year (noncash expense but recoupment of capital outlay). The bank that loaned the $40,000 charges a 5.0% interest, so an additional $2000 will be expended for interest expense. On the basis of discussions with other doctors, our physician estimates that 1.0% of gross revenue will not be collected and will be lost to bad debt. Other miscellaneous expenses for marketing, uniforms and laundry for the physician/RN, housekeeping, travel/professional meetings/meals, and CME/licensure/dues are estimated at $23,640. In addition, the physician has been advised to plan for the unexpected, for example, garbage collection is included in rent, but medical waste disposal is not. The budget cushion is calculated as 2.19% of total expenses.

▶ The Master Budget

A scratch budget provides an opportunity to see the entire budget system at work: are revenues greater than, less than, or equal to planned expenditures? A poor budgeting process, one that overestimates output and revenue and/or underestimates cost, may have an enormous impact on an organization. On the basis of our young physician's assumptions, the practice will see 90 patients per week (versus the national average of 107) in the first year, with an average reimbursement of $87.10 per patient (average relative value units (RVU) 2.56 * $34.023 conversion factor) multiplied by 48 weeks a year, so the total revenue will be $376,267.

TABLE 5.4 demonstrates that if the operating assumptions are realized, the practice will lose $65,284. Since this is a sole proprietorship, the loss will reduce the physician's income to $109,716 ($175,000 – $65,284) and could cripple the long-term viability of the practice. The options facing the physician are to increase patient volume, increase revenue, reduce expenses, and/or accept a lower income.

Improving Net Income

The first option to increase net income is to raise prices. As long as price elasticity is less than 1.0, the percentage increase in price exceeds the percentage decrease in output sold, revenue will increase, and expenses should be unchanged. Opportunities for increasing revenue may be severely limited, given the physician's patient mix. First, raising the price may have little impact if the majority of patients are reimbursed by Medicare, Medicaid, or managed care payers. So the physician decides that increasing price is *not* a viable option to reduce the gap between revenues and expenses. A second option is to provide more comprehensive care, which requires more thorough examinations and more tests. While this could increase revenue, it could also reduce the number of patients that can be seen in a day as each patient takes more time. A second consideration that must be recognized is that the service provided must be medically necessary; providing unnecessary care can run afoul of fraud and abuse statutes.

The limited latitude of increasing revenue leaves two options: the first is to increase output, and the second is to reduce expenses. Increasing the number of patients seen can be accomplished by working for more weeks and/or extending practice hours. Increasing

TABLE 5.4 Master Budget for the Physician Practice

Code	Description	Productivity (Budget) Standard	Budget
Object			
4010	Management and clerical staff	$175,000	$175,000
4020	Staff salaries and wages	$56,000 RN + $34,000 reception/billing	$93,600
4110	FICA	6.2% of $113,000 + 1.45% unlimited	$16,704
4120	Health insurance	$6,000 per employee	$18,000
4130	Retirement	5% of wages	$13,430
4140	Unemployment	1.1% of wages	$1,925
4140	Tuition reimbursement	$1,500/employee	$3,000
4210	Clinical supplies	$5.50 per patient	$23,760
4250	Office supplies	$2.00 per patient	$8,640
4310	Rent	$1,500 per month + $600 IT	$25,200
4350	Repairs and maintenance	$4,000	$4,000
4410	Electricity	$200 per square foot	$2,400
4420	Gas	$200 per square foot	$2,400
4430	Water and sewage	$100 per month	$1,200

4440	Telephone	$180 per month	$2,160
4510	Malpractice insurance	$8,000	$8,000
4610	Depreciation	10% of investment, $40,000	$4,000
4710	Interest expense	5% of $40,000	$2,000
4810	Bad debt	1% of gross charges	$3,763
4910	Marketing	$100 per month	$1,200
4920	Uniforms and laundry	$8 * 2 * 48 * 5	$3,840
4930	Housekeeping	$50 * 48 * 5	$12,000
4940	Travel/professional meetings/meals	$5,000	$5,000
4950	CME	$1,000 per year	$1,000
4960	Other expenses	2.16%	$9,330
	Total expenses		$441,552
	Statistics	90 patient visits per week * 48 weeks	$4,320
	Revenue	2.56 * $34.023 * 4,320	$376,267
	Profit		−$65,284

the weeks worked per year by one (from 48 to 49 weeks), given the assumption that 90 patients are seen in a week, will increase revenue by $7839 (90 patients * $87.10), while the total expense will only increase by $770 (mainly because of supplies, $7.50 per visit). Increasing patient visits to improve income highlights the need to understand fixed and variable costs; the majority of the physician's costs are fixed, and a change in the number of patients seen has a large impact on revenue and a small impact on total expenses. Adding an additional week of work to the year is only

expected to reduce the practice loss by $7069, so the physician may seek other options to increase revenue or decrease expenses. Note that adding a week also increases the expected hours of work for employees by one; instead of planning 4 weeks for vacation and sick time, the budget now expects 49 weeks of work.

The second means to attract more patients is to extend practice hours. Extending office hours to 7:00 P.M. or 8:00 P.M. (adding two to three hours per day) or working on Saturdays or Sundays (8 hours per week) would provide greater access to working people and may increase patient volume. Given that staff salaries were based on a 40-hour week for the RN and the receptionist, extended hours will require paying overtime to these staff members or hiring part-time personnel. An additional hour per day across 48 weeks would provide an opportunity to see 240 additional patients per year. Two more patients per day would increase revenue by $174, but overtime would add $67.50 ($42.00 for the RN and $25.50 for the receptionist) to wages (not including the additional FICA or unemployment taxes that must be paid), and additional clinical and office supplies would add another $15.00 in expenses. The net per day income would be $91.50, or $21,960 per year. Given the logistical problems, the physician does not believe that adding an additional hour per day is desirable; however; the physician is contemplating extending office hours one day a week to 8:00 P.M. to accommodate working patients. The potential impact would be an additional 6 patients and $522.60 (6 ∗ $87.10) in revenue per week; the total compensation to employees will increase by $230.34, including fringe benefits, and supply expenses will increase by $45.00. The annual impact of this change will be $11,839 (48 ∗ ($522.60 − 275.34)).

The third option is to reduce expenses, and a quick review of the budget shows that the three largest expenses are staff salaries, clinical supplies, and rent. Reducing any of these is fraught with risk. Reducing wages (and the associated payroll-related fringe benefits) may hamper the physician's ability to attract and retain competent staff. Reducing clinical supplies may not be possible without jeopardizing patient safety (some providers have reused disposable medical supplies). Moving to a lower-cost and less desirable location (or reducing marketing expenses) could have an adverse impact on the physician's ability to attract patients. Like increasing revenue, there appears to be little opportunity to reduce expenses.

The fourth option, accepting a lower income in the short run, appears to be the most likely one. If nothing is done, the physician could accept a first-year income of $109,716 and hope that future increases in patient visits and reimbursement will move the income toward the average income for a family practitioner.

In the end, the physician may have to adopt more than one option; working 49 weeks versus 48 may decrease the loss by $7839, and working an additional 3 hours one day a week would reduce the loss by another $11,839 (48 weeks). While the major expenses are sacrosanct, marginal reductions could be achieved by reducing the retirement contribution by 1.0% ($2686), eliminating tuition assistance ($3000), and cutting travel by half ($2500) for a total expense reduction of $8186. In the first year, our physician may have to accept an income of $137,580 ($175,000 − $37,420 practice loss) and a below-average income in subsequent years while patient volume is built.

The chief problem in producing a good or service for the first time is that it is next to impossible to anticipate all the events that might arise and the resources required to handle them; it should be expected that the scratch budget will be incomplete. Investing more time and effort to accurately determine expenses is worth the effort, considering the impact that overlooked or underestimated expenses will have on the organization's chance of success. Fortunately, few people are called on to prepare a scratch budget; most managers will have the benefit of prior operation, and estimates of future output, revenues, and expenses are easier to generate when they can be projected from past performance.

The prior example used all four methods of estimating expenses to construct a budget: fixed expenditure based on market prices for resources that do change with output, resources that vary directly with output, expenses that vary directly with other inputs, and arbitrary or best-guesses. When expenses are related to output, an incentive to overestimate and overproduce is created to obtain higher funding. When budgets are determined by output, it is important to determine whether output can be controlled by the budget manager, and if so, a system should be instituted to ensure output is not manipulated (Barnum, 1995, p. 28). Goods or services that are not wanted or cannot be sold should not be produced; resources are squandered when the value of output is lower than the inputs consumed to produce it.

When expenses are determined by the use of other inputs, that is, workforce ratios or the number of beds, an incentive is created to overuse these inputs. This could lead to excessive expenditures for labor or overinvestment in capital. The effective use of resources requires that systems be in place to monitor and prevent excess and unnecessary investment in labor or capital (Barnum, 1995, p. 28).

The budget for the physician practice highlights the main benefits of a budget. Budgeting requires an understanding of what it takes to produce a good or service, presents a picture of where the organization will stand at the end of the fiscal year if budget assumptions are met, and provides an opportunity to enhance financial performance by modifying the operating plan before anticipatable problems are encountered. In this case, the physician has an opportunity to increase effort and accept a lower lifestyle before more dramatic changes are forced upon the practice. Obviously, after operating for 6 months or more, our physician will have a better idea of where the practice is heading and may find that more adjustments are needed if the gap between revenues and expenses is greater than anticipated or some of the economies made are not needed, that is, another week can be taken off or more can be contributed to retirement accounts.

▶ Breakeven Analysis

The physician practice budget demonstrates a point: start-up organizations often face a difficult beginning. Breakeven analysis provides a tool to estimate the output required to cover expenses on the basis of the price charged for

the output, the AVC, and total fixed cost (TFC). The primary challenge in utilizing breakeven analysis is the delineation of fixed and variable costs. Equation 5.1 shows that fixed costs are the numerator and price less AVC, that is, the **contribution margin**, is the denominator in the breakeven formula. The contribution margin indicates how much each unit sold contributes toward paying off fixed costs, so the formula calculates the number of units that must be sold to recoup all fixed costs. After fixed costs are met, any additional units sold increase profit by the amount of the contribution margin.

$$\text{Breakeven} = \text{Total fixed cost}/(\text{Price} - \text{Average variable cost}) \quad (5.1)$$

In the table lamp example, the expense budget was constructed assuming that staff salaries and associated fringe benefits (4020 and 4110–4140), supplies (4214–4250), and freight (4810) were variable costs—costs that increase with each unit of output produced. Total variable costs were $375,690, or $75.14 per unit, when 5000 units are produced. The fixed cost is determined by subtracting the total variable cost from the total cost, or $124,709 ($500,399 – $375,690). The breakeven point shows how many units must be sold at a price of $110.13, providing a contribution margin of $34.99 per unit, to recover $124,709 in fixed costs.

$$\text{Breakeven}_{\text{Lamps}} = \$124,709/(\$110.13 - \$75.14)$$
$$= 3564 \text{ units}$$

The table lamp manufacturer must sell 3564 table lamps to recover all costs. **FIGURE 5.2** demonstrates that after the breakeven volume is achieved, each additional table lamp sold increases profit by $34.99. Similarly, the manufacturer will lose $34.99 for every unit it falls short of 3564 (Figure 5.2).

Assume that the table lamp manufacturer decides that once an employee is hired, he or she will not be laid off if the expected volume of sales does not materialize. This type

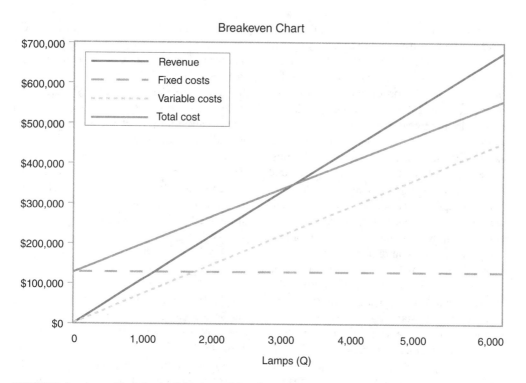

FIGURE 5.2 Breakeven Chart for the Table Lamp Manufacturer

of business practice is designed to retain good employees, and thus staff salaries and related fringe benefits become fixed costs. This business policy more than doubles fixed costs and reduces the AVC by more than $30.00.

$$\text{Breakeven}'_{\text{Lamps}} = \$287,480/(\$110.13 - \$42.58)$$
$$= 4256 \text{ units}$$

Under the no-layoff policy, the organization will have to sell 4256 units to break even or another 692 table lamps to pay all workers their entire salaries and benefits for the year. This more severe analysis should be reassuring to the manufacturer as the 5000-unit forecast can be off by 14.9% ((4256−5000)/5000) and the organization will still be able to pay employees and cover the other fixed expenses. In the physician practice example, the only two expenses that were calculated on the basis of the number of patient visits were clinical and office supplies (4210 and 4250). The breakeven point is 107.1 patient visits per week, assuming

an average level of treatment is provided and 48 weeks are worked per year.

$$\text{Breakeven} = \$409,152/(\$87.10 - \$7.50)$$
$$= 5140 \text{ visits}/48 \text{ weeks}$$
$$= 107.1 \text{ per week}$$

As discussed, the true variable expense is the physician's salary since the physician is the residual claimant on the practice income, he or she will want to understand how the practice operates and how many patients are needed to fulfill their income goals. Breakeven analysis based on accurate budget information lets business managers know what they must achieve to be successful.

Choices, Choices, Choices

One of the jobs of a manager is to decide how output will be produced and what the mix of labor and capital should be. **Operating leverage** measures the extent to which fixed costs are used to produce output. For example, our physician could enter into a long-term fixed contract for computer support or decide to purchase computer support as needed. In the first case, the fixed expense is predictable, and in the second case, although it would be beneficial if no support is needed, the physician will probably pay more for computer support on an as-needed basis. The operating leverage decision is typically envisioned as balancing the cost of workers who can be added or reduced at will against purchasing high-cost equipment that cannot be easily downsized when output falls. While manual methods may be more expensive on a per unit basis than highly automated processes, the uncertainty or variability in demand may favor the higher-per-unit-cost process over the high fixed but potentially lower per unit cost of capital-intensive processes.

Besides labor/capital substitutions, managers have other choices in their use of inputs; they can decide to rent buildings and equipment versus owning or to purchase goods and services versus producing them in-house (e.g., components or housekeeping), which changes the composition of fixed and variable costs. Employing capital versus relying on labor, owning versus renting, and producing versus purchasing increase fixed costs and reduce the manager's ability to balance revenues and expenses. On the other hand, the manager's flexibility is enhanced by relying on labor, rented resources, and outsourcing, which can be reduced or discontinued when demand for output falls.

The choice facing managers is to use resources whose costs can be avoided if estimated output does not materialize versus fixed resources that may lower the average total cost but whose expenses must be paid regardless of output. For example, in the table lamp example, turning the table lamp bases was estimated to require 0.5 person-hours. Assume a computerized lathe can be purchased that will increase the annual fixed costs by $30,000 per year and reduce the time to turn a table lamp base to 10 minutes, saving 20 minutes per table lamp and 1666.5 total person-hours if 5000 table lamps are produced. The AVC would decrease by

$6.27 (−1/3 hour ∗ $18.81 total compensation per hour), and the total compensation would fall by $31,355 per year if 5000 units are produced. The increase in the TFC is less than the reduction in the total variable cost, so total and average total costs decrease. The trade-off, as seen here, is that the breakeven point increases.

$$\text{Breakeven}_{\text{Lamps}} = \$124{,}709/\ (\$110.13 - \$75.14)$$
$$= 3564 \text{ units}$$
$$\text{Breakeven}_{\text{Capital intensive}} = \$154{,}709/(\$110.13$$
$$- \$68.87) = 3750 \text{ units}$$

The choice the entrepreneur must make is to accept more risk due to higher fixed costs in return for lower average total costs. The key issue is the degree of confidence the entrepreneur has in the demand forecast. If 5000 units are probable, increasing fixed costs will increase profit; if less than 4785 units can be sold, the entrepreneur would want to rely on labor. The formula given shows the volume where each production method has equivalent total costs; above this quantity, the capital-intensive production method will be cheaper because of the lower AVC, and below this point, the labor-intensive method will be cheaper because of the lower fixed costs.

$$\text{Breakeven} = \$154{,}709 + \$68.87Q$$
$$= \$124{,}709 + \$75.14Q$$
$$\text{Breakeven} = \$30{,}000 = \$6.27Q$$
$$\text{Breakeven} = 4785 = Q$$

A second way of analyzing the capital/labor choice is to examine the variables that change, that is, marginal analysis. The fixed cost increased by $30,000, and the AVC decreased by $6.27, so $30,000/$6.27 = 4785 units. Marginal analysis again shows that the critical output is 4785 units. Above this quantity, it pays to make a higher investment in equipment; if output is likely to be less than 4785 units, it behooves the organization to use the labor-intensive production method. The entrepreneur/manager should also think about future sales growth; although current sales may not warrant investment in fixed resources, how soon will sales grow to justify higher fixed expenses?

Summary

This chapter demonstrates how an expense budget is created for a new venture. The critical insight needed in budget construction is the relationship between inputs and output. What resources will be needed to run an operation, and how will output change if more or less inputs are used? In this chapter, the emphasis lies on efficiency—determining the minimum amount of resources that can be used to produce a given amount of output. The starting of a new business may be the only time managers truly consider minimum requirements; in successful organizations, expenses are often determined by revenue availability rather than necessity, that is, outlays are based on what can be afforded versus what costs could be.

The chapter constructs a master budget, combining expense estimates with expected revenues to assess where an organization will be at the end of its budget year. If revenues exceed expenses and provide an adequate rate of return, then the budget should be implemented. If revenues are expected to be substantially lower than expenses, owners/managers have an opportunity to reassess operations before resources are committed. The physician in the second example has an opportunity to reconsider hours of operation, prices, and expenses to determine whether revenue can be increased and/or costs decreased to narrow the gap between revenue and expenses.

Breakeven analysis is introduced to assess the uncertainties surrounding starting of a new business. Breakeven analysis determines how many units of output must be sold to recover all costs and allows managers to assess how much difference between expected sales and actual sales can arise before losses are incurred. The next chapter, "Incremental Budgeting," is built on learning by doing: what does management learn from past performance, and how should it change operations to improve financial results? Unlike scratch budgets, incremental budgets are often used to maximize resource allocation rather than seek efficiency. Where scratch budgeting often strives for optimal use of resources, incremental budgeting regularly settles for the status quo and maximizing budgets.

Key Terms and Concepts

Breakeven analysis	Contribution margin	Operating leverage
Business plan	Depreciation	Production function
Chart of accounts	Featherbedding	Total compensation

Discussion Questions

1. Explain the difference between wages and total compensation.
2. Explain the purpose of the chart of accounts.
3. Discuss the four main methods of estimating expenses.
4. The master budget predicts expenses exceed revenues. What actions can be taken to improve net income?
5. What are the three variables in the breakeven formula, and what is the purpose of breakeven analysis?

Problems

1. A physician is considering opening a home health agency to serve patients and others in the community. The physician read that in 2018, the home health industry is expected to earn $5.0 billion on $83 billion in revenue. Create a scratch budget for the physician on the basis of the assumptions given. How is the agency expected to perform relative to the industry?

Total visits: 12,000

Reimbursement per visit: $75

Management and support salaries: $120,000

Staff productivity: 2000 patients per year (8 patients/day * 5 days/week * 50 weeks/year)

Staff wages: $30 per hour for 2080 hours per year

FICA: 7.65% of the total salary

Health insurance: $500 per month per employee

Retirement: 5% of the total salary

Supplies: $7.50 per visit

Travel: 10 miles per visit @ 50¢ per mile

Rent: $2000 per month

Insurance: $1000 per month

Utilities: $24,500

Other: 2% of nonsalary and fringe benefit expenses

Total revenue: $_____

Management and clerical salaries: $_____

Staff salaries: $_____

FICA: $_____

Health insurance: $_____

Retirement: $_____

Supplies: $_____

Travel: $_____

Rent: $_____

Insurance: $_____

Utilities: $_____

Miscellaneous expenses: $_____

Total expenses: $_____

Profit: $_____

Margin: _____%

2. Assume that in problem 1, all costs are fixed except staff salaries, FICA, and retirement, supplies, and travel. Calculate the breakeven quantity.

3. Assume that in problem 1, all costs are fixed except for supplies and travel. Calculate the breakeven point.

4. Estimate your personal revenues and expenditures for the current year. If you do not want to divulge your income, use the $$$ column to complete the % Total Income column and leave $$$ blank.

$$$	% Total Income	
Wages (operating income):	$_____	_____%
Other income (non operating income):	_____	_____%
Total income:	$_____	_____%
Federal income tax:	$_____	_____%
FICA:	_____	_____%
State income tax:	_____	_____%
Sales and property taxes:	_____	_____%

(continues)

$$$	% Total Income _(continued)_
Disposable income (total income):	$_____ _____%
Rent/mortgage:	$_____ _____%
Food (nondurable goods):	_____ _____%
Clothing:	_____ _____%
Telephone:	_____ _____%
Electricity/gas/water:	_____ _____%
Travel expenses, gasoline:	_____ _____%
Entertainment (services):	_____ _____%
Health care:	_____ _____%
Education:	_____ _____%
Furniture, computers (durable goods):	_____ _____%
Pets:	_____ _____%
Total expenses:	$_____ _____%

References

Barnum, H., Kutzin, J., & Saxenian, H. (1995). Incentives and provider payment methods. _International Journal of Health Planning and Management, 10_, 23–45.

Barrow, C., Barrow, P., & Brown, R. (2008). _The business plan workbook_ (6th ed.). Philadelphia, PA: Kogan Page.

Brooks, J. K., & Stevens, B. A. (1987). _How to write a successful business plan_. New York, NY: AMACON.

Crosby, P. (1979). _Quality is free_. New York, NY: McGraw-Hill Book.

Institute of Medicine, Committee on the Learning Health Care System in America. (2013). _Best care at lower cost: The path to continuously learning health care in America_. Washington, DC: National Academies Press.

Medscape. (2016). _Medscape physician compensation report 2016_. Retrieved May 22, 2017, from http://www.medscape.com/features/slideshow/compensation/2016/public/overview#page=2)

Mikesell, J. (1995). _Fiscal administration_ (4th ed.). Belmont, CA: Wadsworth.

Statistic Brain. (2017). _Startup business failure rate by industry_. Retrieved September 22, 2015, from http://www.statisticbrain.com/startup-failure-by-industry

CHAPTER 6

Incremental Budgeting

CHAPTER OBJECTIVES

1. Explain the steps in building an incremental budget.
2. Construct an incremental budget.
3. Describe budget choices, trade-offs, and objectives.
4. Discuss the presubmission review process.
5. Evaluate the strengths and weakness of incremental budgeting.

▶ Introduction

Unlike a scratch budget, where the primary challenge is completeness (does the budget capture all the expenses required to run an operation?), the starting point for an incremental budget is typically current year-to-date (YTD) expenses. Current expenditures provide a comprehensive list of what resources will be needed during the budget year but not the total amount that will be spent in the current year or budget year. Budget preparers face three challenges: (1) estimating the total current year expenses on less than 12 months of data, (2) accounting for changes in the prices of currently used resources in the budget year, and (3) incorporating changes in output or the emergence of new expenses.

Managers typically inherit an operation and its budget from others. A manager may have moved up through the department and may understand the parts of the operation he or she has worked in, or the manager may be brought in from outside and may be unfamiliar with the organization, the department's production process, and/or its budgeting system. In either case, a person inheriting an operation will be unlikely to fully understand all its aspects: what it produces, how inputs are transformed into outputs, and how money has been spent. This problem increases with the size and complexity of the operation; nevertheless, managers are required to prepare the succeeding year's budget.

A good place to begin building a budget is with either current YTD expenditures or the current year budget. The advantage of using the current year budget is that it provides an estimate of the total expected annual cost, while YTD expenditures provide a partial-year total for actual spending. The advantage of using YTD expenditures is that they report actual prices versus budget estimates and capture all changes that were not anticipated in the budget. The problem with both expenditure bases is that they provide an accounting of what *was* spent or anticipated to be spent rather than what *should* be spent.

Both are a record of a production method and resource use, but history does not tell us whether the operation was effective or efficient. Where scratch budgets often overlook costs and understate expenses, incremental (a.k.a. fixed or static) budgets tend to overestimate necessary expenses by incorporating waste into budget allocations. Over time, inefficiencies and waste often grow in organizations. Lean Six Sigma identifies eight types of waste: overproduction, overprocessing, wasted motion, defects, excessive transport, underutilized resources, idle resources, and excessive inventory. Waste becomes accepted practice, increases costs, and lowers output. Managers should be able to identify and reduce waste wherever it emanates, and budgets should assist them in this task.

Prior spending may or may not provide a sound basis for building a tight budget that provides the appropriate level of resources for the output produced, but it does provide a starting point for constructing an achievable budget. At the end of a budget period, the primary question is, are expenses less than, equal to, or greater than the allocated amount? **FIGURE 6.1** highlights an incremental budget's focus on the entry of inputs into a production system and goal of ensuring budgeted expenses are not exceeded.

Incremental budgets are most appropriate when output and revenue projections are relatively certain, that is, the type and quantity of output expected and money flowing into the organization have been and will continue to be stable. Incremental budgeting should be used in environments where there is little chance of dramatic swings in the demand for goods and services and risk that costs may not be recovered. Managers should be capable of producing accurate estimates of future expenses for a known quantity of output within a known budget constraint. The idealistic goal of budgeting to produce the desired outputs at minimum cost, however, receives scant encouragement as inefficiencies may have built up over time in existing systems and obfuscated the link between actual and necessary expenses. Compounding the tendency toward larger-than-necessary budgets is department managers' interest in maximizing the size of their budgets. Operations are easier to manage when employees have more resources than they need and more challenging when working at the bare minimum, where any slippage in performance or disruption could have a noticeable impact on output and cost.

Few managers are asked to construct an expense budget from scratch, so the majority of the time devoted to building a budget is spent adapting prior financial data to future operating plans. Incremental budgeting is primarily a process of identifying what has been

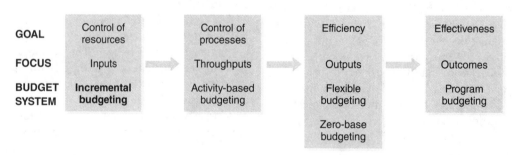

GOAL	Control of resources	Control of processes	Efficiency	Effectiveness
FOCUS	Inputs	Throughputs	Outputs	Outcomes
BUDGET SYSTEM	**Incremental budgeting**	Activity-based budgeting	Flexible budgeting	Program budgeting
			Zero-base budgeting	

FIGURE 6.1 Budgeting Systems

spent (or planned to be spent) and augmenting those expenditures for anticipated price increases.

▶ The Incremental Budgeting Process

Incremental budgeting is a process of identifying an expenditure base and increasing it for anticipated price increases rather than attempting to understand how money was spent or what the relationship is between inputs used and outputs produced (as done in scratch budgeting). If $100,000 is projected to be spent in the current year or was estimated in the budget, a manager may simply request $103,000 for the budget year, assuming that all past expenditures were necessary and will continue to be important and that input prices will increase by 3.0% in the following year.

Incremental budgets can be produced in four steps (**BOX 6.1**). First, determine an expenditure base; this is what was spent in prior periods or budgeted and should be the starting point for the following year's budget. Preparations for the following year's budget generally begin midway through the current operating year, thus creating three choices for the budget base: current YTD expenditures, the current full-year budget, or the last full-year expenditures. When the last full-year data is used as the base, it must be increased for two years

of input price increases. Assuming the 2018 budget is under construction, the last complete year is 2016 and must be increased for 2017 price increases and again for anticipated increases in the 2018 budget year. When YTD expenditures are used, current spending must be annualized to obtain a full-year estimate and increased for anticipated price increases in the budget year, 2017 to 2018. If the current year budget is used, it must only be increased for anticipated price increases in the budget year, 2017 to 2018.

The problem with using the last full-year data or the current budget as the expenditure base is that things may have changed (expenses are no longer needed, new expenses have emerged, etc.) since the year was completed or the budget was finalized, and thus unnecessary costs may be built into the new budget or necessary costs may be excluded. While current year expenditures provide an accurate record of what is being consumed, the key question is, are these expenses needed? If an operation is currently overbudget, should the overage be built into the following year's budget or should the new budget be built around what was thought would be needed?

If department expenses are currently running underbudget, will the lower costs continue? If the lower costs are expected to continue, the new budget should be based on YTD expenses; if the lower costs are unsustainable, the current budget may provide a better base for estimating future expenses. The appropriate expenditure base could vary by type of expense, and a budget could be constructed using all three expenditure bases. The choice of expenditure base should be determined by what occurred, why it occurred, and whether it will continue, rather than which base produces the largest budget.

The second step determines the appropriate rate to increase line item expenditures. The prices of different resources used in the production process will not increase at the same rate, so appropriate indices are needed to incorporate potential expense increase.

> **BOX 6.1** The Incremental Budgeting Process
>
> 1. Identify the expenditure base.
> 2. Identify inflation factors and timing.
> 3. Multiply the expenditure base and the inflation factor.
> 4. Modify for expected changes in output, production processes, and regulatory mandates.

A primary question a manager encounters when building an incremental budget is, what is the magnitude of the inflation factor? How fast are input prices rising, and how fast should they be rising? Consider major expenses such as labor, supplies, and energy; within each major category, there will be multiple rates of price changes. Market wages for skilled and unskilled workers can change at different rates; office, production, and maintenance supplies will not change at the same rates; and prices for energy derived from petroleum, natural gas, and hydroelectric sources may move in opposite directions. **TABLE 6.1** shows the prices for input, the **producer price index (PPI)**, vary widely between the four major types of healthcare providers (not the same as Table 4.1, "Percentage Changes in GDP").

The PPI from August 2012 through August 2013 shows that the change in producer costs in the healthcare industry ranged from a 1.5% increase in hospitals to a −0.2% decrease in home health. While these changes may seem insignificant, examining them over a longer time demonstrates the impact of small changes over multiple years. The index base, column 3, shows the total change over multiple years. Examining the change from December 1993 for industry/product codes 621111–621111-5 (not inclusive) shows that physician practice expenses through August 2013 increased by 60.8% (160.8), pediatrics costs increased by 141.1% (241.1), and one and two physician practice expenses "only" increased by 41.3% (141.3). Within the hospital industry, cost increases are calculated by major diagnostic category (MDC), industry/product codes 622110-101–622110-127, and increased by 1.9% from August 2012 through August 2013. There is wide variation around the average increase: MDC 1 costs increased by 5.4%, while MDC 23 declined by 3.7%, a range of 9.1%.

A second factor that must be incorporated into the budget is when price changes will occur—will prices increase at the beginning of the year, end of the year, or throughout the year? Given that budget maximization is a primary goal of department managers, there is an incentive to make the inflation factor as large as possible and to apply anticipated price increases as early as possible. If input prices are expected to increase in the 7th month of the budget, it behooves a manager to incorporate the price increase into the first month to maximize the budget. The job of finance and senior management, who review and/or approve the budget, should be to determine what is necessary to support operations; their job is not to increase or reduce expenses as much as possible. The budget should provide the appropriate level of resources—no more, no less.

The third step is the easiest: multiply the expenditure base by the expected change in prices for each budget line. If the expenditure base is $1 million and prices are expected to increase by 1.5%, the budget estimate is $1,015,000 ($1,000,000 * 1.015) and the products are totaled for all budget lines. The incremental budgeting approach is a fast and simple means to construct a budget. Incremental budgeting does not require intimate knowledge of the workings of the department and is easily defended. Incremental budgeting assumes that if an expenditure was made last year, it should be continued. The bottom line is that every expenditure made in the last year is not only continued but also augmented to ensure that the same level of resources can be purchased, given anticipated price increases.

The third step produces a budget assuming only input prices have changed, while the fourth step recognizes that other factors may change: it will be extremely rare that an organization or department will do everything in the future exactly as it did in the past and inputs will simply cost more. Adjustments should be made for changes in the quantity or quality of output produced or changes in production processes or regulatory mandates (such as the Occupational Safety and Health Administration [OSHA] and the Environmental Protection Agency [EPA]) that will affect expenses.

TABLE 6.1 Producer Price Index

Industry and Product	Industry/Product Code	Index Base	Index April 2013	Index July 2013	Index August 2013	% Change to August 2013 from August 2012	% Change to August 2013 from July 2013
Offices of physicians	6211	12/96	133.2	133.8	133.8	0.5	0.0
Offices of physicians	62111	12/96	133.2	133.8	133.8	0.5	0.0
Offices of physicians, except mental health	621111	12/93	143.6	144.2	144.2	0.4	0.0
Primary services	621111-P	12/93	143.8	144.4	144.5	0.5	0.1
One and two physician practices	621111-4	12/93	140.8	141.5	141.3	0.7	-0.1
General/family practice	621111-411	12/93	150.4	153.4	152.3	0.7	-0.7
Internal medicine	621111-412	12/99	129.2	129.2	129.2	0.5	0.0
General and specialty surgery	621111-413	12/99	111.9	112.6	112.4	0.9	-0.2
Pediatrics	621111-414	12/93	241.1	241.8	241.1	2.2	-0.3
Obstetrics/gynecology	621111-415	12/93	140.5	140.5	141.2	0.5	0.5
Other specialty	621111-419	12/99	122.2	122.6	122.3	0.3	-0.2
Multispecialty group practice	621111-5	12/93	160.0	160.4	161.2	-0.2	0.5

(continues)

TABLE 6.1 Producer Price Index *(continued)*

Industry and Product	Industry/ Product Code	Index Base	Index				% Change to August 2013 from	
			April 2013	July 2013	August 2013	August 2012	July 2013
Home healthcare services	6216	12/96	130.0	130.1	130.2	−0.2	0.1
Home healthcare services	62161	12/96	130.0	130.1	130.2	−0.2	0.1
Home healthcare services	621610	12/96	130.1	130.2	130.2	−0.2	0.0
Primary services	621610-P	12/96	126.1	126.2	126.3	−0.2	0.1
Public payers	621610-3	12/03	110.6	110.7	110.8	−0.8	0.1
Medicare payers	621610-31	12/96	126.4	126.4	126.6	−1.8	0.2
Non-Medicare public payers	621610-32	12/03	113.2	113.5	113.4	0.3	−0.1
Private payers	621610-4	12/03	108.5	108.5	108.5	1.8	0.0
Hospitals	622	12/92	184.1	184.7	184.6	1.5	−0.1
General medical and surgical hospitals	6221	12/03	133.8	134.2	134.2	1.5	0.0
General medical and surgical hospitals	62211	12/03	133.8	134.2	134.2	1.5	0.0
General medical and surgical hospitals	622110	12/92	184.6	185.2	185.2	1.5	0.0
Primary services	622110-P	12/92	188.4	189.0	189.1	1.7	0.1
MDC 1: Nervous system	622110-101	06/08	111.2	111.5	111.7	5.4	0.2

MDC 3: Ear, nose, mouth, and throat	622110-103	06/08	114.1	114.1	114.1	2.9	0.0
MDC 4: Respiratory system	622110-104	06/08	115.6	116.3	116.2	0.6	-0.1
MDC 5: Circulatory system	622110-105	06/08	112.4	112.8	112.7	2.2	-0.1
MDC 6: Digestive system	622110-106	06/08	116.1	116.1	116.2	-0.9	0.1
MDC 7: Hepatobiliary system and pancreas	622110-107	06/08	105.6	106.2	105.1	0.5	-1.0
MDC 8: Musculoskeletal system and connective tissue	622110-108	06/08	115.7	116.7	116.6	2.1	-0.1
MDC 9: Skin, subcutaneous tissue, and breast	622110-109	06/08	121.0	121.4	121.5	4.3	0.1
MDC 10: Endocrine, nutritional, and metabolic system	622110-111	06/08	114.6	114.6	114.6	2.8	0.0
MDC 11: Kidney and urinary tract	622110-112	06/08	115.9	116.0	116.0	-1.1	0.0
MDC 12: Male reproductive system	622110-113	06/08	99.0	100.5	100.5	-0.1	0.0
MDC 13: Female reproductive system	622110-114	06/08	124.2	124.3	124.5	2.1	0.2
MDC 14: Pregnancy, childbirth, and the puerperium	622110-115	06/08	116.4	117.0	117.9	5.2	0.8
MDC 15: Newborns and other neonates	622110-116	06/08	115.4	115.4	113.8	-0.1	-1.4
MDC 16: Blood, organs, and immunological disorders	622110-117	06/08	128.3	128.1	128.1	5.4	0.0
MDC 17: Myeloproliferative diseases and disorders	622110-118	06/08	103.1	103.1	103.1	4.5	0.0
MDC 18: Infectious and parasitic diseases	622110-119	06/08	109.8	109.9	111.1	-0.5	1.1
MDC 20: Alcohol/drug use and induced mental disorders	622110-122	06/08	120.0	120.0	120.0	3.4	0.0

(continues)

TABLE 6.1 Producer Price Index *(continued)*

Industry and Product	Industry/Product Code	Index Base	Index			% Change to August 2013 from	
			April 2013	July 2013	August 2013	August 2012	July 2013
MDC 21: Injury, poisoning, and toxic effects of drugs	622110-123	06/08	108.3	109.2	109.1	−0.4	−0.1
MDC 23: Factors influencing health status	622110-125	06/08	116.4	115.6	115.7	−3.7	0.1
MDC 24: Multiple significant trauma	622110-126	06/08	125.3	125.3	125.3	4.0	0.0
MDC 25: Human immunodeficiency virus infection	622110-127	06/08	108.6	108.6	108.6	4.1	0.0
Other diseases and disorders	622110-128	06/08	109.4	109.4	110.8	0.7	1.3
Nursing care facilities	6231	12/03	131.3	131.9	131.6	0.8	−0.2
Nursing care facilities	62311	12/03	131.3	131.9	131.6	0.8	−0.2
Nursing care facilities	623110	12/94	199.1	200.2	199.7	0.8	−0.2
Primary services	623110-P	12/94	200.1	201.2	200.7	0.8	−0.2
Public payers	623110-1	12/94	189.8	190.6	190.1	0.2	−0.3
Medicaid payers	623110-101	06/12	100.7	101.2	100.9	0.6	−0.3
Non-Medicaid public payers	623110-102	06/12	99.5	99.7	99.7	−0.5	0.0
Private payers	623110-3	12/94	216.6	218.2	217.9	1.8	−0.1

These adjustments may have a small impact on the total budget, but the failure to make these adjustments will ensure that projected expenses will be either too high or too low. If output is expected to grow by 1.0%, all variable expenses should increase proportionately on top of any price increase, but fixed expenses should not be affected. The budget may not be understated by much if no volume adjustment is made for a small increase in output, but if past budgets were reasonably efficient, it will probably guarantee that the department will overrun its budget. If prior budgets contained "fat," missing the new expenses will probably not make the department overrun its budget, since it has a cushion to absorb small increases in expenses.

An increase in output that will substantially increase expenses should be budgeted, for example, a 5.0% increase in output probably cannot be accommodated by reorganizing operations and economizing. Managers should be able to anticipate output and other changes and incorporate their financial impact into the budget rather than explaining why their departments and the organization failed to achieve the financial plan after the fact.

Beyond minor quibbling over the inflation factor, which may be as trivial as whether paper supplies should increase by 3.0% or 4.0%, incremental budgeting minimizes conflict. Few questions are raised over the necessity of continuing historical resource use (if it was necessary in the past, it is assumed to remain necessary) or supplementing the budget for increases in output (an increase in output should increase expenses). Managers work diligently to incorporate even small increases in output into higher budget requests, while ignoring large and small declines in output that should translate into smaller budgets.

Incremental budgeting minimizes conflict between the chief executive officer (CEO) and the board of directors, senior managers, and department managers over resource allocation. It maintains the status quo and avoids perpetual conflict over what the organization's priorities should be—past priorities remain priorities. It avoids conflict among between the CEO, board members, and senior executives over whose constituents should be served—those served in the past continue to be served. Incremental budgeting minimizes squabbling among managers over whose department should be funded by continuing past funding levels. It eliminates the anxiety of managers and employees over how to deal with budget reductions, who the company will let go, what perks will be reduced, etc. Past priorities, constituents, and departments receive a constant level of support. Managers, employees, suppliers, and customers/clients have the same ability to purchase resources after accounting for inflation and receive the same benefits—no one is worse off. Contention may arise over rates of increase rather than over whether resources and funds should be reallocated. It is easy to see why budget players choose an uneasy budget peace with constant support over interminable warfare and seek small, marginal budget increases.

This type of budgeting is called incremental since expenses are increased (incremented) from year to year to account for changes in input prices in order to provide managers with relatively constant access to resources. Departments continue to receive sufficient funding to purchase the same amount of inputs and produce the same amount of outputs they did in prior periods. This type of budgeting is also called fixed or static in that after the budget is finalized, budget allocations do not change, that is, the budget is neither increased nor decreased because of changes in output. Managers obtain a fixed set of resources, hours, supplies, equipment, and space to complete their tasks. Managers can comfortably make decisions and take action plans, knowing how much money they have to achieve the goals set for their departments.

Incremental budgeting can be the optimal method for assembling financial information when the following assumptions hold: First, prior production methods were effective and efficient. Second, the goods and services produced fulfill the need or desire they were designed for. Third, inputs were fully and effectively employed and managed to secure the greatest possible output. This assumption may be the least tenable; as noted in Chapter 5, some believe that up to one quarter of healthcare resources are wasted. Finally, output is relatively stable, or if not constant, the change in output can be predicted with a high degree of certainty. A stable change in output allows managers to plan capacity increases for the following and upcoming years and avoid last-minute accommodations to deal with unexpected increases or decreases in output.

Incremental budgets are internally focused on department expenses over the following fiscal year, a one-year horizon. Budget decisions are specified in terms of inputs required. While it may be preferable that budget allocations be specified as the number of workers, supplies, and equipment needed (physical units), the budget is often built on the total dollars spent in each object code (monetary aggregates). The goal for department managers is to meet their budgets or get as close to spending everything that was budgeted without going over. Bonuses and other compensation are often tied to coming in on- or underbudget. A graduated bonus based on total cost savings would, however, provide a better incentive to encourage efficiency and reduce waste.

The fundamental unit of analysis or concern is inputs, specifically input expense. Incremental budgeting asks three questions: What types of inputs were used in the past? How many units of each were used? What was their cost? The first two questions can be ignored, however, and managers can simply augment the amount spent in prior periods (the expenditure base) to produce the expense budget. Does it matter if four people are employed, two high-skilled (at $66,667) and two low-skilled workers (at $33,333), at a total cost of $200,000, or three high-skilled people? The number of workers is irrelevant if the expected

wage increase is 3.0% for all workers; the estimated wage expense for the budget year will be $206,000 ($200,000 * 1.03) regardless of the number or type of people employed. Who is employed makes a difference if different classes of labor receive different wage increases. If high-wage earners are slated for a 4.0% increase, the expected salary expense will be $207,333 ([$133,334 * 1.04] + [$66,666 * 1.03]), an average increase of 3.7%.

The number and type of workers are also important when production methods or output changes, as the impact on the expense budget will differ on the basis of whether a high- or a low-skilled employee is added to or subtracted from the production process. While not essential for creating an incremental budget, managers should understand the types of inputs used and the quantities of each in their production processes. This knowledge will increase their understanding of how resources are being consumed and what these resources produce that can be used to improve operations.

Instead of simple augmentation, an informed manager should ask the following question: Will the same production process and mix of inputs be used in the upcoming budget period as prior periods? Can output be expanded and per unit costs reduced by substituting higher- or lower-priced inputs? Adding a higher-skilled and higher-paid employee while subtracting lower-skilled and lower-paid employees could lower per unit costs, but the answer depends on productivity. **Productivity** is output per worker.

It is economically desirable to use an input costing 10% more than the price of a substitute if its productivity is more than 10% higher, all other things remaining constant. For example, a worker paid $7.25 an hour produces three units per hour, while a higher-skilled worker paid $11.00 an hour (52% more) produces 5 units per hour (67% more). The productivity of the lesser-paid worker is three units per hour, while the higher-paid worker produces 5 units in the same amount of time. Since the higher-paid worker produces 67% more output but is only paid 52% more, it is cheaper to employ the higher-skilled and higher-paid worker.

Another way of examining this issue is the cost per output produced; the wage component is $2.42 per unit ($7.25 / 3 units) for the lower-paid worker and $2.20 ($11.00 / 5 units) for the higher-paid worker. The increase in productivity more than compensates the organization for the higher wage paid to the more skilled worker. A third way of envisioning the issue is three high-skilled workers can produce the output of five low-skilled workers. The total wage cost is $33.00 ($11.00 * 3) versus $36.25 ($7.25 * 5), while output is a constant 15 units (5 units/hour * 3 workers or 3 units/hour * 5 workers). The **marginal rate of technical substitution** is the rate at which one input must be increased while a second is decreased to maintain constant output. In this example, it is the number of low-skilled workers who must be substituted for high-skilled workers—1.67 (5 / 3). Managers should employ resources to equalize the marginal products and prices of each input: $MP_a / P_a = MP_b / P_b = \cdots = MP_n / P_n$.

Higher-paid workers should be employed at current wage rates. Changes in wages over time may warrant a different mix of workers. If demand for high-skilled workers increases, driving their wage to $13.00 (or $2.60 per unit produced), the production process should be shifted to lower-skilled and lower-paid workers. Production processes should be flexible to utilize the lowest-cost method of production, while maintaining product quality. Consider the impact of an increase in the minimum wage in the fast-food industry. At the prevailing wage, $7.25 per hour, restaurants may find it advantageous to hire low-skilled workers. If the minimum wage is raised to $15.00 per hour, low-skilled counter workers may be replaced by self-service ordering kiosks and beverage dispensers.

Similarly, healthcare managers are analyzing transcription services to determine whether they should continue traditional on-site transcription or replace it with voice recognition systems or offshore transcription. The input choice centers on the hourly cost of domestic labor versus the cost of voice recognition equipment and maintenance, or the lower cost of foreign labor. Managers should be aware of changes in input prices and be able to act to shift production to the lowest-cost combination of inputs consistent with meeting the needs or desires of customers or clients.

FIGURE 6.2 shows a typical budget form. Managers can be overwhelmed by the magnitude of the expenditures shown in this form. It is easy to get lost in the details and fail to see the structure and organization within the budget when expenses total hundreds of thousands or millions of dollars. Confronted by a budget of, say, $2 million or more, it is easy to throw up your hands and believe you cannot comprehend all the relationships covered in the budget. The job of a manager is to create value by knowing how each input contributes to the goods and services the department produces. The challenge is that each expenditure category may include a multitude of inputs. Object code 4020 (regular salaries) includes multiple individuals with diverse skills; should one person understand everything in the object code and what his or her contribution to the department and organization is? The answer is yes, but it requires effort and cooperation between operating managers and the budgeting and accounting departments.

Aggregate financial data simply records how money is spent; it often does not provide a great deal of information about the inputs used, methods of production, and the interrelationships between inputs. Producers exist to provide effective and pleasing goods and services at competitive prices, and managers need to understand their departments, their processes, and their budgets in order to meet this goal. Budgets are the delineation of the expected operating plan in dollars and cents. The bottom line on a monthly or annual expense report tells a manager whether he or she is over- or underbudget, but it does not tell

Object Code	Description	Last Year 2017	YTD Actual 2018	YTD Budget 2018	Budget Request 2019
4010	Management & clerical staff	$331,200	$176,543	$180,000	_____
4020	Staff salaries & wages	2,066,350	1,235,642	1,105,000	_____
4040	Overtime	33,120	23,833	18,000	_____
4050	Agency & Temporary	374,400	156,115	204,000	_____
4110	FICA	185,946	109,855	99,680	_____
4120	Health insurance	278,760	149,857	151,500	_____
4130	Retirement	121,534	71,801	65,150	_____
4140	Unemployment	26,737	15,796	14,333	_____
4211	Floor medications	22,398	13,589	12,775	_____
4212	Medical instruments	18,596	5,798	9,000	_____
4214	Bandages, gauze...	9,741	5,643	5,110	_____
4216	Latex gloves, gowns...	52,899	32,145	29,383	_____
4216	Sterile wipes	5,211	2,659	2,555	_____
4250	Office supplies	8,452	4,268	4,599	_____
4280	Cleaning supplies	1,202	569	500	_____
4350	Biomedical repairs/maintenance	5,244	3,869	3,000	_____
4410	Electricity	2,453	1,156	1,200	_____
4440	Telephone	5,794	2,645	2,880	_____
4930	Housekeeping	138,240	72,000	72,000	_____
4940	Travel/professional meetings/meals	35,789	14,523	17,850	_____
4950	CME	8,425	3,688	4,600	_____
4960	Other expenses	4,953	1,258	1,655	_____
		$3,737,444	$2,103,252	$2,004,769	

FIGURE 6.2 Budget Request Form

the manager why the operation is spending more or less than expected. The department in Figure 6.2 is overbudget by $98,193 (4.9%) for the first 6 months of 2018. The ability to track expenses by object codes allows managers to begin to identify why they are over- or underbudget and where operations should be assessed and possibly improved.

The chart of accounts tree (**FIGURE 6.3**) allows managers to visualize where their expenses arise and whether they can be and should be controlled. When last year's expenses, 2017, are diagrammed in a chart of accounts tree, it is obvious that the lion's share of this department's expenses are labor related (92.2%: 75.7% wages + 16.5% fringe benefits). The largest expenses outside of salaries and benefits are housekeeping (3.4% of total expenses) and supplies (3.1%, with disposable gloves and gowns constituting 49.7% of the total supply expense). Any serious attempt at cost control must address salaries and fringe benefits, as attempts to reduce office supplies or other low-expenditure areas will have a limited impact, if any, on the overall financial situation.

While the chart of accounts tree and the pie chart (**FIGURE 6.4**) help a manager visualize where expenses arise, the budget request form (or monthly variance report) allows a manager to determine what expenses are higher than the budget and focus the search on where costs can and should be reduced. If operations are over-budget, the budget request form shows whether it is due to labor, supplies, housekeeping, utilities, or other items. Given that labor accounts for 92.2% of total expenses, the budget request form allows managers to determine whether the higher-than-expected expense is the result of changes in the cost of managers, regular staff, overtime, or temporary labor. Of course, judgment of a budget manager's performance should not be based on the sole criterion of whether he

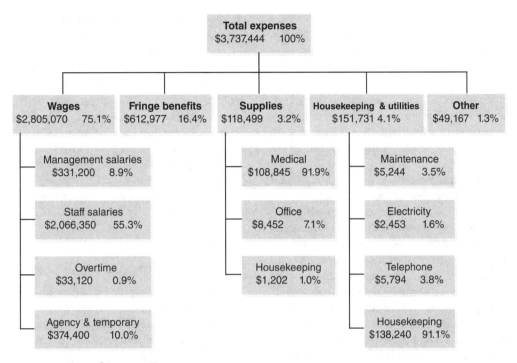

FIGURE 6.3 Chart of Accounts Tree

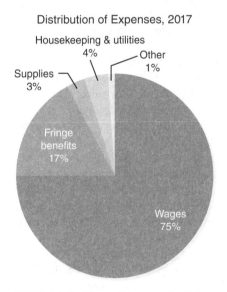

FIGURE 6.4 Pie Chart of Expenses for 2017

controllable; managers should be held responsible only for unneeded and controllable increases in expenses, not for uncontrollable increases necessary to meet customer expectations.

There are many reasons a manager should not be held responsible for higher-than-expected expenditures for labor, such as increased workload, or higher-than-expected wages that he or she did not negotiate. On the other hand, if labor expenses increase because of poor staff oversight, resulting in unbudgeted regular hours, overtime, and/or the use of temporary help, the manager should be accountable. Likewise, higher supply expenditures must be traced to specific items before the overage can be determined to be the result of higher prices or inefficient use of resources. Managers should not be held accountable for changes in prices or volume beyond their control but should be held responsible for poor use of resources.

A person putting together a scratch budget has to identify cause-and-effect relationships between the resources budgeted and the

or she comes in on- or underbudget. Performance assessments should be based on whether deviations from the budget are required and outputs expected. There was no blind acceptance of the status quo (because there was no status quo to rely on), but rather, inputs were employed to fulfill a specific function and achieve a definitive end. Creating a budget from scratch is rare, but understanding cause-and-effect relationships is essential to explain variations in operations (to be discussed in the chapter "Variance Analysis") and improve performance.

The relationship between a budget and output is analogous to a car and motion. Cars, a set of inputs, are purchased to provide movement and other benefits, outputs. What parts are responsible for movement, what parts are responsible for comfort, and what parts are for appearance? Is the price paid for these inputs worth the satisfaction derived from them? Assume the first-order choice for transportation is between a Lexus and a Geo. After a vehicle is selected, second-order decisions require the purchaser to determine whether he or she wants a six-cylinder or a four-cylinder engine, leather seats or cloth upholstery, and standard car audio or iPod-enabled, eight-speaker Bose audio, among other choices. One person will purchase the expensive set of inputs (six-cylinder Lexus with leather seats and a Bose system) because the value of luxury transportation exceeds the cost of the inputs. Another person only wants basic transport and chooses the lower-priced set of features that will reliably move the person from point A to point B. When purchasing a car , consumers do not have to understand the operation of internal combustion engines to compare the values of different cars and options. Similarly, managers need not understand the science of production to compare the values of inputs and outputs.

Of course, car buyers should understand economics enough so that after indulging in amenities, they have enough funds left to put gas in the tank and get to where they want to go. Similarly, managers should understand the contribution inputs play in producing outputs; they need to know what they are purchasing, what its relationship with output is, and whether

they have sufficient funds to reach their goals. Figure 6.3, the chart of accounts tree, conveys this information better than Figure 6.2, the budget request form. The chart of accounts tree not only better represents the data by showing the hierarchical structure of the budget but also emphasizes the relationships between expenses. Knowing what is being spent on various inputs allows managers to investigate the questions of what each input contributes to the production process and whether the expenditure is worth it. The first object of managerial attention should always be the largest, controllable expenditures.

Starting the Budgeting Process

The budget-building process begins with the receipt of budget information, forms, and instructions. Managers are asked to submit the following year's budgets prior to the completion of the current year, given the overlapping time frames of budget preparation and management. To facilitate preparation, budget managers receive information similar to Figure 6.2. The budget request form provides the major information needed to prepare the budget. It generally contains four parts: the object of the expenditure, the amount spent in the last completed fiscal year (2016), the amounts spent and budgeted in the current budget year (2017), and blanks for inserting the budget requests for the upcoming year (2018).

The object of the expenditure (object code and description) is what monies are spent on or what inputs are purchased. The classification scheme should walk the fine line between providing too much and too little information. Too much information occurs when managers cannot identify relevant trends because the information contains too much detail. Office supplies could be broken down into pens, pencils, highlighters, various types of paper, envelopes, paperclips, etc., and each could have its own object code; however, the cost of recording and tracking this level of detail should be weighed against its expected benefit.

OfficeMax may need to track this level of information to control inventories, but a department may not spend enough on any of these items to justify separating them into distinct codes. In Figure 6.2, roughly $100 per month is spent on cleaning supplies (object code 4280) versus $172,000 in staff salaries (object code 4020); the magnitude of expenditure should dictate that more attention be devoted to salaries than supplies. Too much data or excessive detail for small expenditure items can impede rather than facilitate management.

Too little detail occurs if a manager cannot identify resource use or exercise control over resources because information on the use of resources is too highly aggregated, that is, all expenses of a single type are rolled up into a single category. For example, object code 4020 may include wages paid to registered nurses (RNs), licensed practical nurses (LPNs), and nurse assistants (NAs), obscuring the driver behind deviations in budgeted and actual expenditures. Is a cost overrun the result of lower-paid NAs being absent and their duties being performed by RNs? Was a budget saving the result of NAs performing the duties of RNs, and is this substitution acceptable or does it create a potential liability?

Sometimes, the combination of disparate inputs into a single object code is an explicit strategy to render the data unintelligible; some organizations blend executive salaries and secretarial salaries in the same object code. If object code 4010 pools executive and secretarial salaries, it becomes impossible to determine the average executive salary by taking the total salary pool and dividing it by the number of executives; instead, all that can be discerned from the data is the average executive and secretarial salary, a significantly lower number. Similarly, if all medical supplies are rolled into a single object code, it would be impossible to determine whether floor medications, medical instruments, bandages, gloves and gowns, or sterile wipes produced a budget overrun and who should be brought in to control expenses, since each group of supplies may be used by

mutually exclusive groups of employees. In this case, medical supply expenses exceed the budget by 1.7%, but this total masks the fact that gloves, gowns, and sterile wipes increased by almost 10.0% and that these increases were offset by a 35.4% lower expenditure on medical instruments than planned. The question managers and employees should ask is whether these increases were necessary and the decrease appropriate. Without examining the components of change, managers and employees will be blind to how the department is performing.

In establishing the chart of accounts, that is, the level of reporting detail, the accounting department attempts to balance the cost of control versus the benefit of control. This is a dynamic decision. Changes in production processes and information systems will affect the benefits and costs of controlling resources. Changes in production processes and input prices will reduce the importance of certain inputs (declining use and/or lower prices) and increase the importance of others (higher use and/or higher prices). Effective management needs less information on resources declining in importance and more information on those that constitute a larger portion of the costs of production. Managers should take an active role in recommending the level of detail they need to do their job effectively, and recognize when changes in productive methods require changes in accounting. Accounting, being distanced from production, may not be able to detect operational changes that recommend or require changes in financial reporting systems. Expanded reporting on expenses will become more economical as the cost of collecting, analyzing, and storing data decreases and provide better information for managers to control their departments.

There should be separate object codes for each input that has a significant impact on a department's operations and expense. In times of budget crunches, managers frequently devote their time to, and employees are subjected to, controlling inconsequential items, such as pencils, pens, and copier paper, which, even if their cost were totally eliminated, would have a marginal impact on the department's expenses. In Figure 6.2, office supplies constituted only 0.2% ($8,452/$3,921,882) of the spending in 2016; unfortunately, these small-impact items are often targeted for scrutiny as they may be the items that are reported and easy to manage. It is easier to see someone wasting 12 pencils a week than wasting 12 hours. The focus given to obvious and trivial items deflects attention from fundamental items. The squandering of 12 hours per week has a minimum cost of $87.00, while 12 wasted pencils cost $2.28 or less. Labor has a greater impact on operational expenses than pencils, but the accounting system often does not provide sufficient information to identify wasted labor.

Fortunately, the increased capabilities of information systems are leading us to demand a higher level of information support. Managers of the future should be able to determine what level of aggregation they need or desire in a report and structure their monthly or annual reports to serve their goals.

The second part of the budget request, column 3, is often the amount spent in the object code for the last completed year. While this information may be one year removed from current operations, it provides managers with an understanding of how much was spent over the course of a year for each line item. This information is particularly useful in conjunction with the current year budget and actual expenditures to understand the timing of expenses that are not incurred evenly over the course of a year.

The third and fourth parts are a comparison of YTD expenditures, column 4, with the YTD budget, column 5. The importance of this comparison is in determining the accuracy of the budget and/or the effectiveness of management. If a department is overbudget, does this indicate the budget underestimated needs or a lack of control over resources? If a department is underbudget, is it because of overestimation of resource needs or superior management of resources?

The fifth part, column 6, contains blanks for entering the budget request (expenditure base * inflation factor). In addition to the historical financial information, the budget package may include instructions on how the budget should be constructed, the expenditure base(s) for budget projections, inflation factors, and a budget calendar with dates for submission, review, feedback, resubmission, if required, and approval.

Selecting an Expenditure Base

There are three expenditure bases commonly used to estimate the amount of funds needed to acquire resources in the upcoming budget year: YTD actual expenditures, the current year budget, and the last full year of data. Each has advantages and drawbacks.

The advantage of YTD actual is that it is an accurate and up-to-date record of what was spent in the current fiscal year. Unlike using the prior year's data, there is no need to estimate price increases, that is, what last year's inputs would cost at this year's prices. This is the amount spent for the output produced. YTD actual has the advantage of known current input use (number of units purchased), current input prices, current production methods, and current output—it is an accurate picture of current production.

The primary disadvantage of YTD actual is that it is only partial-year data and does not present a complete picture of costs for an entire year. As stated earlier, financial planning requires knowing what resources are required prior to the start of the budget year. In many cases, the following year's budgets are submitted when only 6 months of the current year have been completed; thus YTD requires **annualizing**, estimating total expenses for the year when less than 12 months of data is available. Annualizing takes partial-year totals, calculates a monthly average, and multiples the monthly average by 12 to produce an annual total, assuming the monthly average continues.

A second disadvantage is the timing of expenditures: current expenditures may over- or understate annual expenses due to when costs are incurred and reported and/or cyclical patterns or swings in production. For example, if more than 50% of expenses or output arises in the first 6 months of a year, the early months will be more expensive than the later months and using them as the expenditure base will overstate the required expenses in the second half of the budget year.

In situations in which year-end funding may be cut, astute managers may accelerate purchases to ensure they receive their allocated resources, making the early months of a fiscal year disproportionately costly. On the other hand, managers often create a budget cushion by postponing nonessential purchases. If unexpected expenses are incurred and budget targets can be met by foregoing nonessential expenditures, these expenditures are eliminated. If no unexpected expenses arise, the nonessential purchases can be made in the final months of the budget to ensure unspent funds are minimized; rule #3 of winning the budget game is *always spend your entire budget*. When discretionary expenses are shifted to the later months of a budget year, annualizing early months' expenses understates resource needs.

The second question is, does production take place evenly over the year? If only 6 months of data is available, does the expense cover half of the expected yearly output? Simply doubling expenses for the first 6 months will overstate budget needs if more than half of the total anticipated production occurs in the first half of the year. If the majority of production occurs in the latter half of the year, doubling the expenses made in the first 6 months will not provide adequate funds to support production. For example, retail outlets that estimate their annual sales on the basis of January through June would significantly underestimate sales as 14.2% sales occur in December versus an average of 7.8% in January through November. The understatement

of jewelry sales would be even greater as 18.2% of sales occur in December versus 7.4% in the other months, that is, jewelry sales increase by 146% in December (United States Census Bureau, 2015).

A simple extrapolation of expenditures overestimates resource needs when purchases are accelerated and underestimates input requirements when purchases are postponed. For example, when employee tuition reimbursement is limited to a fixed amount, employees may take classes in the first half of the year and exhaust their benefits. Doubling the amount used in the first half of the year would overstate the budget, given the limit. Conversely, if maintenance contracts are paid in the second half of the year, doubling the first-half expense misses these expenditures and understates the budget. Third, actual expenses may reflect nonrecurring changes, that is, temporary increases or decreases in expenditures. Extraordinary events (unexpected breakdown in equipment, extended absence of one or more employees, etc.) that increase (or reduce) current expenses may arise, which probably will not be repeated in the budget year. These items need to be added to or subtracted from the budget to accurately estimate necessary expenses.

When partial-year data is used as the expenditure base for the following year's budget, it must be annualized to approximate resource costs for a 12-month period. There are two ways of annualizing: the first method factors up current YTD expenditures on the basis of how many months of data is available, and the second calculates an average monthly expenditure.

$$\text{YTD expenditure} * 12/\text{Number of months of current data} = \text{Projected actual} \quad (6.1)$$

$$\text{YTD expenditure}/\text{Number of months of current data} * 12 \text{ months} = \text{Projected actual} \quad (6.2)$$

$$(\text{Average monthly expenditure} * 12 \text{ months} = \text{Projected actual})$$

Equation 6.1 multiplies the current YTD expenditure by 12 (months) divided by the number of months of reported data. If current expenditure for an object code in the first 6 months of the year is $600,000, then extrapolating the total for the entire year simply requires multiplying the current figure by 12/6. If $600,000 was spent in the first half of the year, $1,200,000 is estimated for the entire year.

Equation 6.2 divides the current expenditure by the number of months of data reported in order to produce the average monthly expenditure, that is, $600,000/6 = $100,000 average monthly expenditure. The average monthly expenditure is then multiplied by 12 to project the total for the year. Both formulas assume no acceleration or postponement of costs and constant output across the year, and both arrive at the same figure. Many people see Equation 6.2, average monthly expenditure, as more intuitive.

A comparison of YTD actual expenditures and the YTD budget may also be informative. Are current expenses above or below budget, and if so, why? If there are differences between actual and budgeted expenses, any excess spending or savings should be investigated to determine whether the following year's budget should be increased or decreased to improve its accuracy. Budgets should be adjusted upward or downward for legitimate reasons (downward by budget reviewers and approvers for overt attempts to maximize budgets).

The second expenditure base that could be used is the current full-year budget. While the budget request form (Figure 6.2) displays the YTD budget, if the budget is to be used as the expenditure base, a manager could simply pull the full-year budget and use it to estimate the following year's budget. The advantages of using the current full-year budget are that it provides a full year of data and does not reflect temporary fluctuations. It does not require any calculation to determine what full-year expenditures should be on the basis of what was spent to date, nor does it require consideration of the timing of expenditures. The chief problem is that it represents the prior year's estimate of input prices, output, and production methods. The chief advantage of the full-year budget over current YTD expenditures is that expenditures are subject to month-to-month fluctuations and over the course of a year low and high input use and output periods offset. The full-year budget prevents managers from gaming the expenditure base by shifting when expenditures are made or output is produced. The primary disadvantage of the prior year's budget is that it is old. Budget estimates are based on prices, output levels, and production methods that are 18 months older than current operations, so it may not reflect current input prices, output, or methods.

The third expenditure base could be the last full-year actual (or the last 12 months spanning the current year and the preceding year). The advantage of using the expenses in the last completed year is that they constitute full-year data and no calculation or consideration is required about the timing of expenditures. The disadvantage of using the last full year of expenses is its age, input use, prices, output, and production methods may be up to two years out of date. If you are constructing the 2019 budget and it is July 2018, the last full year is January through December 2017, and information from January 2017 will be two years old when the 2019 fiscal year begins. Using information spanning two different fiscal years (July–December 2017 + January–June 2018) circumvents some of the age problem; the oldest information, July 2017, is only one year out of date, while June 2018 reflects current input price, output, and production methods.

Budget preparers may have the option of using a combination of expenditure bases, that is, selecting a base that provides the most appropriate estimate of future resource needs for each line item. After examining the advantages and disadvantages of each expenditure base that could be used to estimate the budget, it should be clear that regardless of whether your goal is to estimate an efficient budget that provides only needed resources or produce the largest-possible budget, different bases may be used for different types of expenditures. Assume that the organizational policy has established the use of the annualized YTD actual as the base for budget projections but a significant nonrecurring event has resulted in a temporary unpaid leave of absence of one of the department supervisors. Use of the current year expenditures would underestimate salaries and wages, but the full-year budget would provide a better estimate of what expenses should be under "normal" operating conditions. If petroleum prices have spiked because of an environmental disaster or a war in the Middle East (nonpredictable events), use of the last full year of actual expenditures or the current year budget may provide the best estimator of future energy costs. On the other hand, the prior year's actual expenses may be the best base for the budget if current expenditures include large, unanticipated, and nonrecurring expenses and budgeted changes in input process and/or output have not been realized. Astute managers may cherry-pick the base for each object code on the basis of which one supports the highest budget allocation in lieu of organizational policy.

▶ Building an Incremental Budget

The following section presents an example of constructing a budget for a nursing unit, North 2 Medicine. The CEO has requested that all departments submit their 2019 operating budgets by August 31, 2018. The 2019 fiscal year begins on January 1, 2019. To assist departments in preparing their budgets, the YTD expense report (Figure 6.2) was distributed 6 weeks prior to the submission deadline.

The economic outlook for the healthcare industry is continuing financial pressure due to restrictive Medicare and Medicaid reimbursement, given the slow economic growth. Given the financial pressure, salary increases for all personnel, including management, should be budgeted at 3.0%. Administration realizes that this increase may not please all employees, but managers are encouraged to remind their employees that this increase is more than twice the rate of increase in the consumer price index (CPI). The salary increase will appear in the first month of the budget year (full-year versus partial-year increase). Health insurance costs are expected to increase by 6.0%. An across-the-board increase of 2.0% should be used for all supplies (object codes 4210–4280), with the exception of floor medications (object code 4210), which should be budgeted at 5.0%. A 4.0% rate increase for electricity recently passed by the Citizens Utility Board takes effect in October 2018 and thus impacts the entire budget year. All other nonspecified expenses should be budgeted for a 1.0% increase (**FIGURE 6.5**).

Overall, the budget request seeks 3.1% more than the projected actual for 2018 ($4,334,682 versus $4,204,121); however, the 2018 budget is 16.1% above the expenses incurred in 2017 ($4,334,862 versus $3,733,358).

Despite the main assumption that no major changes in output or production methods have taken place, incremental changes in each are often added into the budget on an ad hoc basis. If output, patient days, was expected to increase by 1.0% due to a growing and aging population, it would be reasonable to increase the budget request for variable expenses by an additional 1.0%. Similarly, if technology changes reduce (increase) the amount of time nurses must spend at the patient bedside without corresponding reductions in other areas, this change should reduce (increase) labor requests. Modifying budgets for changes in actual output will be discussed in the chapter "Flexible Budgeting."

Modifications to the budget, step 4, are biased toward incorporating cost-increasing changes and ignoring changes that reduce the amount of resources needed. Supplemental

	A	B	C	D	E	F	G	H	I
1	Chapter 6 - Incremental Budgets			22					
2									
3	Figure 6.5 - Completed Budget Request								
4							Projected	1 +	Budget
5	Object		Last Year	YTD Actual	YTD Budget	Annual-	Actual	Inflation	Request
6	Code	Description	2017	2018	2018	-ization	2018	Factor	2019
7	4020	Staff salaries & wages	$331,200	$176,543	$180,000	12/6	$353,086	1.03	$363,679
8	4030	Management & clerical staff	2,066,350	1,235,642	1,105,000	12/6	2,471,284	1.03	2,545,423
9	4040	Overtime	33,120	23,833	18,000	12/6	47,666	1.03	49,096
10	4050	Agency & Temporary	374,400	156,115	204,000	12/6	312,230	1.03	321,597
11	4110	FICA	185,946	109,855	99,680	12/6	219,711	1.03	226,302
12	4120	Health insurance	278,760	149,857	151,500	12/6	299,714	1.06	317,697
13	4130	Retirement	121,534	71,801	65,150	12/6	143,602	1.03	147,910
14	4140	Unemployment	26,737	15,796	14,333	12/6	31,592	1.03	32,540
15	4210	Floor Medications	22,398	13,589	12,775	12/6	27,178	1.05	28,537
16	4212	Medical instruments	18,596	5,798	9,000	12/6	11,596	1.02	11,828
17	4214	Bandages, guaze...	9,741	5,643	5,110	12/6	11,286	1.02	11,512
18	4216	Latex gloves, gowns...	52,899	32,145	29,383	12/6	64,290	1.02	65,576
19	4218	Sterile wipes	5,211	2,659	2,555	12/6	5,318	1.02	5,424
20	4250	Office supplies	8,452	4,268	4,599	12/6	8,536	1.02	8,707
21	4280	Cleaning supplies	1,202	569	500	12/6	1,138	1.02	1,161
22	4350	Biomedical repairs/maintenance	5,244	3,869	3,000	12/6	7,738	1.01	7,815
23	4410	Electricity	2,453	1,156	1,200	12/6	2,312	1.04	2,404
24	4440	Telephone	5,794	2,645	2,880	12/6	5,290	1.01	5,343
25	4930	Housekeeping	138,240	72,000	72,000	12/6	144,000	1.01	145,440
26	4940	Travel/prof. meetings/meals	35,789	14,523	17,850	12/6	29,046	1.01	29,336
27	4950	CME	8,425	3,688	4,600	12/6	7,376	1.01	7,450
28	4960	Other expenses	4,953	1,258	1,655	12/6	2,516	1.01	2,541
29			$3,737,444	$2,103,252	$2,004,769		$4,206,505		$4,337,317
30									

FIGURE 6.5 Completed Budget Request

staff and resource requests may be made for a higher volume, changes in production methods, and/or regulatory mandates. Managers should explicitly note the changes in the narratives they submit with their budget requests and the additional personnel or resources required rather than simply increasing their budget requests and trying to slip the increase through the budget approval process. Large budget increases are easy to identify and easier to reject when money is tight. Increases based on documented changes in production processes are not as easy to reject. The output for North 2 Medicine is assumed to be constant, so no expense modifications were made to the budget.

The Budget Game

If budget instructions do not specify the expenditure base to use, managers may want to use the base that maximizes their budgets. Notwithstanding explicit game playing, managers should examine all available information to ensure nothing is overlooked. For example, if the YTD actual expense is significantly lower than the budget, is it due to an enduring change in production methods, a temporary reduction in input prices, and/or nonrecurring savings? The key words are "enduring," "temporary," and "nonrecurring." Can lower costs be expected in future periods? If higher-than-expected costs have been incurred, are they the result of a temporary shortage and price spike of key inputs or a one-time retooling of production processes? Efficiency demands that budgets be altered for permanent changes and left unchanged for one-time or temporary events.

After an expenditure base is identified, the second major decision is to determine how much the base should be adjusted for changes in input prices in the budget year. Since an incremental budget is being created, the assumption is that input use and the number of outputs will be similar to the base period; however, any known adjustments to resource use should be added to or subtracted from the base. Typically, the budget office will provide guidelines on the increases planned for each expenditure category. Senior management, finance, and/or human resources will establish a range for salary increases (internally determined), while other input price changes will be determined externally, for example, energy (electricity, natural gas, heating oil, etc.), postage, and supplies. High staff turnover may indicate inadequate salaries and force the organization to provide higher salary increases than it would otherwise choose in the absence of market pressure. Employee turnover may, however, be an indicator of other problems in the organization, such as poor management, that are not remedied by higher wages. Internally set increases should keep pace with the general wage increases in the area to prevent an exodus of employees.

The economy, industry, and geographic area will play a large role in determining the level of price increases, and this information can be centralized in the budget office. Assuming the general rate of increase for producer prices is specified for all expenses, department managers will probably understand the markets for their particular inputs better than either the budget office or senior management and may want to use a higher-than-specified rate when the recommended rate is less than expected price changes. For example, the pharmacy director should know the rate of increase for pharmaceuticals has averaged 2% higher than the hospital PPI over the past five years and, thus, use of the lower specified rate would understate true resource needs when constructing the pharmacy budget.

On the other hand, the centrally specified inflation factor may be larger than the anticipated rate of inflation. In this case, the budget manager knows that past price increases for rent, given a glut of vacant office space, have, and probably will continue to, lag general rates of inflation. In this situation, it is a rare manager who will opt to use a lower, more accurate inflation factor. Any departures from budget directives need to be explicitly noted;

managers who attempt to slip through higher rates of increase will be detected.

A third choice is when an inflation factor should be applied. Generally, price increases are applied in the first month of the budget year, but in the presence of union or supplier contracts, there may be defined months when wage or price increases take effect. When this is the case, the inflation factor should be applied to the appropriate month. Many employers give raises on the anniversary of an employee's hire date, and when this occurs, raises should be spread across the budget year and not instituted on the first of the year. For example, a 3.0% raise for six employees hired in February, April, June, August, October, and November would have a net impact of 1.5% on the salary budget; however, if the salary increase was applied starting January 1, it would increase salaries by the full 3.0%.

An open and upfront budget request provides an opportunity for managers to demonstrate their knowledge of their operations and their environmental constraints. For example, the head nurse in the intensive care unit (ICU) may be able to demonstrate a high turnover and an inability to hire new nurses at the organization's current pay rate. This could be supported by pay information from other institutions to justify incorporating higher pay increases than budgeted for department employees. Likewise, a department manager may have been informed by a supplier that a significant price increase is scheduled for a major supply item; the increase should be noted, explained, and incorporated into the budget.

After the base, inflation factor, and timing of increase are determined, the third step is mathematical: multiplying base expenditures by expected price changes (base * (1 + inflation rate)). The fourth, and final, step modifies the budget estimates for changes in output, production processes, or regulation that will affect resource use and costs. After the line item budget requests are finalized, they are added to obtain the total department budget request.

Presubmission Review

Before the budget is submitted, the budget preparer should review his or her work for mathematical accuracy. The budget preparer should verify that all calculations, including projected actual amounts (if required), input price adjustments, and summations, are accurate. Managers do not want to open themselves or their budgets to additional scrutiny due to avoidable mathematical errors.

Second, managers should ensure their budgets comply with budget directives, that is, use the specified expenditure base and inflation factor, submit the budget on time, etc. If the expenditure base or inflation factor does not follow directives, the budget preparer should explicitly note why the base or factor should not be used and what was substituted in its place. Managers who fail to follow budget directives or flaunt directives can expect increased scrutiny from budget reviewers.

Third, the budget preparer should check for reasonableness. A preliminary review may include evaluating the requested budget increase in light of the current year's projected actual or budgeted expense. How high is the increase? Will the increase call attention to itself? One of the first things budget reviewers look at is year-to-year percentage increases, so managers should anticipate questions and be prepared to respond when large increases are requested. Conversely, managers should be confident that operations can be carried on within the constraints of their budgets. Managers may know that market conditions and anticipated input price changes may exceed "suggested" inflation rates, output may increase, or costlier production methods will be introduced. If any or all of these factors arise, prior expenditures (budgeted or actual) may be a poor base for estimating the budget. The budget preparer is ultimately responsible for the reasonableness of the budget (can expected performance be achieved within the budget constraints?) and meeting the budget once it is approved.

Strengths of Incremental Budgeting

Incremental budgets provide a stable monetary target for managers. Managers know exactly the total amount of resources they are allocated, can see on a monthly basis whether they are over- or underbudget, and can determine which expenses are overbudget to guide actions to meet their budgets. The second strength of an incremental budget is that its ease of calculation reduces the time and cost of budget preparation. Third, it focuses management and employee attention on input use. The budget directive and managerial incentive are clear—do *not* exceed your budget. Finally, an incremental budget allows managers to focus on major changes from the base year to the budget year. Managers do not have to justify every dollar spent and how the departments function but can focus on significant changes in output, production methodology, and/or programs and how they affect input use and expenses (**BOX 6.2**).

Weaknesses of Incremental Budgeting

One of the chief weaknesses of an incremental budget is that it does not focus on effectiveness (accomplishing a task) or efficiency

---

BOX 6.2 Strengths of Incremental Budgeting

1. Incremental budgeting provides a clear and stable monetary target for managers.
2. It simplifies and minimizes the cost of budget preparation.
3. It focuses employee attention on input use.
4. It focuses the managers' attention on major changes, output, production methodology, and/or programs, from the base period to the budget year, and how they impact input use and expenses.

(minimizing cost per unit or maximizing output from a set of inputs). An incremental budget discourages the examination of the totality of a department's operation and tends to institutionalize past practices and discourage efficiency. Budgets must be spent, or superiors will assume that too much money was allocated, and so future budgets may be reduced. Incremental budgets encourage expenditure rather than efficiency. They encourage staying within budget and provide minimal incentives for improvement.

The second weakness is that budget allocations are not tied to actual output or quality; departments experiencing a greater demand for their services receive the same budget increase (expenditure base ∗ inflation factor) as those seeing a lower demand for their services. Ironically, incremental budgeting often rewards departments with declining output, while demanding higher performance from a constant set of inputs in departments with an expanding volume. Departments faced with a demand for higher output where the budget is fixed may reduce the quality of care provided in order to enable a higher volume of care to be delivered from a constant set of resources (**BOX 6.3**).

Third, incremental budgeting provides minimal incentives for managers to consider alternative production methods. Incremental budgets implicitly accept (by funding) current production methods, so managers need not stay abreast of emerging developments in use of inputs, new equipment, or methods. The fourth weakness is that an incremental budget has a one-year focus (a weakness shared with most other budgeting systems), which encourages short-term action, possibly to the detriment of long-term interests. Finally, incremental budgeting encourages managers to overestimate output to maximize their budgets. Given the difficulty of accurately estimating future output (discussed in Chapter 4) and considering that, once set, the budget probably will not change with changes in actual output, overestimation of

---

BOX 6.3 Weaknesses of Incremental Budgeting

1. Incremental budgeting focuses on input use rather than effectiveness or efficiency.
2. Budget allocations are not tied to actual output or quality.
3. It provides minimal incentives to pursue alternative production methods.
4. It focuses on the short term—a 1-year time horizon.
5. It provides incentives to overestimate output.

---

output should be expected. Given the motivation of managers to meet their budgets and the uncertainty surrounding prediction of future output, the incentive to overstate output to maximize budgets is the key weakness in incremental budgeting.

Incremental budgets should be used in efficient, nonrevenue-generating departments when output is measurable and stable or predictable and/or in unalterable or sacrosanct programs where funding cannot or will not be cut. These conditions require a stable environment with minimal change in demand, funding, and/or technology or production methods. Incremental budgeting may also be appropriate when managers lack budgeting expertise or information on output.

The four budget-building steps, (1) identifying an expenditure base, (2) identifying a rate of increase for input prices, (3) multiplying the expenditure base by the inflation factor, and (4) modifying the request for anticipated changes in output and production methods, indicate that budgeting is a straightforward computational problem, but this is not the case. If this were true, it is clear that a single person could create a budget for a multibillion-dollar organization. Budgeting requires what Friedrich Hayek referred to as "knowledge of the particular circumstances of time and place" (Hayek, 1945). Managers bring to the table their knowledge of how things are changing in their area of expertise, innovations in production methods, new opportunities that can be capitalized on, and new regulations being considered or enacted and the costs they will impose on the organization (or what benefits they will bring). It is precisely because the information required to effectively allocate resources is absent or contradictory that people build budgets rather than computers. Managers must assemble their best guesses as to what people will want in the future, what prices the resources will command in the future, and what the optimal methods of production are. Their mastery of the "knowledge of particular circumstances of time and place" will be evident in the budgets they produce.

▶ Evaluating Performance

The primary purpose of a budget is not to detail what will be spent in the future but, rather, to improve the effectiveness of management. Were actual expenses greater than, equal to, or less than budgeted expenses, and should they be? In incremental budgeting, managers are rewarded or receive superior performance evaluations when their expenses are less than budgeted. Conversely, managers who go overbudget have to explain, at a minimum, why they went overbudget, may receive a poor performance review, and ultimately can lose their position if the overage is deemed excessive. Will the evaluation of management be based on line item control or global budgeting? Does a budget preparer have discretion to shift expenditures from one line item to another? If authority is decentralized, managers have an incentive to maintain efficiency by offsetting an overage in one expense line by spending less in another line. If authority is centralized, managers cannot respond to increased expenditures in one line item by reducing spending in one or more

other line items; we should expect that global department expenditures will regularly overrun their budgets.

Budgets should be used as tools to improve performance. Given that the incentive in incremental budgeting is to spend the entire budget, a superior performance evaluation and compensation system should reward managers and employees for bringing expenses in below the budget. The most obvious mechanism would be to distribute a percentage of budget savings to workers. Gain sharing is different from profit sharing. In gain sharing, workers receive a percentage of cost savings, that is, 75% of cost savings are distributed to workers, whereas in profit sharing, they receive a percentage of any profit earned. Both mechanisms give employees a stake in the performance of the organization, but gain sharing is easier to tie to the performance of employees, that is, employees know the cost of producing a good or service and know and have the ability to reduce costs. In profit sharing, the profit earned depends on factors beyond the control of most employees, for example, demand for the product and performance of management. In gain sharing, payments received by employees are viewed as being earned through their cost-reducing actions, while profit sharing is sometimes seen as an entitlement arising with employment.

An effective gain-sharing program requires an easy-to-understand gain-sharing formula based on lower (1) department cost, (2) labor cost per output, or (3) percentage of labor cost to total revenue (in labor-intensive industries). Second, the plan should augment wages; it should not create a system where workers must do more to maintain their current compensation. Gain sharing should provide an incentive for employees to do more. When output increases or cost per unit decreases, employees should receive their base salaries and additional pay based on a percentage of their salaries, a flat payment per worker fee, or a payment per hour. Employees should be involved in setting up the plan, including establishing performance targets and compensation to be earned for meeting and exceeding the targets. Fourth, the product/service mix should be stable; a fluctuating output mix may obscure gains achieved. A gain-sharing program should identify the current labor cost per output and stipulate how much of any reduction will be distributed to employees. Assume the current cost is $20 per unit and is reduced to $18, if the gain share was 75%, $1.50 in additional compensation per hour would be distributed to workers and $0.50 would be retained by the organization (or distributed to owners in for-profit organizations).

Long-term improvement requires that future budgets be reduced as budget savings are introduced, but this feature creates at least two problems: First, will managers and employees pursue cost-saving improvements for a one-time bonus if future budgets will be cut? One possible solution is to provide multiyear, declining-percentage shared-saving distributions to workers. Second, will managers and employees take undesirable actions to reduce costs that undermine the goods and services? Shared-saving programs should also monitor other factors such as sales, returns, and defects to ensure that short-term savings are not achieved by jeopardizing long-term success.

▶ ## An Example of Incremental Budgeting: The Medicare Trust Funds

Assume you must budget Medicare expenditures for 2016, an exercise perfectly suited for incremental budgeting as the primary goal is to estimate the total monetary outlay. **TABLE 6.2** presents Medicare expenditures from 1990 through 2015. If you were budgeting Medicare expenditures, you would note the total and its

three components: hospital (Part A), physician and outpatient (Part B), and pharmaceutical (Part D) expenditures. Compound growth rates for the total and its components are provided in the last row.

You could rely on the 7.3% overall increase in total expenditures and budget $694,690 billion $\left(\$647,356\text{M}_{2015\,\text{base}}*1.073\right)$ for 2016. This would overstate expenditures, given that the total expenditures jumped with the beginning of the Part D program in 2006 and only Part A has grown by less than 5.0% over the past 10 years. A better method would estimate the growth in each component and sum it all up as ($275,693M [Part A] $*$ 1.050) + ($279,950M [Part B] $*$ 1.076) + ($91,714 [Part D] $*$ 1.084). Fifteen-year compound growth rates (2000–2015) were used for Part A and B expenditures and a 9-year rate was used for Part D since the program began full operation in 2006. The sum of the components, $690,129M, is $4,562M lower than $694,690M calculated using total expenditures and highlights the desirability of disaggregating data when variables of different magnitudes increase at different rates. Until 2015, Part A was the largest component of Medicare, and it was increasing at the slowest rate. In 2000, Part A was 42.5% larger than Part B, but the higher growth rate of Part B resulted in physician and outpatient expenditures accounting for the largest share of Medicare expenditures in 2015.

FIGURE 6.6 demonstrates that Medicare expenditures have steadily increased since 1990, with a one-time decline in 1998. Hospital expenditures, Part A, leveled off after 2012, but physician and outpatient and pharmaceutical expenditures continued to increase rapidly. Accuracy in budgeting is needed as expenditures are financed through four sources: Federal Insurance Contributions Act (FICA) payroll taxes, general revenue, premiums, and interest. Medicare expenditures in 2015 exceeded income by $3,534M, and as premiums and interest are in decline, deficits must be plugged by increases in payroll taxes

TABLE 6.2 Medicare Expenditures (in Millions)

Year	Part A	Part B	Part D	Total
1990	$66,785	$44,118	$0	$110,903
2000	$132,803	$93,180	$0	$225,983
2004	$172,649	$139,300	$440	$312,389
2005	$187,456	$153,553	$1,098	$342,106
2006	$198,164	$170,460	$44,342	$412,967
2007	$209,466	$183,678	$50,252	$443,395
2008	$225,568	$183,514	$53,892	$462,974
2009	$239,348	$205,857	$57,868	$503,073
2010	$245,445	$215,327	$62,496	$523,268
2011	$257,556	$226,280	$66,010	$549,846
2012	$263,861	$240,427	$68,484	$572,772
2013	$270,105	$248,234	$72,932	$591,271
2014	$270,513	$266,513	$82,012	$619,038
2015	$275,692	$279,950	$91,714	$647,356
Compound growth rate	4.99%	7.61%	8.41%	7.27%

and transfers from general revenue. In 2016, $20.2B was transferred from general revenue to Medicare and thus reduced the funding available for other federal departments.

The bottom line for Medicare should be no change in trust funds; revenues equal expenditures with no profit or loss. However, Medicare trust funds have been decreasing since 2008 and are putting increasing pressure on the federal budget. The decline in the trust funds has eroded, and will continue to erode, interest income, and the government will have to determine how the program can be brought to a sustainable basis. The government has one of two choices: increase revenue and/or decrease expenditures. If revenue

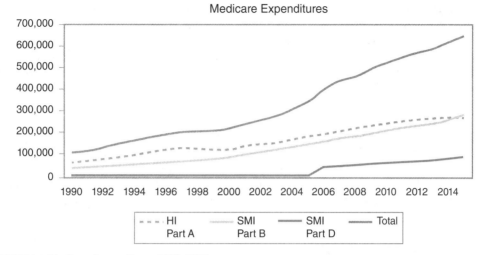

FIGURE 6.6 Medicare Expenditures, 1990–2015

is increased, will it come from higher federal income taxes (general revenue), earmarked payroll taxes (FICA), premiums, or some combination? Attempts to reduce expenditures are shouted down as "healthcare rationing," but it is easy to see that Medicare, as currently structured, is unsustainable, as total expenditures increased by 7.3% annually from 2000 through 2015, while the U.S. economy grew by 2.2%. The goal of budgeting should be to highlight imbalances between expenditures and income, whenever and wherever they arise, and motivate decision-makers to effective, sustainable corrections.

Summary

This chapter focuses on the most basic type of budgeting—that of keeping an existing operation rolling for another year with no major changes in activity. The focus of incremental budgeting is to control the use and cost of inputs. Incremental budgeting can be completed in four steps: identify the expenditure base for object codes, identify expected changes in input prices, multiply the expenditure base by the inflation factor, and add or subtract resources for known or anticipated changes. Summing the object codes produces the budget request.

Incremental budgets are appropriate for stable environments—those without major fluctuations in demand, income, or production methods. An incremental budget would be undesirable in situations in which it is either impossible to meet the budget (the work cannot be produced within the financial constraints invoked) or too lax (the budget provides too little incentive for the efficient use of resources). The trade-off is value versus cost; a budget should encourage value maximization, and when the financial targets are impossible to meet, managers will face undesirable choices when it becomes apparent that revenues and/or expenses will not meet expectations. Managers will have to make spur-of-the-moment decisions instead of proactively building a deliberate plan. When budgets are too lax, resources are wasted and poor practices are institutionalized. In either case, costs may be higher than needed—the choice facing managers is to invest time early building good budgets or invest more time later trying to pick up the pieces of poor budgets.

The goal of incremental budgeting is to ensure resources are used wisely. In the real world, budgets often result in ensuring that all allocated funds are spent (to avoid unspent monies from being removed from future budgets), and managers seeking to preserve their funding levels are often less concerned with what they get for an expenditure than ensuring the flow of future funds. To avoid this dilemma, evaluation of incremental budgets should be shifted from whether actual expenditures were less than or equal to the budget to whether budget savings can be shared with managers and employees to encourage efficiency. The sharing of cost savings would incent managers and employees to identify and reduce overproduction, overprocessing, unnecessary motion and transport, defects, underutilized and idle resources, and excessive inventories. There are better ways of achieving efficiency, but gain-sharing programs, at least, alter the most dysfunctional incentive provided by incremental budgets. The chapter "Flexible Budgeting" will take us further along the road to efficiency by tying budget allocations to output rather than inputs.

Key Terms and Concepts

Annualizing	Producer price index (PPI)	Productivity
Marginal rate of technical substitution		

Review Questions

1. Explain the steps in constructing an incremental budget.
2. Explain how a manager can unnecessarily increase or pad his or her budget.
3. When should an incremental budget be employed?
4. Explain the strengths and weaknesses of incremental budgeting.
5. Describe gain sharing and explain how gain sharing can be employed to encourage efficiency.

Problems

1. Assume your nursing unit must provide services for 489 patients per month and these services can be provided by LPNs earning $25.48 per hour ($53,000 per year) or NAs earning $14.90 per hour ($31,000). An LPN can manage six patients per day, and an NA can handle four patients. (A) Who should be employed to deliver care, and what will be the expected monthly cost for those services? (B) Assume a shortage of NAs in the local market increases their wage to $17.58 per hour ($36,566 per year). What will be the expected monthly cost for providing care for 489 patients after the salary increase?

2. A hospital has opened an urgent care center to siphon off some of the more common reasons for emergency room visits that do not require emergent care. The budget report, BudgetCh06, Problem 6.1 tab, shows the urgent care center's expenses for 2017 and the actual and budgeted expenses for the first 7 months of 2018. The CEO has requested that all department heads submit their 2019 operating budgets by Wednesday, March 1, 2017. The 2019 fiscal year begins on January 1, 2019. The 2019 budget should be based on actual expenses incurred during the first 7 months of 2018.

Object code	Description	2017	Actual 2018	Budget 2018	Budget 2019
4010	Physician salaries	$960,000	$585,306	$576,800	_____
4020	Nursing staff salaries	$1,380,000	$857,157	$829,150	_____
4030	Management and clerical salaries	$780,000	$466,971	$468,650	_____
4110	FICA	$238,680	$143,397	$143,407	_____
4120	Health insurance	$390,000	$238,760	$234,325	_____
4130	Retirement	$124,800	$76,763	$74,984	_____
4140	Unemployment	$31,200	$18,323	$18,746	_____
4211	Medications	$148,152	$91,687	$89,015	_____
4212	Medical instruments	$102,792	$64,287	$61,761	_____
4214	Bandages, gauze, etc.	$57,468	$34,140	$34,529	_____
4216	Latex gloves, gowns, etc.	$40,416	$24,476	$24,283	_____
4216	Sterile wipes	$26,820	$15,780	$16,114	_____
4250	Office supplies	$115,200	$69,388	$69,216	_____
4280	Cleaning supplies	$39,048	$23,103	$23,461	_____
4310	Rent	$144,000	$89,251	$86,520	_____
4350	Maintenance	$13,764	$11,245	$8,270	_____
4410	Electricity	$10,788	$6,684	$6,482	_____
4420	Gas	$18,504	$11,215	$11,118	_____
4430	Water and sewage	$6,756	$4,225	$4,059	_____
4440	Telephone	$3,228	$2,004	$1,939	_____
4930	Housekeeping	$36,000	$21,694	$21,630	_____

(continues)

Object code	Description	2017	Actual 2018	Budget 2018	Budget 2019
4940	Travel/professional meetings/meals	$7,908	$4,744	$4,751	_____
4945	Professional insurance	$22,380	$15,669	$13,447	_____
4950	Education and Training (CME)	$29,856	$17,994	$17,938	_____
4960	Other expenses	$57,732	$35,955	$34,687	_____
		$4,785,492	$2,930,217	$2,875,283	_____

CME, continuing medical education.

Salary and fringe benefit (object codes 4000–4199) increases for all personnel should be estimated at 4.0%, except for health insurance (object code 4120), which is expected to increase by 8.0%. Input price increases for supplies and other costs (object codes 4200–4960) should be increased by 3.0%, except for medications (5.0% increase) and profession insurance (10.0%). All increases are effective January 1, 2019.

3. Recalculate the budget in problem 2, assuming patient visits are expected to increase by 2.0% in 2019. The following expenses should not be increased for the expected patient volume increase: management and clerical salaries, rent, travel/professional meetings/meals, and professional insurance. What is the new budget request? How much did the volume-adjusted budget request increase over the original request?

4. You are budgeting staff salaries and wages (object code 4020) for the urgent care center. Calculate the budget request using last year's budget, the current year budget, and YTD actual as the expenditure base. Which base provides the highest allocation, which the lowest, and what is the total difference in the budget request between the highest and the lowest base?

5. Assume you have the discretion to select the expenditure base to use for each object code. Select the base that maximizes your budget. What is the total budget request? How much of an increase in the new budget over the one calculated in problem 2 using YTD actual expenses?

References

Hayek, F. A. (1945). The use of knowledge in society. *American Economic Review, 35*(4), 519–530.

United States Census Bureau. (2015). *FFF: The 2015 holiday season*. Retrieved November 2, 2016, from https://www.census.gov/newsroom/facts-for-features/2015/cb15-ff25.html.html

CHAPTER 7
Flexible Budgeting

CHAPTER OBJECTIVES

1. Explain the steps in building a flexible budget.
2. Estimate budget standards for variable costs.
3. Construct a flexible budget.
4. Restate the flexible budget for actual output.
5. Evaluate the strengths and weaknesses of flexible budgeting.
6. Incorporate nonproductive/nonvalue-adding activities into the budget.

▶ Introduction

After a budget is produced and approved, managers are expected to produce the forecasted output, while remaining at or below budgeted expenses. When expenses come in overbudget, managers are often required to explain why spending exceeded the budget and take action to ensure they do not continue to consume more resources than they were allocated. The budget provides half the information managers need to identify why they spent more or less than budgeted. The other half, what was actually spent, must be compared to the budget to determine whether variances are acceptable. Are managers providing proper oversight to inputs, processes, and outputs? Are expenses running significantly overbudget, and will overruns jeopardize the goals or existence of the organization?

While incremental budgets are easy to produce, they do not shed much light on operations, given the changes that can arise between when the budget was assembled and when production occurs. Budget variances arise due to changes in prices, efficiency, intensity, and volume. Operations consume more resources than they are budgeted when input prices increase, efficiency is reduced (taking more time to complete a task or redoing tasks that were not preformed properly the first time), the intensity of treatment increases (more tasks are required to produce an output), and/or the volume of patients treated (output) increases. Incremental budgeting systems do not facilitate identification of variances, but flexible (i.e., performance) budgets incorporate changes in patient volume into expense calculations and can also account for changes in the intensity of work required due to sicker patients.

While incremental budgets provide a simple means to estimate future expenses, they do little to facilitate control over operations. Incremental budgeting has many advantages, but it also has glaring deficiencies. Incremental budgeting is most appropriate for efficient operations where output and revenue do not fluctuate and production methods are stable. Unfortunately, these conditions rarely hold in the real world. While the public statements of most organizations, including healthcare providers, indicate they are producing the maximum amount of output possible for the resources they consume; a short talk with front-line workers or observation of operations reveals a multitude of ways output could be increased, quality improved, and costs reduced. Advocates of Lean report that major increases in productivity (20%–80%), reductions in inventory (50%–90%), shorter process times (50%–99%), lower space requirements (30%–50%), and lower overhead (10%–30%) were achieved when Lean principles were implemented (Protzman, Mayzell, & Kepchar, 2011, p. 3).

Even when maximum efficiency is achieved, it may not continue because of fluctuations in output and the introduction of new production processes. Continual changes in output and production technologies challenge managers to appropriately adjust staffing and other resource levels. The failure to adjust resource use to output produces excessive staffing and wasted time during slack periods and inadequate staffing and poor performance at peak periods. Organizations facing large fluctuations in output with inefficient processes need a dynamic budget system to focus employee attention on opportunities to improve performance and reduce cost.

Flexible budgets focus on efficiency and output compared to an incremental budget's emphasis on total expense and input use (**FIGURE 7.1**). Flexible budgeting says that resources should not be fixed 6 months prior to the start of the budget year on the basis of what managers think will be produced, but rather, resource use should depend on what is actually produced during the fiscal year. Actual output cannot be known with certainty until after the close of the budget period, so a preliminary flexible budget is created. But the budget to which department managers are held accountable is determined retrospectively on the basis of actual output. Expense allocations in a flexible budget increase when output (or intensity) is higher than projected and decrease when output is lower than estimated. Flexible budgeting adds uncertainty to management as the ultimate spending constraint cannot be known in advance. Unlike incremental budgeting, the budget to which managers will be held accountable varies with the difference between forecasted and actual output. This uncertainty requires more vigilance from management but has the advantage of automatically supplying additional resources when output increases.

The key to flexible budgeting is understanding how costs should change with fluctuations in output. The performance of managers

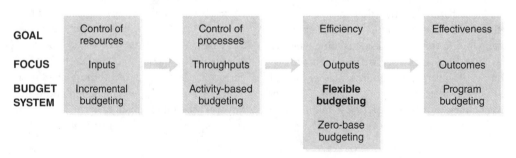

GOAL	Control of resources	Control of processes	Efficiency	Effectiveness
FOCUS	Inputs	Throughputs	Outputs	Outcomes
BUDGET SYSTEM	Incremental budgeting	Activity-based budgeting	**Flexible budgeting**	Program budgeting
			Zero-base budgeting	

FIGURE 7.1 Budgeting Systems

and departments is judged on their ability to manage the cost per output rather than meeting a total budget constraint. Flexible budgeting creates a moving target; managers will be evaluated against a budget constraint that can only be known *after* production occurs. Flexible budgets clearly specify what each unit of output should cost and provide more resources when output increases and cut budgets when output falls. In competitive markets, it is imperative managers and the budgeting and accounting systems understand what additional resources are required to produce one more unit of output and what resources will not be needed if output declines.

While the estimate of budget year output remains a key to constructing the budget, a second critical factor is the identification of variable and fixed costs that should and should not change with fluctuations in output. Resources and costs directly related to output should increase when actual output exceeds forecasted output and decrease when actual output does not meet the forecast. It is easy to see that Ford Motor Company must purchase five more tires, one engine block, one windshield, and roughly 16 hours of labor for every car it manufactures. On the other hand, many of Ford's costs will be unaffected by increases or decreases in output and these fixed costs (the cost of occupying space or the temperature of the facilities) should only change when input prices change.

It is more difficult to see how a healthcare provider's resource use should change as the number of patients treated increases or decreases, given the nondeterministic nature of healthcare treatment. One more patient may not impose any additional costs on the provider, beyond the medical supplies used, given the different condition of patients, different medical practice styles, and current utilization of resources. Healthcare organizations may not incur any additional expenses for labor, administration, accounting, occupancy, or utilities when an additional patient is seen, and

they may be able to increase output by dozens, if not hundreds, of patients before some costs increase.

▶ The Flexible Budgeting Process

In many ways, an incremental budget is a highly unnatural and artificial approach to life. Incremental budgeting assumes managers can look into the future, that is, determine what outputs will be demanded, how much consumers are willing to pay for a good or service, what resources will be needed to produce the output, and what the cost will be to acquire the resources, and nothing will upset these assumptions. An incremental budget is similar to a personal budget for someone on a fixed income. Any unexpected expense must be handled by adjusting the person's existing set of expenditures; for example, a large, unfunded auto repair may require reductions in planned entertainment, furniture, or other purchases to stay within the income.

"Unfunded" is the key word; people on fixed incomes often set aside part of their incomes for major expenditures like auto repairs or vacations. Problems arise if the amount set aside is insufficient to meet a higher-than-anticipated expense or the need for the expenditure comes sooner than expected. In both cases, the individual will not have sufficient resources set aside to meet the required outlay. In the first case, the problem arises from the inability to anticipate cost and in the second the inability to set aside enough income (fully fund the expense) in a short period. Life, health, home, and auto insurance are means to set aside funds to meet high-cost, infrequent events. One key to success is the ability to handle unexpected contingencies: a business that consumes every dime of its income may be unable to survive events that dramatically increase expenses or reduce revenues.

Flexible budgeting is most appropriate when income is directly related to output; higher output facilitates sales that increase revenue, and lower output results in less sales and revenue. A higher demand for output not only increases costs but also provides the means to fully or partially meet the higher expenses. In a personal budget, this is analogous to buying more goods and services when you work overtime and reducing planned expenditures when your hours are cut.

A budget that recognizes that revenue is tied to output should also acknowledge that department expenses will increase as output increases and vice versa. Given the need to tie expenditures to revenue, it is essential to identify what expenses do and do not change with changes in output. The use of personal expenses again helps illuminate the challenge. In a personal budget, there are expenses that cannot be changed in the short run and spending that can be immediately altered. If your income substantially increases or decreases, you could immediately alter the amount of money spent on food, clothing, entertainment, and utilities, while housing, transportation, and medical care may not be immediately changeable. If your income drops, you could immediately purchase less expensive food items, eliminate clothing and entertainment expenditures, and turn down your thermostat. Your mortgage or rent expense may not be alterable in the short run, reducing medical expenditures may not be desirable, and traveling to and from work will not get any shorter, but side trips could be reduced. The nature of your expenditures confronts you with a limited set of options to respond to reductions in income. When your income increases, you may make the purchases you previously thought you could not afford—Parkinson's law rides again.

The option set is broader for organizations where production and sales translate directly into income. Organizations that sell their products to customers automatically generate higher revenues to cover the cost of higher production. Whether higher output and sales generate sufficient revenues to cover **marginal or incremental cost** is the challenge these organizations face. Assuming customers want higher output and they are willing to pay a price that exceeds the average variable cost, all incremental costs will be covered as output increases. When revenues increase with increases in output, the budget system should augment expense allocations; when output and revenues decrease, expenses should be cut.

Flexible budgeting assumes that input use and expenses vary directly with changes in output and that marginal costs can be identified. The third assumption is that future output cannot be determined with sufficient precision to create an accurate incremental budget. Like incremental budgeting, flexible budgeting is focused on the department and its internal operation over the next year—a 1-year horizon. Resource allocations in the preliminary budget are estimated using forecasted output, but the final budget is retroactively determined on the basis of actual output. The primary incentive in a flexible budget is to maintain or increase efficiency, that is, hold the cost per output constant or reduce it.

The Budget Building Process

Constructing a flexible budget requires nine steps (compared to the four steps needed to create an incremental budget), beginning with defining the output measure and estimating the output quantity. **BOX 7.1** lists the nine steps in constructing a flexible budget.

The output measure should have a direct and significant impact on the type and amount of work performed, that is, it should predict resource consumption. While a hospital may define output as total inpatient admissions for purposes of estimating revenue, departments such as nursing or ancillary units require a higher level of granularity. A nursing unit output measure may be patient days in order to recognize the impact of changes in the length of stay, that is, costs will be significantly higher for a nursing unit that treats 80 cases per month staying 5 days than an equal number of patients who stay 4 days. Similarly, labs will want to base their workload on the expected number of lab tests rather than the number of patients. Beyond simple admissions or patient days, managers of nursing and ancillary units may want to know the intensity of care that patients will require. The Medicare case mix index (CMI) is a frequently used index to identify hospitals serving patients with more intense medical needs and compare performance across hospitals that treat different patient populations. Increases in the percentage of patients with major complications and comorbidities should increase patient days, the number of lab tests performed, revenue, and a multitude of other factors.

The output measure should be readily available and, if possible, inexpensive to collect. An example of a poor output measure would be hours of operation. While this measure is easy to collect, it may not indicate what is being produced, that is, the number of patients treated. In addition, while this measure affects costs, it may be incapable of measuring the variability of output. In the extreme case, a medical practice could extend operating hours, incur higher payroll expenses, but see no additional patients. After defining the output measure, output (Q) must be estimated for the budget year.

Step 2 requires identifying how work is to be accomplished: How many units of labor, capital, and supplies are required per unit of output? What types of inputs are needed, and how will their cost change with changes in output? Are costs fixed, variable with output, variable with other inputs, or step? A nursing unit budget for management and clerical salaries would be fixed versus staff salaries that increase in a stepwise fashion when specified patient/staff ratios are exceeded. Medical supplies should rise and fall with the patient census: during high census periods, patients consume more supplies, and conversely, costs

---

BOX 7.1 The Flexible Budgeting Process

1. Define the output measure and estimate the budget year output.
2. Identify how work will be performed and what inputs will be required.
3. Develop productivity standards (input per output) **for variable costs**.
4. Translate productivity standards into cost standards (dollars per output).
5. Inflate cost standards for expected price increases to produce budget standards.
6. Multiply the budget standards by estimated output to obtain budget allocations.
7. Develop budget allocations **for fixed costs** (administrative salaries, health insurance, rent, etc.) using the incremental budgeting process (select an expenditure base, identify the inflation factor, and multiply the base by the inflation factor).
8. Modify for expected changes in output quality, production processes, regulatory mandates and so on to get a **preliminary budget**.
9. At the end of the fiscal period, recalculate variable costs by multiplying budget standards by actual output to get a **final budget**.

---

fall when fewer patients are hospitalized. How much cost should change can only be determined by understanding the relationships between inputs and output.

After cost behavior is defined, **productivity standards, that is**, input units per output, must be developed for variable and step costs. The budget for variable and step inputs is based on the relationship between how much output a unit of input can produce and how many units of output are expected. Productivity standards are often based on past performance, and similar to the expenditure base, in Chapter 6, the standard could be constructed using data from the last completed fiscal year, the year-to-date

(YTD) actual, or the current-year budget. For staff salaries, a nursing unit would identify how many registered nurse (RN), licensed practical nurse (LPN), and nurse assistant (NA) hours are required per patient day. The head nurse could divide total paid hours by current patient days to determine staff hours

per patient day. For example, if paid RN hours are 26,209 and 6,535 patient days of care have been provided, the productivity standard is 4.01 hours of RN time per inpatient day. The **TABLE 7.1** tab in the BudgetCh07.xlsx file provides the number of RN hours paid in the last completed year and the number of patient days

TABLE 7.1 Calculating Variable Nursing Hours

Summary Output: RN Hours

Regression Statistics						
Multiple R	0.8111					
R square	0.6579					
Adjusted R square	0.6237					
Standard error	159.99					
Observations	12					

ANOVA

	df	SS	MS	F	Significance F	
Regression	1	492,352	492,352	19.23	0.0014	
Residual	10	255,973	25,597.3			
Total	11	748,325				

	Coefficients	Standard Error	t-Stat	P-value	Lower 95%	Upper 95%
Intercept	−1,045.6	737.85	−1.42	0.1869	−2,689.6	598.47
Patient days	5.93	1.35	4.39	0.0014	2.92	8.94

produced. Similarly, the head nurse would calculate the time needed for other staff members and the number of supply items consumed per patient day. Other managers, like a lab manager, would want to establish similar standards on the basis of their output measure and the number of hours and supplies needed, for example, hours per lab test, machine time per test, and supplies per test.

In addition to using historical averages, there are other ways to establish productivity standards, including **benchmarks**, time and motion studies, the high/low method, and **regression**. Benchmarking relies on industry standards to determine how much of an input has been consumed to produce an output. For example, *Almanac of Hospital Financial and Operating Indicators* reports that the average adjusted full-time equivalent (FTE) per occupied bed (patient days $*$ CMI) in 2015 was 3.30 (Optum360°, 2016). Managers can use this average and the 25th and 75th percentiles of 2.75 and 4.05 to assess how effectively they are using their labor resources.

A second method is **time and motion studies**, where an analyst records how much time is used to complete an activity. In the operating room, an analyst could record the time needed to close a surgical incision or the time to complete a surgery, from entry into the surgical suite to transfer to the recovery room. Recording the time for a single activity such as checking vital signs or administering medication is simpler than determining how much staff time is required to provide 24-hour nursing care.

The third and fourth methods are based on historical input use; the historical average used produced 4.01 hours per patient day but assumes all hours are variable, which is not the case as minimum staffing levels are required and administrative positions do not vary with output. The **high/low method** recognizes that a minimum level of resources is required for the minimum output level and calculates the increase in inputs corresponding with higher output. The minimum resource level or fixed component may be mandated by regulation.

For example, a pharmacist may only have enough work to occupy him or her for 6 hours, but regulations require round-the-clock pharmaceutical presence, so the pharmacist must be paid for an entire 8-hour shift.

$$\text{Variable input per unit} = \frac{\left(Y_{\mathrm{H}} - Y_{\mathrm{L}}\right)}{\left(X_{\mathrm{H}} - X_{\mathrm{L}}\right)}, \quad (7.1)$$

where Y_{H} is the inputs used in the highest-output month, Y_{L} is the inputs used in lowest-output month, X_{H} is the output in the highest-output month, and X_{L} is the output in the lowest-output month.

Equation 7.1 produces the variable input component, that is, how many additional units of an input have been used when output increases above the minimum output. The high/low method finds that 7.23 RN hours are needed for every patient day above 499 ((2556 − 1804) / (603 − 499)); the data is available in the Table 7.1 tab in the BudgetCh07.xlsx file. The high/low method assumes that a baseline RN staff level of 1804 hours is needed to serve the minimum number of patients, that is, 499 patient days; for each patient day above 499, the RN hours are expected to increase by 7.23. When 550 patient days are expected, the total RN hours should be 2172.8 (1804 + ((550 − 499) $*$ 7.23)).

The fourth method of calculating the resources needed to produce output is regression. Regression creates a best-fitting line, $Y = \alpha + \beta X$, where Y is the total calculated resource need; α is the intercept, denoting the amount of resource needed when output is zero (the fixed component); and β shows how many units of an input are required to produce one additional unit of output (the variable component, X). Table 7.1 provides the regression output: α states that at zero patient days, the unit will need −1045.56 RN hours, and 5.93 RN hours are needed for every additional patient day produced. The adjusted R^2 reports that 62.4% of the change in nursing hours is explained by changes in the number of patient days delivered. When 550 patient days are expected, the total RN hours should be 2216.2 (−1045.56 + (550 ∗ 5.93)).

The method used to determine the productivity standard affects the expected resource cost, and budget managers may want to aggregate methods to produce a more accurate composite estimate, *or* they could select the most advantageous method to maximize their budget. Given the historical average, the high/low method, and regression produced varying estimates of the impact of patient days on labor hours, a manager may want to use the average; in this case, 5.72 ((4.01 + 7.23 + 5.93) / 3) RN hours would be needed per patient day.

The fourth step translates the productivity standard, input units per output, into an input cost per output, that is, a **cost standard**. If 4.01 hours of RN time are required per patient day on the basis of the historical average, the cost standard will be 4.01 hours ∗ average RN hourly wage. Similarly, if 12 units of supplies are used per patient day, the budget standard is 12 ∗ average supply price. Once cost standards are created for all variable costs, managers should know with a reasonable degree of certainty how their costs change as output increases or decreases. A head nurse should be able to predict how much the total expenses will increase as patient days on a unit increase or how much expenses should decrease if patient days are less than expected. In health care, labor costs are often step costs, which complicates cost estimates: One nurse is required if one patient is on a unit, and he or she may be able to handle six patients at a time; however, if a seventh patient is added to the unit, a second nurse may be required. While 4.01 RN hours per patient day may be the productivity standard, the organization may have to pay a nurse for a 40-hour week regardless of the number of patients served. Similarly, the lab manager may calculate the labor and supply costs per test, but supplies may be the only true variable cost.

The second and third steps, identifying input units and developing a productivity standard, are not essential; cost standards can be based on historical input expense divided by historical output rather than being developed from the number of units used multiplied by input prices. This shortcut eliminates the need to count input units and identify input prices. In **FIGURE 7.2**, if the current budget is used as the cost standard, the organization would budget $375.01 ($1,235,642 / 3,213) per patient day for staff salaries, and this could be the basis for calculating the 2019 budget. A cost standard of $295.98 per patient day was produced using the high/low method and $243.93 using regression (Figure 7.2 tab in the BudgetCh07 .xlsx file). Using cost information (versus input units) is useful for inputs like supplies that include a multitude of different items with different prices. The drawback of using total expense divided by total output to calculate cost standards is it does not allow employees to determine whether the quantity or price of inputs is changing when costs increase or decrease.

Given the cost standard was constructed on historical data, the cost per unit of output produced in the base period must be inflated for expected price increases in the budget year to produce the **budget standard** (cost standard ∗ (1 + expected inflation)). Given a cost standard for staff salaries of $343.92 per patient day and an inflation factor of 3.0%, the budget standard will be $354.23 ($343.92 ∗ (1 + 0.03)). The expectation of incurring $354.23 in staff salaries per patient day assumes that salaries increase by 3.0%, no more or less and the amount of employee time (hours) per patient day does not change, that is, productivity is constant.

Step 6 multiplies the budget standard (step 5) by forecasted output (step 1) for each variable input. Given the budget standard of $354.23 per day and a projection of 6,524 patient days in 2014, the total salary expense for staff should be $2,311,015.

Step 7 calculates the budget allocation for fixed inputs such as administrative salaries, health insurance, and rent, which should not change with changes in output, and uses the incremental budgeting process introduced

Object Code	Description	Step	Last Year 2017	YTD Actual 2018	Bases YTD Budget 2018	Steps 3 and 4 Cost Standard	Projected Actual 2018	Step 5 1 + Inflation Factor	Budget Standard	Step 6 Budget Request 2019
4010	Management & clerical staff	F	$331,200	$176,543	$180,000	12/6	$353,086	1.03		$363,679 Step 7
4020	Staff salaries & wages	V	2,066,350	1,235,642	1,105,000	$343.92		1.03	$354.23	2,311,015
4040	Overtime	V	33,120	23,833	18,000	$5.60		1.03	$5.77	37,645
4050	Agency & Temporary	V	374,400	156,115	204,000	$63.49		1.03	$65.40	426,649
4110	FICA	%	185,946	109,855	99,680	7.65%		1.03		240,287
4120	Health insurance	F	278,760	149,857	151,500	12/6	299,714	1.06		317,697 Step 7
4130	Retirement	%	121,534	71,801	65,150	5.00%		1.03		135,718
4140	Unemployment	%	26,737	15,796	14,333	1.10%		1.03		34,551
4210	Floor Medications	V	22,398	13,589	12,775	$3.98		1.05	$4.17	27,237
4212	Medical instruments	V	18,596	5,798	9,000	$2.80		1.02	$2.86	18,640
4214	Bandages, guaze...	V	9,741	5,643	5,110	$1.59		1.02	$1.62	10,583
4216	Latex gloves, gowns...	V	52,899	32,145	29,383	$9.14		1.02	$9.33	60,854
4218	Sterile wipes	V	5,211	2,659	2,555	$0.80		1.02	$0.81	5,292
4250	Office supplies	V	8,452	4,268	4,599	$1.43		1.02	$1.46	9,525
4280	Cleaning supplies	V	1,202	569	500	$0.16		1.02	$0.16	1,036
4350	Biomedical repairs/maintenance	F	5,244	3,869	3,000	12/6	7,738	1.01		7,815 Step 7
4410	Electricity	F	2,453	1,156	1,200	12/6	2,312	1.04		2,404 Step 7
4440	Telephone	F	5,794	2,645	2,880	12/6	5,290	1.01		5,343 Step 7
4930	Housekeeping	V	138,240	72,000	72,000	$22.41		1.01	$22.63	147,658
4940	Travel/prof meetings/meals	F	35,789	14,523	17,850	12/6	29,046	1.01		29,336 Step 7
4950	CME	F	8,425	3,688	4,600	12/6	7,376	1.01		7,450 Step 7
4960	Other expenses	F	4,953	1,258	1,655	12/6	2,516	1.01		2,541 Step 7
			$3,737,444	$2,103,252	$2,004,769					$4,204,974
	Patient days		6,536	3,295	3,213		6,590			6,524 Step 1
	Per day census		17.9	18.1	17.7	budget	proj.actual			17.9
	Occupancy		89.5%	90.5%	88.3%					89.4%

FIGURE 7.2 Budget Request Worksheet

in Chapter 6. Managers select an expenditure base; annualize partial-year data, if used, to obtain a 12-month estimate; identify an inflation factor; and multiply the annualized expense by the inflation factor to determine the budget for each fixed input object code. The only factor that should affect outlays for these resources is changes in input prices (inflation); there should be no change in the number of units consumed, so there is no need to develop productivity, cost, or budget standards.

The final step in constructing a preliminary budget is the same as in incremental budgeting: managers should modify their budgets for expected changes in expenses. New production methods, work processes, or regulations (waste disposal, reporting requirements, etc.) may be introduced that lead to new steps or expenses or expand or reduce the time required to complete present tasks, which should be incorporated in budget standards or captured in new object codes.

Comparing the flexible budget to the incremental budget originally calculated in Chapter 6, Figure 6.3 shows that the flexible budget allocates 9.2% less resources for staff salaries, $2,311,015 versus $2,545,423, because of the lower forecasted output. Similarly, allocations for the other variable expenses have been reduced by 2.0%–11.0%. The amounts budgeted for fixed inputs are the same as in the incremental budget since their costs are independent of output. Overall, the flexible budget is 3.1% lower than the incremental budget because of the expected decline in patient days. While the budget reduction will not be welcomed by the unit manager or employees, who may see vacancies go unfilled and/or reductions in the use of overtime or agency nurses, the flexible budget should more accurately reflect what costs should be on the basis of what is expected to be produced. The second point needing emphasis is that the preliminary budget allocations may *not* be the budget to which the manager and department will be accountable. The final, flexed budget, step 9, is determined by what is actually produced: If total patient days equal 6,524, the department will have $4,204,974 to deliver care; if patient days exceed 6524, the budget will increase; and if patient days are less than 6524, the budget will be lower.

▶ Restating the Budget for Actual Output

The main objective of flexible budgeting is to create a budget that provides appropriate funding for the output produced. A flexible budget seeks to subtract the main element of uncertainty, predicting output, from budget calculations. Managers' performance should not be praised or criticized because they came in under- or overbudget simply because actual output is less than or greater than what was forecasted in the budget. To neutralize the impact of volume changes, the flexible budget is restated (or flexed) at the end of each budget period to reflect what the budget should have been if output could have been foreseen, and budget standards are met. The restated budget increases when output exceeds the forecast by the volume increase multiplied by the budget standards and decreases by the same amount for every unit actual output falls below forecast. Managers can then be evaluated on their ability to meet productivity standards rather than an inappropriate budget figure that does not reflect work actually performed.

FIGURE 7.3 restates expenses for the first 6 months of 2018 as the actual output, 3295 patient days, is running ahead of the budget forecast of 3213—step 6 in the flexible budgeting process. The flexed budget shows that all fixed costs remain the same as calculated in the preliminary budget and all variable costs as well as the expenses based on other inputs have increased. In 2018, the budget standard for staff salaries is $343.92 per patient day; the original budget estimated 3,213 patient days for a total staff salary expense of $1,105,000. If patient days had been estimated with complete accuracy in the preliminary budget, the salary expense would have been estimated at $1,133,201 for 3,295 patient days. The final budget to which the manager should be held accountable is increased by $28,201 (or $343.92 * 82 unanticipated patient days) to recognize that serving more patients requires higher expenses.

While output was 2.6% (3295 / 3213 patient days) higher than forecasted, the flexed budget only increased by 2.1% ($2,046,769 / $2,004,769) over the preliminary budget because of the presence of fixed costs. Figure 7.3 highlights the advantage of flexible budgeting. The

Object Code	Description	F/V	YTD Actual 2018	Preliminary YTD Budget 2018	Flexed YTD Budget 2018	Difference Flex & Prelim	Difference Act & Flex	% Diff Act & Flex
4010	Management & clerical staff	F	$176,543	$180,000	$180,000	0	-$3,457	-1.9%
4020	Staff salaries and wages	V	1,235,642	1,105,000	1,133,201	28,201	$102,441	9.3%
4040	Overtime	V	23,833	18,000	18,459	459	$5,374	29.9%
4050	Agency & Temporary	V	156,115	204,000	209,206	5,206	-$53,091	-26.0%
4110	FICA	%	109,855	99,680	101,872	2,193	$7,983	8.0%
4120	Health insurance	F	149,857	151,500	$151,500	0	-$1,643	-1.1%
4130	Retirement	%	71,801	65,150	66,583	1,433	$5,218	8.0%
4140	Unemployment	%	15,796	14,333	14,648	315	$1,148	8.0%
4210	Floor Medications	V	13,589	12,775	13,101	326	$488	3.8%
4212	Medical instruments	V	5,798	9,000	9,230	230	-$3,432	-38.1%
4214	Bandages, guaze...	V	5,643	5,110	5,240	130	$403	7.9%
4216	Latex gloves, gowns...	V	32,145	29,383	30,132	750	$2,013	6.8%
4218	Sterile wipes	V	2,659	2,555	2,620	65	$39	1.5%
4250	Office supplies	V	4,268	4,599	4,716	117	-$448	-9.7%
4280	Cleaning supplies	V	569	500	513	13	$56	11.2%
4350	Biomedical repairs/maintenance	F	3,869	3,000	3,000	0	$869	29.0%
4410	Electricity	F	1,156	1,200	1,200	0	-$44	-3.7%
4440	Telephone	F	2,645	2,880	2,880	0	-$235	-8.2%
4930	Housekeeping	V	72,000	72,000	73,838	1,838	-$1,838	-2.6%
4940	Travel/professional meetings/meals	F	14,523	17,850	17,850	0	-$3,327	-18.6%
4950	CME	F	3,688	4,600	4,600	0	-$912	-19.8%
4960	Other expenses	F	1,258	1,655	1,655	0	-$397	-24.0%
	Total Expenses		$2,103,252	$2,004,769	$2,046,045	$41,276	$57,207	2.9%

FIGURE 7.3 Restated 2018 YTD Budget

department's actual expenses were $98,484, or 4.9%, above the preliminary budget; however, $41,276 of this difference is due to the higher volume of patients, so the manager should only be concerned with the $57,307 difference between actual expenses and the flexed, final budget. This difference is primarily due to the increase in staff salaries (object code 4020). The manager should investigate whether the higher cost arose from more staff hours or higher wages.

The downside to budget flexing is that managers are expected to reduce costs when output falls below forecasted volume, so manager vigilance and action are paramount. Managers must be capable of recognizing when output is significantly less than forecasted and be willing to reduce resource use proportionately; reducing input consumption is especially sensitive and challenging if it requires cutting employee hours and income.

Flexible budgeting is a better tool to evaluate managerial effectiveness than incremental budgeting because it recognizes how expenses should change with output. The final budget is not tied to an estimate of output made more than a year before the fiscal year began but incorporates actual output into the final expense allocations. The key problem with incremental budgeting is that the actual output may be greater than the forecasted output but the department is still expected to operate within its budget. Staying within a budget is a difficult, if not impossible, task when resource use increases with output. A manager has the choice of going overbudget and potentially being poorly evaluated or meeting the budget by reducing the inputs used to produce a unit of output. If there was "slack" or "fat" in the budget, staying underbudget may be doable, but if the budget accurately predicted the cost for the planned level of output, the manager must reduce the quality of the output, that is, purchase lower-quality inputs, reduce the time devoted to certain actions (quality control, customer service, maintenance, etc.), and hope for the best. All of these actions may have substantial negative long-term consequences for

the organization, but managers may think they have no other alternative to stay within the budget. The failure of incremental budgets to recognize the reality of production processes is a primary reason budgeting is criticized.

Coming in underbudget is easy when actual output is less than the forecast used to construct the incremental budget. When actual output falls below the forecast, it is clear that less labor, supplies, utilities, etc., should be needed, but the incremental budget allocations remain fixed. A manager with declining output can come in underbudget (spend less than the total amount allocated), and his or her department can also be less efficient (an increase in the cost per unit produced). Budgeting should not be a perverse system that rewards employees for doing less and allows the cost of output to increase.

When actual output is higher than forecasted, meeting demand requires more resources than provided in the budget. In an incremental budgeting system, the department could operate more efficiently (reduce the cost per output) and still fail to meet its budget (spend more than the allocated amount). Restatement of expenses in the flexed budget ensures that the expected level of productivity (or cost per unit) becomes the focal point of employee efforts. Achieving goals, and potentially a superior performance evaluation, should not be made easier by falling output, nor should it be made more difficult by higher demand for the organization's products. Flexible budgeting, by recognizing that expenses should move directly with output, avoids the criticism that the budget is impossible to meet as output increases and unchallenging as output falls.

Flexible budgeting asks the question, did a manager effectively oversee his or her area of responsibility if output and expenses could have been forecasted with complete accuracy? Are actual expenses greater than, equal to, or less than restated expenses? This question can be more accurately answered after establishing what costs should be and restating the budget for differences between actual and forecasted output. Flexible budgeting eliminates the impact of changes in output and isolates the effect that changes in efficiency, input prices, and intensity have on budget variances. The availability of productivity and budget standards on a period-to-period basis should allow managers to recognize inefficiencies, price changes, and/or changes in the type of output produced on an ongoing basis and make adjustments to meet budget targets. Flexible budgeting recognizes that success, increasing demand for the product, should be rewarded with an increase in resources, while failure, falling demand, should be discouraged. Under an incremental budget, it is easy to see why managers may desire and pursue lower output since their salaries and department funding are unaffected and they will have less work.

Strengths of Flexible Budgeting

One of the primary strengths and challenges of flexible budgeting is it requires managers to achieve a deeper level of understanding of the production process. Flexible budgeting ties resources to output and asks what the relationship between inputs used and outputs produced is, or more precisely, how much should output increase when additional resources are committed to the production process? Flexible budgeting requires managers to know why they are consuming resources.

Second, flexible budgeting decentralizes the decision-making process. Senior management does not dictate the set of inputs that should be used or set rigid budget targets managers must meet. Rather, a system is created, hopefully agreed to by the department managers and senior management, that recognizes that resource use should be proportionate to the quantity of output produced and delegates the authority for resource use decisions to line managers (**BOX 7.2**).

Third, flexible budgeting encourages managers to seek ways of becoming more efficient. Will a different set of inputs be more efficient? Are there other production methods that will improve the productivity of inputs? Managers and employees who improve processes by

---

BOX 7.2 Strengths of a Flexible Budget

1. A flexible budget ties input use to actual output produced.
2. It decentralizes the decision-making process.
3. It encourages efficiency.
4. It produces more realistic budgets.
5. It simplifies review and evaluation.
6. It establishes appropriate incentives and empowers managers.

---

increasing productivity and reduce the cost per output should see their compensation increased. Any changes that reduce overprocessing, unnecessary motion and transport, defects, underutilized and idle resources, and inventory (seven of the eight Lean wastes) will reduce the cost per unit.

Fourth, the final budget is not tied to forecasted output and managers are not saddled with an unrealistic budget if output is higher than expected. Budgets grow with increases in actual output but only to the extent required, that is, by the amount of variable expense. Flexible budgets allow and require managers to fulfill their role as facilitators of work; when output is increasing, managers can supply their staff with more resources without seeking approval from superiors. Managers are not tied to a static and unrealistic budget and faced with undesirable options such as reducing product quality to meet a budget. On the other hand, flexible budgeting requires that in their role as stewards of resources, managers monitor what their employees are producing and reduce resources consumption when output declines. Managers are employed for their expertise and ability to control operations; flexible budgeting tests their knowledge and ability to adapt to unexpected changes in output.

Fifth, flexible budgeting focuses review and evaluation on a single measure: the cost per unit. Flexible budgeting recognizes that total cost may increase at the same time as cost per output declines. Managers who reduce the cost per unit should be rewarded over managers who simply reduce costs. Similarly, evaluating performance across time is simplified: is the cost per unit greater than, less than, or equal to the cost per unit adjusted for inflation achieved in prior periods?

Finally, flexible budgeting encourages managers and employees to increase efficiency and provides an easy-to-measure efficiency metric: the cost per output. When the inflation-adjusted cost per unit declines, employees should share the gain. To ensure employees understand that cost-saving efforts will be rewarded, the budget and performance evaluation system must explicitly pursue the same efficiency goal.

Weaknesses of Flexible Budgeting

The first drawback of flexible budgeting is the additional time and cost to prepare and finalize the budget. Initial preparation of the preliminary budget requires a greater understanding of operations and involves more steps than incremental budgeting. Restating the budget at the end of each fiscal period on the basis of actual output to create the final budget requires additional effort. Budget construction is no longer confined to the prospective phase but is required throughout the concurrent and retrospective budget phases. In the author's opinion, working intimately with a budget throughout the fiscal year emphasizes the point that budgeting is a tool to increase the effectiveness of management rather than simply estimate expenses.

Second, budget allocations shrink with decreases in output. This weakness is the flipside of the fourth strength; managers must be cognizant of lower-than-expected output and make the necessary reductions in input use to meet their restated budgets. Real-time information identifying output changes is required; it must be conveyed promptly to managers, and they must have the authority and willingness to make necessary adjustments to input use. Real-time adjustment in input use, especially reducing

resource use, is more difficult than meeting a static budget where the manager "knows" how much money he or she can spend in a budget period. In response to declining demand, managers may have to reduce employee hours to avoid having idle resources. Although reducing input use is necessary when output falls, one must recognize that cutbacks negatively affect employees and other input suppliers and are challenging for even the best managers.

On the other hand, the automatic increase in budget expenses that accompanies increases in output can be a problem if output cannot be sold (more output is produced than demanded by customers) or the revenue generated by sales does not cover marginal costs. A flexible budget may encourage overproduction, one of the eight Lean wastes. Those considering flexible budgeting must determine whether additional output can be sold and whether revenue from the sale of the output is sufficient (or other sources of revenues are available) to cover the additional expenses (**BOX 7.3**).

The third weakness of flexible budgeting is it does not produce a definitive prospective budget since the final budget will only be determined by the actual output after the end of the budget period. The budget is a moving target, and the impact of this weakness is magnified by the potential swings in output. The lack of

---

BOX 7.3 Weaknesses of a Flexible Budget

1. A flexible budget requires more time and cost to prepare and revise than an incremental budget.
2. It shrinks (grows) with decreases (increases) in output.
3. It does not produce a definitive budget since the actual budget will only be determined retrospectively once the actual volume is known.
4. It may not be feasible for an organization whose output is not tied to revenue.

a definitive budget may encourage managers to avoid commitments that could reduce long-term costs but will be uneconomical if demand falls. Flexible budgeting complicates management's job and requires a fast response to changes in output. Managers must assess how volatile output is and whether inputs can quickly be increased or reduced with changes in output.

Although it is logical to tie expenses to output, often output (especially in government and nonprofit agencies) may not impact revenues (think of an all-you-can eat buffet; if people suddenly begin to consume more or shift to more expensive food items, costs will increase, yet revenue will not increase). Organizations producing nonmarket-transacted goods and services using flexible budgeting could find themselves in a situation of increasing output and expenses with unchanged revenues. Managers would be free to increase their use of resources, but there may be no means to cover the higher costs.

Flexible budgeting should be used when the demand for output fluctuates widely from period to period and when revenues move proportionately with output, that is, sufficient funds are generated from sale of the output to defray higher production costs. A third consideration is that there should be no significant changes in production methods or the nature of the product produced that would alter historical productivity and cost standards.

The Budget Game

Any system can be gamed, and flexible budgeting is no exception. A manager attempting to maximize his or her budget must first determine whether future output will increase or decrease before he or she can effectively increase the budget. If the manager expects future output to increase, the easiest way to maximize the budget is to assume all expenses are variable. If all inputs were variable, a 10.0% increase in output would require a 10.0% increase in the budget. As seen in Figure 7.3, where the budget for the first 6 months of 2018 was restated for actual output, output increased by 2.6% but restated expenses only increased by 2.1% because of the presence of fixed costs. While a manager may not be able to sell the "all costs are variable" story, he or she could attempt to establish as many expenses as possible as variable.

After identifying an expense as variable, a second means to increase the budget is to select the highest cost standard. As seen in step 4, translating productivity standards into cost standards, three plausible estimates for the cost of RN services per patient day were calculated: the highest, $343.92, was based on the historical average, while the high/low method and regression estimated the cost at $295.98 and $243.93 per day, respectively. A manager expecting higher output would rather see the budget increase by $343.92 per patient day rather than lower amounts. These incentives are in addition to the budget-maximizing tactics introduced in the chapter "Incremental Budgeting": selecting the largest expenditure base, selecting the highest inflation factors for inputs, and applying the inflation factors to the first period of the budget year.

Managers expecting output to fall would make opposite choices. A manager expecting falling output would maintain all costs are fixed, that is, he or she will be unable to reduce any costs as output falls. While this will not be credible, the budget-maximizing manager would want to establish as many expenses as possible as fixed and thus not subject to reduction if output falls. After expenses are deemed variable, the manager should attempt to establish the lowest-possible cost standard. While the manager facing higher output wants his or her budget to increase by $343.92 per unit of output produced, those facing declining output want their budgets to fall by the lowest-possible amount, or $243.93 per patient day.

The risk faced by a manager who aggressively maximizes his or her budget is that the knife cuts both ways: A manager who has enjoyed large budget increases from overstating the percentage of expenses that are variable and using the highest-possible cost standard should see large budget reductions if output falls.

Similarly, a manager who did not have to reduce the budget when output fell as all costs were deemed fixed should be expected to produce more work with no more resources when output increases. While correctly identifying fixed and variable resources and the amount of variable expenses needed to produce a unit of output is vital to ensuring wise use of resources that will maximize the value of the organization, it is also in the interest of managers whose output varies dramatically to correctly estimate resource needs so that they have sufficient funding whether output is higher or lower than expected.

▶ Combining Flexible and Incremental Budgets

It is easy to see that flexible budgeting is a tool to assess how a department is fulfilling its primary production tasks, but we know that employees and departments must engage in low- or nonvaluing-adding activities. Frank Gilbreth categorized work into four groups:

Therblig 1: Essential or the highest-value work, including assembly, disassembly, or use. It includes activities that transform materials and meet a need.

Therblig 2: Preparation activities that support essential work, including loading, transporting, unloading, and setup.

Therblig 3: Incidental activities, including searching, finding, selecting, and inspecting—work that should be minimized.

Therblig 4: Unnecessary activities, which include planning, thinking, rest, and delay—work that should be eliminated.

Gilbreth's idea was to maximize essential work, optimize preparatory tasks, minimize incidental activity, and eliminate unnecessary and nonvaluing-adding activities (Protzman et al., 2011, p. 115).

Today, Gilbreth's contribution can be seen in **5S**, a five-step process to organize work to optimize output by: (1) **sorting** or decluttering inputs, eliminating unneeded resources and removing little-used resources from work areas; (2) **storing**, that is, a place for everything and everything in its place so that time is not wasted looking for tools and supplies; (3) **shining** or cleaning, to increase visibility and reduce hazards; (4) **standardizing** best practices, identifying evidence-based practices, and establishing them as standard operating procedures everyone follows; and (5) **sustaining**, ensuring improvements are continued and preventing return to prior practices. When 5S is followed, workers do not waste time looking for supplies or tools or wondering what to do; resources are where they should be, and work is defined. 5S minimizes or eliminates obstacles to essential work and maximizes value-adding activities.

By combining incremental and flexible budgeting methodologies, a strong budgeting system can be created that evaluates how departments perform and how much resources are consumed by low- or nonvalue-adding activities. Value-added or required work fulfills three conditions: it is valued by the customer, it produces change (a physical product or service is enhanced), and it is done right the first time. Nonvalue-adding activities may be required, but nonvalued work meets only one or two of the conditions to produce value, for example, medication reconciliation or inspection. On the other hand, unnecessary work does not meet any condition, and idle time produces nothing (Protzman et al., 2011, p. 97). Required but nonvalue-adding activities should be minimized by limiting these activities to the extent possible; this could include making these activities more effective (record-keeping that improves processes versus simply documenting processes and outcomes) and minimizing errors and nonvalue-adding repair and corrective action (do it right the first time). Unnecessary work and idle time should be eliminated.

In a perfect world, everyone would engage purely in value-adding work (and we would be more fulfilled by our work and happier), but this will never happen. The first problem is error; reports suggest that 25% of healthcare expenditures arise because of quality issues such as scrap, rework, and inspection. Few people like redoing their own work or fixing the errors of others, but it is clear that a substantial amount of time is consumed redoing things that were not done right the first time. A second category of nonvalue-adding work includes staff meetings and paperwork that do not produce change and are simply unnecessary work (work that is not valued by the consumer, produces no change, and/or is not done right). A third category of wasted effort is idle time. Idle time may be sought by employees who want to minimize effort or can be imposed upon them by a lack of demand for their work or a lack of inputs required to complete work. The three categories of nonvalue-adding work may constitute a significant percentage of employee time, so the budgeting system should be capable of measuring their magnitude and directing effort to better uses. Philip Crosby (1979) noted that it is easy to ignore the cost of poor quality when you don't know its cost.

Budgets should be capable of identify high- and low-value activities and the time spent in each activity. In the chapter "Scratch Budgeting," productive time was estimated at 1800 hours per year per employee: total time (2080 hours) – vacation (80 hours) – sick time (80 hours) – break time (120 hours = 0.5 hour * (48 weeks * 5 days)). If 90% of available work time is spent in productive activities and 10% in nonproductive activities, 1620 hours are available for productive work. The impact of nonproductive time on the flexible budget is obvious: more minutes per output must be budgeted (↓productivity standard) and the cost per output must increase (↑cost standard). Understanding the relationship between productive and nonproductive work allows managers to determine the financial impact when the amount of time spent on nonproductive activities increases (or decreases) and encourages them to find ways to reduce time spent on nonvalue-adding activities.

Organizations benefit when its managers understand what their employees do, what they produce, and how changes should affect operations. Managers who can reduce rework (Shewhart), wasted motion (Gilbreth), or excessive transport (Ford) can recalculate their budget standards and either increase output with existing resources or reduce their use of resources, while maintaining output. On the other hand, regulations that increase steps, handling, and/or paperwork (think pseudoephedrine regulations) reduce productivity and drive up expenses. The impact of increasing regulation may be especially impactful for administrative positions, but one can see that managers should be able to forecast the impact of government regulations on costs and prices. How much will expense increase if another record keeper must be hired (a fixed cost) or production workers must take more time per unit? The question is not simply one of how costs will be affected but also includes whether customers will be willing and able to pay the additional costs. A combination of flexible and incremental budgeting should make clear the costs and benefits of changing production processes and regulatory mandates.

An example of a recent push that should have a major impact on healthcare costs was the emphasis on handwashing. Assuming a caregiver has 1620 hours he or she can devote to patient care; what is the budget impact if every caregiver washes his or her hands for 30 seconds in hot water after every patient is seen? Assuming each caregiver sees 10 patients an hour (1 every 6 minutes), the total handwashing time would be 300 seconds (10 * 30 seconds), or 5 minutes per hour. The impact of 100% compliance would be a potential loss of 160 hours per year (5 minutes per hour * 40 hours/week * 48 weeks per year). Diligent and thorough handwashing would reduce the number of patients a caregiver could see in an hour by almost one patient. The key issue is whether the higher costs resulting from more systematic handwashing are less than the cost arising from higher infection rates due to bacteria transmitted by healthcare workers. Aiello and Larson (2002), in a systematic review of the literature, suggest a 20% or more reduction in illness for hygiene interventions.

The discussion of hand hygiene is *not* meant to discourage handwashing but rather to recognize the added cost of handwashing. The medical profession and society believe that reducing the possibility of infections is worth the price, but making this decision is easier when the cost is undefined. The benefit of explicitly recognizing cost, a potential loss of 160 hours (or 10% of available productive time) per caregiver per year, is that we should see organizations exploring different means to meet the goals of handwashing. Recognition of handwashing costs has led many providers to install hand sanitizers in every room to save time; employees can use these sanitizers when they enter or leave a patient room and thus combine hand hygiene with moving between patient rooms.

▶ Evaluating Performance

The assessment of performance at the simplest level reduces to whether actual costs per output were greater than, equal to, or less than budgeted. Under flexible budgeting, managers should be rewarded or receive superior performance evaluations when their actual costs per unit are less than the budgeted costs per unit regardless of whether total actual expenses are greater than or less than their original budget. Conversely, managers may spend less than they were allocated in the preliminary budget but incur higher-than-budgeted per unit expenses due to a fall in output; these managers, at a minimum, should have to explain why budgeted productivity and cost standards were not met.

Budgets should be tools to improve performance. The incentives in flexible budgeting to hold unit costs at or below the budget should be incorporated into performance evaluation and compensation systems to reward managers and employees for improving productivity. The most obvious mechanism would be to distribute a percentage of budget savings to managers and workers and reduce future cost standards for these savings.

Given effective and timely resource adjustments by the manager through the budget year to variances, the year-end review should approach the cost per output target set by the budget. If actual expenses exceed those calculated in the flexed budget, a search for cause(s) should be undertaken. Are differences, overruns or savings, due to changes in input prices, efficiency, products, or processes? One issue that does *not* require exploration is volume, as the flexible budget incorporates output changes into the final budget.

▶ An Example of Flexible Budgeting: Medicare Expenditures per Beneficiary

In the chapter "Incremental Budgeting," Medicare expenditures were shown to have increased by 7.3% per year from 2000 through 2015, and that was more than 1.9 times the increase in the gross domestic product (GDP). The high growth in Medicare demands analysis: why is it growing so rapidly, and is the program properly managed? A problem with the focus on inputs (or expenditures) in incremental budgeting is that it ignores changes in output. The U.S. population is aging, more people are retiring, and Medicare enrollment is expanding, but these factors were not considered in the incremental budgeting chapter. To recognize the impact of enrollment growth, average expenditure per beneficiary is a superior output measure to total Medicare expenditures. A good argument can be made that each component should be examined separately (as performed in Chapter 6), and rather than the number of beneficiaries, Part A should examine expenditures per discharges; Part B, expenditures per encounter (visits); and Part D, total prescriptions. However, we will forego this detail.

TABLE 7.2 demonstrates that enrollment growth has averaged 2.23% per year from 2000

TABLE 7.2 Medicare Expenditures per Enrollee

| Year | (In Millions) | | | | (Millions) | (per Capita) | | | |
	Total	Part A	Part B	Part D	Enrollment	Total	Part A	Part B	Part D
1990	$110,903	$66,785	$44,118	$0	34.251	$3,334	$1,963	$1,355	$0
2000	$225,983	$132,803	$93,180	$0	39.688	$5,844	$3,348	$2,496	$0
2001	$248,976	$145,018	$103,958		40.103	$6,370	$3,610	$2,760	$0
2002	$266,773	$153,794	$112,979	$0	40.508	$6,788	$3,813	$2,975	$0
2003	$284,081	$159,796	$124,286		41.188	$7,144	$3,924	$3,221	$0
2004	$312,389	$172,649	$139,300	$440	41.902	$7,723	$4,163	$3,560	$0
2005	$342,106	$187,456	$153,553	$1,098	42.606	$8,278	$4,440	$3,839	$0
2006	$412,967	$198,164	$170,460	$44,342	43.436	$10,179	$4,601	$4,116	$1,461
2007	$443,395	$209,466	$183,678	$50,252	44.368	$10,703	$4,759	$4,313	$1,630
2008	$462,974	$225,568	$183,514	$53,892	45.500	$11,232	$4,996	$4,574	$1,662

2009	$503,073	$239,348	$205,857	$57,868	46.604	$11,702	$5,174	$4,798	$1,730
2010	$523,268	$245,445	$215,327	$62,496	47.720	$11,897	$5,182	$4,907	$1,808
2011	$549,846	$257,556	$226,280	$66,010	48.896	$12,201	$5,305	$5,038	$1,858
2012	$572,772	$263,861	$240,427	$68,484	50.874	$12,234	$5,221	$5,173	$1,840
2013	$591,271	$270,105	$248,234	$72,932	52.504	$12,228	$5,177	$5,177	$1,874
2014	$619,038	$270,513	$266,513	$82,012	54.077	$12,463	$5,033	$5,395	$2,035
2015	$647,356	$275,692	$279,950	$91,714	55.264	$12,744	$5,019	$5,522	$2,203
CGR 2000–15	7.27%	4.99%	7.61%	8.41%	2.23%	5.34%	2.74%	5.44%	4.67%

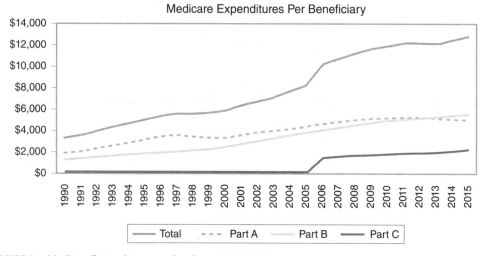

FIGURE 7.4 Medicare Expenditures per Enrollee, 1990–2015

through 2015 and has accounted for 30.7% of the growth in the total Medicare expenditure during this time. The remainder of the increase is due to higher expenditures per beneficiary. Inpatient expenditures, Part A, grew at 2.74% and accounted for approximately 24.2% of the change in the total expenditure per enrollee. Outpatient expenditures, Part B, grew the fastest, increasing by 5.44% annually and accounting for 43.9% of the change in per beneficiary expenditure. The final driver of the higher expenditure was the pharmaceutical coverage, Part D, which grew by 4.67% from 2006 through 2015 and accounted for 32.0% of the change in per beneficiary expenditure.

FIGURE 7.4 graphically illustrates that enactment of Part D provided the major spark to higher Medicare expenditures; per enrollee expenditures jumped from $8,278 in 2005 to $10,179 in 2006, and the $1,461 increase in pharmaceutical benefits accounted for 76.9% of the year-to-year increase. The line chart shows a decline in per enrollee beneficiary Part A expenditures starting in 2013, but the increases in Part B and Part D continue to drive total expenditures higher.

Understanding these changes and evaluating management requires examining the number of discharges, outpatient visits, and prescriptions paid, as well as changes in reimbursement. In the flexible budgeting system, the objective is to control the cost per beneficiary (or discharge, visit, or prescription); the data shows that after subtracting the effect of enrollment growth, the annual increase in expenditure per beneficiary is 5.34%, or 82.7% higher than the growth in per capita GDP. While the increase in per beneficiary expenditure is considerably less than the increase in total expenditures, the problem remains that Medicare expenditures are growing at an unsustainable rate relative to the economy and program changes, including management, benefits, and financing, are needed.

Summary

Flexible budgeting requires greater effort than incremental budgeting, so the choice of a budgeting system must be based on whether the added effort is worth the cost. Flexible budgeting provides better incentives than incremental budgeting, that is, a focus on the cost per output versus simply keeping expenses below the budget, but will managers and workers respond to the incentives and information to improve efficiency?

Flexible budgeting requires two major sets of calculations: the first is the preliminary budget based on forecasted output, and the second is the final budget determined by actual output. The value of budgets is determined by whether managers and employees respond to the information provided and the validity of the data. Were fixed and variable costs correctly identified, and is the variable cost per output (the budget standard) accurate? Flexible budgeting provides obvious incentives toward defining expenses as fixed costs and underestimating budget standards to avoid having to reduce resources as output falls as well as overestimating the variable cost component when output is rising to obtain larger budget allocations. These incentives will be lower in organizations that regularly see output rise and fall, as large variable cost standards that provide windfalls with increasing output cut as deeply when output falls. Managers and employees should be incented to cut per unit costs by seeking ways to reduce overprocessing, unnecessary motion and transport, defects, underutilized and idle resources, and inventories through sharing of savings.

The appropriate environment for the flexible budgeting system is where an organization faces stiff price competition; rapid environment change, changing demand and production methods, and increases in output generate sufficient revenue to cover incremental production costs. Successful implementation of the flexible budgeting system requires organizations to upgrade the financial management skills of their managers. Flexible budgeting requires managers to not only complete tasks but also understand the financial impact of how resources are used.

Key Terms and Concepts

5S	High/low method	Regression
Benchmarks	Incremental (marginal) costs	Time and motion studies
Budget standard	Marginal costs	Therblig
Cost standard	Productivity standard	

Discussion Questions

1. Describe the steps needed to construct a flexible budget.
2. Compare a flexible and an incremental budget.
3. Describe the five ways to calculate productivity standards.
4. How can a manager maximize his or her variable expenses in a flexible budget?
5. When should a flexible budget be employed?
6. Explain the strengths and weaknesses of flexible budgeting.

Problems

1. Calculate productivity and cost standards for the patient accounting department. The Problem 7.1 tab in the BudgetCh07.xls file provides inpatient claims, staff hours, and total staff salaries. Calculate the cost standard for staff salaries on the basis of the fluctuation in inpatient claims and staff hours and salaries using (a) historical average, (b) the high/low method, (c) regression, and (d) an unweighted composite estimate. Explain your results.

2. Your proposed incremental 2019 budget has been rejected (Chapter 6, Problem 6.1). Use the Problem 7.2 file to resubmit it as a flexible budget. Salary and fringe benefit (object codes 4000–4199) increases for all personnel should be estimated at 4.0%, except for health insurance (object code 4120), which is expected to increase by 8.0%. Input price increases for supplies and other

costs (object codes 4200–4960) should be increased by 3.0%, except for medications (a 5.0% increase) and profession insurance (a 10.0% increase). Explain the changes in requested expenses between the incremental budget (Problem 6.1) and your new flexible budget. How much ($ and %) has the total budget changed?

3. Create a flexible budget for the patient accounting department in Problem 7.1. The budget office has analyzed the first budget submission and believes it significantly overstates actual resource needs. Staff salaries per inpatient claim have increased from $15.15 ($600,000 / 39,600) in 2017 to $17.02 ($310,000 / 18,213) in the first 6 months of 2018 and were incrementally budgeted at $17.07 ($638,600 / 37,400) for 2019. The proposed 2019 budget presents an increase of 12.7% over 2017. To achieve greater efficiency, you are directed to resubmit your 2019 budget using flexible budgeting with inpatient claims as your output measure. Use 2017 as the base year (the cost standard) and the project staff cost per claim allowing for a 3.0% salary increase. Management salaries should be increased by 4.0%.

Use the Problem 7.3 tab in the BudgetCh07.xlsx file to submit your 2019 flexible budget for 37,400 expected claims on the basis of the per unit expenses achieved in 2017, allowing for a 3.0% increase in office supplies (object code 4250), a 1.0% increase in telephone expenses (object code 4440), and a 5.0% increase for electricity (object code 4410). The post office has

recently announced a 3-cent increase ($0.46 to $0.49) in postage rates, which must incorporated into your revised budget. Federal Insurance Contributions Act (FICA) and other fringe benefits should be calculated as 7.65% and 20%, respectively, of total budgeted salaries. Management salaries (object code 4030), telephone expenses (object code 4440), and electricity (object code 4410) should be budgeted incrementally since these are fixed expenses that do not vary with volume.

4. Assume 2019 has ended. Using the Problem 7.3 tab in the BudgetCh07. xlsx file, recalculate the flexible budget using actual claims that were higher than expected (37,831 versus 37,400 forecasted). Actual expenses are shown. Evaluate managerial performance.

5. Assume 2019 has ended. Using the Problem 7.3 tab in the Budget Ch07.xlsx file, recalculate the flexible budget using actual claims that were higher than expected (35,564 versus 37,400 forecasted). Actual expenses are shown. Evaluate managerial performance.

References

Aiello, A. E., & Larson, E. L. (2002). What is the evidence for a causal link between hygiene and infections? *Lancet Infectious Diseases, 2*(2), 103–110.

Crosby, P. B. (1979). *Quality is free.* New York, NY: McGraw-Hill Book Company.

Optum360°. (2016). *2017 Almanac of hospital financial and operating indicators.* Salt Lake City, UT: Author.

Protzman, C., Mayzell, G., & Kepchar, J. (2011). *Leveraging lean in healthcare.* Boca Raton, FL: CRC Press.

CHAPTER 8

Zero-Base Budgeting

CHAPTER OBJECTIVES

1. Explain the steps to build a zero-base budget.
2. Construct a zero-base budget.
3. Compare zero-base budgeting, zero-base review, and target-base budgeting.
4. Evaluate the strengths and weaknesses of zero-base budgeting.
5. Explain the interrelationships between decision packages and performance audits.

▶ Introduction

A budget is the financial specification of the operating plan of an organization—what products will be produced, what resources will be consumed, and the expected inflow and outflow of funds. While every organization has an operating plan, the work of most organizations is due to evolution rather than planning. Contrary to earlier assumptions that work was necessary and performed efficiently, work is typically based on past practice rather than scientific study. Inefficient, ineffective, and inconsequential work is institutionalized and continued because of tradition rather than necessity. Previously examined budgeting systems contain the flaw that they gave too much credence to the past—what was previously done and spent drove future budgets.

Zero-base budgeting (ZBB) does not start with the assumption that an organization is efficient or that the value of its output exceeds the cost of resources consumed. ZBB assumes that everything an organization does should be justified *prior* to receiving funding. ZBB also does not assume that prior processes should be continued and the budget can be eliminated, that is, zeroed out, if managers cannot justify their operations. Where incremental and flexible budgeting assumes that existence presupposes value to the organization, ZBB asks whether existing resources can be used more effectively to maximize the value of the organization by eliminating or reducing one or more operations and reallocating resources to other uses.

ZBB parallels strategic planning by asking fundamental questions about the organization's mission, goals, and programs and ranking expenditures and outputs according to their contribution to the organization. Success under ZBB is not measured as meeting a budget (incremental) or reducing the cost per output (flexible), because neither of these efforts necessarily adds value to the organization. An organization may spend no more money than what was budgeted and/or produce a good or service at the lowest-achievable cost without producing anything that people need, want, or are willing to pay for. ZBB assesses the value of expenditures—what role the activity or output plays in achieving the organization's mission— and introduces competition between alternative uses of resources. ZBB focuses directly on waste created by overproduction: should output be reduced or eliminated? ZBB creates competition for resources to benefit high value-creating activities and encourages improvement, including increasing the value of output produced (effectiveness), reducing the cost of production (efficiency), or both. ZBB is a system to dynamically shift resources to uses that create the highest value.

Texas Instruments implemented ZBB in the late 1960s to control overhead costs where output and quality were difficult to quantify, that is, expense centers. In the early 1970s, ZBB was introduced in the state of Georgia because of the difficulty in evaluating the efficiency and effectiveness of government programs that lacked profit signals (Pyhrr, 1973, p. 157). Although **FIGURE 8.1** categorizes ZBB as being primarily concerned with efficiency, the goal of ZBB is to develop a system where managers are encouraged to reduce cost per

output *and* increase the value of outputs produced by increasing or improving outcomes. Managers should think about what end users want or need in order to improve the usefulness of products and maximize the value of the organization. ZBB spans the breath of operations, starting with what is produced (design), how it is produced (throughput), and how it is delivered to end users (service) and ending with how the product is used or what benefit it bestows on customers or clients (outcome). While acceptable performance under flexible budgeting may be reduced to two dimensions, maintaining the cost per unit and meeting quality standards, ZBB is forward looking and asks whether value to end users can be increased by producing a set of more highly valued goods or services and/or introducing new production methods.

The economic principles of opportunity costs and diminishing marginal returns form the foundation of ZBB. Are there better ways of using resources to maximize output or outcomes? Managers are encouraged to think about and identify alternative means of accomplishing the same tasks (i.e., centralization versus decentralization, in-house versus purchased service, etc.). After selecting the lowest-cost method for performing work that meets quality standards, the second question is, how much output should be produced? The level of activity should be decided by economics: output should be expanded until the resources used in production could yield greater value in other uses.

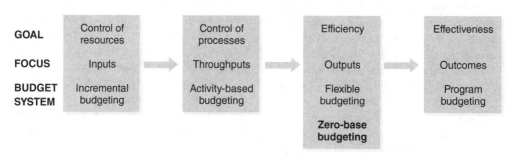

FIGURE 8.1 Budgeting Systems

The law of diminishing marginal returns holds that past a certain point, the more you have of something, the more the value of each additional unit will fall. Regardless of what you are producing or consuming after a certain point, its value diminishes. The more you eat, the less satisfaction you receive from the additional food consumed. As more health-care activities are created, the value of each additional activity falls. It is assumed the initial items consumed or produced meet the most pressing needs. After they are consumed, additional units of the same items are used to satisfy less important needs or desires; hence, later units produce less value or lower satisfaction. In medicine or public health, efforts should be targeted at individuals at the most risk. As health screenings and preventive care are extended to lower-risk groups, the value of these activities decreases at an increasing rate. Similarly, in production processes, if more units of one input, such as labor, are added, while other inputs are held constant, the marginal product will decrease.

In ZBB, managers are tasked with identifying the costs and benefits associated with different production methods and levels of output where the relationship between benefits and costs should determine the production method and the level of output that will be funded.

TABLE 8.1 shows how diminishing returns affect the level of output decisions based on the desirability of vaccination for different population groups. The table splits the population into high-, medium-, and low-risk groups, where the only difference is their susceptibility to contracting a disease. In the high-risk group, 1 person in 10 is likely to contract a disease; in the medium-risk group, 1 in 20; and among low-risk individuals, 1 in 100. The cost of vaccination is $40.00 per person.

Table 8.1 shows that the cost per avoided case increases dramatically as susceptibility falls. Identifying which groups should be vaccinated requires determining the benefit of vaccination. This example assumes that the benefit of vaccination is to avoid time away from work and that the average worker salary is $200 per day. If less than 2 days of work will be lost to illness, no group should be vaccinated, as the less-than-$400 benefit is lower than the $400 cost. If 2–4 days may be lost, the only group that should be vaccinated is the high-risk group: the benefit ranges from $400 to $800 and equals or exceeds the $400 cost. If 4–9 days may be missed, the high- and medium-risk groups should be vaccinated, and all groups should be vaccinated if 10 or more days are expected to be lost. The cost per output is probably understated as enticing medium- and low-risk groups to be vaccinated will require more effort and cost compared to high-risk individuals as the lower-risk groups know that their potential benefit is lower than that of the high-risk group and may be unwilling to accept the

TABLE 8.1 Vaccination, Risk, and Diminishing Returns				
	Susceptibility	Total Cost (*n* = 100)	Output (avoided cases)	Cost/Output
High risk	10/100	$4,000	10	$400
Medium risk	5/100	$4,000	5	$800
Low risk	1/100	$4,000	1	$4,000

time and transportation costs to be vaccinated. A more sophisticated analysis would increase the expected benefit by including avoided medical costs and attempting to place a monetary value on pain and suffering.

The goal of ZBB is to allocate resources to their most valued uses—those uses that produce the greatest benefit per dollar invested. If resources are not allocated to maximize the value of the organization, ZBB should identify higher-value activities where resources should be increased and less important areas where funding should be cut back. ZBB is *not* about expanding total resource use but is about creating greater value from existing resources, although the same methodology can be used to allocate new funds as they become available. ZBB highlights competing uses for an organization's resources and the fundamental trade-offs involved in funding an activity—funding one activity precludes others. The output of ZBB is the explicit recognition of value created by activities and the identification of where expenditures should be expanded, contracted, or terminated.

To maximize value, managers must be cognizant of environmental changes and changes in consumer tastes and preferences, understand the impact of these changes on output (increasing the importance of some activities, while decreasing the importance of others), and incorporate these changes into operations and budgets. ZBB continues the progression toward better budgeting by incorporating a greater understanding of operations and external factors (prices consumers are willing to pay or benefits created, including reduced future costs) into budgeting and day-to-day management started in flexible budgeting.

▶ Zero-Base Budgeting

ZBB returns to the fundamental reason organizations exist to guide resource allocation decisions. Pyhrr (1973, p. 2) notes that planning identifies the output desired, while budgeting identifies the inputs required. While incremental and flexible budgeting systems enshrine the past, prior resource use dictates future resource use, ZBB returns to the first question of what the organization wants to produce. This question is *not* answered by projecting output quantities from history (Chapter 4) but returns to fundamentals by asking what the organization wants to be and what set of activities will maximize its value. Who should the organization produce goods and services for, what should be the characteristics of the outputs, and how much output should be produced? When ZBB is performed correctly, it challenges current and accepted practices by returning to the fundamental questions of what should be produced, how it should be produced, and how much output should be produced.

The first assumption of ZBB is that managers should justify every dollar spent. The simple fact that a function was performed earlier does not provide sufficient justification for its continuation at current funding levels or for its continuation at all. Changes in the environment (economic, social, demographic, and technologic) and consumer preferences can dramatically alter the need or desire for goods and services. The March of Dimes was founded to advance polio treatment. When the Salk vaccine eliminated the need for polio research, the organization changed its mission to ending premature birth, birth defects, and infant mortality. ZBB frames resource use questions as if the organization is starting anew and not performing a task, should it be undertaken? ZBB attempts to re-instill the scratch-budgeting ethos and urgency: are activities essential and worth their cost? Every activity, output, and input decision is questioned: is X essential to meeting current goals (versus historical goals), and is the benefit derived from X greater than its opportunity cost?

The second assumption is that there is always an alternative means to complete an activity, that is, many roads to the same destination. At the most basic level, the question is, should an activity be performed or foregone?

Is there a compelling reason to undertake an activity, and does the activity increase the value of the organization? The second question is, should the activity be performed in the manner it has been performed, and has the most effective and least cost method been identified and implemented? The final question is, how much of the activity should be undertaken? Owners and managers face many choices on organizational size: do they want limited output (a niche market), large output (mass market), or something in between? Given diminishing returns, at what level does increased output reduce the value of the organization? Austin and Cheek (1979, pp. 10–11) identified and diagrammed the three primary questions managers must answer on objectives, methods, and scale (**FIGURE 8.2**).

The first decision managers make is selecting objectives, that is, planning. The choices are to continue to pursue current objectives, eliminate one or more current objectives, pursue new objectives, or some combination. Reducing the size of programs is not a planning consideration—the scale of programs is a funding or allocation decision made at the third level. The second-level decision asks, how will objectives be pursued? For current objectives, this may entail maintaining existing methods or introducing new methods. Austin and Cheek (1979) describe the selection of method as an organizational decision. The third-level decision, allocation, addresses the scale or size of the operation: will output be increased, maintained, or reduced?

Figure 8.2 perfectly expresses the change from incremental and flexible budgeting to ZBB. The former budgets pursue the following path: **Current objectives (planning) → Current methods (option 1) → Current output (100% allocation)**; other objectives, methods, and/or output levels are not typically considered. Previous budgeting systems support the status quo. The goal of ZBB is to recognize and create competition between alternatives objectives, methods, and levels of output. Given the specification of costs and outputs, ZBB allocates resources based on the value or benefit created per dollar expended. In for-profit organizations, operationalizing this rule is straightforward; if there is demand for additional output from product line A and it produces a 10%

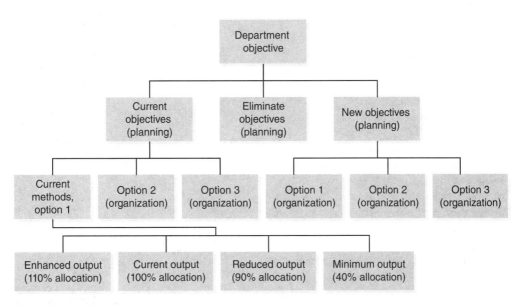

FIGURE 8.2 ZBB Decisions: Objectives, Methods, and Scale

return on investment (ROI), while product line B produces a return of 5%, product line A should be expanded (increasing supply and driving down price) by removing resources from product line B (decreasing supply and increasing price). The optimal point is reached when expansion of product line A and reduction in product line B produces comparable returns, for example, 7.5% is produced in each product line.

Quantification of benefit is more difficult in fields where value is not measured in dollars, but the calculation remains the same. Public health officials should ask whether expanding prenatal care generates more value than existing immunization, sexually transmitted disease (STD) control, or restaurant inspections, as measured by maximizing avoided future healthcare expenditures. The goal of primary care may be to maximize quality-adjusted life-years (QALYs), allowing expenditures across different programs to be evaluated on the basis of how many additional years of life each produces and at what cost.

The goal of ZBB is to ensure that the expansion of activities and programs that produce the highest value per dollar expended is budgeted at the expense of lower-benefit outputs. Organizations should expand high value-creating activities by reducing the scale of or eliminating lower-benefit activities. Redistribution of existing funds versus simple competition over the rate of increase facilitates the flow of funds between departments, and departments are not guaranteed the same amount of funding (or even continued existence) from year to year. Competition between departments and the potential loss of funding are designed to encourage employees to find better methods of performing work by improving their output (making it more attractive and/or desirable to consumers) and reducing operating costs. Not all work should be continued; ineffective and/or inefficient operations that fail to respond to environmental changes deserve to see their resources transferred to superior activities and programs.

Structure and Design

ZBB focuses on activities and functions rather than departments. ZBB envisions a department as a set of activities that produce various outputs versus a single output. A change in perspective opens up a possibility of endless combinations of activities that could be performed and goods and services that could be produced. The budget is no longer a take-it-or-leave-it decision: a complete set of activities and outputs is purchased instead of a menu of choices. The logic is identical to going to a restaurant, where a patron can purchase any combination of beverages, appetizers, salads, entrées, vegetables, potatoes, and/or desserts. Astute restaurants, like other budgeting systems, attempt to maximize revenue by offering package deals, where patrons can obtain a set of food items at a reduced price to induce them to spend more money than they would if they ordered individual items.

ZBB provides managers with an à la carte menu. The first step recognizes a goal: why does the organization exist, and what should it produce? The next steps examine how the system works and could work. After the system and alternatives are understood, discrete **decision packages** are developed that describe options and costs. When we go out to eat, the prime goal is to satisfy hunger: do we want Surf and Turf for $29.99 or Monterey Chicken for $12.99? Decision packages, like menu choices, explain what a department could produce, how it will produce it, and what the cost of resources required will be. Decision packages also identify what will be produced and the quantity of output, including outcomes, activities/projects, personnel, supplies, and capital expenditures. Pyhrr (1973, p. 6) sees the primary items in a decision package as (1) objectives, (2) consequences of elimination, (3) performance measures, (4) alternative production methods, and (5) benefits and costs.

Instead of funding a department as a whole, assuming everything the department does is worth continuing, ZBB recognizes that many departments produce various outputs, some are more valuable than others, and each output receives inputs and costs from other operations. Departments are divided into different processes that contribute to the outputs produced. Managers are first required to specify what their departments do by activity and provide a rationale for the process: why it is performed (i.e., its purpose), what it achieves, and how it ties to the larger goals of the organization. ZBB provides an opportunity to evaluate the accuracy of past projections, since the majority of current expenditures are grounded in the past: are expenditures producing the expected output or outcomes under which they were originally justified?

Managers must also specify alternative means of achieving the same output, the cost of the current activities (not solely departmental cost as contributions and costs are received from other departments), the cost of alternative performance methods, performance measures, and the consequences of nonperformance. ZBB is a radically different approach to budgeting, which asks fundamental questions about what an organization does, what its production methods are, and whether the activity needs to be performed at all. The questions of how things are performed and the comparison of current methods with alternative production processes are routinely overlooked in traditional budgeting systems.

ZBB is more outward and forward looking and goal directed than incremental or flexible budgeting systems. ZBB requires that all expenditures be explicitly linked to the organization's mission and goals. In the forefront of ZBB are the questions of why the organization is doing things and how much customers value activities. Where flexible budgeting is inwardly and historically directed (what it has cost the organization to produce a good or service) and measures success by the ability to minimize the cost per output, ZBB encourages managers to explore more efficient production methods by introducing a system that looks ahead to see where resources could be more effectively used. ZBB incorporates an **external scan** into the budgeting process to monitor environmental changes and direct new activities.

Budget choices are specified in terms of outputs: should an activity or project be undertaken, what does it cost to perform the activity, what benefit does the organization receive from the activity, and how do the marginal costs and benefits of the activity change when the scope of the operation expands or contracts? The specification of outputs portrays budget choices based on cost–benefit or cost-effectiveness ratios (CERs). Ratios are calculated for each output and different quantities of each good or service so that decision packages can be compared. How do the benefits and costs of different activities (A versus B) and different levels of output for a single activity ($A_{1current output}$ versus $A_{2expanded output}$) compare? Comparisons can also be made between different activities with different levels of output: is $A_{1current}$ a better use of resources than $B_{2expanded}$, or is $A_{2expanded}$ a better use of resources? Like other budgeting systems, expenditures are budgeted on a 1-year horizon.

Finally, ZBB establishes incentives for efficiency and flexibility in resource allocation. When costs and benefits are explicitly recognized, it is easy to rank activities from high to low; managers wishing to maximize organizational value select the highest-value and forego lower-value activities. ZBB encourages managers to reduce the costs and/or increase the benefits of their activities to increase the cost–benefit ratio and enhance the desirability of the activity over other endeavors. The use of cost–benefit ratios increases the probability that funds will flow to departments improving their performance and reduce their chance of budget cuts. A clear system of funding based on benefits produced and costs consumed is established, which produces competition among alternate activities.

The Budget-Building Process

Step 1 in ZBB determines objectives. The determination of objectives is more likely to be the duty of senior management, but ZBB forces lower-level managers to address how their operations advance organizational goals. ZBB is a conscious effort to reduce silo thinking, where managers are primarily concerned with their areas of responsibility, and force them to explain how the work of their departments contributes to the value of the organization. Common objectives include maximizing profit, number of patients (customers or clients) seen, or population health.

Step 2 describes current operations: what activities are undertaken, and how does each activity and its output contribute to the achievement of organizational objectives? The description should illuminate what the department does and for whom, how much total resources are consumed, what their cost is, and what outputs are produced. Like step 1, step 2 is a conscious effort to avoid assumptions of what workers believe they are doing and develop greater understanding of what the department actually does. Step 2 encourages means (what is done) and ends (for what purpose) thinking. Managers should describe the consequences if current activities are discontinued: who or what would be impacted and by how much?

Step 3 explores alternative means of conducting each activity. What alternative productive methods exist, how do other organizations operate, and what outcomes do they achieve? Can an activity be centralized or decentralized to lower cost, and should the activity be produced in-house or purchased from an outside vendor? Exploring alternatives is designed to identify the lowest-cost method of performing an activity and avoid thinking that current methods are the best or the only methods. After developing and examining options, managers should select the lowest-cost method that can produce the desired objectives (**BOX 8.1**).

After objectives, current processes, and alternatives are evaluated, managers develop decision packages, that is, different levels of output and service and their accompanying costs. A decision package includes activities, purpose, costs, alternative performance methods, performance measures, consequences of nonperformance, and benefits. **FIGURE 8.3**

BOX 8.1 The Zero-Base Budgeting Process

1. Establish objectives.
2. Describe current operations.
3. Identify alternative means of performance.
4. Develop decision packages.
5. Rank the decision packages.
6. Compile a final budget.

---

shows a standard ZBB decision package form. Activities are discrete subprocesses within a department and force managers to examine their operations and define their major activities. Decision packages should highlight how output will be affected by changes in funding. Will the percentage change in output be greater than, less than, or equal to the percentage change in resources used?

Assume a human resources (HR) department carries out four primary tasks: recruitment and employment, training and development, compensation review and management, and disciplinary action. The HR manager must first divide total resources among these four areas to describe operations (what is produced), consider alternative means of delivery, and determine current funding levels (what inputs are consumed to perform each activity, how many activities are undertaken, and what they cost). After the four major activities are identified, the manager must determine how outputs and goals will be impacted if current activity levels are increased or decreased.

The most challenging part of describing current activities is to define the benefits obtained by the organization. Revenue-producing activities are the easiest to rank; a list is produced that identifies revenue, cost, and ROI: does the activity generate more revenue than cost? When not all activities can be supported, activities with the highest ROI are selected until funds are exhausted.

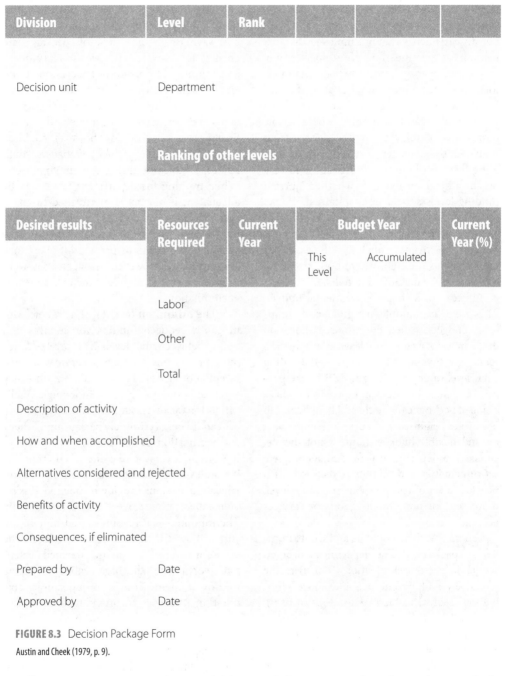

Division		Level	Rank			
Decision unit		Department				

Ranking of other levels		

Desired results	Resources Required	Current Year	Budget Year		Current Year (%)
			This Level	Accumulated	
	Labor				
	Other				
	Total				

Description of activity

How and when accomplished

Alternatives considered and rejected

Benefits of activity

Consequences, if eliminated

Prepared by   Date

Approved by   Date

FIGURE 8.3 Decision Package Form
Austin and Cheek (1979, p. 9).

For nonrevenue-generating activities like HR, the output measures could be the length of time to hire (weeks), the number of training sessions delivered, the number of salary reviews undertaken and/or the length of time to complete the reviews, and the number of disciplinary actions taken and/ or the length of time to complete each. For three activities (recruitment, compensation management, and disciplinary action), the benefit is timeliness. Attempts to decrease resources would slow processes and add costs due to extended vacancy, employee dissatisfaction, or continuation of nonperforming employees. Managers must explain how performance and output would change if funding is increased or decreased. In training, an increase (decrease) in funding would enable more (less) employees to be educated and prepared; the manager is tasked with quantifying the contribution training makes toward organizational goals and whether current funding levels should be maintained. Unlike revenue-generating departments, ranking of nonrevenue-generating departments depends on cost-effectiveness analysis—the cost per output versus the ROI, where both costs and benefits can be quantified in dollars.

Instead of a single departmental budget, ZBB produces multiple, marginal, and cumulative budgets so that the resource allocation decision is not a take-it-or-leave-it proposition (generally take-it) but a matter of deciding what level of activity is best. ZBB is like grocery shopping; one does not have to purchase a side of beef but can purchase 2 lb of beef, 2 lb of chicken, eight ears of corn, etc. Incremental and flexible budgets limit, if not dictate, choice. If a department is funded, a complete set of activities and outputs is received. ZBB provides a set of choices—buy the same level, more, less, or none of the goods or services currently received.

In theory, there could be an infinite number of packages for a department ordered sequentially, from elimination (0 of n) to the lowest level of output possible above elimination (1 of n) to increased output (n of n). Assume a heart transplant program performs 60 surgeries per year. The output could range from 0 transplants to 70 or more—potentially more than 71 decision packages (too much detail to be useful). The output could be specified in multiples of 10: 0, 1–10, 11–20, and so on (nine packages or another ordering system). For the HR department, five decision packages are constructed:

Elimination (0 of 4) reports the cessation of all activities (zero output) and 100% cost savings. Assume decision packages are created for two HR functions, recruitment and training. Elimination of recruitment and employment activities is not possible, given staff turnover and the lack of desirability for department managers to initiate and manage hiring processes. Training, however, could be eliminated, and department managers could be responsible for training their employees. While training for department tasks may be adequately, if not better, performed by managers, training on organizational-wide issues may be less effective. A formal decision package may not have to be prepared if operations are terminated; however, managers may want to produce one to highlight the consequences of elimination.

The **minimum level (1 of 4)** reports significantly reduced funding for services and output below current levels. This level of funding supports only products or services deemed essential or critical. For recruitment, this may entail only one job posting in a single publication for vacancies and less thorough vetting of candidates (criminal background check and verification of education) but no checking of employers or references. For training, it would reduce the number and frequency of education sessions provided—one live session videotaped for employees who cannot attend. The minimum level assumes that output and cost will be at their lowest-possible level. The question is, are the activities deemed "essential" worth what the organization is paying to provide them? This is an opportunity cost question; the cost of providing one service (e.g., training) may be reduced to increasing funding to hire better candidates (and thus reducing the need for training and education). The minimum funding level could be set at 60%, 70%, or some other percentage of current funding.

The **reduced level (2 of 4)** highlights the impact of marginal reduction on funding and output (e.g., 20% reduction in funding).

The reduced level assumes that a department will provide less than the current level of output but more than the minimum level. For recruitment, this may include multiple job postings in a single publication over 2 weeks and more thorough vetting of candidates (criminal background checks, verification of education, and reference checks with current and former employers). For training, it will reduce the number and frequency of education sessions provided—one live session per shift plus a video recording. The reduced-level decision package includes total costs, but evaluation and ranking are based on marginal costs and outputs; that is, the reduced-level package specifies the increase in cost and output above that specified at the minimum reduced level.

The **current level (3 of 4)** reports the status quo—no change in funding or output. The current level assumes that the department continues to provide the current level of output at the same cost (given input price increases). Currently recruitment involves posting of jobs in the local paper for 14 days and one or more postings to relevant professional newsletters. Vetting of candidates includes criminal background checks, verification of education, and reference checks with current and former employers and one reference. Training provides two live sessions for first shift employees and one session for the evening and night shift employees, plus a video recording. The current-level decision package again includes total cost and output, but evaluation and ranking are based on marginal costs and output— the increase in cost and output above that provided at the reduced, 80% level.

The **enhanced level (4 of 4)** highlights the impact of increasing funding to support expanded output (e.g., 20% budget increase). The enhanced-level question asks the "what if" question: if a department could receive additional funds (not limited to inflation-based budget increases), what could it produce with the additional funds? The funding increase could be 5%, 10%, or any amount above current

levels. In addition to current recruitment activities, the HR department may propose rebuilding its website and developing computer-based assessments tests for common positions with frequent hiring. In addition to current training opportunities, the manager may propose developing and offering new topics and/or expanding off-site training opportunities. Like the current level, the enhanced decision package includes the total cost, but its ranking is based on marginal costs and outputs, that is, the increase in cost and output above the current level.

Assume the managers in training and recruitment have prepared the decision packages shown in **TABLE 8.2** based on funding at 60%, 80%, 100%, and 120% of the current level. Note that recruitment cannot be zeroed out because of retirements, resignations, and terminations, so elimination is 40% of current funding. Both managers describe how training and recruitment activities could be increased with a 20% funding increase. The training manager details how the number of sessions, participants, and topics will expand with funding. Similarly, the recruitment manager describes how job postings and background checks will increase with funding. The benefit of these activities declines as the program expands, as the most important training sessions and background checks (criminal > educational > current employer > references) are tackled first and less important activities are only pursued if funding is available. Senior management decides the value of training activities versus recruitment to the organization.

TABLE 8.3 summarizes the expected costs and benefits from training activities. The benefits of training activities were weighted by senior management, and marginal benefit and cost calculations can be found in the **TABLE 8.4** tab in Chapter08.xlsx. In Table 8.3, column 2 details the number of people who could be trained at each funding level, and column 3 shows the total and marginal benefits expected from training. Current training activities

TABLE 8.2 Training and Recruitment Decision Packages

	Elimination	Minimal	Reduced	Current	Expanded
Training benefits	0 topics	20 topics	25 topics	**30 topics**	35 topics
	0 sessions/ topics	1 session (first shift)	3 sessions (all shifts)	**4 sessions (all shifts)**	4 sessions (all shifts)
	0 total sessions	20 sessions	75 sessions	**120 sessions**	120 sessions
	0 participants	1400 participants	2150 participants	**2750 participants**	3150 participants + off-site training
Training costs	$0 (0%)	$150,000 (60%)	$225,000 (90%)	**$250,000 (100%)**	$275,000 (110%)
Recruitment benefits	Internal and website posting	Internal, web, and one weekly advertisement	Internal, web, and two weekly advertisements	**Internal, web, and two publications for 2 weeks**	Internal, web, and two publications for 2 weeks
Elimination impossible because of turnover	Criminal background check and verification of education	Criminal, education, and current employer	Criminal, education, current employer, and previous employer	**Criminal, education, current and previous employer, and single reference**	Criminal, education, current and previous employer, and all references
	2 checks/ applicant	3 checks/ applicant	4 checks/ applicant	**5 checks/ applicant**	7 checks/ applicant
	1000 applicants	1000 applicants	1000 applicants	**1000 applicants**	1000 applicants
	2000 checks	3000 checks	4000 checks	**5000 checks**	7000 checks + website rebuild + computer assessments
Recruitment costs	$100,000 (40%)	$150,000 (60%)	$200,000 (80%)	**$250,000 (100%)**	$300,000 (120%)

TABLE 8.3 Marginal Analysis of Training Activities

Decision Package	Total Benefit (#Trained)	Total Current Benefit (%) Marginal Benefit (%)	Total Cost (% of Current Cost)	Marginal Cost (%)	Cost Effectiveness Ratio (Marginal Benefit/ Marginal Cost)
Eliminate (0 of 4)	0	0.0 0.0	–	–	–
Minimum (1 of 4)	1,400	59.3 59.3	$120,000 (60%)	60	0.99
Reduced (2 of 4)	2,150	84.7 25.4	$160,000 (80%)	20	1.27
Current (3 of 4)	2,750	100 15.3	$200,000 (100%)	20	0.76
Enhanced (4 of 4)	3,150	108.5 8.5	$240,000 (120%)	20	0.42

(3 of 4) produce 100% of current benefits and require $200,000 to deliver, that is, 100% funding. Columns 4 and 5 document funding levels: the minimum training level requires 60% of current funding, and every program expansion requires a 20% increase in funding. The table demonstrates how marginal benefit declines as the number of people trained and topics increases.

Column 6 calculates the CER (marginal benefit/marginal cost) to rank decision packages, that is, prioritize activities within and between departments. At the minimum training level (1 of 4), the CER is 0.99 (59.3% of total current benefit / 60% of total current cost). Increasing the scale of operations to the reduced level (2 of 4) increases the output by 25.4% and the cost by 20.0%, a CER of 1.27, and returning

to the current level (3 of 4) increases the output by 15.3% and the cost by 20.0%; a CER of 0.76. ZBB is based on the idea of diminishing marginal returns: as the scale of a program increases, the output increases at a diminishing rate and the costs increase at an increasing rate.

Step 5 ranks packages in order of importance to the organization, that is, the rankings should reflect the organization's priorities. After the decision packages are produced, they are ranked from the highest benefit to the lowest. Note that no higher level (2 of *n*) can be introduced into the list before the minimum level (1 of *n*) is in place. The organization cannot obtain the benefits from reduced training activities (1.27) before the minimal training level (0.99) is funded. In comparing activities across functions, the question is,

	CER		CER	
Decision Package (Trained)	**Training Priority**		**Recruitment Priority**	
Eliminate (0 of 4)	–	–	1.82	#1
Minimum (1 of 4)	0.99	#2	0.67	#5
Reduced (2 of 4)	1.27	#3	0.60	#6
Current (3 of 4)	0.76	#4	0.38	#8, reduced
Enhanced (4 of 4)	0.42	#7, expanded	0.29	#9, not funded

TABLE 8.4 Ranking Training and Recruitment Decision Packages

does the enhanced level of training with a CER of 0.42 exceed the returns of other currently funded activities, and should it be undertaken by removing funds from other functions or departments? On the other hand, is the current training activity with a CER of 0.76 less than the returns available from other currently unfunded activities, and should funds be removed from training and distributed to other functions or departments?

The HR director could possibly review 20 decision packages, 5 for each major activity (recruitment and employment, training and development, compensation review and management, and disciplinary action) and assess whether funding levels are appropriate. ZBB is designed to assist directors in determining whether the mix of activities within their departments is optimal, for example, should more resources be employed in HR for recruitment or training? At higher levels of management, similar assessments determine whether funding levels to HR, accounting, research and development

(R&D), and other departments are optimal. ZBB facilitates continual assessment of performance and funding within and across departments.

The last step is the compilation of the final budget. The final budget is determined by matching the organization's resource constraints with prioritized activities. Activities are funded in order of their CERs: activities with the highest ratios are budgeted first, and lower-value activities are funded until funds are exhausted. Theoretically, it is possible that one activity's minimum level may have a lower ratio than another's enhanced level and the former would be eliminated to provide funds for the expansion of the later activity.

Table 8.4 ranks the training activities examined in Table 8.3 with recruitment activities to allocate funding in the HR department. The HR director places the highest priority on posting job vacancies, performing criminal background checks, and verifying education on all job applicants, a CER of 1.82. The second, third, and fourth priorities are training,

CERs 1.27–0.76. Expanding recruitment activities to include contacting current and previous employers, package rankings #5 and #6, are seen as the next best resource uses. If funds remain, they would be committed to expanding training to the enhanced level.

ZBB attempts to clarify budget choices in areas where alternatives cannot be easily measured in dollars and cents. Table 8.4 indicates that training activities should be expanded and recruitment should be scaled back. The HR director places a higher value (0.42) on enhanced training (4 of 4) than (0.38) on the current recruitment activities (3 of 4), so funds should be shifted from recruitment to training. If additional funding should become available, recruitment could return to its current level of activity and resume contacting a single personal reference prior to employment; conversely, if revenue declines, training activities should be cut back to their current level.

County Health Department Example

Assume a county health department providing infection control (epidemiology), restaurant inspection, STD services, water testing, health education, vaccinations, the Women, Infants, and Children (WIC) program, health screenings, and pest control services decides to reevaluate its service and funding levels. The department employs 130 workers and has a budget of $10.5 million. The manager of each area is instructed to create three decision packages: a minimum level to perform only essential or legally mandated services, a budget to support current operations, and a third package to expand operations. The nine budget managers need to specify what will be provided (the programs), how many people will be served, and what resources will be required. **FIGURE 8.4** provides a synopsis of the decision packages in four areas; the complete data set is available in Chapter08.xlsx in the Figure 8.4 tab. The objective or criterion for evaluating and ranking the decision packages is the expense per person served and drives the competition between programs introduced by ZBB. An alternative method of ranking health department activities using a cost–benefit ratio approach could use the costs avoided by each program as the benefit.

The question is, should funding to a program be increased to enable it to produce

	Zero Base	Reduced	Current	Enhanced
Infection Control (IC)	**IC0**	**IC1**	**IC2**	**IC3**
Program	No Inspection	10 employees	13 Employees	16 Employees
Population Affected		1,600	400	200
Expense		$770,000	$230,000	$231,000
Cost per Person Served		$481	$575	$1,155
Restaurant Inspection (RI)	**RI0**	**RI1**	**RI2**	**RI3**
Program	No Inspection	Every 2 years	Annual	Every 6 months
Population Affected		1,800	900	600
Expense		675,000	675,000	1,350,000
Cost per Person Served		375	750	2,250
Sexual Transmitted Disease (ST	**STD0**	**STD1**	**STD2**	**STD3**
Program	None	On demand MWF	On Demand M-F	On demand M-S
Population Affected		1,000	200	75
Expense		720,000	480,000	240,000
Cost per Person Served		720	2,400	3,200
Water Testing (H2O)	**H2O0**	**H2O1**	**H2O2**	**H2O3**
Program	No Testing	Weekly Public	Daily Public Supply	Private Wells
Population Affected		12,000	9,000	3,000
Expense		1,100,000	1,000,000	700,000
Cost per Person Served		92	111	233

FIGURE 8.4 Public Health Department Programs

desirable, nice-to-haves, or luxury outputs, while reducing resources to another program to its essential or critical funding level? Do the desirables, nice-to-haves, or luxury outputs produce greater value for the organization than the current output of another area?

The objective is to maximize the number of citizens served, so the cost-effectiveness measure is the change in population affected divided by the change in expenses or the marginal cost per person served. Figure 8.4 demonstrates that as the program size increases, expenses increase faster than output, that is, diminishing returns accelerate. The next step is to rank the 27 packages from the lowest cost per person served to the highest. No current level can be ranked prior to funding the minimum level, and no expanded service can be ranked higher than its current level (**TABLE 8.5**).

Austin and Cheek (1979, p. 33) note that department managers are responsible for the substance of decision packages and senior management for ranking packages according to their congruence with organizational strategy and goals. The magnitude of work for an organization is shown in **FIGURE 8.5**. The Health Department is one of four divisions within the county government, and division directors (the second level of the organization) must rank all the decision packages produced by their managers. The director of the health department must rank the 27 packages produced by his or her area managers and produce a budget for the office. The county executive must rank the 28 budgets from the health department with the 13 packages from public safety, 10 from social services, and 16 from general administration, and produce a budget for his or her office, that is, 69 packages.

TABLE 8.5 Public Health Department Preliminary Program Rankings

Program	Cost per Person	Program Cost	Population Served	Total Budget	
PC[a]	$50	$297,500	6,000	$297,500	
PC[b]	$53	$52,500	1,000	$350,000	
H_2O[a]	$92	$1,100,000	12,000	$1,450,000	
H_2O[b]	$111	$1,000,000	9,000	$2,450,000	
PC[c]	$117	$350,000	3,000	$2,800,000	Expansion
HEd[a]	$188	$750,000	4,000	$3,550,000	
Vac[a]	$210	$630,000	3,000	$4,180,000	
H_2O[c]	$233	$700,000	3,000	$4,880,000	Expansion
HEd[b]	$250	$250,000	1,000	$5,130,000	

HSc[a]	$283	$510,000	1,800	$5,640,000	
HEd[c]	$333	$166,667	500	$5,806,667	Expansion
Vac[b]	$350	$420,000	1,200	$6,226,667	
RI[a]	$375	$675,000	1,800	$6,901,667	
IC[a]	$481	$770,000	1,600	$7,671,667	
Vac[c]	$525	$210,000	400	$7,881,667	Expansion
IC[b]	$575	$230,000	400	$8,111,667	
STD[a]	$720	$720,000	1,000	$8,831,667	
RI[b]	$750	$675,000	900	$9,506,667	
HSc[b]	$1,046	$340,000	325	$9,846,667	
IC[c]	$1,155	$231,000	200	$10,077,667	Expansion
HSc[c] (last program funded)	$1,360	$170,000	125	$10,247,667	Expansion
RI[c]	$2,250	$1,350,000	600	$11,597,667	
WIC[a]	$2,399	$1,600,000	667	$13,197,667	Elimination
STD[b]	$2,400	$480,000	200	$13,677,667	Reduction
WIC[b]	$2,594	$319,040	123	$13,996,707	Reduction
STD[c]	$3,200	$240,000	75	$14,236,707	

PC, pest control; H_2O, water; HEd, health education; Vac, vaccination; HSc, health screening; RI, restaurant inspection; IC, infection control; STD, sexually transmitted disease; WIC, Women, Infants, and Children.

[a] Minimum
[b] Current
[c] Expanded

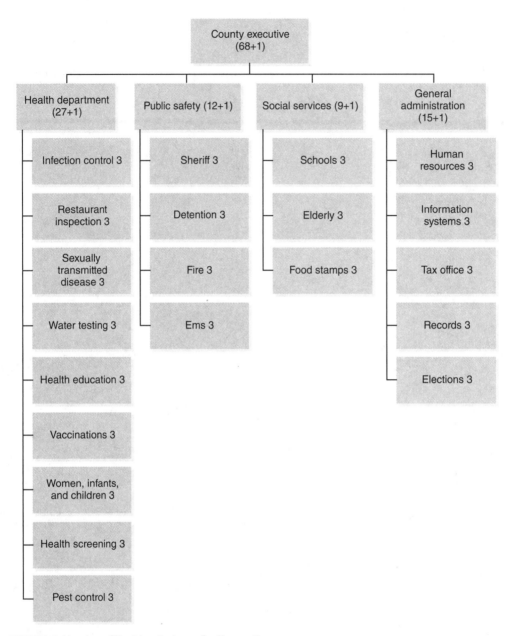

FIGURE 8.5 Number of Decision Packages for County Government

The program rankings in Table 8.5 show that five departments are designated for increased funding to allow them to provide expanded services, while one department, WIC, stands to be eliminated. The director of the public health department has stated that the WIC program will be continued, given the amount of federal money that is received to operate the program and the assistance it provides for low-income mothers and children. Under federal regulation, all WIC programs must meet minimum requirements, which is the current level that the department provides, so no reduction is possible. The current WIC program cost per person was arbitrarily set at $1 versus its actual cost of $2400 to ensure its inclusion in funded programs. **TABLE 8.6** shows the re-ranking based on the forced inclusion of the current level of the WIC program.

The final step is the compilation of the final budget. The final budget is determined by matching the organization's resource constraints with the prioritized activities. Table 8.6 provides a cumulative total for the ranked packages and draws a line at the point where the resource constraint is met. The last program to be funded is the minimal level of the STD[a] program. Every

program continues to be funded, and four programs (pest control, water testing, health education, and vaccinations) are slated for expansion. Three programs (restaurant inspection, health screenings, and STDs) may be reduced to their minimum levels to fund the four programs identified for expansion. The department budget for this set of programs could be reduced from $10,500,000 to $10,431,667 (−0.65%), while expanding the number of people served from 45,225 to 51,367 (+13.58%). ZBB allows managers to reevaluate what their organization does and what it achieves in light of changing needs for its products and services and the efficiency of providing these services.

TABLE 8.6 Public Health Department Final Program Rankings

Program	Cost per Person	Program Cost	Population Served	Total Budget	
WIC[a]* (non-eliminable)	$1	$1,600,000	667	$1,600,000	
PC[a]	$50	$297,500	6,000	$1,897,500	
PC[b]	$53	$52,500	1,000	$1,950,000	
H_2O[a]	$92	$1,100,000	12,000	$3,050,000	
H_2O[b]	$111	$1,000,000	9,000	$4,050,000	
PC[c]	$117	$350,000	3,000	$4,400,000	Expansion
HEd[a]	$188	$750,000	4,000	$5,150,000	
Vac[a]	$210	$630,000	3,000	$5,780,000	
H_2O[c]	$233	$700,000	3,000	$6,480,000	Expansion
HEd[b]	$250	$250,000	1,000	$6,730,000	
HSc[a]	$283	$510,000	1,800	$7,240,000	

(continues)

TABLE 8.6 Public Health Department Final Program Rankings *(continued)*

HEd[c]	$333	$166,667	500	$7,406,667	Expansion
Vac[b]	$350	$420,000	1,200	$7,826,667	
RI[a]	$375	$675,000	1,800	$8,501,667	
IC[a]	$481	$770,000	1,600	$9,271,667	
Vac[c]	$525	$210,000	400	$9,481,667	Expansion
IC[b]	$575	$230,000	400	$9,711,667	
STD[a] (last program funded)	$720	$720,000	1,000	$10,431,667	
RI[b]	$750	$675,000	900	$11,106,667	Reduction
HSc[b]	$1,046	$340,000	325	$11,446,667	Reduction
IC[c]	$1,155	$231,000	200	11,677,667	
HSc[c]	$1,360	$170,000	125	$11,847,667	
RI[c]	$2,250	$1,350,000	600	$13,197,667	
STD[b]	$2,400	$480,000	200	$13,677,667	Reduction
WIC[b]	$2,594	$319,040	123	$13,996,707	
STD[c]	$3,200	$240,000	75	$14,236,707	

	Zero-Base Budget	Current Budget	Change (%)
Budget	$10,431,667	$10,500,000	−0.65
Population served	51,367	45,225	13.58

*Program cost per person set to $1 to ensure funding.

▶ Variations on Zero-Base Budgeting

While ZBB never achieved widespread use, it gave rise to two variations that could benefit all organizations. The idea that all expenditures should be justified is sound, but analyzing every expense every year is probably not worth the effort. The first variation, **zero-base review**, moves away from an annual review of all expenditures to 5-year or longer reviews, while **target-base budgeting** focuses analysis only on discretionary expenses and ignores nondiscretionary (mandated by law) spending. Both variations reduce the scope of analysis and simplify the ZBB process.

Zero-Base Review

Even if managers choose to rely primarily on an incremental or flexible budgeting system to provide line item projections of expenses on an annual basis (due to ease, inability to cut expenses, or other reasons), ZBB techniques should be used periodically to evaluate whether resources are being used effectively. Too much spending is left unquestioned in incremental and flexible budgeting systems; low-value operations are continued simply because they were funded in the past, alternative resource uses are not explored because of a lack of funds, and managers receive little or suboptimal performance incentives. Meeting the budget to fulfill incremental budgeting goals provides little incentive and often encourages squandering of resources (use it or lose it), while the emphasis on maintaining or reducing the cost per output under flexible budgeting provides a partial incentive to increase organizational value.

Zero-base review employs the assumptions, structure, and process of ZBB but is not performed annually. Zero-base review may target each division or department on a periodic basis, possibly every 5 years, and requires directors and managers to develop decision packages, in addition to normal budget requirements. The goal is to capture the insight that ZBB can provide into priorities, methods, and scale to improve resource allocation. If zero-base review is implemented on a rotating 5-year system, the entire budget does not have to be justified every year—20% of managers would be required to provide information beyond normal budget requirements, and assumptions and past practices can be regularly questioned.

Zero-base review recognizes the utility of questioning all expenses to identify costs that produce less than their expected result, are no longer necessary, or were never needed to reduce waste, while eliminating the need to perform this analysis every year. Zero-base review assumes that the majority of benefits from a ZBB process can be obtained at a lower cost if reviews are not done annually. The knowledge that operations will regularly undergo a thorough review and historical funding levels will not be guaranteed should encourage managers to innovate, reduce costs, and improve goods and services produced.

Target-Base Budgeting

A second variation of ZBB is target-base budgeting, which relies on the same basic procedures as ZBB but is only used to evaluate discretionary funds. For example, in 2015, the total federal spending was $3700 billion: mandatory (entitlement) spending and interest comprised $2500 billion, leaving only $1200 billion in discretionary spending. Performing ZBB analysis on mandatory expenditures that can only be reduced by changing law may be futile (Congressional Budget Office, 2016). If target-base budgeting was implemented by the federal government, it could be limited to the 32.4% of total expenditures that are subject to annual appropriations, like defense (15.7%), education (2.4%), and transportation programs (2.4%). Organizations may choose to rely primarily on an incremental or flexible budgeting system to provide line item projections of expenses on an annual basis but use a target-base approach to evaluate and fund new projects and expansions.

The primary assumptions underlying target-base budgeting is that the majority of expenditures cannot be altered but competition for discretionary funds can be created. The competition for funds is directed by senior management priorities. Discretionary funds could be the result of increasing revenue, that is, revenue growth exceeds expenditure growth, providing discretionary funds or the result of cutting expenditure budgets, for example, a 2.0% across-the-board cut. The "free" funds can then be bid upon: what new activities can a department provide that will add the greatest value to the organization?

Department managers develop operating budgets as usual (base plus inflation) or to the target (base minus 2.0% set aside) and then develop requests to capture the discretionary funds. Requests for discretionary funds highlight new activities that will be undertaken if additional resources are available, tie the proposed activities to the organization's mission and goals, and specify marginal cost. There is an obvious incentive for managers to overestimate outcome and underestimate costs to secure funding. These requests are then submitted to senior management for ranking. New program/activity requests are ranked (high to low yield), and monies are allocated on the basis of their contribution to the organization until the discretionary funds are exhausted.

The strengths of target-base budgeting are it does not require justification of the entire budget, thus requiring less paperwork, and it encourages innovation, competition, and efficiency. On the other hand, its weaknesses include institutionalizing past performance (rather than a critical review), and it can encourage gaming. Managers may not propose new activities but rather rename existing programs to capture discretionary funds—old wine repackaged in a new bottle.

Notwithstanding the weaknesses of target-base budgeting, it provides a useful structure to evaluate how budget expansions and marginal fund reallocations should be handled.

Strengths of Zero-Base Budgeting

ZBB provides a number of benefits over traditional budgeting systems. First, it does not rest on historical goals and practices but requires explicit recognition of current priorities and how processes operate and contribute to organizational objectives. The detailing of activities within a department allows ZBB to identify whether multiple departments are doing the same work, whether redundancy is justifiable, and who has the best process based on output and cost. Senior management may obtain a better perspective of the value of centralization; it may be more efficient to centralize the functions when multiple departments spend significant resources on the same or similar activities.

An obvious benefit of ZBB is the expanded information and choices it can illuminate. When activities are defined within a department, it is easy to see that the budget decisions are not all-or-nothing choices, but that activities and programs can be funded individually and low-benefit work can be reduced or eliminated. Outputs are ranked according to cost, and this ranking does not ask, "is this output worth the cost?" but rather "how much do various sets of output cost?" In for-profit organizations, the primary question is, will price cover the cost of production? ZBB is often used for "nonmarket" outputs, where it is not a question of whether costs are covered but rather whether the organization is getting the maximum value from the resources it employs. A flexible budget with a cost cap may be best for market-transacted outputs; outputs will only be funded if their price exceeds their cost.

While the budget is created from the bottom up, senior management is provided with

1. It formalizes priorities: senior management sets the agenda, and department managers determine how the objectives can be met.
2. It develops operational data: what is done, how it is done, and what the alternative methods are.
3. It identifies redundant activities. By basing the decision packages on activities, multiple departments performing the same activities or producing the same or similar outputs can be easily identified.
4. It provides distinct budget choices.
5. Budget construction occurs from the bottom up: managers propose various levels of input use and expected outputs, and senior management selects the mix of outputs to meet the organization's objectives.
6. It creates competition between programs and an incentive to produce the greatest outcomes at the lowest cost.

more detailed information on what departments do and what their costs of operations are, and can evaluate their performance in light of organizational goals. The greatest benefit ZBB can provide is to establish competition between departments for resources. Managers should be encouraged to become more customer centered, cost conscious, and innovative to protect, if not expand, their budgets when they understand the incentives ZBB introduces (**BOX 8.2**).

Weaknesses of Zero-Base Budgeting

ZBB has never achieved widespread use because of several weaknesses. The primary weakness is excessive paperwork. There are theoretically an infinite number of decision packages that can be generated from a single operation, that is, output at 110% of the current level, 109%, 100%, 90%, and so on, with a distinct budget for each output level. The level of detail required to specify what is needed to produce a good or service for each decision package may approach the complexity seen in scratch budgeting.

The second weakness is the limited potential for change. Robert Anthony (1977) declared, "Zero-base budgeting is a fraud," noting that in Georgia, a zero base meant that departments retained 80% of past spending, so only expenditures above 80% of the current funding were reviewed. Only 2 of 13 department heads stated that ZBB may have reallocated resources, and all 32 budget analysts reported no major shift of resources (21 reported no shift of resources, 7 reported some reallocation, and 4 were uncertain). Anthony also accurately noted, "the worth of programs cannot be determined by reading a two-page form." The problem cited in Georgia for the lack of ZBB-driven change was that federal regulations specifying minimum program requirements did not permit, or were interpreted as prohibiting, expenditure reductions.

Like other budgeting systems, ZBB can be gamed. Managers have an incentive to inflate the cost of the minimum (or essential) level services and thus enhance the attractiveness of scope-expanding activity by understating the cost of expansion. For example, the total cost to produce 30 units may be $150, or an average of $5.00 per unit. When preparing the minimum or essential decision package, the manager may report the cost of the first 20 units as $120, or $6.00 per unit; the next 10 units (the current output level) would then cost $30, or $3.00 per unit. By inappropriately front-loading costs, managers enhance the attractiveness of maintaining the current level of output by underreporting its true cost. The front-benefit ploy can also enhance the attractiveness of expanding activities beyond the current level, that is, the cost for an additional

10 units (from 30 to 40) may be $10, or a marginal cost per unit of $1.00.

The Air Force's B3 bomber program is currently slated to cost $60 billion and produce 80–100 planes. It provides an example of how costs can be front-loaded to enhance the desirability of program expansion (Henegan & Petersen, 2015). The current projection produces an average cost of $600 million per jet. Assuming R&D costs are $30 billion and produce two planes, the marginal cost of producing the next 98 jets would be $306 million ($30 billion / 98 units). Congressional approval should be more likely when the per unit cost is quoted at $306 million rather than $600 million. The question is, are reported cost true, or have they been manipulated by managers to obtain additional funding? See **BOX 8.3**.

ZBB can be used anywhere a cost–benefit relationship can be identified (Pyhrr, 1973, p. 19). Fruitful areas of application include overhead (administration, marketing and sales, R&D, etc.), production support services (maintenance, supervision, and engineering and design), and capital expenditures. ZBB is less appropriate for direct or nondiscretionary production costs where clear physical relationships exist between inputs and output (engineering costs); it is most appropriate for discretionary costs in nonprofit and government organizations.

BOX 8.3 Weaknesses of Zero-Base Budgeting

1. It requires extensive paperwork and time to prepare.
2. It is ineffective when managers have limited ability to control spending: can programs be reduced or eliminated?
3. It encourages gaming by inflating the cost to provide a minimum level and reducing the marginal cost of expansions.

ZBB requires a greater understanding of operations; unlike flexible budgeting, it is not concerned with the cost per output but rather focuses on the use and costs of different activities that could produce an output. This perspective is more dynamic as managers can dissect and scrutinize operations to identify alternative means to accomplish activities and produce output. In further breaking with the past, not only may different production processes be pursued, but the size of the department and the amount of activity performed may also change. ZBB is designed to redirect resources to departments that operate effectively and efficiently by reducing or eliminating the budgets of low-benefit departments. The zero says it all; a low-yield department may see its budget eliminated (i.e., zeroed out) if other managers make a compelling case that they can use resources more effectively to advance the organization's goals and objectives.

▶ Evaluating Performance

Unlike flexible budgeting, which is primarily concerned with the question of whether actual per unit costs are greater than, equal to, or less than budgeted, ZBB explores whether activities should be continued even if costs have been pushed to their minimum. Beside the questions of efficiency and quality, ZBB assesses whether the good or service is needed or desired and whether resources should be transferred to other uses that can produce more highly valued outputs.

Given the incentive in ZBB to maximize the value of output and the organization, the performance evaluation and compensation system should reward managers and employees for increasing customer and client satisfaction, in addition to managing costs and quality. The obvious mechanisms would base salary increases or bonuses on customer satisfaction ratings or, in for-profit organizations, an increase in market valuation (stock prices).

Given effective and timely adjustments by managers, the year-end review should approach the targets set by the budget. If expenses, quality, volume, and customer satisfaction do not meet the targets set in the budget, a search for cause(s) must be undertaken. Are the variances due to higher input prices, lower efficiency, changes to products or processes, or shifts in customer preferences?

Zero-Base Performance Audits

ZBB suggests that major benefits will accrue to organizations that make the effort to implement it, but like many claims, more may be promised than delivered. The question is, how can an organization improve its use of resources, as described by the decision packages and their rankings? **Zero-base performance auditing** is a form of operational auditing that focuses on the claims made in decision packages and determines whether activities were conducted as promised and whether the expected costs and benefits were realized (Austin & Cheek, 1979, p. 30).

The five primary items in a decision package are objectives, consequences of elimination, performance measures, alternatives, and benefits and costs. As auditing will only occur on funded packages, the consequences of elimination can be ignored, and for clarity, benefits and costs should be treated as separate items. The operational audit should assess whether the objective was realized and, if not, whether the objective was viable. The second question is, was a complete set of alternatives considered? Were other means of production given serious consideration or simply a perfunctory review? Are the manager and staff open to new ways of doing things? The third and fourth questions are, if a complete set of alternatives was presented, did the manager select the best approach and was the approach followed?

Decision package	Performance audit
Objective	Is the objective viable?
Alternatives considered	Was a complete set of alternatives considered?
Approach taken	Was the best approach taken?
Expected costs	Were costs less than or equal to the budget?
Expected benefits (results)	Were expected benefits realized?

The final two questions, were expected costs and benefits realized, analyze whether the expected output was produced, if it performed as expected, and whether it cost more or less than expected. Obviously, many factors can affect output, its value, and costs; the performance audit seeks to separate controllable and noncontrollable factors in order to assess managerial performance and correct future budget requests for bias.

The Air Force provides another example of how things work out compared to how they were planned. The F-22 fighter was budgeted for 648 planes at $139 million per plane, but the Air Force received 188 jets (29% of the planned output) at a cost of $412 million each (an increase of 296%). Henegan and Petersen (2015) quote Pentagon officials, who again claimed that they have learned from past mistakes, but massive cost overruns continue to bedevil government projects in general and defense procurement in particular. Zero-base performance auditing assesses whether the claims made in the decision packages budgeted are followed and whether the expected benefits are obtained. Retrospective review is an essential component to ensure that managers do not make unrealistic claims and that they strive to realize the claims they make in their budgets. Audits, like zero-base performance review, that expand the scope of factors beyond benefits and costs to encompass objectives and processes would benefit any organization.

After ZBB was initially embraced as the next big thing in finance, it fell into disfavor; however, it is once again drawing attention. Bain and Company look to ZBB as a means of redesigning processes and reducing costs by examining every aspect of a business and considering what activities should be undertaken and how they should be performed (Cichocki, 2012). The approach parallels Lean Six Sigma, and the goal is to design optimal workflows and detailed procedures to standardize work. Tamara Rosin (2015) posed the question, should more healthcare providers adopt ZBB in response to reduced reimbursement, bundled payments, and higher patient deductibles and copayments? It seems clear that the financial challenges facing healthcare providers will require them to evaluate not only how efficiently they use their resources but also what type of care they will offer.

▶ **An Example of Zero-Base Budgeting: Medicare Part A**

Chapters 6 and 7 examined Medicare expenditures. Chapter 6 reviewed total expenditures, and Chapter 7 focused on expenditures per enrollee to identify the impact of enrollment growth and expenditure growth per enrollee on total outlays. Using a ZBB approach, Medicare Part A expenditures can be analyzed by what is delivered (i.e., cost per enrollee per patient in each of the 26 major diagnostic categories [MDCs]). TABLE 8.7 shows the author's estimate of how Part A expenditures are divided across the 26 MDCs. The estimates are based on the Part A outlays in 2010, the simple average for diagnosis-related group (DRG) weight (2013) and the percentage of inpatient discharges by MDC (Kansas Hospital Association, 2013).

Table 8.7 shows that the expenditure per discharge varies from $7,455 for alcohol/drug

TABLE 8.7 Medicare Part A Expenditures by MDC

MDC	Average DRG Weight	Arithmetic Mean LOS (days)	Kansas (%)	Total Expenditure/ MDC (000)	Total Discharges	Average Expenditure/ Discharge (000)
Pre-ungroupable	6.364	12.580	0.06	$376,755	7,405	$50.881
1. Nervous	1.987	4.382	8.01	$15,701,549	988,514	$15.884
2. Eye	1.052	3.041	0.11	$114,222	13,575	$8.414
3. ENT	1.212	3.088	0.89	$1,064,491	109,835	$9.692
4. Respiratory	1.515	4.527	16.09	$24,050,145	1,985,667	$12.112
5. Circulatory	2.925	4.741	18.83	$54,338,712	2,323,810	$23.383
6. Digestive	1.797	4.920	10.61	$18,812,268	1,309,380	$14.367

7. Hepatobiliary	1.980	5.276	2.21	$4,317,528	272,736	$15.830
8. Musculo-skeletal	2.251	4.448	13.46	$29,900,291	1,661,099	$18.000
9. Skin	1.472	4.282	2.21	$3,210,235	272,736	$11.770
10. Endocrine	1.720	4.280	3.37	$5,718,545	415,892	$13.750
11. Kidney	1.703	4.298	6.93	$11,646,678	855,231	$13.618
12. Male reproductive	1.237	3.201	0.48	$585,616	59,237	$9.886
13. Female reproductive	1.507	3.709	0.45	$668,986	55,535	$12.046
14. Pregnancy	0.803	2.474	0.00	$0	0	$0.000
15. Newborn	2.395	7.543	0.00	$0	0	$0.000
16. Blood	1.801	4.413	1.30	$2,309,608	160,433	$14.396
17. Myelopro-liferative	2.374	5.882	0.64	$1,498,937	78,982	$18.978
18. Infectious	2.171	5.755	6.29	$13,471,878	776,249	$17.355
19. Mental diseases	1.072	4.096	1.93	$2,041,598	238,181	$8.572
20. Alcohol/drug	0.933	4.817	0.18	$165,615	22,214	$7.455
21. Injury/poison	1.540	3.931	0.94	$1,428,137	116,005	$12.311
22. Burns	4.777	8.133	0.05	$235,684	6,171	$38.195
23. Factors	1.247	4.057	4.77	$5,868,979	588,666	$9.970
24. Trauma	3.405	6.266	0.16	$537,608	19,746	$27.227
25. HIV	2.324	5.983	0.01	$22,934	1,234	$18.584
Average	2.060		99.98	$198,087,000	12,338,532	$15.488

LOS, length of stay.

rehabilitation treatment to $50,881 for patients classified as ungroupable. If the objective of Medicare is to maximize the number of inpatient discharges, while reducing expenditures, MDCs could be ranked according to their average expenditure per discharge. Low-cost MDCs would be ranked higher than high-cost MDCs if healthcare rationing were required to reduce costs. **TABLE 8.8** displays the MDC rankings to maximize discharges and limit expenditures.

The cost per discharge increases rapidly, beginning with MDC 5, circulatory. Assuming that Medicare decides to restrain expenditures by limiting coverage a ZBB approach may recommend excluding high-cost MDCs, such as circulatory, trauma, burns, and ungroupable, from covered benefits. This change would reduce expenditures by 28.0% and paid discharges by 19.1%, or 80.9% of patients could be covered at 72.0% of current spending. Obviously, Medicare will not determine healthcare

TABLE 8.8 Medicare Part A Expenditures by MDC (Lowest to Highest Cost per Discharge)						
MDC	**Average DRG Weight**	**Arithmetic Mean LOS**	**Kansas (%)**	**Total Expenditure/ MDC (000)**	**Total Discharges**	**Average Expenditure/ Discharge (000)**
20. Alcohol/drug	0.933	4.817	0.18	$165,615	22,214	$7.455
2. Eye	1.052	3.041	0.11	$114,222	13,575	$8.414
19. Mental diseases	1.072	4.096	1.93	$2,041,598	238,181	$8.572
3. ENT	1.212	3.088	0.89	$1,064,491	109,835	$9.692
12. Male reproductive	1.237	3.201	0.48	$585,616	59,237	$9.886
23. Factors	1.247	4.057	4.77	$5,868,979	588,666	$9.970
9. Skin	1.472	4.282	2.21	$3,210,235	272,736	$11.770
13. Female reproductive	1.507	3.709	0.45	$668,986	55,535	$12.046
4. Respiratory	1.515	4.527	16.09	$24,050,145	1,985,667	$12.112
21. Injury/poison	1.540	3.931	0.94	$1,428,137	116,005	$12.311
11. Kidney	1.703	4.298	6.93	$11,646,678	855,231	$13.618

10. Endocrine	1.720	4.280	3.37	$5,718,545	415,892	$13.750
6. Digestive	1.797	4.920	10.61	$18,812,268	1,309,380	$14.367
16. Blood	1.801	4.413	1.30	$2,309,608	160,433	$14.396
7. Hepatobiliary	1.980	5.276	2.21	$4,317,528	272,736	$15.830
1. Nervous	1.987	4.382	8.01	$15,701,549	988,514	$15.884
18. Infectious	2.171	5.755	6.29	$13,471,878	776,249	$17.355
8. Musculo-skeletal	2.251	4.448	13.46	$29,900,291	1,661,099	$18.000
25. HIV	2.324	5.983	0.01	$22,934	1,234	$18.584
17. Myelopro-liferative	2.374	5.882	0.64	$1,498,937	78,982	$18.978
5. Circulatory	2.925	4.741	18.83	$54,338,712	2,323,810	$23.383
24. Trauma	3.405	6.266	0.16	$537,608	19,746	$27.227
22. Burns	4.777	8.133	0.05	$235,684	6,171	$38.195
Pre-ungroupable	6.364	12.580	0.06	$376,755	7,405	$50.881
14. Pregnancy	0.803	2.474	0.00	0	0	$0.000
15. Newborn	2.395	7.543	0.00	0	0	$0.000

coverage based on the cost to treat patients, but this type of analysis could be used to examine why treating circulatory, trauma, burns, and ungroupable patients is so expensive and devise new treatment methods to lower costs. This type of analysis could also be used to analyze the effectiveness of treatments (DRGs) within an MDC, that is, if two or more treatments produce similar patient outcomes,

should coverage be limited to the most cost-effective treatment? Chapter 9 takes this analysis one step further by examining outcomes. The current analysis of Medicare expenditures is incomplete as it does not report the change in health status (benefit of treatment) only the treatment cost. High-cost MDCs may extend life expectancy and/or improve the quality of life more than low-cost MDCs.

Summary

ZBB deviates from incremental and flexible budgeting as it harkens back to planning to ask, should existing activities continue to be performed? Even when activities cannot be eliminated, ZBB questions whether their scope should be expanded or contracted and whether there are better ways to perform a function and achieve an end. The primary focus of ZBB is outputs produced and the activities required to produce them. ZBB peers inside black box production processes to ask how outputs are produced and whether resources can produce higher value in alternative employments. The focus on alternative production methods distinguishes ZBB from other budgeting systems—it asks whether a different set of resources and/or production system can lower costs and increase the value of the organization.

In ZBB, managers must produce multiple budgets reflecting different levels of output and sets of resources, which increase their understanding of departmental processes and organizational goals. ZBB introduces competition into the budgeting process, where managers who produce greater benefits for the organization can obtain larger budgets, while those who fail to meet the organization's objectives or are inefficient see their budgets shrink. ZBB changes the competition within an organization from the question of the year-to-year increase in the budget to whether an activity will receive the same level of funding as it has in the past. ZBB recognizes that consumer tastes and preferences as well as production technologies are ever-changing and that past performance should not be the key determinant for continued funding.

The ZBB approach is valuable to any organization where operating premises are not regularly challenged. ZBB offers valuable insight into alternative ways of running an operation, given the constant changes in an organization's operating environment, which include a rapidly changing demand for goods and services and changes in information and production technologies. While ZBB is a time-consuming process and may not be desirable for annual use, zero-base review and target-base review offer comparable means of obtaining the benefits of ZBB by evaluating departments on a less frequent basis or applying the process to discretionary or new expenditures.

ZBB is most appropriate for organizations that lack the profit incentive (nonprofit and government organizations) and overhead departments in for-profit organizations where quantity and quality are not easily measured. Success under ZBB requires organizations to question how they operate, develop their managers' financial skills, devote more time to developing multiple budget packages, and be willing to fundamentally question how their resources are used. ZBB is a budgeting system that challenges the status quo.

Key Terms and Concepts

Decision package	Target-base budget	Zero-base performance audit
External scan	Zero-base budgeting	Zero-base review

Discussion Questions

1. Describe the steps needed to construct a zero-base budget.
2. Compare a zero-base budget with flexible and incremental budgets.
3. What steps can a manager take to maximize his or her budget in a ZBB system?
4. When should a zero-base budget be employed?
5. Explain the strengths and weaknesses of ZBB.
6. Describe the difference between ZBB and zero-base review and target-base review.

Problems

1. A community health center is currently operating from 7:00 A.M. to 11:00 P.M., Monday through Friday. The manager has constructed five decision packages. The first calls for closure; the second, the minimum level, reduces hours to 8:00 A.M. through 5:00 P.M. (40 hours per week); the reduced level operates from 7:00 A.M. to 7:00 P.M. (60 hours); the current level maintains the current 80 hours per week; and the enhanced level adds 8 hours on Saturday (88 hours). The clinic receives $92 per patient seen. The following table shows the manager's estimates of patients seen under each set of operating hours. Calculate the marginal cost, total and marginal revenues, and the cost–benefit ratio (marginal benefit/marginal cost). What is your recommendation for operating hours? Should hours be increased or reduced from current hours?

Decision Package	Patients	Total Cost	Marginal Cost	Total Revenue	Marginal Revenue	Cost–Benefit Ratio
Eliminate (0 of 4)	0	$0	_____	_____	_____	_____
Minimum (1 of 4)	120	$8,000	_____	_____	_____	_____
Reduced (2 of 4)	144	$12,400	_____	_____	_____	_____
Current (3 of 4)	184	$16,800	_____	_____	_____	_____
Enhanced (4 of 4)	208	$19,200	_____	_____	_____	_____

2. The ambulatory care division of an integrated health system is evaluating its four departments (a multidisciplinary physician practice, same-day surgery, outpatient clinic, and home health practice) to determine whether it is maximizing the value of healthcare services it could provide under its $6,800,000 budget. All four departments are operating at their current level, and each manager has been told to create a budget, including revenues, expenses, and number of patients that can be seen if the budget is increased and decreased. Substantial changes in patient volumes have been seen with a large increase in demand for same-day surgery and a modest decline in the outpatient clinic. The output measure that the departments will be evaluated and ranked on is revenue generated per dollar of expense. The health system recognizes that the outpatient clinic, although generating less revenue than its expenses, provides an outlet for the emergency room (ER), and has estimated that two of every five clinic patients would end up at the ER and

generate substantial uncompensated costs. Avoided ER costs are included as a benefit (revenue) of the clinic to recognize its contribution to the health system.

Using the Problem 8.2 tab in BudgetCh08.xlsx, calculate the revenue/expense ratios for all the decision packages and rank them from highest to lowest. Assuming a budget constraint of $6,800,000, should any departments be expanded or contracted? How many

patients can be served under ZBB versus the current budget?

3. Calculate the marginal revenue/marginal expense ratio for each decision package. Note the current budget is $22,370,000 revenue, $20,000,000 expense, and $2,370,000 profit. Using ZBB, should any program's funding be increased or decreased by $500,000 (i.e., total expenses remain at $20,000,000)? What will be the total revenue, total expense, and total patients in the new budget?

General Surgery	−$500,000 Reduced	Current	+$500,000 Expanded
Revenue	$9,600,000	$10,180,000	$10,730,000
Expense	$8,000,000	$8,500,000	$9,000,000
Patients	9,000	10,000	11,000
Cardiology	Reduced	Current	Expanded
Revenue	$7,700,000	$8,240,000	$8,750,000
Expense	$7,000,000	$7,500,000	$8,000,000
Patients	5,500	6,000	6,400
Oncology	Reduced	Current	Expanded
Revenue	$3,640,000	$3,950,000	$4,350,000
Expense	$3,500,000	$4,000,000	$4,500,000
Patients	3,400	4,000	4,500

	MR/MC		Program Cost	Cumulative Budget
Priority	**Program**	**Ratio**		
First	_____	_____	_____	_____
Second	_____	_____	_____	_____
Third	_____	_____	_____	_____
Fourth	_____	_____	_____	_____
Fifth	_____	_____	_____	_____
Sixth	_____	_____	_____	_____
Seventh	_____	_____	_____	_____
Eighth	_____	_____	_____	_____
Last	_____	_____	_____	_____

MR, marginal revenue; MC, marginal cost.

4. The county health department examined in Figures 8.4–8.7 has calculated avoided costs for each of its nine programs. Calculate the cost–benefit ratio for each of the 27 decision packages and compile the final budget based on an increase in the health department's budget to $10,900,000 (or a decrease to $10,000,000).

References

Anthony, R. N. (1977). Zero-base budgeting is a fraud. *Wall Street Journal*, April 27, 1977, 26.

Austin, L. A., & Cheek, L. M. (1979). *Zero-base budgeting: A decision package manual*. New York, NY: AMACOM.

Cichocki, P. (2012). Radical redesign through zero-based budgeting. Retrieved May 11, 2017, from http://www.bain.com/publications/articles/radical-redesign-through-zero-based-budgeting.aspx

Congressional Budget Office. (2016). *The federal budget in 2015: A closer look at discretionary spending*. Retrieved from https://www.cbo.gov/sites/default/files/114th-congress-2015-2016/graphic/51112-discretionaryspending.pdf

Henegan, W. J., & Petersen, M. (2015). Air Force's plan for new stealth bomber could bring thousands of jobs to Southland. Retrieved October 27, 2015, from http://www.latimes.com/business/la-fi-bomber-contract-20151027-story.html

Kansas Hospital Association. (2013). Percentage of Inpatient Discharges by MDC. Retrieved January 14, 2015, from http://www.kha-net.org/dataproductsandservices/stat/hospitalutilization/inpatientdischargesbymdc/

Pyhrr, P. A. (1973). *Zero-base budgeting*. New York, NY: John Wiley & Sons.

Rosin, T. (2015). Should more health systems adopt zero-based budgeting. Retrieved May 11, 2017, from http://www.beckershospitalreview.com//finance/should-more-health-systems-adopy-zero-based-budgeting.html

CHAPTER 9

Program Budgeting

CHAPTER OBJECTIVES

1. Explain the steps to build a program budget.
2. Construct a program budget.
3. Evaluate the strengths and weaknesses of program budgeting.
4. Explain the purpose and performance of the Oregon Health Plan.

▶ Introduction

The major shift that program budgeting makes away from the three systems previously discussed is its primary concern for effectiveness and outcomes. Do expenditures and activities produce the desired result? Program budgeting is less concerned with what is done, staying within the budget (incremental budgeting), minimizing the cost per output (flexible budgeting), or determining what outputs should be produced (zero-base budgeting), to focus on what is accomplished. Like zero-base budgeting, program budgeting is designed to promote competition for resources.

Program budgeting is designed to fulfill the organization's mission (maximize profit, population health, education, etc.) and is explicitly a priority-setting mechanism. Program budgeting differs from other budgeting systems as it is often used to centralize resource allocation decisions versus the bottom-up approach of previous systems. Program budgeting recognizes that desired outcomes often require the coordination of resources across departments and moves away from single-year, department-centered budgets in favor of multiyear, outcome-centered planning. Program budgeting subordinates the interests of departments to the larger goals of the organization and is a means of setting long-term direction rather than estimating expected expenditures by object code (**FIGURE 9.1**).

The preeminent users of program budgeting are the U.S. Department of Defense and the National Health Systems of the United Kingdom, Australia, and Canada. While the coupling of medicine and military seems incongruent, each uses program budgeting for similar reasons. Both activities are performed by public agencies facing defined spending constraints, with multiple demands for service that must be prioritized. The nuclear deterrence triumvirate of air-, land-, and sea-based warheads is an oft-cited example of program

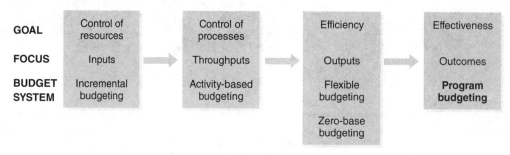

GOAL	Control of resources	Control of processes	Efficiency	Effectiveness
FOCUS	Inputs	Throughputs	Outputs	Outcomes
BUDGET SYSTEM	Incremental budgeting	Activity-based budgeting	Flexible budgeting	**Program budgeting**
			Zero-base budgeting	

FIGURE 9.1 Budgeting Systems

planning, where the outcome, national security, can be achieved in multiple ways and investment decisions are made to achieve an end in the most cost-effective manner. Similarly, national health systems aim at maximizing the health of the citizenry by allocating funds between patients, providers, and types of care (acute, chronic, and preventive).

▶ Program Budgeting

According to Brambleby (1995), program budgeting serves five functions: simplification, clarification of past expenditures, planning, coordination, and communication. These are standard roles of a budget, but as program budgeting is often undertaken at the government level and the amount of money at play dwarfs the resources of even the largest organizations, simplification and clarification are sorely needed. In national health systems, such as in the United Kingdom and Canada, program budgeting is used to distribute 5.0% and 9.0% of the total gross domestic product, while the U.S. defense department spent $582 billion in 2015. When hundreds of billions of dollars are spent, simplification is vital to grasp why money was spent and what was purchased (similar to the task of the chart of accounts). Budgets specify the financial plan that managers expect to follow to achieve organizational goals and, once finalized, are a tool to assess and manage day-to-day operations. The last function, communication, is essential to provide transparency for public spending. While for-profits and nonprofits address a relatively small range of interests, public budgets should serve all members of society. Public agencies should clearly define how funds are allocated and should be ready to justify their spending.

Ruta, Mitton, Bate, and Donaldson (2005) state that program budgeting answers five questions: First, what is the total funding constraint? Second, how are funds currently spent (i.e., what is purchased and what is received)? Third, what new funding opportunities have arisen, what are their benefits and costs, and which are desirable expansions? Fourth, can existing services be provided more efficiently to release funding for other purposes? Question 4 addresses **technical efficiency**, a situation in which output cannot be increased by increasing the use of one input and decreasing the consumption of another. Fifth, if desirable expansions cannot be funded through efficiency gains, should existing services be reduced to fund desired expansions? The final question addresses **allocative efficiency**, a situation in which a good or service is produced up to the point where marginal benefit equals marginal cost. According to Bate and Mitton (2006), healthcare funds have been allocated on the basis of history, decibels (who could shout the loudest), or epidemiology. Program budgeting adds effectiveness, efficiency, necessity, fair use of public money, and public values to the decision-making process.

Program budgeting attempts to assemble logical groupings of resources to perform activities and achieve outcomes rather than simply maximizing output. The recognition that outcomes (improved health, national security) are not momentary achievements but require multiyear, if not continual, effort frees planners from the short-run, 1-year perspective to focus on long-term results and consequences. Program budgeting is a systematic process to identify the best means to achieve an outcome.

Program budgeting rests on the same economic principles of opportunity costs, diminishing marginal returns, and efficiency as other budgeting systems but adds **equity**, the question of what is a fair distribution of a society's economic goods among its members. The importance of opportunity cost is elevated over its use in other budgeting systems because of the wider scope of concern program budgeting takes. While zero-base budgeting, in theory, allows funding to be totally eliminated, in practice, it often settles for marginal adjustments in budgets, succumbing to the tendency to enshrine the past. The outcome focus in program budgeting supplies greater weight to the reallocation of funds when one program achieves superior results to another. Few should complain when funds are shifted from program B to program A, if a compelling case can be made that A produces more and/or better outcomes than B using the same amount of funds. Clients, the recipients of goods or services, should be delighted with more or improved outcomes, and the providers of funding should be indifferent if no additional resources are needed. The only opposition to the reallocation of funds should arise from the employees of program B, who stand to lose jobs, funding, and power; this loss, however, should be wholly offset by the support of employees of program A, who will receive higher funding.

Diminishing marginal returns and efficiency play the same roles in program budgeting as they do in other budgeting systems. Diminishing returns warn us that as programs expand beyond a certain point, they generate less benefit per dollar expended. Auctions are processes to reveal valuation and vividly demonstrate the impact of diminishing returns. In an auction, value is determined by the person who is willing and able to bid the most for the good or service. If additional quantities of the good or service are available, they can only be sold at lower prices. Likewise, the value of health programs declines as they are expanded. When influenza vaccines are in short supply, they should be allocated to high-risk individuals, the young and the elderly, who have the greatest probability of sustaining serious injury or death from influenza and should be protected to avoid substantial remedial medical expenses should they contract the flu. As the supply of vaccines increases, they should be allocated to lower-risk individuals, who are less likely to contract the flu or to suffer serious injury if they do. The wastefulness of attempting to vaccinate the entire population is obvious. If society produces enough vaccines for everyone, millions of doses will be discarded as large numbers of the public will refuse to be vaccinated, even if the vaccine is provided at no cost. In 2010, Maggie Fox reported 71 million swine flu doses went unused in the United States (Reuters, 2010).

Efficiency, minimizing the cost per output produced, was the primary measure of managerial effectiveness in flexible and zero-base budgeting. Zero-base budgeting elevated the incentive toward efficiency by introducing the possibility that departments with lower per unit costs could gain resources at the expense of less efficient departments. Program budgeting continues this trajectory, but rather than asking what the cost per output is, it asks what the cost per outcome achieved is. Program budgeting recognizes that organizations must do more than efficiently produce goods and services; they must efficiently produce goods and services that people value.

Program budgeting adds equity to the standard economic principles. Equity asks the questions of what is a fair distribution of a society's economic resources, which groups should be permitted to retain their property, which groups should be given resources, and who should go without. Arguments for equity can be based on equal distribution of resources, equal outcomes, or equality of marginal products. Each measure of equity has positives and negatives, produces winners and losers, and yields a different impact on **social welfare**, the well-being of the entire society. Social welfare is a function of the level of wealth, distribution of wealth, liberty, environmental quality, crime, and spirituality. An individual's conception of what maximizes social welfare is a value judgment. Allocating resources based on the need to equalize outcomes appeals to those who believe that social welfare is highest when the disparity of wealth is minimized. Others prefer allocating resources to maximize wealth without regard to how it is distributed.

The simplest measure of equity, equal shares, would ensure each individual receives the same level of funding. The $3.2 trillion spent on health care in the United States in 2015 would provide each person with $9990 of healthcare goods and services (Centers for Medicare & Medicaid Services, 2015). The obvious problem with equal shares is that some people are in greater need of health care than others and that health gains are greater for some conditions than others.

FIGURE 9.2 shows that 1.0% of the population accounts for more than 20% of the total spending ($161,970 per person) and the top 20% of patients consume more than 80% of all healthcare dollars. At the other end of the spectrum, the bottom 50% of citizens account for only 7.0% of healthcare spending, or $1134 per person. An equal share distribution system would not allocate funds in a manner that would maximize health outcomes, that is, those in most need of care would go without treatment, while people in good health would be given access to more care than they need or want.

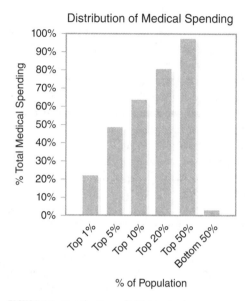

FIGURE 9.2 Distribution of U.S. Medical Spending, 2009

The second equity measure addresses need. Needs-based allocation, or increasing funding proportionately with need, attempts to equalize outcomes. In a needs-based system, patients with the worst medical problems receive the highest funding and healthy individuals receive little. Under a needs-based model, healthcare funding for women should be reduced and shifted to men. According to the Centers for Disease Control and Prevention (CDC), in 2014, U.S. females had a life expectancy of 81.2 years compared to 76.4 years for males (Arias, 2016). Increasing funding for men's health care should increase their life span, while reducing funding for women should have the opposite effect. Reallocation of funds in a needs-based system should end when both genders have an equal life expectancy. A principle problem with needs-based allocation is the impossibility of equalizing health outcomes by increasing spending due to the lack of effective treatment for some conditions.

The third measure of equity allocates funds so that the last dollar spent produces an equal benefit. Equalizing marginal products allocates resources to patients who get the most benefit. In a system designed to maximize health outcomes, young, healthy individuals may receive preventive care in lieu of chronic care for elderly patients. The focus on the young recognizes that these patients may obtain the greatest benefit from health expenditures due to their projected life span. A dollar of healthcare expenditure for a newborn female may produce benefits for another 81.2 years, whereas a dollar of funding for an 80-year-old woman may produce only 1.2 years of benefits. Equalizing marginal products ensures that the outcome of interest is maximized. However, the objection to equalizing marginal products is that it can produce a distribution of resources that is the opposite of needs-based funding.

Program budgeting is built on high-level decision-making based on widely supported goals where outcomes and costs are simultaneously determined. Resource allocations should be supported by explicit analyses of intervention effectiveness and total costs. This brief discussion of equity highlights the need for decision-makers and society to make explicit value judgments: what is fair, what is efficient, and how will the inevitable conflicts between fairness and efficiency be resolved?

Structure and Design

In program budgeting, resource choices are specified in terms of outcomes or ends sought versus inputs or outputs. Performance is evaluated on results rather than inputs consumed or outputs produced. The explicit outcome criterion aims at ensuring that public good is pursued rather than private interest. In for-profit organizations, the profit incentive drives managers and employees to produce goods and services that customers are willing to pay more for than their cost of production. In public organizations, an explicit mechanism is required to replace profit to ensure government workers remain in touch with changing client needs and produce the highest-value goods and services, given the resources available.

Program budgeting recognizes that achieving outcomes often requires contributions from multiple departments, and a mechanism for coordinating the actions of different units is needed to ensure effectiveness and minimize redundancy. In modern health systems, the health of a patient or a population is determined by the actions of various organizations, departments, and individuals. A patient admitted to the hospital interacts with multiple departments during his or her stay and outpatient services and physicians after discharge. Coordination of care is needed because of the fragmentation of care that can arise; bundled payment, clinically integrated networks, and accountable care organizations all attempt to impose a program budgeting structure on the healthcare delivery system.

The shift to an outcome focus allows organizations to engage in multiyear planning. While incremental and flexible budgeting are concerned with the cost of production in a fiscal year, a program budget seeking to maximize population health can take a long view: what preventive services can be delivered this year that may produce future savings, that is, reduce healthcare usage in 5, 10, or more years?

Like zero-base budgeting, program budgeting is based on explicit cost–benefit analysis (CBA) or cost-effectiveness analysis (CEA). CBA assesses two or more means to achieve an end by comparing the ratio of benefits to costs, both denominated in dollars. For example, medical and surgical treatment for heart failure could be assessed by measuring avoided future treatment costs (the benefit) divided by treatment cost. CEA compares two or more means to an outcome, but outcome is not measured in dollars. For example, medical and surgical treatment for heart failure can be compared on the basis of the ratio of expected **quality-adjusted life years (QALYs)** to treatment cost. QALYs measure the effectiveness of healthcare treatment by the change in life expectancy and the degree of health achieved. Fifty percent of people diagnosed with heart failure die within 5 years, so CEA could be used to assess the differences in life expectancy and costs for those surgically and medically treated.

The sea change provided by program budgeting is a better incentive, a focus on ends versus means. Managers and employees operating under a program budget should be motivated to produce more and/or better outcomes. Managers should constantly assess opportunities that increase customer-valued goods and services and resource allocation, that is, eliminating low-value activities, to pursue new opportunities.

The Program Budgeting Process

The first step in the budget construction process is the specification of the desired outcome. Program budgeting aligns itself with the mission of the organization by explicitly incorporating outcomes in the financial plan. While flexible and zero-base budgeting focuses on outputs, or the means to an end, program budgeting directly targets the end. The goal of all organizations is, or should be, to produce goods and services that satisfy the public to retain its support. While the means of generating income may be different for for-profits (voluntary sales), nonprofits (donations), and public organizations (taxes), they all pursue the same goal of maximizing the value of the organization. All three types of organizations must be responsive to the demands of the public to maximize value.

The recognition of the sovereignty of the customer, the belief that consumer preferences determine the type and number of goods and services produced, is the primary driver of the shift from targeting inputs and outputs to outcomes. An organization is not creating value if the good or service it produces does not satisfy its customers. Healthcare organizations should ask whether their resources and processes maximize the health of their patients, a region, or the country, and whether they satisfy patients and resource providers. Production is not the end but the means of satisfying consumers and those providing funding. Systems should

be designed to serve the needs of consumers rather than producers; program budgeting is not concerned with output per se but whether the output produces the desired result.

After the goal is specified, the second step identifies all programs that contribute to the desired outcome. For example, the federal government has various programs to support the poor. Each **program** specifies the major goal of an organization and whom it will serve, and under this umbrella are the **subprograms** that satisfy one end of the major goal, such as housing, nutrition, health care, and education. In each subprogram, there are a variety of **elements** or alternative means to an end. For example, elements under the housing subprogram include public housing, section 8 subsidies, low-interest loan guarantees, etc. The healthcare subprogram includes Medicaid; Veterans Administration (VA); Women, Infants, and Children (WIC); community health centers, etc. The elements of any subprogram may fall in different managerial jurisdictions. For example, Medicaid is in Health and Human Services, while the VA is a stand-alone cabinet-level entity. However, all aim at improving the status of the poor. **FIGURE 9.3** depicts a program to improve the status of poor with its subprograms and elements.

There are multiple subprograms dedicated to improving the status of the poor through improving access to health care and thus the need to assess how different elements perform. How cost effective are Medicaid, public hospitals, and community health centers in improving the health status of the poor, what are their outcomes and costs? Costs must be allocated when a program element produces multiple outcomes. In Figure 9.3, the WIC program supplies nutrition and health care (as well as health-related education) for the poor, and hence, its costs must be allocated across multiple outcomes to accurately determine its cost per outcome.

Experimental medicine is an example of treatment that serves two goals, patient care and research. Experimental medicine, which

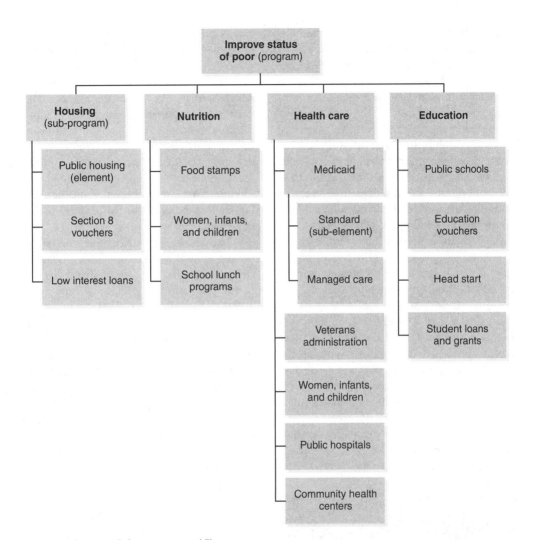

FIGURE 9.3 Program, Subprograms, and Elements

expands our understanding of a disease, does more than simply treat a patient, so its entire cost should not be included as treatment expense but a portion of the cost should be allocated to building knowledge (a complementary outcome). Medical education similarly provides patient care and trains the next generation of providers; the distribution of costs between two complementary outcomes, however, will be subject to debate and possible gaming. Is patient care delivered by residents cost effective? The answer depends upon how costs are allocated. Is over-ordering of tests

and procedures a necessary cost of education or inappropriate and unnecessary treatment? Resident care may appear to be low cost when overuse of tests and procedures is allocated to education. On the other hand, if these costs are assigned to patient care, resident care may be less attractive than other alternatives.

In health care, the program is to improve patient health, and the Medicare diagnosis-related group (DRG) reimbursement system provides an opportunity to evaluate the cost-effectiveness of different treatments. The major diagnostic category (MDC) system denotes different body systems (subprograms) and different means to increase the health of a population. The cost-effectiveness of one MDC versus another and the effectiveness of one DRG (an element) within an MDC can be assessed. Are medical or surgical treatments more cost effective? Within medical and surgical treatments, is one approach better than others? The goal of program budgeting is to determine which methods produce superior outcomes, given their costs. For-profit organizations use program budgeting to assess return on investment (ROI) across divisions and product lines and allocate investment funds on profitability (**BOX 9.1**).

After the goal and means are identified, the third step defines how outcomes will be measured. Program budgeting frees managers to pursue long-term outcomes rather than short-run results. For example, if improved health is measured as 30-day mortality rates, there will be a preference for interventions that have the lowest number of deaths in the 30 days immediately after discharge. If health status is measured as a change in life expectancy, interventions that have higher 30-day mortality rates but substantially higher long-run life expectancies for patients that survive may be preferred. Life expectancy is only one outcome of medical

care; other considerations include the quality of life gained (complete recovery from disease or injury, lowered disability, or lessened discomfort and pain) as well as the pain associated with treatment. ROI was mentioned as the primary outcome pursued by for-profits, but these organizations might also target other outcome measures such as expanding their market share or building customer loyalty. Similarly, government agencies may pursue economic growth, economic stability, and/or an equitable distribution of resources (reduced poverty) as their target outcome.

The fourth step determines the cost of each program. Unlike zero-base budgeting, which examines the alternative means of performing an activity within a department, program budgeting defines the total cost of achieving outcomes without regard to where the cost is incurred. What resources and costs are required to produce outcomes across all involved departments? In all organizations, costs are incurred that provide support to more than one program, for example, overhead administrative costs provide managerial services (leadership, human resource management, financial management, etc.) to more than one program and may contribute to more than one outcome. In health care, it is easy to see that ancillary departments (labs, X-ray, pharmacy, etc.) provide substantial resources to the primary medical product lines (medicine, surgery, pediatrics, etc.), and any analysis of costs must include these "nondepartmental" expenses. To accurately assess the total cost of programs, subprograms, or elements, a mechanism must be developed to allocate distinct departmental costs to each program.

The fifth step evaluates the effectiveness of each element: what outcomes does it achieve? While the ability of a program to produce a desired product should be assessed by customers or clients, in health care, patients may not be capable of accurately assessing treatment choices or the effectiveness of care. In medicine, quality evaluations are often the responsibility of physicians and other healthcare

---

BOX 9.1 The Program Budgeting Process

1. Establish the outcome desired.
2. Identify all programs, subprograms, and elements that contribute to the outcome sought.
3. Define how the outcome is measured.
4. Evaluate the cost of alternative means to achieve the outcome (including overhead costs and costs emanating outside the program).
5. Evaluate the benefits (including the production of complementary outcomes).
6. Calculate CBA/CEA ratios and rank programs.

workers, but self-evaluation produces an inherent conflict of interest, where producers may systematically overvalue the benefits of their programs and underestimate costs.

Medicaid (an element) provides an example of assessment of two different means of delivering care to the poor. Can medical care to the poor (the desired outcome) be provided more effectively and efficiently through the standard Medicaid fee-for-service program (subelement 1) or as managed care (subelement 2)? The fourth step would record the cost per Medicaid beneficiary to determine whether one subelement has a significantly lower cost than the other, and the fifth step would document outcomes such as health status, beneficiary satisfaction, and use of acute and preventive services. Funding decisions should consider what is being achieved, and the cost of reaching the outcome, higher-cost methods, may be justified and warrant funding if they can demonstrate better outcomes than lower-cost alternatives.

The final step, after outcomes and costs have been defined, is an explicit CBA or CEA to calculate the cost per outcome achieved. CBA and CEA create a ratio of benefit (numerator) to cost (denominator) to compare different programs and make resource choices. In CBA, benefits and costs are denominated in dollars; in CEA, benefit is measured as the actual outcome, not dollars but rather number of lives saved, life years gained, etc., to create a ratio of cost per outcome.

$$CBA = \frac{Benefit\ (\$)}{Costs\ (\$)} \quad (9.1)$$

Resource decisions using CBA allocate funds to programs with the highest cost–benefit ratios (CBRs) as long as funds are available. In some cases, organizations may not allocate funds if the CBR < 1.0, that is, the program costs exceed its benefits.

$$CEA = \frac{Nonmonetary\ outcome\ (benefit)}{Costs\ (\$)}$$

$$(9.2)$$

CEA resource decisions allocate funds to programs that produce the desired outcome at the lowest cost, for example, $\Delta QALY\ /\ cost\ (\$)$, until all funds are exhausted. CEA lacks the "bright line," the cutoff rule used in CBA (CBR $\geq$ 1.0), as the outcome has been deemed worthwhile, leaving the only the question of how the goal can be achieved at the lowest possible cost.

Technology assessment is the systematic evaluation of the introduction of new methods or tools for people, society, and the environment. Health technology assessment examines the impact of new or modified healthcare processes. The following formula is used to compare two treatments:

$$\frac{(Outcome\ treatment\ A - Outcome\ treatment\ B)}{(Cost\ treatment\ A - Cost\ treatment\ B)}$$

$$(9.3)$$

The preceding equation emphasizes the change from one method to another and allows immediate rejection of treatments that produce equal outcomes at higher cost or worse outcomes at equal or higher cost compared to existing treatments. The goal of technological assessment is to find treatments that produce better outcomes at equal or lower cost or equivalent outcomes at lower cost. **TABLE 9.1** highlights the nine possibilities of outcome and cost. Options in the southeast area, better or equal outcomes with equal are lower cost, are clearly desirable, whereas those in the northwest area are undesirable. The diagonal provides the two most challenging cases: are better outcomes at higher cost worth it, or should worse outcomes be accepted if they substantially reduce costs? It is these two possibilities that require society and decision-makers to be clear when establishing goals to subordinate cost to outcome or outcome to cost.

At the end of the program budgeting process, programs, subprograms, and elements are ranked from the highest benefit per dollar expended to the lowest. The CBA or CEA rankings should then be used to determine resource allocation: which subprograms or

TABLE 9.1 Outcome and Cost Options			
	Better Outcome	**Equal Outcome**	**Worse Outcome**
Higher cost	Maybe	No	No
Equal cost	Yes	Indifferent	No
Lower cost	Yes	Yes	Maybe

TABLE 9.2 Priority Setting and Portfolio Analysis		
	Low Cost	**High Cost**
High community need	#1—invest	#2
Low community need	#3	#4—disinvest

elements should be funded, and which do not generate sufficient outcomes to justify their continuation?

Portfolio analysis is useful to illustrate program budgeting choices. Portfolio analysis can be used to compare product lines based on their market share and profitability in for-profits or community need and profitability in nonprofits. Organizations can adapt the two criteria to reflect their goals. **TABLE 9.2** ranks program desirability based on community need and cost.

When funds are limited, a rational allocation of resources maximizes outcomes by satisfying the highest needs and the greatest number of people first. Accordingly, the first programs funded would be those that fulfill high needs at low cost (cell 1). Funding the highest-need/lowest-cost programs first maximizes the total benefit. If additional funds are available, funds could be directed to the high-cost and high-need groups (cell 2). While benefits are increased, the high cost limits the number of people who can be served. If funds

have not been exhausted, low-need and low-cost programs could be funded (cell 3) and, finally, low-need and high-cost treatments (cell 4). When choices must be made between programs, low-need and high-cost activities should be first eliminated to provide resources for more desirable ends.

The desirability of funding high-need/high-cost and low-need/low-cost programs may be swapped as it is conceivable that the ability to meet the lower needs of a large number of people may produce more benefit than meeting the high needs of a few people. Quantifying benefit, whether in dollars or in a nonmonetary measure, facilitates the effective allocation of resources and the identification of programs that should be increased or decreased as funds become more plentiful or scarce, respectively.

Brambleby (1995, appendix I) provides an example from Britain's National Health Service (NHS). In the NHS, healthcare spending was allocated on the basis of three criteria: medical specialty (33 classifications), patient age (seven groups), and whether the expenditure supported acute care (local importance) or community care (political imperative).

TABLE 9.3 allows anyone to assess the breakdown of funds between specialties, patient groups (age), and acute versus community (preventive) care in the Hastings Health Authority jurisdiction in 1992–1993. In general surgery, all spending is on acute care and the amount spent increases with age. In pediatrics, roughly two of every three pounds is spent on acute care and 33% is devoted to prevention; of course, pediatric spending decreases with age. Interestingly, Brambleby (1995) reports that management overhead was evenly allocated to acute and preventive care despite health expenditures being heavily skewed toward acute care. While this breakdown could be used to determine whether funds can be reallocated to improve overall health, its primary purpose

is to ensure an equitable distribution of funds between patient groups and healthcare providers.

Over time, public needs and funding levels change due to variations in the economy (increases or decreases in sales or tax collections), and low-need and high-cost programs should be the first to be cut back if new programs with superior ability to meet community needs are created or funding is reduced. Program budgeting provides a rational mechanism to expand services when funds increase and contract services when the current level of activities is no longer optimal or cannot be sustained. Most of the literature emphasizes that program budgeting has been used to contract spending and suggests that it rarely has been employed to reallocate resources. Maintaining the relevance of the program rankings requires managers to stay abreast of changes in need as well as production costs.

TABLE 9.3 Distribution of Funding in the National Health Service (£000s)

Age (years)	0–4		5–14		...	85 +	
Medical Specialty	Acute	Community	Acute	Community	...	Acute	Community
1. General surgery	£79	0	£117	0		£741	0
2. Urology	£3	0	£18	0		£1,931	0
3. Orthopedics	£74	0	£209	0		£7,731	0
⋮							
15. Pediatrics	£1,879	£850	£568	£276		0	0
⋮							
33. Management overhead	£38	£38	£72	£72		£21	£21

Example: Hospital Service Line

Step 1: Establish the outcome desired. An urban, publicly supported hospital has run chronic operating losses and must trim its services lines to meet its fixed budget. Its most recent loss amounts to $6.5 million (operating margin −3.4%), and the county commissioners have mandated that the operating loss must be reduced by $3.0 million in the upcoming year, while maximizing health services provided to the poor.

Step 2: Identify all programs that contribute to the outcome sought. The hospital currently has six primary service lines (programs): heart and vascular services, medicine, musculoskeletal, oncology, surgery, and women's health. Each service line has multiple specialties (subprograms), for example, medicine covers 14 specialties (elements), while oncology has 2. The six service lines provide 42 specialties in all.

Step 3: Define how the outcome will be measured. Given that service to the poor is the primary mission, each service will be evaluated on the number of poor patients seen (versus the total patients seen). Additional factors to be considered when ranking programs include utilization, outcomes, staff recruitment, profitability (loss), and availability of alternative providers.

Step 4: Evaluate the cost of alternative means to achieve the outcome (including overhead costs and costs emanating outside the program). TABLE 9.4 provides the average cost per case in each program, total patients served, poor patients served, total cost, and percentage of cost recovered.

Step 5: Evaluate benefits (including the production of complementary outcomes). As the goal is to maximize treatment to the poor and the amount of care that can be delivered is a function of service line profitability, eliminating the service line with the greatest loss per poor patient served will maximize resources available to other lines (TABLE 9.5).

TABLE 9.4 Patient Volume and Financial Performance by Service Line

Service Line	Cost/Case	Total Patients	Total Poor	Total Cost	Cost Recovery (%)
Heart and vascular	$36,400	430	310	$15,652,000	92
Medicine	$11,600	2,007	1,545	$23,281,200	102
Musculoskeletal	$28,000	717	430	$20,076,000	82
Oncology	$29,600	287	258	$8,495,200	88
Surgery	$23,500	1,577	1,246	$37,059,500	100
Women's health	$15,400	1,003	802	$15,446,200	93
		6,021	4,591	$120,010,100	

TABLE 9.5 Service Line Rankings

Service Line	Cost/ Case	Total Patients	Total Poor	Total Cost	Loss	Loss/ Poor Patient
Musculoskeletal	$28,000	717	430	$20,076,000	−$3,613,680	−$8,404
Heart and vascular	$36,400	430	310	$15,652,000	−1,252,160	−$4,039
Oncology	$29,600	287	258	$8,495,200	−1,019,424	−$3,951
Women's health	$15,400	1,003	802	$15,446,200	−1,081,234	−$1,348
Surgery	$23,500	1,577	1,246	$37,059,500	0	$0
Medicine	$11,600	2,007	1,545	$23,281,200	465,624	$301
		6,021	4,591	$120,010,100	−$6,500,874	

Step 6: Calculate CBA/CEA ratios and rank programs. Ranking the six services lines by loss per poor patient served shows that the musculoskeletal program has the highest loss. Eliminating the musculoskeletal service, assuming the patients can obtain care from other providers, will reduce the operating loss by $3,613,680 and the number of poor patients seen by 430. The loss per poor patient served in musculoskeletal services is twice the loss seen in heart and vascular services, meaning that two poor patients can continue to be served for every one patient reduction in musculoskeletal services. This elimination is desirable as it saves more money than by eliminating heart and vascular, oncology, and women's health ($3,613,680 versus $3,352,818 [$1,252,160 + 1,019,424 + 1,081,234]) and impacts fewer people (430 versus 1370 [310 + 258 + 802]).

Given that a $3 million reduction in loss was sought, management may choose to examine the five musculoskeletal subspecialties (orthopedics, pain management, physical medicine, podiatry, and spine) to determine whether one or more should be retained. If continuing financial difficulties require additional trimming of service lines, heart and vascular and oncology services should be considered for reduction, assuming alternative providers are available. The analysis demonstrates that services serving the greatest number of poor patients as well as moving the organization close to a financial breakeven are medicine, surgery, and women's health.

Program budgeting is a tool for senior managers to assess what an organization should do versus what it is doing. It is well suited for budget expansions, contractions, and reallocations as it is built on cost–benefit or cost-effectiveness measures, which rank and produce a concise (but probably contested) list of high- and low-value programs, activities, and/or products. The need for such a tool is essential in dynamic environments with changing consumer demands, production methods, and input prices and where profit incentives are absent.

Strengths of Program Budgeting

The primary benefit of program budgeting is its focus on results: ends are the sine qua non, and without results, resources cannot be justified. The focus on results and a knowledge of how they are measured should, in turn, focus employee efforts on producing goods and services that maximize the outcomes sought. The second and third benefits derive from the first: goods and services should be delivered to the highest-benefit groups (allocative efficiency), and efficient production methods should be sought (technical efficiency). The focus on the benefits and costs of a program through the CBR or CER should drive managers and employees to identify people who will obtain the greatest benefit from a program to increase the numerator and to simultaneously employ the lowest-cost production methods to reduce the denominator (**BOX 9.2**).

The final strength of program budgeting is it puts managers on notice that resources cannot be taken for granted and that funding can be reallocated to departments producing better outcomes at lower cost. Competition for resources should encourage managers to monitor changes in consumer needs and implement new production techniques that improve outcomes and/or lower costs (all other things remaining equal).

Weaknesses of Program Budgeting

The primary weaknesses of implementing an effective program budget are cultural and administrative. Given that outcomes often require coordination across departments and that organizations frequently have trouble working across department lines, not to mention division lines (e.g., quality problems are always caused by someone else), program budgeting may require a degree of interdepartment cooperation that is unrealizable. While this is a weakness, healthcare payers are increasingly recognizing that health care must be coordinated across departments and organizations to ensure that desired patient outcomes are achieved and efficient care is delivered, and new reimbursement mechanisms are propelling this change (**BOX 9.3**).

The other weaknesses deal primarily with accounting issues: How are benefits measured, how should overhead costs be allocated to departments or programs, and how should programs costs be allocated when multiple outcomes are produced? Outcomes can be pursued and measured clinically as changes in life expectancy, severity, complications and iatrogenic illness, acute clinical stability, and/or physical functioning. Clinical measures appeal to caregivers but outcomes should also be assessed from the patients' perspective on satisfaction and quality-of-life issues and from the societal perspective of resource use, given the large contribution workers and taxpayers make toward covering healthcare costs. Decision-makers need to be clear when setting outcome measures and priorities to ensure that program rankings reflect the values of resource

---

BOX 9.2 Strengths of Program Budgeting

1. Defines, measures, and focuses employee attention on outcomes.
2. Encourages allocative and technical efficiency.
3. Introduces competition for resources.

BOX 9.3 Weaknesses of Program Budgeting

1. Administrative problems arising from program boundaries spanning multiple managerial jurisdictions.
2. Measuring and achieving outcomes.
3. Allocation of costs when programs fulfill more than one goal.
4. Allocation of overhead costs.

providers and consumers. The numerous measures of healthcare outcomes ensure ongoing conflict as partisans find the outcome measure that provides the highest ranking to their favored program and use it as ammunition to call for higher funding.

The allocation of direct costs when programs fulfill more than one goal provides a second opportunity to game the ranking process. As stated earlier, program costs can be manipulated when a program produces more than one outcome. A public agency with a high cost per recipient served can argue that a secondary outcome it produces is public education and that 10%, 20%, or more of the total cost should be reallocated from client services to public education to reduce its cost-to-client ratio.

Finally, there is the question of what percentage of overhead costs a program should carry. Managers of customer- and client-serving programs are always concerned about the percentage of overhead their departments must carry and how it affects their perceived performance, that is, an increase in expenses diminishes the financial attractiveness of their programs. This concern reaches its zenith if the higher expense places a program into the unfunded territory and the manager believes he or she is receiving insufficient support services for the expense allocated. For example, a program may be allocated $100,000 for general administration (or information technology, human resources, accounting, etc.) and the manager and employees may believe they do not receive $100,000 in service. Overhead allocation is generally based on simple, easy-to-collect measures such as total revenue, number of employees, and floor space occupied, and the subsequent distribution of overhead expenses based on these measures may have little correlation to services received. Accounting issues open the door for astute budget managers to promote the outcome measure, cost distribution between two or more simultaneously produced outcomes, and overhead allocation basis that elevate their programs' ranking.

The Budget Game

As seen in all the budgeting systems reviewed, the criterion to secure funding establishes incentives to maximize budgets by focusing on or at least presenting the appearance that the department is pursuing the key objectives of the organization. In program budgeting, the key objectives are maximizing outcomes and minimizing costs; unfortunately, budget managers can manipulate or misrepresent outcomes to appear in line with desired goals rather than putting forth the effort to improve outcomes or reduce costs. A prime example of manipulating results arose in the No Child Left Behind act, where the Atlanta and Chicago school districts were caught cheating on student achievement tests. In both cities, teachers were changing incorrect student answers to obtain higher test scores without actually educating their pupils. In Atlanta, at least eight school administrators were sentenced to prison for their role in the cheating scandal (Lowry, 2015).

The manipulation or outright fabrication of outcome data highlights the necessity of objective, third-party assessment of outcomes. The preferred assessment would be by the customers or clients of the goods or services produced, but when that is not possible, the outcome measure must be definitive and data should be collected from visible sources resistant to manipulation by self-interested parties.

Without actually reducing costs, program costs can be minimized by ignoring costs incurred in the department or the contributions and costs generated outside the department that advance the program goals. As discussed, selective use of accounting may allow managers to manipulate program costs by selecting an outcome measure that minimizes the cost per outcome, dividing department costs over multiple, simultaneously produced outcomes, or minimizing allocated overhead costs. Each of these ploys attempts to minimize the cost per outcome measure and elevate a program's ranking without actually increasing or improving outcome or reducing costs.

▶ Evaluating Performance

Program budgeting provides a seismic shift in evaluating performance from a department perspective to an outcome orientation. In previous budgeting systems, measurement of performance was primarily internal, conducted and judged within the department or organization. Evaluation of program outcomes should involve external parties, that is, customers and clients. Purchasers and users of goods and services should be the people who determine whether the output meets their needs and whether the service associated with its purchase or use is appropriate.

The voice of the customer (VOC) is a process for assessing the needs and requirements of customers and clients. The VOC extends satisfaction surveys in that they elicit customer comments on currently provided goods and services and are also used to determine customer desires, expectations, and dislikes at the product design stage. Aghlmand, Lameei, and Small (2010) provide a case study of maternity care that prioritized patient wants using the VOC process and found that healthcare outcomes (mother and child well-being) were the most highly valued outcomes (from a list of 20 treatment factors), while patient education ranked low.

The VOC process specifies customer desires and should be the starting point for performance evaluation: what products are produced, are desired features being provided, and is the customer satisfied? The second step is to determine program costs: what does it cost to produce the product? The final step determines whether costs are allocated in conformance with customer preferences: are highly valued products adequately supported in the budget and should effort and expense be shifted from low-value to higher-value products?

In some cases, a VOC analysis may not be required, and an organization with an increasing market share can confidently assume it is meeting customer desires. An organization operating as a monopoly, whether a government organization, legally instituted monopoly, or due to the inability of the market to support more than one provider, should have a proactive process to determine whether it is satisfying its customers or clients. Program budgeting, steps 1, 3, and 4, define performance assessment. Steps 1 and 3 establish the desired outcome and how it will be measured, while step 4 defines cost; these elements are restated in the following value equation:

$$\text{Value} = \frac{\text{Outcome}}{\text{Cost}} \qquad (9.4)$$

The preceding equation quantifies value as the ratio of outcome and cost. Evaluation can be simplified to whether outcomes were greater than or less expected and whether more or less expenses were expended. **TABLE 9.6**

TABLE 9.6 Outcome, Cost, and Program Value Cost			
Outcome	**Lower than Budget**	**As Budgeted**	**Higher than Budget**
Better than expected	Superior	Superior	To be determined
As expected	Superior	As expected	Substandard
Less than expected	To be determined	Substandard	Substandard

categorizes performance into four groups: superior, as expected, substandard, and to be determined, based on outcome and cost. Cell 5 defines expected performance: the department produced the expected outcome and met its budget. Superior performance occurs when outcomes are better than expected and costs are lower or equal to budget (cells 1 and 2) or expected outcomes are achieved, while costs are held below budget (cell 4). Substandard performance requiring improvement includes lower-than-expected outcomes with budgeted or overbudgeted costs (cells 8 and 9) or expected outcomes produced at higher-than-expected costs (cell 6).

Cells 3 and 7, to be determined, require analysis as performance may be better or worse than expected. Value, according to Equation 9.4, will be higher if the increase in outcome is greater than the increase in cost in cell 3. For example, a 20% increase in outcome divided by a 10% increase in cost (120% outcome/110% cost) would indicate better-than-expected, superior performance. Lower-than-expected, substandard performance arises if the increase in outcome is less than the increase in cost. If the reduction in outcome is less than the fall in cost (cell 7), for example, a 10% reduction in outcome and a 20% reduction in cost would mean that 90% of the benefit is obtained at 80% of the expected cost, that is, superior performance.

While the complication of multiple outcomes and other issues may deny program budgeting the mantle of definitiveness, that is, one, and only one, allocation of resources maximizes outcomes, its usefulness in presenting budget choices should be recognized as well as its potential to improve budgeting practices. The purpose of a budget is to establish expectations; program budgets with their specification of outcomes not only provide a mechanism for ranking programs during the planning and expense estimation phases but also provide the metrics needed to evaluate performance during the budget year for purposes of facilitating and controlling and for year-end accountability.

▶ An Example of Program Budgeting: Medicare Part A

Returning to the analysis of Medicare Part A, the limitation of prior budgeting perspectives should be clear: we should not be concerned with expenditures but rather with whether spending improves health. What we expect to receive from healthcare expenditures is longer and better lives; accordingly, we will measure the desired outcome as cost per enrollee per QALY.

Assume you are the inpatient healthcare czar of the United States. Currently, your department oversees approximately 33 million admissions annually (total, not just Medicare) and reimburses hospitals $827,617 million for these admissions. Because of high federal deficits, you have been directed to cut inpatient expenditures by 10%. You decide that future funds, $744,855 million, will be allocated to each MDC by the median dollar expenditure per QALY, ranked from lowest cost to highest cost. This allocation system ensures that the greatest benefit is achieved for the greatest number of people; however, once the budget is exhausted, patients in diagnostic groups below the cutoff will not be funded, although they can purchase care using private funds. **TABLE 9.7** lists 13 MDCs, the number of cases, the cost per case, and the cost per QALY.

After ranking each MDC by the cost per QALY and calculating the total cost to meet the need in each diagnostic category (cases * cost per case) and the cumulative outlays, it is clear that after the budget cut, only the first 12 MDCs and 94.3% of neoplasm cases can be funded and remain within the budget. The 178,784 neoplasm cases that cannot be funded may be shifted to the following fiscal year. The program budget deletes funding for respiratory system conditions due to its high cost per QALY.

TABLE 9.7 MDC Cases, Cost per Case, and Cost per QALY

Disease Category	Median Cost/ QALY	Number of Cases	Cost per Case
16. Blood and blood-forming organs	Cost savings	297,942	$22,400
5. Circulatory	$14,000	9,184,513	$36,400
14. Perinatal conditions	$5,800	1,569,212	$10,000
6. Digestive	$9,000	2,828,798	$22,400
10. Endocrine, nutritional, etc.	$10,000	1,015,365	$21,400
12/13. Genitourinary	$16,000	2,895,854	$15,400
18. Infectious and parasitic	$4,400	512,318	$27,000
21. Injury and poisoning	$2,000	375,666	$19,200
19. Mental	$6,200	2,796,921	$13,400
8. Musculoskeletal	$3,500	2,019,681	$28,000
17. Neoplasms	$20,000	3,119,247	$29,600
1. Nervous	$11,800	2,282,190	$24,700
4. Respiratory	$40,500	4,098,925	$18,900
		32,996,632	

The logic behind CEA can be seen in Tables 9.7 and 9.8. Dividing cost by the median cost per QALY provides the number of QALYs expected to be gained by the treatment. For example, in the injury and poisoning MDC, an additional 9.6 life years is expected from treatment ($19,200/$2000) versus 0.47 years ($18,900/$40,500) from respiratory care. A dollar transferred from respiratory care to injury and poisoning treatment generates 20.6 times (9.6 years/0.47 years) the

benefit in the QALY. The shift between neoplasm and respiratory care is also significant: one dollar of neoplasm care is expected to yield 1.48 ($29,600/$20,000) QALY, and a dollar transferred from respiratory to neoplasm care would yield more than three times the benefit (1.48/0.47 = 3.17).

The relevant question is what set of programs (MDC) produces the most benefit for the sick. **TABLE 9.8** is a broad-brush approach, and we know that within each MDC, there are

TABLE 9.8 MDCs Ranked by Cost per QALY and Total Budget Outlay

New Budget					
		$744,855,300,990			
MDC	**Median Cost/QALY**	**Number of Cases**	**Cost per Case**	**Cost**	**Cumulative Budget**
16. Blood and blood-forming organs	Cost savings	297,942	$22,400	$6,673,900,800	$6,673,900,800
21. Injury and poisoning	$2,000	375,666	$19,200	$7,212,787,200	$13,886,688,000
8. Musculoskeletal	$3,500	2,019,681	$28,000	$56,551,068,000	$70,437,756,000
18. Infectious and parasitic	$4,400	512,318	$27,000	$13,832,586,000	$84,270,342,000
14. Perinatal conditions	$5,800	1,569,212	$10,000	$15,692,120,000	$99,962,462,000
19. Mental	$6,200	2,796,921	$13,400	$37,478,741,400	$137,441,203,400
6. Digestive	$9,000	2,828,798	$22,400	$63,365,075,200	$200,806,278,600
10. Endocrine, nutritional, etc.	$10,000	1,015,365	$21,400	$21,728,811,000	$222,535,089,600
1. Nervous	$11,800	2,282,190	$24,700	$56,370,093,000	$278,905,182,600
5. Circulatory	$14,000	9,184,513	$36,400	$334,316,273,200	$613,221,455,800
12/13. Genitourinary	$16,000	2,895,854	$15,400	$44,596,151,600	$657,817,607,400
17. Neoplasms	$20,000	3,119,247	$29,600	$92,329,711,200	$750,147,318,600
4. Respiratory	$40,500	4,098,925	$18,900	$77,469,682,500	$827,617,001,100
Current budget		32,996,632			$827,617,001,100
Program budget through neoplasm		28,897,707			$750,147,318,600
					−$5,292,017,610
					−178,784 neoplasm cases

multiple DRGs to evaluate. The Oregon Health Plan demonstrates how one state rebuilt its Medicaid system by evaluating health care at the treatment level. There may be treatments within the blood and blood-forming organ MDC that have a higher cost per QALY than treatments in the respiratory system that went unfunded. Additionally, Table 9.8 specifies average cost, and we know that certain groups of patients will be more or less responsive to treatment and their cost per outcome will systematically vary, so the analysis may need to be undertaken on the basis of treatment and patient. Likewise, we can ask the same question regarding the elements: which element in a subprogram produces the most benefit? After these questions are answered, we can ask the allocation questions: Should dollars be reallocated from one subprogram or element to another? Should low-performing subprograms or elements be discontinued?

The Oregon Health Plan

In 1989, Oregon wanted to fundamentally change how health services purchased by the state for Medicaid recipients were made. Oregon wanted to expand the number of people served and reduce the number of medical services covered. The problem with the historical allocation of Medicaid spending was the lack of coverage for low-income individuals and denial of life-saving treatment, while millions of dollars were spent on less effective treatments for less serious conditions (Bodenheimer, 1997, p. 661).

The Oregon plan was built on six principles: First, Medicaid should cover everyone below the poverty line. Second, medical treatments should be prioritized on the basis of effectiveness. Third, funding should be allocated to the most effective treatments first, and lower-priority services would be provided as funds allow. Fourth, reimbursement to healthcare providers should not be reduced. Expansion of medical coverage should be

driven solely by reallocation of funds rather than forcing lower payments on providers. Fifth, managed care organizations should be used to facilitate patient–provider interactions to improve access, increase quality, and reduce cost. Finally, all treatments on the prioritized list covered by Medicaid should establish the minimum benefit package for employer health plans (**TABLE 9.9**).

Seventeen categories of health needs were identified and ranked. Acute and fatal conditions with the possibly of full recovery were ranked first, followed by acute and fatal conditions that are treatable. At the bottom of the list (#17) were chronic and nonfatal conditions. Thirteen criteria were assessed to determine benefits, including life expectancy, quality of life, CEA, and the number of people served. The final list ranked fatal and full-recovery conditions first; followed by maternity and fatal but incomplete recovery in second and third places, respectively; and in last place were conditions where no improvement was expected.

Given the expected cost savings with the program, Oregon increased the population covered by Medicaid from 57% to 100% of those below the federal poverty line. The Medicaid population increased by 39%, and the uninsured population fell to 12% from 14%. The total cost increased by 36% from 1993 to 1996, but this compared favorably with a nationwide increase of 30% that accompanied an 11% increase in Medicaid recipients.

Afterword: An economic downturn in Oregon resulted in changes to the plan in 2003. Enrollees were split into a Plus plan for those eligible under federal Medicaid coverage and a Standard plan for those eligible under Oregon rules. Enrollees in the Standard plan saw four changes: first, fewer healthcare services were covered, that is, to reduce costs, the coverage for dental, mental health, and other services was dropped. Second, copayments were added. Third, premiums were raised. Finally, an exclusion period was added for those who

TABLE 9.9 Oregon's Prioritized List of Covered Conditions and Treatments

The Top Four

1. Pregnancy; treatment: maternity care

2. Birth of infant; treatment: newborn care

3. Preventive services, birth to 10 years of age; treatment: medical therapy

4. Preventive services, over the age of 10, treatment: medical therapy

Two Above/Two Below the Cutoff Point

497. Ptosis (acquired) with vision impairment; treatment: ptosis repair

498. Chronic sinusitis; treatment: medical and surgical treatment

Cut-off

499. Keratoconjunctivits and corneal neovascularization; treatment: medical and surgical treatment

500. Selective mutism; treatment: medical/psychotherapy

The Bottom Four

689. Respiratory conditions with no or minimally effective treatments or no treatment necessary; treatment: evaluation

690. Genitourinary conditions with no or minimally effective treatments or no treatment necessary; treatment: evaluation

691. Musculoskeletal conditions with no or minimally effective treatments or no treatment necessary; treatment: evaluation

692. Gastrointestinal conditions and other miscellaneous conditions with no or minimally effective treatments or no treatment necessary; treatment: evaluation

failed to pay their premiums. Wright, Carlson, Allen, Holmgren, and Rustvold (2010) report that between March and December 2003, after changes were implemented, enrollment fell from 88,874 to 47,957, a drop of 46%. By November 2005, only 24,000 remained enrolled in the Standard plan, and the uninsured rate in Oregon had risen to 17% (2010, p. 2316).

Summary

Program budgeting is a method of setting priorities and harkens more toward planning and less toward the line-by-line specification of resources. More than any other budgeting system, program budgeting recognizes that inputs and outputs are simply means to achieve an outcome. Effectiveness is the primary driver; efficiency is always desirable, but there is little sense in producing a good or service no one wants or benefits from at the lowest-possible cost.

Program budgeting requires employees to focus on what the organization is trying to achieved, how the organization operates, including what inputs are purchased and what they achieve, and what alternatives exist— different methods of achieving the current goals and/or existence of other possible goals. CBA or CEA provides a succinct encapsulation of the metrics and objectives of program budgeting and encourages managers to improve outcomes and reduce costs.

The challenges to program budgeting include difficulty in defining nonmonetary outcomes and allocating costs to outcomes when a program produces more than one outcome. Once metrics are established, it should be easy to calculate the cost per outcome, but after this is completed, another challenge arises, that of shifting resources based on CBA or CEA. It is easy to see that recipients of government funds and producers will fight tooth and nail to avoid reductions in their benefits or level of funding. Unless economic growth picks up in developed countries, we should expect to see increasing competition for government funds and can only hope that economic analysis and program budgeting guide future decisions.

Key Terms and Concepts

Allocative efficiency	Programs, subprograms, and	Social welfare
Equity	elements	Technical efficiency
Portfolio analysis	Quality-adjusted life year	Technology assessment
Program budget	(QALY)	Voice of the customer (VOC)

Discussion Questions

1. What are the primary differences between program budgeting and incremental, flexible, and zero-base budgeting?
2. Describe the steps needed to construct a program budget.
3. What steps can a program manager take to enhance the probability that their program is funded?
4. When should a program budget be employed?
5. Explain the strengths and weaknesses of program budgeting.

Problems

1. The following table provides the cost per case for four medical treatments and the change in health status expected in QALYs. Calculate the cost per QALY and rank the treatments from lowest to highest cost per QALY.

Treatment	Cost per Case	QALY
A	$10,000	2
B	$10,000	4
C	$20,000	6
D	$20,000	8

2. The medical director of a large health insurer, 100,000 enrollees with a premium income of $500,000,000, has a preventive care budget of $10,000,000 (2% of premium income). BudgetCh09.xlsx, Problem 9.2 tab provides a list of preventive care services in declining order of cost-effectiveness, their prices, and the number of members who could benefit from each service, assuming only 40% of eligible persons will seek preventive care. What types of care should be offered to subscribers for free, or where should the medical director draw the line?

3. A nonprofit hospital board is contemplating service line reductions because of declining reimbursement. The board disagrees on what the hospital's goal should be. Group A believes the hospital should maximize the number of patients seen, group B believes the hospital should maximize health by funding the service lines that maximize the QALY, and group C believes profit should be maximized. Assuming the board believes that it will only have $114,000,000 million in funding, create three program budgets: one to maximize the number of patients seen, maximize the QALY, and maximize profit (BudgetCh09.xlsx, Problem 9.3 tab). Which service lines should be eliminated or reduced under each budget? If they are reduced, calculate by how much (%) the program will be reduced. Complete the following table and discuss the trade-offs between the three budgets.

Service Line	Patients	Per Case Reimbursement	Cost	QALY
Medicine	1,400	$18,000	$17,000	10
Cardiology	1,200	$34,000	$32,500	6
Surgery	1,000	$27,000	$26,500	8
Oncology	800	$30,000	$29,250	5
Obstetrics	600	$10,000	$11,000	20
Pediatrics	500	$7,000	$6,250	40
Psychiatry	500	$8,000	$8,600	12

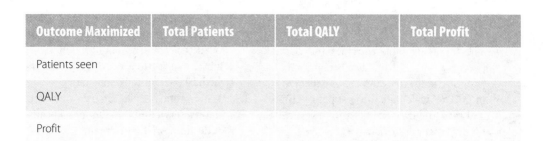

Outcome Maximized	Total Patients	Total QALY	Total Profit
Patients seen			
QALY			
Profit			

References

Aghlmand, S., Lameei, A., & Small, R. (2010). A hands-on experience of the voice of customer analysis in maternity care in Iran. *International Journal of Health Care Quality Assurance, 23*(2), 153–170.

Arias, E. (2016). *Life expectancy for non-Hispanic black males has been changed from 72.2 to 72.0 to correct a transcription error.* Retrieved November 16, 2016, from http://www.cdc.gov/nchs/products/databriefs/db244.htm

Bate, A., & Mitton, C. (2006). Application of economic principles in healthcare priority setting. *Expert Review of Pharmacoeconomics & Outcomes Research, 6*(3), 275–284.

Bodenheimer, T. (1997). The Oregon health plan: Lessons for the nation. First of two parts. *New England Journal of Medicine, 337*(9), 651–655.

Brambleby, P. (1995). A survivor's guide to programme budgeting. *Health Policy, 33*(2), 127–145.

Centers for Medicare & Medicaid Services. (2015). *NHE fact sheet.* Retrieved May 30, 2017, from https://www.cms.gov/research-statistics-data-and-systems/statistics-trends-and-reports/nationalhealthexpenddata/nhe-fact-sheet.html

Lowry, D. (2015, April 30). Sentences reduced for 3 in Atlanta cheating scandal. *USA Today.* Retrieved October 21, 2015, from http://www.usatoday.com/story/news/nation/2015/04/30/atlanta-educators-resentenced/26643997/

Oregon Health Plan Administrative Rules. (2013). Retrieved October 26, 2013, from http://www.oregon.gov/oha/herc/PrioritizedList/10-1-2013%20Prioritized%20List%20of%20Health%20Services.pdf

Reuters. (2010, May 4). *U.S. has 71 million unused flu vaccine doses.* Retrieved November 16, 2016, from http://uk.reuters.com/article/flu-vaccine-usa-idUKN0318959620100503

Ruta, D., Mitton, C., Bate, A., & Donaldson, C. (2005). Programme budgeting and marginal analysis: Bridging the divide between doctors and managers. *British Medical Journal, 330*(7506), 1501–1503.

Wright, B. J., Carlson, M. J., Allen, H., Holmgren, A. L., & Rustvold, D. L. (2010). Raising premiums and other costs for Oregon health plan enrollees drove many to drop out. *Health Affairs (Millwood), 29*(12), 2311–2316.

CHAPTER 10

Activity-Based Budgeting

CHAPTER OBJECTIVES

1. Explain activity-based costing.
2. Explain the steps in building an activity-based budget.
3. Construct an activity-based budget.
4. Evaluate the strengths and weaknesses of activity-based budgeting.
5. Discuss the process, potential results, and challenges of using activity-based costing to examine healthcare processes.

▶ Introduction

The common approaches to constructing a budget based on inputs, outputs, and outcomes have been discussed, but each fails to recognize the multitude of tasks needed to produce goods and services. A department seldom performs a single task but performs a collection of activities completed by different individuals who need to be effectively managed. Individual inputs are seldom devoted to a single activity; workers are employed in a number of tasks, and supplies and equipment are used to achieve a number of different ends. A department can be conceived in the same manner as a football team: the team is divided into offensive, defensive, and special teams with specialized duties. Players are delegated specific roles within each group: offensive players are expected to throw the ball, catch the ball, run with the ball, and provide

blocking. Some members of the offensive team are cross-trained to perform two or more duties, depending on what the situation (strategy and actions of the opposing team) calls for. Running a football team requires ensuring the right inputs are in the right place—an incremental budgeting approach.

Simply having every position filled does not ensure success, so coaches track output: points for (offense) and points against (defense)—a flexible budgeting approach. At a higher level of detail or a finer level of granularity, quarterbacks are evaluated on the basis of passing yards, the rate of pass completions, and the number of touchdowns and interceptions thrown. Defensive linemen are evaluated on the number of tackles and sacks made. Tracking output measures enhances the ability of the coach to evaluate how the team and individuals are performing and to make necessary adjustments.

Developing a program budget for a football team would require defining the desired outcomes: is the goal having more wins than losses and postseason success (a championship), maintaining fan support, or generating more revenue than expenses? After the desired outcome is established, the team can draft or trade for the players it believes will accomplish the desired goal at the lowest cost. The team's investment decision may lead to drafting a star player to fill the stands or a role player to fill an offensive or defensive weakness. Incremental, flexible, and program budgets provide information on performance, but at the most basic level, an organization, like a team, must manage activities to achieve success.

Activities are the heart of any operation, and how well or poorly they are performed determines whether outputs are produced efficiently (outcomes are achieved) and whether the organization succeeds. If a quarterback has a low pass completion rate (and the team is losing more games than it is winning and attendance is declining), what is the problem? Are incomplete passes due to poor throwing or receiving mechanics, poor target selection, inadequate time to throw (and throwaways to avoid sacks), or an inappropriate game strategy and offensive system? The potential reasons for a low pass completion rate span the quarterback, receivers, offensive line, the defensive line of the opposing team, and the coaches and their strategies. Performance improvement requires identifying and correcting the appropriate cause(s): who, what, and how.

Activity-based budgeting (ABB) recognizes that costs arise from activities, and whether a good or service is embraced by customers depends on competent completion of work. Creating an ABB requires more detail than incremental, flexible, or program budgets, as the number of activities vastly exceeds the number of inputs, outputs, or outcomes. ABB (**FIGURE 10.1**) focuses on how work is performed, emphasizing the old adage "A system is only as strong as its weakest link." By focusing on facilitation and control, the concurrent phase of budgeting, ABB enables managers to identify and improve weaknesses and prevent small dysfunctions from having a disproportionate impact on organizations.

▶ Activity-Based Costing

At the dawn of the Industrial Revolution, Adam Smith observed and documented the advantage that specialization of labor played in maximizing output. Smith noted that a single man employed in pin making could produce 20 pins per day. Smith concluded that 18 distinct activities were required to produce a pin, including drawing the wire, straightening the wire, cutting, pointing, grinding for the head, producing the head, attaching the head, whitening, and packaging. When the 18 activities were divided among 10 men, allowing each man to focus his attention and effort on one or two tasks, they produced 48,000 pins per day, or 4,800 pins per day per man (Smith, 1977, 8–9).

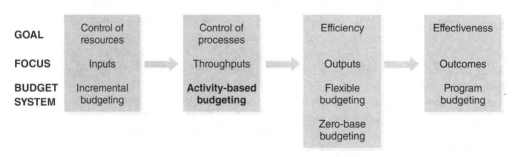

FIGURE 10.1 Budgeting Systems

Task specialization propelled a productivity increase of 240 times (4800 / 20).

Smith's story is about designing production processes and controlling activities. Smith recognized that maximizing output and managing an operation are significantly easier when jobs are understood and there is minimum transition between tasks. Task shifting reduces worker productivity and increases costs in three ways. The first is the time lost transitioning from an activity in one place using one set of tools to another operation requiring different equipment in another location. Time is consumed by each relocation or tool change, and the total cost of task transitioning increases with the number of times per day a worker changes activity. The minimum time is determined by the physical distance that must be traversed and amount of setup or preparation required.

The second and third inefficiencies relate to how men behave. Smith notes that men saunter between tasks. The first inefficiency defines the minimum time required to transition from one task to another; the second is the cost of ineffective management. Ineffective management allows transitions that should take 2 minutes to grow to 3, 4, or more minutes. The third inefficiency arises from the time it takes a man to refocus his attention and effort on a new task and reach a high and consistent level of performance. The cost of transitioning between tasks cannot be identified if we do not understand how long an activity should take. If we understood how much time a job should take, it would be easy to add up all the tasks performed and multiply the number of tasks by the time per task to determine productive time. Productive time could then be subtracted from the total hours paid to identify, and hopefully minimize, nonproductive time.

Idle resources are the most visible source of loss, but value is lost for many other reasons. When analyzing production processes, tasks should be divided into necessary and avoidable work. Value is increased when the time engaged in the former is increased and in the later reduced. Lean, relying on Gilbreth's

therbligs, divides activities into four classes (Protzman, Mayzell, & Kepchar, 2011, p. 115): essential (assemble), preparatory (transport), incidental (search, select, inspect), and eliminable (think/plan, delay, rest). Essential tasks are the "point of the sword," where goods and services are produced; preparatory and incidental activities enable production but do not add to a customer's perception of value. Eliminable activities such as idleness add nothing but cost to operations.

Activity-based costing (ABC) is designed to produce useful cost information. Only by understanding activities can managers accurately assess costs for products, customers, and channels and effectively coordinate resources. Cokins (2001) includes ABC as part of a new improvement paradigm that moves accounting away from a policing role to one of aiding decision-making by providing accurate, relevant, and timely information to managers. This shift parallels Deming's thought on management: management should not concern itself with oversight but rather facilitate work and remove obstacles to success. The goals of the new improvement paradigm described by Cokins (2001, p. 2) include:

Management of processes rather than inputs

Elimination of waste, including idleness, overprocessing, unnecessary motion, and excessive transport

Improvement in processes to deliver better, faster, and cheaper outputs and outcomes

Downward delegation of decision-making

The goal of ABC is to trace costs to outputs and customers. Indirect costs are equal to or greater than direct costs in some organizations and industries. While direct costs can be traced straight to products, indirect costs are allocated on readily available measures (revenue, units produced, etc.) that may not correlate with services received. Given the magnitude of indirect costs in most organizations, the accuracy of product costs and their contribution to the organization's financial performance are often unclear. Brimson and Antos (1999, p. 52) believe 80%–90% of costs should be directly traceable to activities (versus allocated). In addition to overhead allocation problems, we should not assume that the direct costs of similarly classified outputs are the same. For example, the Healthcare Common Procedure Coding System (HCPCS) 99201 specifies a brief physician visit for a new patient (or Diagnosis-related group [DRG] 127, a congestive heart failure admission), but not all 99201 visits cost the same. The time per visit and the cost of a visit will vary systematically by the type of patient seen, and pricing all visits as if they had the same cost will result in low-cost patients subsidizing high-cost patients.

Health care has long relied upon questionable bookkeeping practices that do not facilitate management or cost control. Pricing in health care has been, and continues to be, primarily concerned with revenue maximization, and as a result, prices of individual services as well as their reported costs bear little resemblance to the actual costs of care. A review of the two major types of cost systems, job order costing and process (absorption) costing, is in order, given the lack of emphasis given to cost accounting in health care. In **job order costing**, the cost of individual outputs is determined by the amount of resources used in their production; therefore, similar outputs that consume more (less) resources can be identified and their prices increased (decreased) accordingly. In **process (or absorption) costing**, all outputs are assumed to be roughly equivalent and the total cost of resources consumed is allocated to individual products on a pro rata basis (total cost / total output = cost per unit). This method of allocation produces reasonable cost estimates when outputs are equivalent (produced in batches of standardized output such as books or continuous processes such as petroleum refining) but fails spectacularly when outputs consume different levels of resources.

Health care has largely ignored job order costing in favor of process costing. Given the different needs of patients, payers, and disease groups and provider practice patterns, a process costing system can seriously distort cost information and hamper management. Process costing understates the cost of low-volume, high-complexity outputs and overstates the cost of high-volume, standardized products.

The difference (and impact) of job order and process costing can be understood by comparing gall bladder surgery and transmission repair. An automobile repair business uses job order costing and charges car owners on the basis of the amount of time a mechanic spends with their cars and the parts needed for repair. On the other hand, a hospital charges a flat fee per day of hospitalization or service, for example, drawing blood. While surgery may be billed on the amount of time spent in the operating room (OR) (the surgeon fee, however, is typically a flat rate) and medical supplies are charged on what is actually given to the patient, a large percentage of hospital costs assume that every patient (or patient day, therapy session, etc.) is equal, so patients who take minimal staff time are assumed to cost the same as patients requiring maximum care. Healthcare costing and pricing systems have undermined the industry's ability to understand actual costs and manage operations.

Routine costs (room and board) are regularly allocated on crude measures that fail to recognize how resources are used, and ancillary costs are often determined by their prices rather than an understanding of work performed and costs incurred. Traditionally, total department costs were divided by total department revenue to produce a cost-to-charge ratio, and this ratio was subsequently multiplied by the price of each individual service to determine its cost (total department costs / total department revenue * charge description master price). Given how costs are calculated, it is difficult or impossible to determine how costs vary by patient, diagnosis, payer, and/or provider. For example, do older patients cost more than younger patients to treat for the same service, and if so, how much more? Does a particular third-party payer provide a disproportionate share of a provider's higher-need and higher-cost patients, and should the payer be charged more for the care provided to their patients? Given fixed reimbursement systems, healthcare managers should understand how costs vary by patient type, physician, and/or third-party payer to ensure that patients and third-party payers are appropriately charged for resources consumed.

The goal of ABC is not the allocation of costs but rather tracing costs (what resources were purchased) to the tasks the resource was purchased for and tracing activities to specific outputs, customers, providers, or channels. ABC returns to the insights provided by Frederick Taylor's time and motion studies and the specificity of job costing. According to Cokins (2001, p. 15), ABC pursues two goals: the first, and subordinate, goal is to understand costs, and the second, and primary, goal is to use cost information to effectively manage operations.

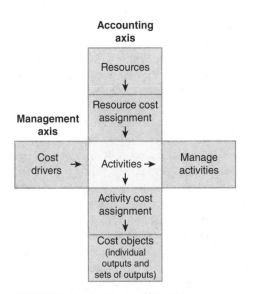

FIGURE 10.2 The Activity-Based Cost Management Framework (Cokins, 2001, p. 15)

Data from Consortium of Advanced Manufacturing-International.

The accounting axis (*y* axis) in **FIGURE 10.2** is designed to determine the cost of products and the sensitivity of costs to products, production processes, and customers. The accounting axis requires managers to trace input costs to activities and activities to cost objects—specific products purchased by identifiable purchasers and produced and handled through specific processes. The goal is to recognize costs imposed on the organization because of special handling requirements that increase product costs and, when possible, charge higher prices for these products.

The five-step cost-tracing process starts with the traditional expense view: what **resources** were purchased, divided into the common categories of salaries, supplies, equipment, etc. In terms of management, the only control this view provides is on the cost per input: is the organization paying too much per unit to acquire resources? ABC starts with what resources were purchased, but instead of simply dividing total resource acquisition costs by total output (the method used in process costing) to determine cost per output, it asks the more organic question of what the resources were purchased to do. The first step requires managers to define the activities expected to be fulfilled by the purchased resources.

The second step is **resource cost assignment**; this process answers why the organization purchased a resource and what it received in return. Resource cost assignment requires the number of activities performed by a resource to be quantified. The expected output is the cost per activity. There are two ways to arrive at activity cost. The time and motion study approach asks what is the minimum time necessary to perform an activity. The minimum time would be multiplied by the input price of the resource to determine a cost standard. If time and motion studies indicate an activity should take 15 minutes for a worker to complete, the labor cost of the activity would be 15/60 minutes * hourly wage: if the wage is $20, the labor cost per activity is $5.00.

A second method calculates the percentage of time an employee spends in an activity and multiples this percentage of time by the employee's annual salary and divides the product by the number of activities. For example, a worker earning $20 per hour has an annual salary of $41,600 ($20/hour * 2,080 hours). If 70% of the worker's time is devoted to an activity, 70% of his or her salary, or $29,120, would be the total labor cost of the activity. The cost per activity would be $5.60 ($29,120/5,200) when 5200 activities are performed in a year. The advantage of this approach over time and motion studies is the recognition that achievable costs ($5.00) are not often realized because of nonproductive time and activities. In this example, the actual cost incurred per activity is 12% higher because of delays, idle time, rework, and/or other factors.

Resource cost assignment provides information to managers to determine whether their cost per activity is excessive. Managers should use this information to compare themselves against competitors or industry benchmarks to determine whether too many labor hours or supplies are being consumed to produce an activity. One of a manager's prime duties is to ensure his or her department's activities are efficient, that is, cost per activity is at a minimum.

The third step, **activities**, addresses what the organization does. What was the total number of activities undertaken, and was this level of activity necessary? Did the organization perform effectively in terms of the number of activities performed? If excessive activities were undertaken, was it because of the need to redo work that was not done correctly the first time or overprocessing? On the other hand, additional activities could be undertaken because of the demands of customers or providers, for example, tests are rerun because the patient or physician doubts the results and/or wants further confirmation.

The fourth step, **activity cost assignment**, tracks how many activities are performed and what costs arise for each cost driver. A **cost driver** is an event that gives rise to one or more activities, that is, it is an event that causes work to be undertaken and resources to be consumed. Any product is a set of activities driven by customer requirements, and ABC attempts to identify why the activities are performed, how many activities are needed, and how much cost is involved.

The final step in the cost determination process is tracing activity costs to **cost objects**, that is, for whom or what are activities performed? At the finest level of granularity, the patient is a cost object and ABC mimics a job costing system that attempts to determine as accurately as possible the resources consumed to treat a particular patient. Do certain types of patients or physicians require special handling, for example, "stat" tests, which increase costs, and are the added costs paid by the patient or passed on to all patients? In health care, patient-specific data may not be useful for managing patient care processes, but ABC should be used to trace costs to groups of patients such as those being treated by a particular doctor, those reimbursed by a specific third-party payer, or those with a distinct diagnosis. Managing resource consumption by groups of patients may be vital to a provider's long-term success.

Brimson and Antos (1999, pp. 11–12) provided a perfect example of the change in perspective provided by ABC for a claims-processing department. The first two columns of **TABLE 10.1** provide the traditional accounting view, where resources are aggregated by object code (what type of resource was purchased); columns 3 through 6 reinterpret the chart of accounts by focusing on why resources were acquired and what they produced. In this example, $1,571,515 of salaries and other expenses are tied directly to inpatient billing and account collection activities and $76,403 is untraced to work and output.

ABC provides information to judge whether the cost of the activity is excessive or inadequate and whether the volume of the activity is too great (rework, duplication, or

TABLE 10.1 Activity-Based Costing and the Translation of the Chart of Accounts

Expense	Cost		Activity	Cost/Output	Quantity	Cost
Salaries	$675,432		Bill	$18.00	36,543	$657,774
Fringe benefits	$195,875		Answer inquiries	$4.00	8,523	$34,092
Supplies	$25,643		Rebill rejected claims	$36.00	2,076	$74,736
Telephone	$42,909		Charge audits	$175.00	812	$142,100
Information technology	$76,598		Unpaid account turnover (collection agency)	$1009.00	591	$596,319
Occupancy	$18,153		Post payments	$2.00	33,247	$66,494
Collection agency fees	$596,319		Overhead			$76,403
Travel	$16,989					
Total	$1,647,918		Total			$1,647,918

unnecessary) or insufficient (inefficiency and idleness) by focusing on the question of why inputs were purchased (versus what inputs were purchased) and what was produced by the inputs. The first two columns of Table 10.1 show $1,647,918 was spent processing inpatient claims. Claim processing includes initial billing, charge audits, and turning unpaid accounts over to collection agencies but from traditional accounting statements, a decision-maker gains little insight into what the organization does or how it performs.

The ABC translation details the six major processes, the quantity of output each process produces, and the cost of each unit of output. The ABC translation demonstrates the highest-cost activities are initial billing ($657,714, or 39.9% of total costs), turning unpaid accounts over to collection agencies ($596,319, or 36.2%), and charge audits ($142,100, or 8.6%). These three activities account for 74.7% of total costs, and any serious effort to improve performance and reduce costs must focus on these three processes.

The most expensive processes per unit of output produced are turning unpaid accounts over to collection agencies ($1,009 per unit) and charge audits ($175 per unit). Cost reduction efforts can take two tracks: the first determines whether the cost per activity can be lowered, and the second determines whether the number of activities can be reduced. In this example, a manager should examine what can be done to improve in-house collection rates and thereby reduce the number of accounts turned over to collection agencies or reducing collection agency fees. Assume claims can be divided into two groups, or cost objects: surgical patients and medical patients. Do surgical patients have a higher rate of rejected claims and charge audits? If so, the patient accounts manager should investigate the causes of rejected claims and charge audits, for example, high rates of charge or coding errors, and institute improvements to avoid rebilling and auditing costs.

A third strength of the ABC perspective is the clear identification of overhead

(or nonproductive time). In Table 10.1, only 4.6% of the total cost ($76,403/$1,647,918) is traced to nonoutput-related activities. When managers understand what their employees do (processes or what resources are purchased to produce), how many units of output are produced, and how much each activity costs, they will be more capable of pinpointing and reducing waste. The goal of ABC is to provide organic information on how organizations work, whom they serve, and how customers are served. ABC traces costs to work performed versus traditional cost allocation, which allocates costs on broad measures (revenue generated, total, undifferentiated output, number of employees, etc.) that may not reflect how costs are incurred.

The management axis (x axis) provides a business process or operation view and challenges managers to control cost drivers and activities. Costs are driven by the demand for activities (cost drivers) and the actual activities performed. Managers should either reduce demand by customers for cost-increasing activities such as customized (versus standard) outputs, higher-quality and reliability outputs, and faster delivery or ensure the costs of these services are paid by the users and not passed on to others.

As discussed previously, cost drivers are the reason there is work. **Cost drivers** are events that trigger activity, and managers should control the demand for their resources as well as the resources themselves. A single cost driver, a particular product (price), customer/patient (revenues), or channel (% of business), drives multiple activities, so managing demand is a primary management task. Can managers change the demand function, redesign products, redirect customers, or change processes to reduce the need for activities?

Management's job, after cost drivers are assessed and controlled, is managing day-to-day **activities**: the range and number of tasks and functions performed and their effectiveness and efficiency. Reducing the range of activity performed can lead to greater specialization and effectiveness and lower costs. Reducing the number of activities undertaken requires minimizing error and rework and/or eliminating low-value or unnecessary activities. A third means of lowering cost is to identify better means of working, that is, reducing the amount of time needed to complete an activity.

The end sought is superior **management of activities**. While traditional accounting may indicate whether an organization's financial performance is subpar, it provides little insight into the cause(s) of the problem. ABC is designed to facilitate performance improvement. ABC allows managers to determine whether suboptimal financial performance is due to inefficiency, intensity of demanded activity by cost objects, and/or poor pricing of products. Efficiency can be improved and costs lowered by reducing the cost per activity or the number of activities undertaken. Management's attention should focus on reducing nonvalue-adding work, errors requiring rework, and/or idleness. When an organization is efficient, managers may still be able to improve performance by reducing the intensity of under- or noncompensated activities demanded by cost drivers. If customers are unwilling to reduce the intensity of activity they demand, prices should be increased. Prices should be set to ensure customers carry the full cost of activities they demand.

The key to ABC is determining the number and cost per activity (**TABLE 10.2**, columns 4 and 5). Kaplan and Anderson (2004) label the two methods of resource cost assignment as traditional ABC, which uses total time estimates to drive the cost per activity rate, and the time and motion approach, or **time-driven ABC**. The total time estimate method asks employees to estimate the percentage of time per day (week, year) they spend in various activities. Assume a physician defines the three major revenue-producing activities as examining patients, performing procedures, and seeing patients in the hospital. The physician estimates that 50% of the time is spent in seeing patients in the office, 30% performing procedures, and 20% making hospital rounds. Assuming the physician earns $200,000, the salary is prorated across the activities, and the prorated cost is divided by the quantity of each activity produced.

While this method can provide reasonable estimates of the actual cost per activity, its primary drawback is that workers regularly attribute 100% of their time to productive work. That is, workers do not report nonproductive time; nonproductive time is included in the percentages attributed to activities. A second problem is employees may not be capable of accurately estimating activity times, and

TABLE 10.2 Traditional Activity-Based Costing

Task	Estimated Time (%)	Time Allocated Cost	Quantity of Activity	Cost per Activity
Patient exams	50	$100,000	5,029	$19.88
Procedures	30	$60,000	878	$68.34
Hospital rounds	20	$40,000	470	$85.11
Total	100	$200,000		

this difficulty grows with the number of tasks employees perform in a day. We know workers do not spend 100% of their day in productive activities, so the overestimation of productive time inflates cost rates, while the accuracy issue will increase the rates of activities whose times are overestimated and understate costs for under-estimated activities. Kaplan and Anderson (2004) recommend using time-driven ABC to rectify these problems.

Time-driven ABC returns to the insights of Frederick Taylor and scientific management to construct cost estimates. A centerpiece of scientific management was the use of time studies to determine the amount of time needed to complete a task. Time studies performed by Taylor broke jobs into elementary movements, discarded useless movements, selected the quickest and best movements, and, finally, recorded the times of skilled workers. Taylor added additional time to the calculated time standard to account for unavoidable delays, performance of new workers, and rest periods (Wren, p. 126). Taylor broke with his forerunners, such as Charles Babbage, by emphasizing the time a task should take versus the average time the task did take. **TABLE 10.3** shows the transition to time-driven ABC; instead of backing into time estimates, it begins with the expected time per activity and multiplies time per output (column 2) by total output (column 3) to calculate the total time that should be spent in an activity (or productive time). The difference between the time that should have been consumed by activities and total hours paid is nonproductive time. The identification of nonproductive time, unfortunately, does not mean that this time can be redirected to productive activity. For example, understanding and responding to government regulations may not benefit anyone, but organizations must submit required reports or face penalties.

Like employee estimates of times, the results of time studies will not produce definitive standards for the time per task. The first problem is one of generalizability: are the times collected 1 day (week, month, and so on) reflective of other days (weeks, months, and so on), and/or are the performance times of one employee or group of employees generalizable to other employees? The second issue is the **Hawthorne effect**—employees being observed modify their normal behavior. Closely supervised workers

TABLE 10.3 Time-Driven Activity-Based Costing					
Task	**Time/Output (minutes)**	**Quantity of Output**	**Total Minutes**	**Total Cost**	**Cost per Activity**
Patient exams	12	5,029	60,348	$72,544	$14.43
Procedures	45	878	39,510	$47,495	$54.09
Hospital rounds	15	470	7,050	$8,475	$18.03
Other	–	–	59,472	$71,486	–
Total			166,380	$200,000	

Notes: Physician minutes/year: 59 hours/week * 60 minutes/hour * 47 weeks = 166,380 minutes.
Cost/minute: $200,000 / 166,380 = $1.2021.

may improve their performance as a reaction to being observed. In spite of these difficulties, ABC should produce superior information than existing cost accounting systems.

Table 10.3 demonstrates a substantial portion of our physician's time, 35.7%, is spent on activities other than patient exams, procedures, and hospital visits. By highlighting the time spent on "Other" activities, time-driven ABC adds another opportunity for improvement: can the time spent on potentially nonrevenue-generating activities be reduced to increase the output of reimbursable patient exams, procedures, and/or hospital visits? Managers who are effectively utilizing their resources, for example, 80% or more productive time versus more than 20% nonproductive time, may see little need to evaluate their operations. On the other hand, the physician in Table 10.3 may ask, "Why am I spending more than one-third of my time on 'Other' activities?" Is this time-generating revenue, is it a necessary but nonrevenue-producing activity, or is it truly unproductive time?

ABC supplies a wealth of financial and operational information to organizations willing to supplement traditional accounting methods. Accounting processes are routinely designed to serve the interests of accounting professionals rather than managers. Cost allocation in health care was built on easily collected measures that were selected to maximize revenues. The cost allocation methods and measures were not designed to accurately reflect resource use. ABC, on the other hand, focuses on how costs are incurred to increase effectiveness and efficiency. ABC traces resources and their cost to work performed, identifies activities and workers, and recognizes variation in output and customers and how these variations affect cost. The goal is better decision-making and management based on a more accurate understanding of costs and profitability (**BOX 10.1**).

Cooper and Slagmulder (2000) note that ABC is a perfect starting point for a budgeting system by identifying the need for future

> **BOX 10.1** Benefits of Activity-Based Costing
>
> 1. Embeds the process view.
> 2. Provides a realistic view of workloads.
> 3. Places responsibility and accountability on employees to manage their activities, cost per job, and cost per output.
> 4. Identifies variation in the quantity of output and costs between the budget and actual operating results.
> 5. Increases the accuracy of product costing and demonstrates how different products and activity requirements drive costs.
> 6. Improves the ability to monitor and control work.
> 7. Identifies under- and overuse of resources.

resources, in addition to its ability to identify accurate costs and sources of profitability, and encourage efficiency by increasing the visibility of activity costs. Traditional budget systems can be characterized as input expense → output → product cost. In ABB it is output → activities → resource → product cost, that is, ABB starts with planned outputs, defines the activities and inputs needed to produce those outputs, and ends with product cost.

▶ Activity-Based Budgeting

ABC provides the cost per activity—one of the critical elements to constructing an ABB. Like other budgeting systems, the forecast of output is a second key element in defining resource requirements. Unlike other types of budgets, an activity-based budget is constructed on the basis of the tasks employees complete and is more focused on supporting management than estimating expenses. The third element is the number of activities required per output;

ABB offers managers the ability to move from how many activities *are* undertaken to how many *should* be required. An activity-based budget can be constructed in nine steps; see **BOX 10.2** (Brimson & Antos, 1999, p. 103).

Structure and Design

While previous budgeting systems were characterized as being internally focused (inputs used and outputs produced by an organization) and externally focused (results produced for customers), ABB concentrates on activities. That is, what resources are required per activity, what is the cost per activity, and how many

---

BOX 10.2 The Activity-Based Budgeting Process

1. Identify current resources, for example, paid full-time equivalent (FTE), total compensation, and cost per hour.
2. Define required activities (what were resources were purchased for) and activities per output.
3. Estimate the budget year output.
4. Calculate the quantity of expected activity: Activities/Output (2) * Forecasted output (3).
5. Define required resources per activity, for example, hours, supplies, and machine time per activity.
6. Calculate total required resources: Total expected activity (4) * Input/activity (5), for example, total person-hours for an activity.
7. Calculate the total expected resource cost per activity: Cost/Input (1) * Needed inputs (6), for example, Cost per hour * Total person-hours (one activity).
8. Summarize total inputs required ($\Sigma 6$) and the expected cost for all activities ($\Sigma 7$).
9. Compare current (1) and required resources (8) and adjust work and/or resources for excessive and insufficient demand.

---

activities are needed per output? ABB requires a shop floor understanding of the production process. It has a 1-year time horizon like most budgeting systems.

As seen in ABC, ABB focuses on outputs produced and the variation in activities required for each output. ABB recognizes the distortion that occurs when managers assume products are similar. While Henry Ford is often claimed to have stated, "You can have any color car as long as it is black," in the era of mass customization, few industries can assume their outputs are the same and have identical costs. In health care, managers should recognize that the cost per admission or patient day will vary with the patient seen, the patient's condition, when he or she arrives for care, the employees providing care, and other factors. When the impact of these factors is understood, managers can take the first steps toward improving the effectiveness and efficiency of the health delivery system. The goal of ABB is to improve products, reduce product costs, and set appropriate product prices. The means to achieve these goals is supplying management with information on the number of activities performed, the effectiveness and efficiency of activities, and margins earned.

The Activity-Based Budgeting Process

ABB starts like other budgeting systems by identifying available resources, step 1. What resources are currently employed; for labor, this includes the number of employees, total compensation, and cost per hour. **TABLE 10.4** shows $1,939,442 was expended for wages and benefits in the first 6 months of 2018 for a nursing unit, 52 employees received paychecks, the number of regular hours (management and staff) was 50,960, and 670 overtime hours were paid (2602 for agency nurses); the average cost per labor hour was $35.76. For supplies and other expenses, the number of units used and the cost per unit is unavailable so only total

TABLE 10.4 Inventory of Resources and Costs

Object Code	Step 1 Description	Type of Cost	YTD Actual 2018	Hours	Total Expense	Total Paid Hours	Exp./Unit
4010	Management and clerical staff	F	$176,543	5,200	$1,939,442	54,232	$35.76
4020	Staff salaries and wages	V	$1,235,642	45,760			
4040	Overtime	V	$23,833	670			
4050	Per diem/agency nurses	V	$156,115	2,602			
4110	FICA	%	$109,855				
4120	Health insurance	%	$149,857				
4130	Retirement	%	$71,801				
4140	Unemployment	%	$15,796				
4210	Floor medications	V	$13,589				
4212	Medical instruments	V	$5,798				
4214	Bandages, gauze, etc.	V	$5,643				
4216	Latex gloves, gowns, etc.	V	$32,145				

(continues)

TABLE 10.4 Inventory of Resources and Costs *(continued)*

Object Code	Step 1 Description	Type of Cost	YTD Actual 2018	Hours	Total Expense	Total Paid Hours	Exp./Unit
4218	Sterile wipes	V	$2,659				
4250	Office supplies	V	$4,268				
4280	Cleaning supplies	V	$569		$64,671	Total supplies	
4350	Biomedical repairs/ maintenance	F	$3,869				
4410	Electricity	F	$1,156				
4440	Telephone	F	$2,645				
4930	Housekeeping	V	$72,000		$79,670	Total housekeeping/ utilities	
4940	Travel/professional meetings/meals	F	$14,523				
4950	Education and training	F	$3,688				
4960	Other expenses	F	$1,258		$19,469	Total other	
			$2,103,252				

FICA, Federal Insurance Contributions Act.

cost incurred is available. The inventory of resources is *not* the starting point for building a budget but, rather, is used to assess how efficiently current resources are employed.

Step 2 details output at a finer level of granularity than a traditional budget. Where an incremental budget would simply take current year-to-date (YTD) expenses and annualize and increase them for inflation and a flexible budget would be content driving expense estimates on total patient days, assuming every patient day demands the same amount of resources, that is, the cost standard increased for inflation, ABB divides patient days into the activities performed for patients. Step 2 begins by identifying the activities that are performed and then quantifying the number of activities that should be performed on the basis of who is receiving care (Table 10.4).

The first part is descriptive; a patient day requires the following activities: checking of vital signs, dispensing of medications, care coordination and communication with other caregivers, patient hygiene, etc. Part two is quantitative: how often are vital signs checked, how often should they be checked, and how many medications does or should a patient receive in a day? On the basis of history, a manager could document that patients on his or her unit receive an average of 10 medications per day. The budgeting and quality question is, is this the appropriate level of medication based on generally accepted medical practice? If not, should patients receive more or less medication? If the average utilization rate is "correct," how much variation exists between patients and providers, do some patients require more or less than the average, and do some doctors overprescribe or underprescribe? The question of the correct activity rate is a prime concern for the budget, but it also affects the effectiveness of treatment and patient safety.

Step 2 is the starting point for recognizing differences in care on the basis of the type of patient treated. Assume it has been documented that patients over the age of 65 receive twice the number of medications compared to patients under 65 (13.34 versus 6.67) per day and are twice as likely to call a nurse or other caregiver for problems. The type of patient treated is a cost object, and a change in the composition of patients may have a profound impact on the total number of hours needed to treat patients and the pharmaceutical costs. If the percentage of older patients increases, more time will be needed to handle their concerns and dispense medications; conversely, an increase in younger patients may free up staff time for other duties. Managers using ABB for the first time may want to build their budget on the number of activities currently performed; as their operational and financial acumen grows, they may start exploring whether the current level of activity is warranted.

Step 3 estimates expected output. Returning to the nursing unit examined (Chapter 7), the unit expects to provide 6524 days of patient care in the budget year. The head nurse estimates that 50% of patients in the upcoming year will be over the age of 65. The cost drivers, therefore, are the number of patients over 65 and under 65. If the 50/50 split occurs, the unit will provide 3262 days of care for each group. The reader should note that unlike other budgeting processes, there is no need for modification for mandates, as any additional work should be included in activities (step 3) and/or the required resource per activity (step 6).

Given the activities per output, step 2, and forecasted output, step 3, step 4 calculates the total number of activities expected in the budget year. On the basis of the actual number of medications dispensed in the first 6 months of 2013, 10 per patient day, and a forecast of 6524 patient days in the upcoming fiscal year, 65,240 medications are expected to be administered in the budget year. The total number of activities expected for the eight remaining patient care activities is shown in column 4 of **TABLE 10.5**.

TABLE 10.5 Estimated Total Budget Year Activity

Step 2 (Descriptive)	(Quantitative)	Step 3	Step 4
Activity	Per Output	Expected Output	Total Activity
Checking of vital signs	6	6,524	39,144
Dispensing of medications	10	6,524	65,240
Care coordination and communication	1	6,524	6,524
Patient hygiene	3	6,524	19,572
Patient educations and concerns	1	6,524	6,524
Handwashing	75	6,524	489,300
Movement/to/from	75	6,524	489,300
Shift handoffs	2	6,524	13,048
Other	1	6,524	6,524

Step 5 defines required resources per activity: how many labor hours, supplies, machine time, space, etc., are required for each activity performed? Determining the total cost of medication administration requires knowing how much staff time is necessary to deliver medicines, the pharmaceutical costs, building (occupancy) costs, etc. Resource requirements can be developed using staff estimates of the time they devote to an activity or a time study (time per activity and the number of activities per cost driver). The easiest approach relies on staff estimates, the percentage of time devoted to an activity, and the number of activities performed. The staff estimate approach suffers from the assumption that time is fully utilized and "bakes" into the resource requirement current inefficiencies and/or underutilization. The staff estimates that 10.4% of time is spent

administering medications, or 10.9 minutes are needed per medication administered. The following ABB, **TABLE 10.6**, uses the time estimate approach where 10.4% of staff time is estimated to have been spent dispensing medications, 12.5% checking vital signs, and the remaining for seven activities, totaling 100.0%.

A time study approach records the starting and ending times of activities and develops productivity standards. Time studies allow managers to more accurately identify nonproductive time; the difference between total hours paid and the amount of time needed to complete tasks is nonproductive time (paid hours − Σ(time standard * activities) = nonproductive time). Assume the industry average, a benchmark, for delivering medications is 8 minutes; the unit is current taking 10.3 minutes, and the difference should be explored. Why is

Activity				Step 5	
	Time Estimate (%)	2018 YTD Hours	2018 YTD Activities	Hours per Activity	Minutes per Activity
Checking of vital signs	12.5	6,779.0	19,770	0.343	20.6
Dispensing of medications	10.4	5,649.2	32,950	0.171	10.3
Care coordination and communication	20.8	11,298.3	3,295	3.429	205.7
Patient hygiene	6.3	3,389.5	9,885	0.343	20.6
Patient educations and concerns	8.3	4,519.3	3,295	1.372	82.3
Handwashing	7.8	4,236.9	247,125	0.017	1.0
Movement/to/from	15.6	8,473.8	247,125	0.034	2.1
Shift handoffs	4.2	2,259.7	6,590	0.343	20.6
Other	14.1	7,626.4	3,295	2.315	138.9
	100.0	54,232.0			

TABLE 10.6 Input Requirements per Activity

departmental dispensing time longer than the industry, and can process changes save time?

Step 6 calculates needed resources by multiplying total expected activity (step 4) and inputs required per activity (step 5). For example, if staff estimates that 0.171 hours (10.3 minutes) are needed to administer each medication and 65,240 medications are expected in the budget year, 11,185 hours will be needed to provide medications. Supplies are a different "animal" as each line item ties to a specific activity: medical instruments to vital signs, floor medications to dispensing of

medications, gloves and gowns to handwashing (patient safety), office supplies to "Other," and all else to patient hygiene. Their cost, rather than physical units, is divided by activities to determine the cost per activity.

The expense rates for housekeeping and utilities could be based on square footage, but since patient rooms are relatively the same size, costs were traced to the percentage of staff time devoted to each activity to determine the total expense per activity. The rationale is that if 10.4% of staff time is devoted to dispensing medications, then 10.4% of occupancy costs (housekeeping, depreciation, etc.), where medications are delivered, should be traced to the same activity. Other expenses were allocated using the same procedure.

If the industry average is used, 8 minutes, and 65,240 administrations are expected, the hospital would need 8699 staff hours to dispense medications. Readers should note that ABB calculates that 11,185 hours are needed to dispense medications versus 8,699 if the industry benchmark is used. The sources of the difference between these two estimates, that is, staff productivity, could be current process inefficiencies, inaccurate time estimates by staff, differences in patients served, differences in defining the activity (are handwashing and

documentation part of administering medications, or are they separate activities?). In this example, documentation is included in the time estimate but handwashing is not.

The total labor cost to perform an activity, step 7, requires multiplying the resource cost (step 1) and total resource requirement (step 6). Step 1 determined an average wage of $35.76 per hour; with a 3% increase, the budget rate would be $36.83. Multiplying by total hours, 11,185, produces a cost for dispensing medicines of $412,004. In the spirit of ABB, illustrated in **TABLE 10.7**, the alternative calculation would multiply budgeted activity, 65,240, and the calculated cost per medication dispensed, $6.32, to obtain $412,004. The author

TABLE 10.7 Estimate of Labor and Supply Costs

| Activity | 2019 Budget Activities (4) | Step 6 (4 * 5) | | | Step 7 (1 * 6) |
		Hours per Activity (5)	Total Hours	Cost per Activity	Total Labor Costs
Check vital signs	39,144	0.343	13,422	$12.63	$494,405
Dispense medications	65,240	0.171	11,185	$6.32	412,004
Care coordination and communication	6,524	3.429	22,370	$126.30	824,008
Patient hygiene	19,572	0.343	6,711	$12.63	247,202
Patient educations and concerns	6,524	1.372	8,948	$50.52	329,603
Hand washing	489,300	0.017	8,389	$0.63	309,003
Movement/to/from	489,300	0.034	16,778	$1.26	618,006

Shift handoffs	13,048	0.343	4,474	$12.63	164,802
Other	6,524	2.315	15,100	$85.26	556,205
			107,378		$3,955,238

	2018 Hour rate	$35.76	*Step 1*
	Budget rate (+3%)	$36.83	

	2018 Hour rate	$35.76

	Budget rate (+3%)	$36.83

Activity	2019 Budget Activities (4)	2018 YTD Expense	2018 YTD Activities	Cost per Activity	Inflated Rate	Total Supply Cost
Check vital signs	39,144	5,798	19,770	$0.29	$0.30	$11,824
Dispense medications	65,240	13,589	32,950	$0.41	$0.42	$27,713
Care coordination	6,524		3,295			$0
Patient hygiene	19,572	8,871	9,885	$0.90	$0.92	$18,091
Patient educations	6,524	32,145	3,295	$9.76	$10.05	$65,556
Hand washing	489,300		247,125			$0
Movement/to/from	489,300		247,125			$0
Shift handoffs	13,048		6,590			$0
Other	6,524	4,268	3,295	$1.30	$1.33	$8,704
		$64,671				$131,888

prefers the second method as it highlights the work being performed and the cost per activity. The second half of Table 10.7 traces supply expenses to activities. Price increases for supplies are expected to increase by 3%, so the 2018 rates are increased accordingly. Different input price increases can be incorporated for each line item, for example, medical instruments and pharmaceuticals.

Step 8 summarizes total resource requirements, labor, supplies, machine time, etc., across all activities for the budget. ABB calculates the needed resources to perform the nine activities identified in step 2 by summarizing resources needs (Σstep 6) total hours, units, space, etc., and totaling all activity costs (Σstep 7) to determine total expected expense (**TABLE 10.8**).

Given $3,955,238 is budgeted for total compensation, this amount must be divided between salaries (staff, management, overtime, and agency/temporary) and fringe benefits (FICA, health insurance, retirement, and unemployment). The total labor expense can be allocated to each line item using the proportions in YTD actual (**TABLE 10.9**). Similarly,

TABLE 10.8 Estimate of Total Resource Costs

Activity	Labor	Supplies	Building	Other	Step 8 Total Cost
Checking of vital signs	$494,405	$11,824	$20,310	$4,963	$531,502
Dispensing of medications	$412,004	$27,713	$16,925	$4,136	$460,777
Care coordination and communication	$824,008	$0	$33,849	$8,272	$866,129
Patient hygiene	$247,202	$18,091	$10,155	$2,482	$277,930
Patient educations and concerns	$329,603	$65,556	$13,540	$3,309	$412,007
Handwashing	$309,003	$0	$12,693	$3,102	$324,798
Movement/to/from	$618,006	$0	$25,387	$6,204	$649,597
Shift handoffs	$164,802	$0	$6,770	$1,654	$173,226
Other	$556,205	$8,704	$22,848	$5,583	$593,341
	$3,955,238	$131,888	$162,477	$39,704	$4,289,307

TABLE 10.9 Line Item Budget Estimates

Object Code	Description	Type of Cost	YTD Actual 2018	Major Expense Total	%	ABB Expense Total	2019 Budget
4010	Management and clerical staff	F	$176,543	$1,939,442	9.10	3,955,238	$360,036
4020	Staff salaries and wages	V	1,235,642		63.71		2,519,930
4040	Overtime	V	23,833		1.23		48,604
4050	Per diem/agency nurses	V	156,115		8.05		318,376
4110	FICA	%	109,855		5.66		224,036
4120	Health insurance	%	149,857		7.73		305,614
4130	Retirement	%	71,801		3.70		146,429
4140	Unemployment	%	15,796		0.81		32,214
4210	Floor medications	V	13,589	64,671	21.01	$131,888	27,713
4212	Medical instruments	V	5,798		8.97		11,824
4214	Bandages, guaze, etc.	V	5,643		8.73		11,508
4216	Latex gloves, gowns, etc.	V	32,145		49.71		65,556

(continues)

TABLE 10.9 Line Item Budget Estimates   *(continued)*

Object Code	Description	Type of Cost	YTD Actual 2018	Major Expense Total	%	ABB Expense Total	2019 Budget
4218	Sterile wipes	V	2,659		4.11		5,423
4250	Office supplies	V	4,268		6.60		8,704
4280	Cleaning supplies	V	569		0.88		1,160
4350	Biomedical repairs/ maintenance	F	3,869	79,670	4.86	$162,477	7,890
4410	Electricity	F	1,156		1.45		2,358
4440	Telephone	F	2,645		3.32		5,394
4930	Housekeeping	V	72,000		90.37		146,835
4940	Travel/professional meetings/ meals	F	14,523	19,469	74.60	$39,704	29,618
4950	CME	F	3,688		18.94		7,521
4960	Other expenses	F	1,258		6.46		2,566
			$2,103,252		400.00	$4,289,307	$4,289,307

4950 CME should read Education and training.

the total expected expense for supplies, house-keeping, and other expenses would be allocated across the relevant object codes on the basis of their current proportions).

The last step compares available (step 1) and required resources (step 8), allowing managers to determine whether they are employing too many or too few resources for the output they expect to produce. Using a time estimate approach ensures the operation will appear efficient as "Other" activities will include productive work as well as nonproductive time. If time standards were developed from time and motion studies and show the department produces too few activities, given the number of hours paid, the manager should increase work and/or reduce resources to balance inputs and output. ABB may indicate staff is overworked and more resources are required to maintain output. Unlike this example, where labor was rolled into a single category, Brimson and Antos (1999, p. 116) prepared an example that calculated resource use and need for two different groups of workers and found

one group was overworked, while the other has spare time. In their example, the solution is clear: shift appropriate activities from the overworked group to the underutilized workers. For example, if registered nurses (RNs) are overworked, while licensed practical nurses (LPNs) have spare time, activities currently performed by RNs that could be handled by LPNs should be shifted until workloads are balanced.

TABLE 10.10 provides a hypothetical example of comparing current and required resources using industry benchmarks. The primary challenge the department apparently faces is overuse of labor: the industry standard is 14.4 hours per patient day, and the department is consuming 16.6 hours, or 13,562 (14.3%) more hours than expected. The discrepancy is that labor dollars are only $205,238 (5.4%) overbudget, suggesting that more, lower-skilled and paid employees may be employed; a second reason for the higher-than-expected use of labor could be sicker-than-average patients on the unit.

TABLE 10.10 Budgeted and Required Resources						
Resource	**Budgeted Units**	**Benchmark Units**	**Excess/ (Deficiency)**	**Budgeted $**	**Benchmark $**	**Excess/ (Deficiency)**
Labor	108,160	94,598	13,562	$3,955,238	$3,750,000	$205,238
	16.6 hrs/ pat.day	14.5 hrs/ pat.day	2.1 hrs/ pat.day			
Supplies	–	–	–	$131,886	$150,000	−$18,114
House keeping, etc.	–	–	–	$162,477	$180,000	−$17,523
Other expenses	–	–	–	$39,704	$35,000	$4,704
Total	–	–	–	$4,289,305	$4,115,000	$174,305

On the positive side, supply use and housekeeping costs are lower than expected. A reference point is essential to evaluating the efficient use of resource, while comparison over time allows managers to determine whether their departments are doing better or worse than history; industry benchmarks provide an opportunity to compare resource use against the industry average or best-in-class performers.

An Alternative Approach to Activity-Based Budgeting

As seen in the calculation of supply rates, it is often difficult to identify input units. While the type and quantity of floor medications (object code 4210) are tracked as they are administered, other supplies such as medical instruments (object code 4212) and gloves and gowns (object code 4216) may not be meticulously tracked. How many different medical instruments are subsumed in object code 4212, what are their input prices, and how many were consumed? When supplies or other resources are not closely tracked, steps 5 and 6, defining the units of a resource needed to produce an activity and total resources needed, can be skipped in favor of simply calculating a resource cost per activity rate, step 7. **TABLE 10.11** restates nursing unit resources for the first half of 2018 in terms of what the department receives from its resource (versus what the resource is). Columns 1 and 2 show the standard chart of accounts approach, where line items are rolled up into homogeneous expenses categories such as salaries, fringe benefits, and supplies (**BOX 10.3**). Column 3 denotes the expected activities, and column 4 shows the percentage of time staff estimates spent on each activity (or time standards could have been developed and used). Column 5 calculates the total cost to perform an activity (% of time * total expense).

Column 6 provides the actual count of current activities, hopefully captured in an information system or, if not available, an

> **BOX 10.3** An Alternative Activity-Based Budgeting Process
>
> 1. Estimate the budget year output.
> 2. Calculate current activities per output.
> 3. Calculate the total cost per activity.
> 4. Calculate the budget: Output (1) * Activity / output (2) * Cost (inflated) / activity (3).
> 5. Decompose the total budget into line items: Total budgeted expense * Historical % of spending per line item.
> 6. Modify for mandates.

estimate of the number of activities performed in the current year. The use of estimates recalls scratch budgeting (Chapter 5), where managers of a to-be-created organization ask, "How many activities are required to complete a task?" The use of actual counts, the historical approach, reports how many activities were undertaken to complete a task. Column 7 reports the average number of activities per patient day, YTD activity/YTD patient days. The drawback in the historical approach is that unnecessary activities may have been undertaken in the past performance and waste may be baked into budget projections. In this case, are 75 trips to and from patient rooms per day appropriate, and will better scheduling or mandated rounding allow staff to perform multiple tasks at a single visit and reduce the time spent walking to and from patient rooms? On the other hand, were the 19,770 checked vital signs, 6 per day, enough for the number of patients treated, or was checking excessive?

Column 8, YTD cost per activity, is the quotient produced by dividing the total YTD activity cost (column 5) by YTD activities (column 6). Given the staff estimate that 12.5% of the time is devoted to checking vital signs and 19,770 vital signs were checked, the cost per activity rate is $13.30. This example assumes all expenses are driven by the same factor that accounts for labor use; more sophisticated

TABLE 10.11 Calculating the Cost per Activity

1. Resource	2. Total Expense	3. Activity	4. Time (%)	5. Total YTD Activity Cost	6. YTD Activities	7. Activity per Output	8. Cost per Activity
			YTD Output	**3295**			
Salaries and wages	$1,415,590	Checking of vital signs	12.5	$262,907	19,770	6.00	$13.30
Fringe benefits	$347,309	Dispensing of medications	10.4	$219,089	32,950	10.00	$6.65
Supplies	$64,671	Care coordination	20.8	$438,178	3,295	1.00	$132.98
Utilities	$7,670	Patient hygiene	6.3	$131,453	9,885	3.00	$13.30
House keeping	$72,000	Patient concerns	8.3	$175,271	3,295	0.51	$53.19
Other expenses	$19,469	Handwashing	7.8	$164,317	247,125	75.00	$0.66
	$1,926,709	Movement/to/from	15.6	$328,633	247,125	75.00	$1.33
		Shift handoffs	4.2	$87,636	6,590	2.00	$13.30
		Other	14.1	$295,770	3,295	1.00	$89.76
			100.00	$2,103,252			

ABC would develop other factors for nonlabor expenses that more closely track their use.

Having established the current-year cost per activity rates for the nursing unit, preparation of next year's budget is shown in **TABLE 10.12**. Step 4 requires the budget preparer to estimate the volume of activity per cost driver (patients above and below the age of 65). Once these estimates are in place, the cost per activity rate calculated in step 3 must be increased for expected price changes. In this example, all expenses are increased by 3.0%; the current-year cost for checking vital signs, $13.30 (column 8 in Table 10.11) is multiplied by 1.03 to arrive at the budget standard of $13.70 (column 5 in Table 10.12). The final step to determining the total budget year expenses is simply a mathematical process of multiplying total budgeted activities and the inflated cost per activity.

Unlike other budget systems that estimate the input expense directly by object code, ABB, in this example, estimated the total department expense, so step 5 divides the estimated expense into specific line items. If the activity cost was composed of a single line item, staff salaries (object code 4020), then compiling the staff salary budget would require only adding up all the calls on staff time. Decomposition of the total expense would not be required if each line item was individually calculated (which would also allow the specification of more appropriate cost drivers for each type of expense); however, detailing activities for each line item may be more trouble than it is worth, so the aggregated cost per activity must be divided into its constituent parts, that is, labor, supplies, and utilities.

In this example, all expenses were rolled up to produce the total expected cost for the nursing unit, so after the total budget is determined, it must be divided into the 22 line items. When all costs are rolled up into a single cost per activity rate, the budget can be unrolled by multiplying the total expected expenditures by the current expense distributions (line item expense/total cost). **TABLE 10.13** takes the total budgeted expense from Table 10.10, $4,289,306, and divides it among the 22 object codes on the basis of their current proportion of the budget. Staff salaries (object code 4020) constitute 58.75% of current salaries and fringe benefits ($1,235,642 / $2,103,252), so 58.75% of the $4,603,977 is allocated to staff salaries in the coming budget year. This allocation method ignores the fact that expenses may not be infinitely divisible, that is, it may not be possible to purchase a fractional input. But in many cases, fractional inputs not only can be purchased (part-time workers), they should also be used to avoid idle resources.

A case can be made like that made in flexible budgeting (Chapter 7) that certain object codes should not be adjusted for volume, that is, management salaries, repairs/maintenance, utilities, etc., which are not affected by changes in output, are immune to changes in cost drivers. This complication should be recognized, but the author prefers to ignore fixed costs to avoid overcomplicating the example.

The last step in the alternative ABB process is similar to other budget systems: new initiatives for which there is no historical data must be incorporated into the budget. Comparing the first example and the alternative approach shows no difference in expected total resource needs or by object code. The rationale for the alternative approach is that data on resource use (number of units consumed and their input prices) may not be readily available, while expense data (total line item expense incurred) is regularly reported and the expense estimation process is simpler. While the simpler method produces similar expense estimates (the prospective budget function), it does not produce the information necessary to manage activities and resources (the concurrent function). The standard, first approach defined how many activities were needed and how much inputs were required, physical units and/or dollar amount, to complete the activity that allows managers to identify deviations between actual and expected performance. The author recommends the alternative approach

TABLE 10.12 Constructing the Activity-Based Budget (Alternative Method)

Total Forecasted Patient Days	6,524						
% Patients < 65	0.5						

Activity	Cost Driver <65	Cost Driver >65	Budgeted Activities	Cost/Activity plus Inflation	Budget	Expense <65	Expense >65
Check vital signs	19,572	19,572	39,144	$13.70	$536,163	$268,082	$268,082
Dispense medications	21,744	43,496	65,240	$6.85	$446,803	$148,919	$297,883
Care Coordination	3,262	3,262	6,524	$136.97	$893,605	$446,803	$446,803
Patient hygiene	9,786	9,786	19,572	$13.70	$268,082	$134,041	$134,041
Patient concerns	2,175	4,349	6,524	$54.79	$357,442	$119,147	$238,295
Handwashing	202,896	286,404	489,300	$0.68	$335,102	$138,956	$196,146
Movement/to/from	202,896	286,404	489,300	$1.37	$670,204	$277,911	$392,293
Shift handoffs	6,524	6,524	13,048	$13.70	$178,721	$89,361	$89,361
Other	3,262	3,262	6,524	$92.46	$603,184	$301,592	$301,592
Total	3,262	3,262			$4,289,306	$4,289,306	$2,364,495
Average expense					$657.47	$590.07	$724.86

TABLE 10.13 Estimating the Budget by Object Code

Total ABB Expense					$4,289,306
Object Code	Description	Last Year 2017	YTD Actual 2018	YTD Actual (%)	2019 Budget
4010	Management and clerical staff	$331,200	$176,543	8.39	$360,036
4020	Staff salaries and wages	$2,066,350	$1,235,642	58.75	$2,519,930
4040	Overtime	$33,120	$23,833	1.13	$48,604
4050	Per diem / agency nurses	$374,400	$156,115	7.42	$318,376
4110	FICA	$185,946	$109,855	5.22	$224,035
4120	Health insurance	$278,760	$149,857	7.13	$305,614
4130	Retirement	$121,534	$71,801	3.41	$146,429
4140	Unemployment	$26,737	$15,796	0.75	$32,214
4210	Floor medications	$22,398	$13,589	0.65	$27,713
4212	Medical instruments	$18,596	$5,798	0.28	$11,824
4214	Bandages, gauze, etc.	$9,741	$5,643	0.27	$11,508
4216	Latex gloves, gowns, etc.	$52,899	$32,145	1.53	$65,556
4218	Sterile wipes	$5,211	$2,659	0.13	$5,423
4250	Office supplies	$8,452	$4,268	0.20	$8,704
4280	Cleaning supplies	$1,202	$569	0.03	$1,160
4350	Biomedical repairs/ maintenance	$5,244	$3,869	0.18	$7,890

4410	Electricity	$2,453	$1,156	0.05	$2,358
4440	Telephone	$5,794	$2,645	0.13	$5,394
4930	Housekeeping	$138,240	$72,000	3.42	$146,835
4940	Travel/professional meetings/meals	$35,789	$14,523	0.69	$29,618
4950	Education and training	$8,425	$3,688	0.18	$7,521
4960	Other expenses	$4,953	$1,258	0.06	$2,566
		$3,737,444	$2,103,252	100.00	$4,289,306

for novices and the standard approach as budgeting expertise increases.

ABB allows managers to see how expenses vary by cost object; in this case, there is a substantial difference in cost between patients under and over 65 years of age because of the different demand for activities by each group. Table 10.12 shows the cost of patients over 65 and under 65 years of age can be calculated using the expected number of activities for each group and the estimated cost per activity. Patients over the age of 65 give rise to $724.86 of costs per day, 22.8% higher, than the $590.07 needed for patients under 65. The higher cost of elderly patients is the direct result of increased staff time to handle their concerns (at $54.79 per concern) and the higher use of medication (at $6.85 per administration). The higher need to handle concerns of patients over 65 years of age and deliver more medicine also increases the number of trips staff make to these patients and handwashing. Similar analyses could be undertaken on the basis of the number of comorbidities a patient presents with, by diagnosis, by provider, or by any other observable trait that could drive resource use.

Table 10.12 allows us to determine the budget impact of a shift in the types of patient treated, that is, cost drivers. If patient days is 6524 but the proportion of patients over 65 increases to 60% (from 50%), ABB estimates that total expenses will increase by $87,937, costs for patients under 65 will decrease by $384,962, and costs for those over 65 will increase by $472,899. Similarly, the impact of increases in the number of patient days on expenses can be calculated: an increase of 100 patient days, assuming 50% of patients will be over and under the age of 65, predicts a cost increase of $65,747.

ABC and ABB are powerful tools for managers to understand what they do and whom they do things for. Armed with this information, managers will be challenged to provide more impactful actions to improve operations. Can they change production by improving efficiency through reducing the amount of a resource needed to produce an activity or reducing the number of activities performed? On the demand side, can managers change customer requirements? Can they discourage customers from demanding high-cost activities? If they cannot influence demand, managers should ensure the prices charged to customers that impose costs on the organization fully cover the added expense.

If current productivity standards (output per unit of input or units of input per activity) are based on current work, ABB cannot provide insight into efficiency. The budget, however, will reflect the impact on expenses for changes in output, the composition of output, and processes. Like a flexible budget, an increase (decrease) in patient days will require more (less) activity and expenses will change accordingly. Similarly, should the composition of output change, the cost drivers, the budget will reflect the higher or lower call for activities and increase or decrease the required resources and expenses. Third, changes in processes, decreasing the number of activities required or seeking more efficient ways to deliver activities (reducing the number of units of a resource needed to deliver service), will reduce expenses. Mandates that require additional services for patients or inefficiency that results in more activities undertaken will increase the amount of resources needed to deliver care and increase expenses. ABB increases the time required to prepare a budget, but by stating budget requirements in terms of work performed, it supplies a wealth of information to managers to enable them to understand how their departments work and what the impact of changes in output, customers, and processes on required expenses is.

The reader should see that ABB returns us to where we started, scratch budgeting. In an ABB system, managers are faced with the questions of how much work should be done and what the minimum resource requirement is that will get the task done. In scratch budgeting, economic necessity, that is, lack of funds, regularly forces start-ups to operate at minimum cost. As organizations prosper, "nice to have it if you can afford it" items become incorporated into their cost structure. Incremental and other budgeting systems institutionalize these costs by increasing them for expected price increases year after year, and inefficiency grows over time. Managers inheriting an operation may never consider why resources were acquired and what they should produce; they may simply assume that if it was needed in the past, it must still be needed. The last thing

a manager wants to do is voluntarily give up resources and then discover the resources were needed to complete work. As consumers and the economy change, traditional ways of doing things are often unsustainable. Organizations may find themselves competing against new and hungry competitors, and those unwilling or unable to change will put themselves out of business. ABB is a way to introduce or re-instill the entrepreneurial spirit into an organization by requiring managers to know their operations thoroughly (Henry Ford is a prime example of an executive who understood his business and every task required to build a car) and establish incentives for them to improve effectiveness and increase efficiency.

Strengths and Weaknesses of Activity-Based Budgeting

The primary strength of ABB is it ties resources to what is actually done to produce goods and services. ABB is built on an operational view of an organization: what is done, what resources are needed to perform tasks, how effective are work activities, and whom the work is done for. This operational view facilitates management; managers can determine whether tasks are necessary, whether excess resources are consumed in accomplishing tasks, whether unneeded or duplicate work is performed, and whether customers are paying appropriately for the services they demand. The ability to evaluate what is being done and for whom highlights the superior cost information ABB supplies. ABB, like flexible budgeting, recognizes the impact changes in the quantity of output have on cost, but beyond flexible budgeting, ABB also recognizes the impact of changes in the number of activities and the resources consumed by these activities on cost.

The primary weaknesses of ABB are the expertise and data needed to understand and operate the system. The primary budget challenge facing healthcare managers is their lack of financial expertise, and the challenge facing finance professionals is their lack of medical training. ABB, with its organic approach (what medical services are employed, and needed, and tying resources to services provided and services to outputs), demands higher understanding and skills from managers and finance professionals. If this challenge is overcome, managers will have a greater understanding of their operations and the ability to maximize output from the resources they employ. The second weakness is data; to make an ABC/ABB system work, more information is needed on how resources are employed (rather than simply purchased), the effectiveness of tasks undertaken, and whom they are working for. The advent of better and cheaper information systems should supply the data necessary to improve budgeting and management.

▶ Activity-Based Costing Case Studies

Cleveland Clinic employed a time-driven ABC project to examine heart value surgery (Donovan, Hopkins, Kimmel, Koberna, & Montie, 2014). This study highlights the opportunities and difficulties associated with using ABC. The authors note that Cleveland Clinic uses a "patient-encounter view of financial performance" to supplement the traditional accounting view to inform business plans, evaluate service lines and market areas, reduce costs, and improve quality. Heart surgery was analyzed because of the high volume of patients receiving mitral valve repair and aortic valve replacement.

The first step created process maps: 43 distinct care processes were mapped for valve surgery. To accurately map processes, the ABC team needed to identify the right caregivers, and this touches on two of the primary difficulties of employing ABC, (1) the knowledge of multiple people whose primary jobs are not financial must be tapped, and (2) major organizational resources must be committed to yield results. Process mapping included

identifying who performs work and what the average time to complete tasks is. The mapping process yielded insight into previously ignored, unbilled activities that could be improved. After identifying who performs the work, what the wage rates are, and how long it takes, cost standards were developed.

The analysis yielded insight into redundant activities (overprocessing, unnecessary wait times, and wasted motion and transport) and the recognition of how long it takes for various actions: 110 minutes to see patients, 90 to review records, 45 to order tests, and 40 to review test results. The results identified the duplication of work by different staff members and set the stage for developing standards, for example, scheduling staff, equipment, and rooms should take no more than 30 minutes. The analysts concluded that administrative and support services accounted for 6%–7% of the total cost of valve surgery and that the total cost of services was 10% lower than estimated in the existing cost accounting system.

A primary reason for the lower cost estimate was that the existing system included unused capacity costs. This finding requires comment: costs will only be lower if the expense of unused capacity is reduced either by eliminating the excess capacity or by redeploying those resources to other uses. If neither action is taken, the finding is merely academic, that is, total cost and output will be unchanged, and the analysis yields no benefit. While Cleveland Clinic gained insight into its care processes, at this point, it is unclear whether the analysis yielded any financial benefit.

The Cleveland Clinic project demonstrates how budgets should be constructed. First, identify high-volume activities. The **Pareto 80/20 rule** suggests that 20% of activities will account for 80% of the cost. Second, map work processes for the essential 20% (who performs and for how long). Third, calculate costs, and finally, improve the process. Dissecting processes is a costly and arduous task, but one can see that true management requires knowledge of what is occurring and what should occur. Building a budget based on activities performed is an essential tool for managers to use to fulfill their roles as facilitators and controllers of processes.

Haas and Kaplan (2017) used time-driven ABC to examine variation in treatment costs for total knee arthroplasties across 29 hospitals. They found that costs were 61% higher at the 90th percentile compared to the 10th percentile, that is, hospitals in the top 10% of costs were substantially more expensive than hospitals in the bottom 10%. This finding motivated an exploration of how and why the cost varied so much. Haas and Kaplan identified and measured the variation in 13 cost categories ranging from total personnel cost to standardized post-acute-care costs. The use of cost indexes prevented identifying the major cost components in total dollars but allows the reader to see which categories of cost had the greatest variation. The largest variation was seen in bone cement costs and standardized personnel cost during follow-up visits; the ratio of the 90th to the 10th percentile was 17.4 and 5.9. The least variation was seen in standardized personnel costs during hospitalization and standardized personnel costs: 1.8 and 1.9.

Understanding where costs differ gives providers an opportunity to examine their processes and reduce excessive costs. Haas and Kaplan also explored the impact of discharge status on costs. They found that hospitals with the highest post-acute-care cost discharged patients to inpatient rehabilitation 24% of the time versus 4%–7% of the time for hospitals below the 75th percentile. Correspondingly, only 4% of patients in the top 25th percentile were discharged to their homes versus 17%–44% in other hospitals. Hospitals with the lowest cost, in the bottom 25th percentile, discharged 44% of the patients to their homes and 4% to inpatient rehabilitation and had the lowest rate of readmission (2% versus 3% for other hospitals). Haas and Kaplan demonstrate that if costs are going to be controlled, providers must understand the care process and be

willing to change how they treat patients. Hospitals with the highest costs sent 53% of their patients to inpatient rehabilitation or skilled nursing care versus 14% in hospitals with the lowest costs. Conversely, the lowest-cost hospital discharged 86% of its patients to their homes or with home health compared to 46% in high-cost hospitals. Whether high-cost hospitals should follow the example of low-cost hospitals must be considered in light of who they are treating, are their patients older and sicker, and the outcomes each achieve.

▶ Recap and Summary of Budgeting Systems

The chapter "Financial Planning and Management" noted that the budgeting process starts with planning; proceeds to estimation of revenues and expenses, facilitation and control, and concludes with evaluation. The journey through the different budgeting systems highlights the need to match the primary objective with the optimal tool, that is, the means should serve the desired end. Planning (determining where an organization should go, what it will produce, and whom it will serve) recommends a zero-base or program budget. Both are geared toward critical evaluation of current processes, setting the direction, and reallocating resources. This type of decision-making is the responsibility of senior managers, who should be assisted by finance and operating managers.

The first phase of the budgeting process per se is the estimation of expenses and revenues. Incremental and flexible budgets are the easiest methods of estimating resource needs by object codes. The assumption of "no change is needed" in incremental budgeting makes it the easiest and most widely used budgeting method as well as the most appropriate as long as the assumption holds. An incremental budget utilizes the straightforward procedure of increasing prior-year expenditures for infla-tion for each object code to create a budget; however, changes in consumer preferences, production technology, input prices, and other things may make continuation of historical practices undesirable.

The greatest weakness in incremental bud-geting is that it often dismisses changes in out-put. Flexible budgeting addresses this weakness by making the final budget contingent upon actual output produced rather than forecasted output. Flexible budgets create more realistic models of production systems that recognize fixed and variable costs and how expenses should change when output is higher or lower than forecasted. Flexible budgets provide bet-ter incentives than incremental budgets. The primary incentive in an incremental budget is to meet the budget—neither over- or under-spending; the flexible budget, by establishing the expected cost per unit, encourages effi-ciency. Managers and workers operating under a flexible budget may receive bonuses if the actual cost per unit is less than the budget stan-dard, that is, they have incentives to find better and less costly ways of producing outputs.

The second phase of the budgeting pro-cess is managing to the budget and requires managers to facilitate and control work pro-cesses. While flexible budgeting can encour-age efficiency, it does not provide the insight of an activity-based budget: what resources are needed and how many, who is expected to per-form a task, and how long should it take? ABB provides the essential elements for managers to identify why budget targets are not met, were higher- or lower-priced inputs employed, did tasks take longer or less time to complete, were steps unnecessarily repeated, and/or were new steps added or current steps deleted? Both flexible and activity-based budgets adjust for output, but only ABB provides the necessary information to determine how a production process is varying from the financial plan, so managers can make adjustments to ensure operations for the year meet the budget.

The final budgeting phase is evaluation: did the operation meet its budget? While an activity-based budget may be the most cum-bersome to calculate, the wealth of informa-tion it provides in the final phase facilitates evaluation. By defining activities, ABB pro-vides the essential basis to determine why costs are higher or lower than expected. In the final analysis, senior management should deter-mine what the organization needs most: is it planning, estimation of expenses, concurrent facilitation and control of processes, or retro-spective accountability for financial perfor-mance? How senior management answers this question will determine which budget system or systems should be employed, and the bud-get systems selected will determine employee performance.

Summary

Budgeting complexity and realism increases with the quantity of items considered. In incre-mental budgeting, the focus is on the number of inputs consumed, and the biggest expense, labor, is easily counted. In some organizations, the total number of employees can be counted on one hand; in most departments, total staff-ing will be less than 100 full-time employees. When the focus shifts to flexible budgeting, output must be counted. For example, in a sole-physician practice with five employees, 140 patient visits per week of varying intensity may be provided (or 6720 patient visits per year). Obviously, it is easier to build a budget based on a staff of 5 rather than an anticipated output of 6720 patient visits.

Program budgeting adds another element of complexity by asking, what did the patient visit (output) achieve? Did the patient's health improve, and was the patient satisfied with the care he or she received? The question of out-come requires collecting and analyzing data beyond the immediate patient encounter. ABB further refines budgeting by recognizing that each output requires multiple activities and that each input, more often than not, performs more than one activity. A typical physician visit includes most, if not all, of the following activities: chart review, a history and physical, a physical examination, specimen collection, diagnosis and review of options, and treatment (injection and/or prescription). ABB leaps from quantifying the cost of 6720 visits to estimating the cost of performing up to 40,320 activities. While simplified budget systems can fulfill the prospective role of estimating revenues and expenses, they do not adequately support the concurrent management role or facilitate retrospective evaluation of operations. Only ABB provides the information necessary to understand what an operation is doing and should be doing and control the demand for resources and what resources produce.

The question managers should be able to answer is, does their operation consume more or less resources than it should for the output it produces and the outcomes it achieves? Resource use and cost can be too high if input price or volume is higher than expected; any budget system can provide this information. In addition, ABB can determine whether individual activities increased in cost because of inefficient provision (taking too much time), ineffectiveness (having to repeat processes because of unacceptable performance), or increased customer demand (intensity). ABB foreshadows the chapter "Variance Analysis," which defines why actual expenses differ from budgeted expenses by examining changes in prices, volume of output, efficiency of processes, and the intensity of work performed.

Key Terms and Concepts

Activity-based budgeting (ABB)
Activity-based costing (ABC)
Activity cost assignment
Cost driver

Cost object
Job order costing
Pareto rule
Process (absorption) costing
Resource cost assignment

Scientific management
Time and motion studies
Time-driven activity-based costing

Discussion Questions

1. Explain the two axes of the activity-based cost management framework.
2. Explain the difference between job order costing and process costing.
3. Describe the differences between traditional ABC and time-driven ABC for determining resource costs.
4. Explain the steps required to construct an activity-based budget.
5. Explain the strengths and weaknesses of ABB.

Problems

An ophthalmology practice is analyzing its outputs, cost, and prices to determine whether changes are needed. The practice provides five types of eye surgery: lasik, photorefractive keratectomy, lens implants, cataract surgery, and vitrectomy. Current output costs are based on total practice costs of $2 million and the physician's assessment in 2016 of how much time is devoted to each type of surgery (surgery is performed twice a week, or 768 hours per year are devoted to surgery).

1. Calculate the cost per output, given the physician's time estimate. Do current prices cover costs?
2. A time study was recently performed to determine the average minutes per surgery. Calculate the new cost per output based on minutes. Compare the costs determined by estimating the percentage of time spent and the time study. How and why have the costs changed? What is the cost of nonproductive time?

Surgery	Price	Time (%)	Quantity	Cost/Output
Lasik	$800	30	847	_____
Photorefractive keratectomy	$700	20	491	_____
Lens implants	$1,000	25	523	_____
Cataract surgery	$900	15	264	_____
Vitrectomy	$1,200	10	239	_____

Surgery		Minutes Total Per Case Minutes	% Total Time	Total Cost	Cost/ Output
Lasik	13	_____	_____	_____	_____
Photorefractive keratectomy	10	_____	_____	_____	_____
Lens implants	22	_____	_____	_____	_____
Cataract surgery	18	_____	_____	_____	_____
Vitrectomy	26	_____	_____	_____	_____
Nonproductive time	–	_____	_____	_____	_____
Total		46,080		$2,000,000	

3. Construct an activity-based budget based on the cost per output calculated in problem 2 with a 3% inflation factor, the forecasted output given, and assuming nonproductive time can be reduced to $300,000.

Forecasted (cost / output * 1.03)			
Surgery	**Quantity**	**Budget Standard**	**Budget**
Lasik	865	_____	_____
Photorefractive keratectomy	500	_____	_____
Lens implants	530	_____	_____
Cataract surgery	270	_____	_____
Vitrectomy	245	_____	_____
Nonproductive time			$300,000
Total			_____

References

Brimson, J. A., & Antos, J. (1999). *Driving value using activity-based budgeting*. New York, NY: John Wiley & Sons.

Cokins, G. (2001). *Activity-based cost management*. New York, NY: John Wiley & Sons.

Cooper, R., & Slagmulder, R. (2000). Activity-based budgeting: Part 1. *Strategic Finance, 82*(3), 85–86.

Donovan, C. J., Hopkins, M., Kimmel, B. M., Koberna, S., & Montie, C. A. (2014). How Cleveland Clinic used TDABC to improve value. *Healthcare Financial Management, 68*(6), 84–88.

Haas, D. A., & Kaplan, R. S. (2017). Variation in the cost of care for primary total knee arthroplasties. *Arthroplasty Today, 3*, 33–37.

Kaplan, R. S., & Anderson, S. R. (2004, November). Time-driven activity-based costing. *Harvard Business Review, 82*, 131–138.

Protzman, C., Mayzell, G., & Kepchar, J. (2011). *Leveraging lean in healthcare*. Boca Raton, FL: CRC Press.

Wren, D. A. (1979). *The evolution of management thought*. New York, NY: John Wiley & Sons.

PART 3

Financial Management Tools

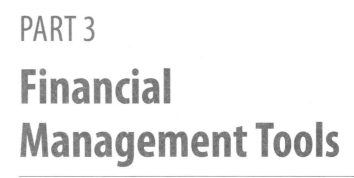

Part 2 dealt with constructing budgets that would facilitate planning, estimating revenues and expenses, and facilitating and controlling performance. Part 3 focuses on interpreting performance. Variance analysis examines the *differences* between actual and expected performance, and ratio analysis assesses an organization's performance relative to other organizations and/or its own prior performance. Capital budgeting and cost–benefit or cost-effectiveness analysis shift emphasis from departments or organizations to analyze the desirability of specific investments or programs.

The chapter "Variance Analysis" provides the critical linkage between budgeting and management to ensure budgeting is more than a one-time exercise in estimating expenses. Variance analysis focuses day-to-day management on achieving the operational plan defined in the budget and provides the tool for year-end evaluation: did managers meet or exceed financial targets? Variance analysis first identifies the expenses management should pay attention to, that is, large and controllable costs. Holding managers accountable for deviations in expenses they cannot control is pointless and unjust. Variance analysis provides the starting point for explaining the differences between actual operating results and the budget: Were deviations due to changes in price, efficiency, intensity, and/or volume? Were the variances significant, controllable, positive, or negative, and should action be taken? Although a variance may be uncontrollable, it does not mean that nothing should be done: Compensating changes in other areas may be desirable when a large, unfavorable variance arises, and conversely, additional opportunities can be pursued when favorable variances arise. While variances cannot tell why more or less resources were consumed than expected, they provide a starting point for investigation. For example, efficiency could decline because employees engage in nonvaluing-adding activities or managers allow employees to be idle, use more resources than necessary, or make excessive errors.

The chapter "Ratio Analysis and Operating Indicators" assesses performance (like variance analysis) but focuses on organizational rather than departmental performance. There are four major types of ratios focusing on different areas of performance or capability. Profitability ratios evaluate overall management performance: is financial performance increasing, decreasing, or stable, and how does it compare to the industry and/or similar organizations? Turnover ratios assess the productivity of assets: how much revenue is earned on invested assets? Liquidity ratios provide insight into the capacity of the

311

organization to meet its short-term liabilities, and capital structure ratios assess the use of debt to finance assets, the ability to satisfy long-term debt obligations, and the ability to secure additional financing at reasonable interest rates.

Ratios provide the starting point for assessing performance, but drilling down to the causes of low profitability or productivity often requires the use of operating indicators. Operating indicators provide the metrics to determine whether prices are too low or costs are too high. In the latter case, costs may be too high because of high input prices, low productivity of labor and/or capital, long lengths of stay (LOSs), etc. Identifying necessary actions using ratios and operating indicators requires understanding how and why performance has changed over time and knowing how other organizations perform. Improving performance is easier when opportunities are identified and targets are not only achievable but being achieved by competitors.

The chapter "Capital Budgeting and Time Value of Money" evaluates whether high-cost assets that produce a stream of revenue over time should be purchased. Unlike operating budgets, expenditures on high-cost assets are infrequent, and given the long lives of these investments, a higher level of scrutiny is given to these decisions compared to resources whose use can be adjusted from period to period. In the operating budget, if a one-dollar expenditure generates a dollar in revenue, it can be said to break even, but a one-dollar investment that produces a dollar in revenue two or more years in the future does not recoup its investment because of the declining purchasing power of money. While analyzing a capital expenditure requires the same skills as constructing an operating budgeting, to project output and estimate revenues and expenses, revenues and expenses received one or more years in the future must be reduced to current purchasing power to determine whether future returns are sufficient to warrant investment.

The chapter "Cost–Benefit and Cost-Effectiveness Analysis" discusses the means to organize information for assessing current operations and forming future operations. While cost–benefit analysis (CBA) measures benefits and costs in dollars to determine whether an activity should be undertaken, cost-effectiveness analysis (CEA) begins with the assumption that a particular end should be pursued, and is used to identify the alternative that produces the desired result at the lowest cost. Program evaluation differs from CBA and CEA as it is often retrospective rather than prospective. Program evaluation requires understanding the original need and the alternative means to fulfill the need to assess how the program implemented is performing, including its expected outcomes and costs and whether the need has changed. Program evaluation is a tool to assess the current effectiveness and efficiency of operations, while CBA and CEA are designed to ensure future investments are directed to the best alternatives.

These chapters provide essential skills for managers to assess current performance and identify areas for improvement. Variance and ratio analyses document differences in actual performance from the budget and other organizations for setting targets. Capital budgeting and CBA/CEA evaluate future investment to determine whether they are worth undertaking, while program evaluation provides a wide-ranging framework to assess operations and outcomes.

CHAPTER 11

Variance Analysis

CHAPTER OBJECTIVES

1. Explain the role of variance analysis in financial management.
2. Calculate cost and volume variances.
3. Calculate and interpret efficiency, intensity, and price variances.
4. Identify variances to be investigated.
5. Analyze, discuss, and assess financial performance.

▶ Introduction

The purpose of building a budget is to define where an organization wants to go and what resources it needs to get there. Whether budgets improve processes and performance or they don't depends on the degree to which managers use budgets to guide resource consumption. The concurrent management phase is where the "rubber hits the road": it is the test of foresight, budgeting, and managerial ability. The energy put into budget construction is wasted if goals are not internalized by employees and the budget is not used as an operational guide.

Does the budget make the transition from estimating revenues and expenses to a tool managers use to facilitate and control operations? Do managers reference the budget when reality differs from budget assumptions, and are resources increased or decreased when output exceeds or falls behind projections? Even when output projections are on target, it is rare that actual revenues and expenses equal the budget, so managers should be able to explain the differences between expected and realized inflows and outflows. The first question is, "Is actual financial performance better than, equal to, or worse than expected?" The second question is, "By how much do actual results vary from expectations, and is the difference a matter of concern?" If the difference is large enough to warrant concern, the final question is, "Why is there a difference?"

At the organizational level, the first question can be reduced to "Is actual net income greater than, equal to, or less than budgeted net income?" When actual profit exceeds budgeted profit, a positive and favorable variance occurs. Variances are generally calculated as actual amounts minus budgeted amounts, but it is likely the reader may see variances calculated as budget minus actual. The reader should not focus on whether variances are positive or negative but rather whether they are favorable or unfavorable. Regardless of whether budgeted amounts are subtracted from actual amounts or vice versa, the reader should be able to identify whether the variance is favorable or unfavorable. Actual revenues exceeding budgeted revenues is desirable, and actual expenses exceeding budgeted expenses is undesirable. When actual revenues *and* expenses exceed the budget because of higher sales, this may be good or bad, depending on the magnitude of the change. If costs increased by 5% and revenue by 10%, the organization is better off; if the increase in costs exceeds the increase in revenue, the organization is worse off (**TABLE 11.1**).

Accounting information should be used by managers to control their departments and move the organization toward higher net income (revenue minus expenses) and equity (assets minus liabilities). The first question is whether a change from the budget makes the organization stronger (generates a larger surplus or smaller deficit) or weaker (reduces the expected surplus or produces a larger deficit). The second question recognizes that not all variances are worth devoting attention to. Understanding small variances, measured in absolute dollars or as a percentage of the budget, whether favorable or unfavorable, may not generate sufficient benefit to warrant devoting managerial time to discovering their cause or controlling them. On the other hand, large variances require understanding and action due to their potential impact on the viability of the organization. This chapter is devoted to determining whether variances are due to changes in price, volume, efficiency, or intensity and whether these factors are controllable. *The discussion is limited to expenses to simplify the presentation as the majority of managers have little control over revenues, but the same reasoning applies to the analysis of revenue variances.*

Variance analysis is a management tool to improve operations by determining the reason(s) for deviations between actual and budgeted operating expenses. Variance analysis should be performed monthly, when accounting reports are released after the close of each accounting period, so timely corrective action can be taken. Monthly budget reports do not allow managers to rectify what has already occurred but provide them with an opportunity to identify and correct past problems that may continue to have an adverse financial impact on operations in future periods.

The efficacy of variance analysis is determined by the budget (does the budget define efficient operation?), the timeliness and extent of data available, the manager's analytical ability to identify problems, and whether he or she has the willingness and authority to alter operations. Information gained through variance analysis should be used to refine actual operations and/or improve the resource allocation process—the prospective and concurrent budget functions. A manager's main duty is to ensure his or her department is advancing organizational objectives within the constraints of available resources.

TABLE 11.1 Budget Variances and Favorability		
	Revenue	**Expense**
Favorable (↑ net income)	Actual revenue > Budgeted revenue	Actual expense < Budgeted expense
Unfavorable (↓ net income)	Actual revenue < Budgeted revenue	Actual expense > Budgeted expense

Variance analysis is the first step in determining the reason(s) for higher- or lower-than-expected resource use. Operating expenses may be higher than budgeted because work is not being performed as planned or the budget was insufficient to fund the current level of operations. Assuming the budget provided sufficient resources for the work expected, variance analysis should identify why higher-than-budgeted expenses were incurred and guide the process of achieving greater efficiency in the future. Variance analysis should identify the major reason(s) for budget variances and guide the search for actionable causes. Variance analysis may lead to the conclusion that the budget was simply too low to support the quantity of goods or services being produced. If the budget did not supply sufficient resources, the expense estimation process should be evaluated and adjusted to ensure future budgets provide the appropriate funding for expected output.

When expenses are underbudget, variance analysis should identify the reason(s) for lower-than-expected resource use. Has a reduction in input prices or a change in the production process reduced the cost of producing the good or service, and are these levels of performance and cost sustainable? Of course, the budget may have overstated necessary expenditures and provided more than enough resources for the actual output produced. Budget surpluses can also arise when necessary services are ignored, that is, corners are cut or a lower-quality product is produced. Knowing why operations are running underbudget is essential to planning, budgeting, and day-to-day management.

Budget variations may result from period-to-period fluctuations, and a current budget deficit may be followed by a surplus of similar magnitude in a subsequent period or vice versa. The timing of many expenses is often based on the external billing cycle of suppliers and the internal order processing/payment cycle of the organization. Although managers are certain the expenses will be incurred, the timing of payments may be unknown. Differences in the timing of expenses between the budget and the monthly accounting statements should be recognized so that extensive time is not spent investigating differences that are purely temporal or offsetting.

Managers not only engage in strategic behavior to increase their budgets but also are strategic in committing funds. Some managers spend or commit funds early in a budget year if they suspect budget reductions may occur. Early commitment ensures funds cannot be reduced during the budget year. Managers who commit funds as early as possible will show budget overruns in the initial months of the fiscal year that are subsequently offset by surpluses later in the year. Expenditures are simply shifted into the early months of the fiscal year and out of later periods, while total budgeted expenditures remain constant.

The opposite strategy postpones early period expenditures as a contingency for unplanned expenses. Managers may delay discretionary expenditures to year-end to ensure budgets are met. If an unforeseen event increases expenditures on one or more line items above the amount set in the budget, the overrun can be offset by reducing or foregoing purchases of nonessential items. Expendable or unnecessary items initially delayed may not be purchased or may be purchased in lower than anticipated quantities to meet the overall budget target. If actual expenses meet the budget, managers then spend their more discretionary funds; that is, if budget targets are met in the first 10 months of a year, managers can confidently commit their discretionary funds.

Variance analysis is a tool to decide whether operations or the budget should be altered and, if so, what actions can and should be taken. Monthly variance reports provide the raw information for managers to enact effective control through the budget year. Retrospective analysis of full-year performance should determine whether monthly information was acted upon and the desired goals were achieved.

The insight provided by variance analysis is limited by the data available. When only cost and a gross output measure are available, managers can only determine whether a difference between actual results and the budget is due to (a) producing more output or (b) spending more on inputs. Spending more on inputs, or a cost variance, can arise from (a) an increase in the price of inputs, (b) poor use of inputs so more resources are needed to complete a task or produce an output, or (c) a change in the characteristics of the output require additional inputs to meet the revised product standards. Determining whether inputs are being underutilized or output requires additional resources requires information on the amount of inputs consumed and the activities need to produce outputs.

The units of some inputs, like labor, are easy to quantify: the payroll department knows the total paid labor hours, and managers can easily determine whether hours per output are increasing or decreasing. When hours per output are increasing, it may not be clear whether the increase is due to lower productivity or a need for more staff time due to sicker patients. Changes in the use of other inputs, like supplies, are more difficult to determine. Supplies within an object code are often an aggregation of high- and low-priced items, and it is difficult or impossible to tell whether changes in cost are due to changes in prices, the total units consumed, or a shift between high- and low-priced supplies.

The second issue, how many units of a resource are needed to produce an output, is often difficult to determine in health care. As seen in Chapter 4, providing care for a patient in diagnosis-related group (DRG) 216 typically requires a length of stay (LOS) of 13.8, but patient needs differ, and it may be difficult to determine on a case-by-case basis when the LOS is excessive. On the other hand, if a hospital's average LOS for all its DRG 216 patients is significantly higher than 13.8 days, it may indicate the care process should be reviewed with an eye toward decreasing the LOS. The

validity of the "our patients are sicker, so our LOS is longer" argument can only be taken so far as Medicare adjusts for differences in the level of illness; patients without major complications or comorbidities (DRG 217) and those without any complications or comorbidities (DRG 218) should have a shorter LOS: 9.0 and 6.6 days, respectively.

The relationship between inputs and outputs in health care cannot be as rigidly defined as other industries. For example, automakers know precisely how many parts are required per car and can quickly determine whether excessive resource consumption is occurring. Ford knows immediately when it produces 10,000 vehicles but consumes 52,516 tires that 2,516 tires were wasted. However, a hospital with 10,000 admissions may be unable to determine whether 52,516 patient days were appropriate or whether patients should have been discharged earlier. This is the cost challenge in health care; healthcare managers need variance analysis to determine why their expenses vary from the budget, and this requires the ability to identify changes due to input prices, efficiency, intensity of the care delivered, and the number of patients served. The first variance analysis example will be demonstrated on the basis of minimal information (cost and output), and a second, more involved example incorporating input units consumed and activities performed will explore the impact of changes in efficiency and intensity on costs.

▶ Cost and Volume Variances

Traditional variance analysis reduces the differences between actual and budgeted expenditures to changes in input costs and output quantities and provides a starting point for learning how to evaluate performance. Variance analysis links budget construction to management and evaluation of operations. Budgets should not be one-time estimating events to be subsequently ignored, but they should be used throughout the fiscal year to guide and evaluate and control operations.

Budgets are developed to estimate and provide sufficient resources to accomplish the organization's overall mission and goals and the tasks delegated to each department. Budgets are constructed around the inputs that should be used (incremental), the cost per output (flexible or zero-base), the cost per outcome (program), or the cost per work performed (activity-based). The same basis used to build a budget should be used to dissect actual operating results when they differ from the financial plan.

At the most elementary level, a budget specifies how much it should cost to produce a defined quantity of output. The budget should specify the output that will be produced, the quantity of output expected, a plan of what inputs will be needed, the amount of each input required to produce the expected output, and input prices. Expense variances arise for four main reasons: changes in input prices, the use of more or less inputs (changes in efficiency), the need to devote more or fewer activities to produce outputs (changes in intensity or type of output produced), and the production of more or less output (changes in the volume of output produced).

Variance analysis is a management tool and a tool to evaluate management. To fulfill both roles, inputs that managers can affect and those that cannot be changed must be identifiable. It makes little sense to institute extensive reporting and analysis of inputs that cannot be changed, and it would be unjust to hold managers responsible for deviations in noncontrollable expenses.

Understanding what can and cannot be changed is essential to achieving efficiency. Variance analysis focuses on variable expenses that should and do change with expansion and contraction of output. Input use or expenses expected to be unaffected by changes in output include management salaries, insurance, rent, and depreciation. Analysis of fixed

inputs and fixed costs should not consume a large amount of managers' time, given their unchanging/unvarying nature and lack of controllability.

Variable inputs having a direct relationship with output, that is, expenses that increase with the expansion of output and fall as output declines, include production salaries, supplies, and utilities. Monitoring and controlling variable inputs should consume the majority of a manager's attention and time. Are resources being used properly, should resource consumption be cut back (increased), and, if so, by how much as output falls (rises)? Managers should be evaluated and rewarded on their ability to manage controllable resources. A primary role of accounting and information systems is to provide managers with the information they need to make timely resource use decisions.

Before a manager is praised or blamed for a budget variance, two questions must be answered: Is the variance favorable or unfavorable, and is the expense controllable? Expenses coming in underbudget are favorable; were these expenses reduced by instituting better processes, more effective management, better purchasing decisions, and/or securing long-term contracts to insulate the organization from input price increases? Expenses may also fall for reasons unrelated to management, such as reductions in input prices due to market surpluses (increase in resource availability or decrease in demand). Reductions in the demand for the organization's output will also reduce expenses, but managers should not receive credit for their products falling out of favor with consumers.

Expenses coming in overbudget are unfavorable, and managers should be held accountable for variances arising from the lack of or ineffective management, including the incompetence of employees, excessive waste, idleness, theft of resources, and/or lack of arms-length price negotiation in contracting resources, including no-bid and sweetheart contracts. Unfavorable and uncontrollable factors that increase expenses include higher demand for the organization's products (of course, if higher demand produces additional revenue that exceeds the additional expenses, it is positive for the organization), input market shortages resulting in higher prices, and extraordinary events (**TABLE 11.2**).

The point is to give credit and blame where each is due. When expenses do not match the operating plan, it should first be determined whether the variance is favorable or unfavorable and second whether the manager could control the resource. Uncontrollable events should be recognized and communicated to ensure their impact on current operating results and future budgets can be accommodated.

Variance analysis in this example divides differences between actual operating results and the budget into changes in input costs and changes in output. **Cost variances** arise when the actual cost for an input is greater than or less than its budgeted cost per output, for example, $200 in registered nurse (RN) labor was planned per patient day but $220 is incurred. This variance identifies the amount of the total budget variance that is due to differences in the projected and incurred costs of a resource. The $20.00 cost difference per day may be due to changes in input prices (wages)

in the time between when wages were estimated and when RNs were paid, lower productivity (more time to complete a task), or the need to commit more resources per output (more time due to sicker patients).

The cost variance is calculated as follows:

$$\text{Cost variance} = (\text{Actual cost/actual output} - \text{budgeted cost/budgeted output}) * \text{actual output} \quad (11.1)$$

Why would RNs be paid $220 per patient day rather than the $200 estimated in the budget? This is the cost per output, so it could arise from paying more for a resource or using more resources; it does not arise from producing more output. Actual input prices may deviate from the budget for many reasons: unrealistic (overly optimistic or pessimistic) price estimates, changes in market conditions, or introduction of different production processes in the period between when expenses were estimated and when production occurred. Likewise, the substitution of higher-skilled and better-compensated employees, use of overtime (time and a half pay) versus regular time, and labor shortages will also increase the cost of inputs. If a change in the production process requires that higher-priced inputs be

TABLE 11.2 Budget Variances, Controllability, and Action		
	Favorable	**Unfavorable**
Controllable	Give credit -Better management (less waste/idleness) -Introduction of better processes -Better price negotiation	Hold accountable -Lack of management -Outdated processes -Sweetheart, no-bid contracts
Uncontrollable	Acknowledge -Decline in output -Input market surpluses	Acknowledge -Increase in output -Input market shortages -Extraordinary events

substituted for lower-priced inputs, an unfavorable variance will arise. The necessity of using higher-priced inputs may result from the unavailability of the previously used inputs, an attempt to increase quality, or a safety/environmental mandate. Surpluses or shortages of resources may decrease or increase prices of currently used resources. For example, recent changes in the supply and demand for oil have contributed to the volatility of gasoline and heating oil prices and rendered many budget projections unrealistic. When input prices are falling, it is easy for managers to meet their budgets; however, when input prices rise, it may be impossible for them to meet their budgets.

Variance analysis narrows the potential causes of budget overages and assesses whether managers could control the expenses, that is, are higher salaries (cost per hour) due to injudicious awarding of pay increases or overtime or a reasonable and necessary attempt to retain employees or fill vacancies? Managers should not be held responsible for budget overruns if the higher cost per hour is due to market pressure or the need to schedule overtime to ensure continuity of patient care. If the overrun is due to unmerited salary increases or unneeded use of overtime, it should be used to evaluate and change management performance.

The other reason is that more RN hours per output are being consumed. If more hours are required because of lower productivity, the head nurse should be held accountable. If additional time is required because patients are sicker, as evidenced by an increase in the Medicare case mix index (CMI), the head nurse should not be held accountable. The problem with traditional variance analysis using cost per output to determine the price variance is that it cannot differentiate between paying more for resources and using more resources.

Changes in prices are the only reason actual fixed expenses should be greater than or less than budgeted. Measures of efficiency,

intensity, or volume should be irrelevant since the quantity of a fixed expense should be constant and changes in productivity, type of output produced, and/or amount of output should not call forth more resources or require less resources.

Volume variances arise when actual output is greater than or less than forecasted output. Output projections may be inaccurate, given the 18-month lapse between budget construction and the end of the budget year, and lead to higher or lower expenditures than planned. Consumer demand for a product will change with changes in its price or its expected future price, purchasers' income and wealth, prices of substitute and complementary goods, and tastes and preferences. One or more of these variables may change in a short period, so understanding the impact of output changes on input use and costs is essential. Volume variances quantify the impact of output changes on input expenses, that is, how much should input expenses increase or decrease if output increases or decreases?

The volume variance for a variable cost is calculated as follows:

$$\begin{aligned} \text{Volume variance} = {} & (\text{Actual output} \\ & - \text{budgeted output}) \\ & * \text{budgeted cost per output} \quad (11.2) \end{aligned}$$

The volume variance recognizes that actual expenses should increase (decrease) by the budgeted cost per output for every additional unit of output produced above (below) forecasted output. If 1200 admissions are projected but 1235 occur and each admission requires 30 hours of RN time at an average wage of $20 per hour, the increase in output should increase RN salary expense by $21,000 (35 admissions * 30 hours/admission * $20/hour). If admissions are 35 less than forecasted, labor expense should be $21,000 underbudget. This assumes that labor is increased or decreased with changes in output—an assumption that may carry greater weight in the case of resources like pharmaceuticals and medical supplies. If RN hours do not change with output, then wages should not change, that is, RN salaries would be similar to managers' salaries, who are paid on salary rather than the number of hours worked. Higher or lower admissions should have no budget impact on fixed costs like rent, insurance, and interest expense.

The generic reasons for differences between actual and budgeted output include unrealistic forecasts and unanticipated changes in demand, marketing, and/or competitor prices. Hospitals may see higher admissions from increases in readmissions, medical and technological advancements, changes in insurance coverage (reductions in out-of-pocket expenses or changes in provider networks that funnel more patients to their institutions), and/or service line reductions by competitors.

Variance analysis is traditionally conducted by object code, as illustrated by **TABLE 11.3** that provides the labor expense for a hospital dietary department for one month. The hospital has 300 beds and averages a 70% census, so the budget was constructed assuming 210 patients would receive 3 meals per day, or 18,900 meals would be served in a 30-day month. Table 11.3 shows the operating plan has not been met as expenses are 8.8% overbudget but the overrun is driven, in part, by an erroneous volume estimate—actual admissions and patient days are higher than forecasted.

Variance analysis depends on available data; in some cases, the only measure of output available is admissions. In this example, output is measured at a higher level of granularity, that is, patient days; however, this level of detail does not allow price, efficiency, or intensity variances to be calculated. Additional insight can be gleaned through variance analysis when information on the quantity of inputs used and the number of activities provided is available, as demonstrated in the next example. Traditional variance analysis revolves around the identification of total, cost, and volume variances; the advantage *and* drawback of this approach are its reliance on gross or macro-output measures.

The total labor variance is the difference between actual and budgeted expense *and* the sum of the cost and volume variances. Calculating both formulas and reconciling any difference ensure the analyst has not made a mathematical error.

$$\text{Total variance} = \text{Actual expense} - \text{Budgeted expense}$$

$$\$3,800 = \$47,000 - \$43,200$$

The cost variance identifies the difference between the budgeted and actual cost per output produced and multiplies this difference by actual output.

TABLE 11.3 Actual Operating Results and Budget Estimates

	Actual	Budgeted	$ Difference	% Difference (%)
Labor expense	$47,000	$43,200	$3,800	8.8
Admissions	1,297	1,260	37	2.9
Patient days (output)	6,615	6,300	315	5.0

$$\begin{aligned}
\text{Cost variance} &= (\text{Actual cost/actual output} - \text{budgeted cost/budgeted output}) * \text{actual output} \\
&= (\$47,000/6,615 \text{ actual patient days} - \$43,200/6,300 \text{ budgeted patient days}) \\
&\quad * 6,615 \text{ actual patient days} \\
&= (\$7.1051/\text{actual patient day} - \$6.8571/\text{budgeted patient day}) \\
&\quad * 6,615 \text{ actual patient days} \\
&= \$0.2480 \text{ unplanned cost per patient day} * 6,615 \text{ actual patient days} = \$1,640
\end{aligned}$$

The cost variance shows the labor cost per patient day for meal preparation is $0.25 higher than budgeted. Given 6615 patient days were provided, the higher cost per day accounts for $1640, or 43.2%, ($2140/$3800) of the labor expense overrun.

The remainder of the expense variance, 56.8%, must be explained by higher-than-expected output. The volume variance identifies the difference between budgeted and actual output and multiplies this amount by the budgeted cost per output.

$$\begin{aligned}
\text{Volume variance} &= (\text{Actual output} - \text{budgeted output}) * \text{budgeted cost/output} \\
&= (6,615 \text{ actual patient days} \\
&\quad - 6,300 \text{ budgeted patient days}) * \$43,200/6,300 \text{ budgeted patient days} \\
&= 315 \text{ unplanned patient days} * \$6.8571/\text{budgeted cost per patient day} = \$2,160
\end{aligned}$$

The volume variance shows 315 more patient days were provided than forecasted and the budget anticipated each patient day required $6.86 of labor. If the output forecast had been correct, the 315 unanticipated patient days would have increased budgeted labor expense by $2160; the change in output explains 56.8% ($2140/$3800) of the total labor variance.

$$\begin{aligned}
\text{Total variance} &= \text{Cost variance} \\
&\quad + \text{Volume variance} \\
\$3800 &= \$1640 + \$2160 \\
100.0\% &= 43.2\% + 56.8\%
\end{aligned}$$

Traditional variance analysis could lead to an erroneous conclusion that the $3800 budget deficit was due to higher input prices (especially when the cost variance is called a price variance) and higher volume. That is, the department paid $7.11 per patient day versus a budget of $6.86, and the higher cost accounted for 43.2% of the total variance. The remaining 56.8% is attributable to higher output: 315 additional patient days produced at the budgeted cost of $6.86 per day. Traditional variance analysis does not provide a complete picture of operations, because it fails to differentiate between *paying* more for an input and *using* more inputs to produce the budgeted output or requiring more services due to a change in the budgeted output.

The important question is, "Is the output produced and input productivity the same as what was expected and budgeted?" The output may require more or fewer activities or more or less resources per activity to complete the job, for example, administration may require dietary to shift from processed foods to locally grown produce to improve the taste and nutritional value of meals and support local farmers. Preparing fresh food often takes more time than using preprocessed foods and increases the cost per meal. If the output or food preparation process has not changed, are employees taking more (or less) time to accomplish the same tasks? Obviously, patient days do not adequately track the output of the dietary department, and labor expense does not fully illuminate labor use; more data is needed on output and productivity to identify changes in the intensity or efficiency of work performed.

▶ Efficiency, Intensity, and Price Variances

The fundamental problem with traditional variance analysis is that the cost variance conflates changes in productivity, intensity of resources needed, and prices. The consolidation of these three factors is often the result of insufficient data. Variance analysis is limited to cost and volume variances when managers only have access to the amount spent per line item and total output. Greater insight into how processes are operating requires information on the number of inputs consumed and the number of activities needed and undertaken to produce an output. The following example demonstrates how cost variances can be divided into efficiency, intensity, and price components when data on inputs and activities performed is available.

Efficiency variances arise when actual input use per activity is greater than or less than the budgeted input use per activity. Efficiency variances measure the ability of systems to transform inputs into activities that produce outputs. Unlike changes in input price or output, resource productivity is the area where managers should have the greatest control—hence the need to understand how to identify and act on inefficiencies as they arise. **FIGURE 11.1** shows a generic system model, with the ellipse documenting the boundary between the producer and the external environment. Managers have limited control over

the prices of inputs purchased outside the organization and the quantity of output sold. Managers should control the production process within the organization and the number of inputs consumed to perform activities as well as the number of activities undertaken to produce a product.

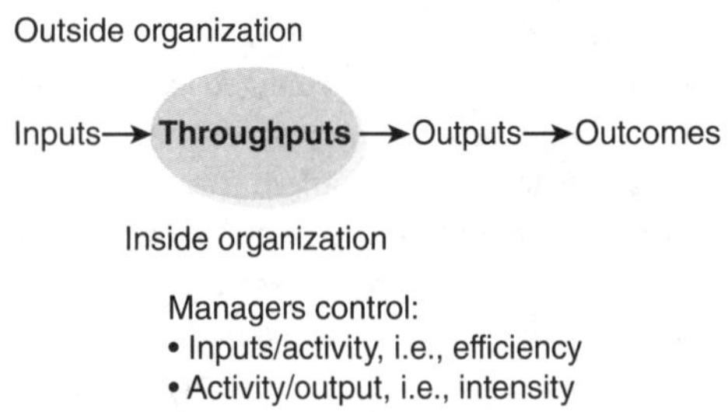

TABLE 11.4 provides the additional data needed to calculate efficiency, intensity, and price variances—the number of staff hours paid (inputs consumed) and meals prepared (activities undertaken) during the budget period. Labor hours paid increased less than patient days increased (4.5% versus 5.0%), suggesting an increase in efficiency, while meals prepared increased more than patient days (6.8% versus 5.0%), suggesting an intensity increase, that is, more meals per day. The questions is, were these meals ordered by the patient or physician, or is the increase due to wasted meals?

The efficiency variance allows the number of activities to vary, so the necessity to expend more resources to produce more activities is not confused with an inability to produce outputs with the minimum amount of inputs, that is, the department budgeted 2,880 hours to produce 18,900 meals, or 0.1524 hours per meal (9 minutes and 8 seconds). The monthly payroll report shows 3010 hours were paid; this could be the result of producing more meals at 9 minutes and 8 seconds per meal or increasing the time per meal to 9 minutes and 57 seconds if the budgeted number of meals (18,900) was produced.

Efficiency is constant if the time to complete an activity, that is, prepare a meal, does not change. An increase (decrease) in the time per meal suggests lower (higher) efficiency. The reader should note the impact of higher output: when patient days increase, more meals should be prepared and more resources should be consumed to prepare them; the increase in volume may but should not be a factor in calculating the efficiency variance. Increases (decreases) in output will explain changes in efficiency if activity rises (drops) and the same

Outside organization

Inputs→ **Throughputs** →Outputs→Outcomes

Inside organization

Managers control:
• Inputs/activity, i.e., efficiency
• Activity/output, i.e., intensity

FIGURE 11.1 A System

TABLE 11.4 Actual Operating Results and Budget Estimates with Inputs Consumed and Activities Performed

	Actual	Budgeted	$ Difference	% Difference (%)
Labor expense	$47,000	$43,200	$3,800	8.8
Admissions	1,297	1,260	37	2.9
Patient days (output)	6,615	6,300	315	5.0
Meals prepared (activity)	20,191	18,900	1,291	6.8
Hours paid (input)	3,010	2,880	130	4.5

level of variable resources are consumed, that is, the time per meal must decrease (increase) if the number of meals prepared increases (drops) with no change in staffing, that is, paid labor hours. Managers should adjust variable resource use directly with changes in volume and when they do changes in output will have no impact on efficiency. The reasons more resources (labor, supplies, energy, etc.) per output will be used than budgeted include unrealistic budget standards, more complex products, poor use of resources, waste and theft, poorly planned workflows, bottlenecks, lack of accountability, and/or ineffective management.

Intensity variances arise when the actual number of activities required to produce an output is greater than or less than the number of activities planned per output. In this example, fulfilling dietary requirements (achieving nutritional effectiveness) is the primary goal of serving three meals per patient per day, but managers should recognize the secondary purpose of providing satisfaction, that is, the meals should be tasty, served at the correct temperature, and visually appealing. Meals prepared (activities) should fulfill the

purposes for which they were undertaken, and if they do not produce the desired result, they may need to be redone. A cold, unappetizing meal could meet nutritional standards, but if it is so unappealing that the patient sends it back or refuses to eat, costs will increase if a second meal must be prepared or the ultimate objective of restoring a patient's health may be undermined by inadequate caloric intake.

Changes in intensity may require more resources to produce an output. For example, in a nursing unit, a sicker patient will require more attention from staff and increase the number of hours consumed per patient day and/or a longer LOS to recuperate, that is, a 6-day LOS was forecasted but the actual LOS is 7 days. Healthcare managers often cannot control the intensity of care required but should ensure sufficient resources are available to provide required treatment. LOS (discharge orders), the number of tests and procedures, and meals are dictated by physicians; the manager's role is not to judge the appropriateness of physician orders but, rather, to see they are carried out promptly, effectively, and efficiently.

The reasons for higher intensity (needing more activities than planned in the budget) include unrealistic budget standards, production of higher-quality output, different patient or product mix, and mandates (e.g., minimum legislated LOS). Longer-than-expected LOSs may be driven by sicker populations (should be reflected in changes in the CMI), physician performance, inability to find alternative care settings, and legislative mandates. If duplicate tests are required because initial tests were faulty or the results were lost, it is the manager's job to ensure the quality of work in his or her department. Managers should be capable of quantifying shifts in intensity to ensure they are held accountable only for resource use in their control.

Price variances arise when the actual price of resources is greater than or less than the budgeted price. Price variances focus on the cost per input rather than cost per output used in Equation 11.1. Input prices may increase (or decrease) due to uncontrollable changes in the supply and demand for an input, the failure of managers to seek the best prices, or unwarranted overtime or salary increases.

Efficiency, intensity, price, and volume variances examine particular aspects of an operation by holding other factors constant. In the dietary example, the volume variance is only concerned with how many more (fewer) patient days are provided than were planned; it uses standard rates (cost per output) to calculate how far actual expenses should be over- or underbudget on the basis of the amount of output produced. Factors that would affect the actual cost per output are held constant by the use of standard rates (rather than the budgeted cost), including cost/input (price), inputs/activity (efficiency), and activity/output (intensity) (**TABLE 11.5**).

TABLE 11.5 Types of Variances

Variance	Measures	Controllable/Noncontrollable
Total	Δexpense	
Price	Δcost/input	Noncontrollable: Changes in input supply and demand
		Controllable: Unwarranted raises, overtime
Efficiency	Δinput/activity	Noncontrollable: Change in activity
		Controllable: Change in performance
Intensity	Δactivity/output	Noncontrollable: Activities ordered
		Controllable: Repeated activities that did not meet standards
Volume	Δquantity of output	Noncontrollable: Meeting demand
		Controllable: Overproduction

The measure of output for a nursing unit could be admissions (gross level), and the intensity could be measured as patient days per admission. If the analysis is more refined, output could be patient days and intensity could be a measure of acuity based on care required (pain medication, oxygen, etc.) and patient behavior and ability. When patient days is the measure of intensity, it assumes all patient days are similar, which is obviously untrue. But this assumption is often necessary to work within the confines of available data. The dietary example is based on patient days as the output measure, and meals, the measure of intensity, are assumed to be homogeneous.

The understanding of variances can be illuminated by returning to the system model (Figure 11.1). In a system, the entry of inputs and the production of outputs are clear. Inputs enter the production process from outside the organization, and price variances arise when their prices are more or less than planned. Outputs are the end result of the production process, and expenses change directly with the quantity of output produced, that is, volume variances. Inputs and outputs are easily measured.

The challenge in many production processes is to understand throughputs: how are inputs transformed into outputs? The first step in the production process is to transform inputs into activities: activity-based costing calls this resource cost assignment. What activities are inputs expected to provide, and how many activities can each input produce? Second, how many activities are needed to produce an output, that is, activity cost assignment. Figure 11.1 shows that understanding the production process requires understanding the type and number of inputs required

to produce an activity and the type and number of activities needed to produce an output. Rather than envisioning a system as producing a single output, we should conceptualize production systems as producing intermediate outputs that are subsequently combined to produce a final output. In hospitals, ancillary departments produce tests and procedures and nursing units provide medical and hotel functions that are combined to produce a patient day or an admission.

The system model allows us to visualize the interrelationships of variances. Total cost is a function of input prices, the effectiveness of the transformation of inputs into medical services, the effectiveness of the transformation of medical services into health outputs, and the volume of outputs produced. The following formulas illustrate these relationships:

$$\text{Total cost} = (\text{AVC} * Q) + \text{TFC} \quad (11.3)$$

where AVC is the average variable cost, Q is the quantity, and TFC is the total fixed cost.

$$\text{Total cost} = \text{Price} * \text{Efficiency} * \text{Intensity} \\ * \text{Volume}$$

$$\text{Total cost} = \text{Cost/input} * \text{Input/activity} \\ * \text{Activity/output} * \text{Output} \quad (11.4)$$

When examining the performance of the dietary unit with budgeted labor expenses of $43,200, we start with how the budgeted expense was estimated. The budget assumed a wage of $15.00 per hour (input price), 0.1524 hours per meal (productivity standard), 3 meals per patient day (activity benchmark), and 6300 patient days (output).

$$\text{Total cost} = \text{Wage} * \text{hours/meal} * \text{meals/patient day} * \text{patient days}$$
$$\$43,200 = \$15.00/\text{hour} * 0.1524 \text{ hours/meal} * 3 \text{ meals/patient day} * 6300 \text{ patient days}$$

Actual expenses were $47,000, and there are four major causes for the $3,800 variance. The following calculations demonstrate how

each of the previously described factors could increase labor expense by $3800 and generate the 8.8% budget variance:

Total cost = $ / hour * hours / meal * meals / patient day * patient days

$47,007* = **$16.32** * 0.1524 * 3.00 * 6,300 ← increase in wage

$47,004* = $15.00 * **0.1658** * 3.00 * 6,300 ← decrease in efficiency

$46,950* = $15.00 * 0.1524 * **3.26** * 6,300 ← increase in intensity

$46,998* = $15.00 * 0.1524 * 3.00 * **6,853** ← increase in volume

*Total variance does not equal $47,000 because of rounding errors.

Each of the four possibilities explains the 8.8% variance and provides different information on the effectiveness of management and its impact on operations. Changes in prices may be uncontrollable, but managers may need to seek out ways of maximizing productivity and minimizing costs. When input prices increase, managers should determine whether lower-priced inputs can be substituted for higher-priced inputs. If higher-priced inputs are more productive, does the higher output per input more than offset the higher input price, reducing the cost per unit? When currently nonutilized inputs fall in price, managers should consider substituting them for current resources, even if they are less productive, if the fall in cost exceeds the reduction in output.

One of the healthcare managers' prime responsibilities, given the proliferation of fixed reimbursement plans, is to increase efficiency. Efficient use of resources is a prime determinant of the financial success of an organization. The time per meal was expected to be 9 minutes and 8 seconds (0.1524 hours); if preparation and delivery time increased to 9 minutes and 57 seconds (0.1658 hours), it would account for the total labor variance. The question, however, would remain: did the 49-second-per-meal increase indicate lower staff productivity (taking more time to perform an activity) or the need to prepare more complicated meals? Identifying how the time per activity changed (or resources used per

activity) is the easy part; determining whether the increase was necessary or inappropriate is more challenging.

The impact of changes on the intensity on costs may be similar to changes in volume. Increases in intensity (the need for more services per patient) may produce higher revenue, that is, an increase in the CMI for Medicare patients or additional tests, procedures, and/or patient days for fee-for-service patients. On the other hand, providing more services per patient day may have no impact on revenue if the additional services are due to deficiencies in the system. In the dietary example, 3 meals per patient per day were expected, and an increase to 3.26 meals per day would explain the total labor variance. After identifying the increase, a manager would have to determine whether it was due to incomplete or faulty work (lack of discharge orders, inability to identify an appropriate discharge destination, or duplicate meals) or due to supplemental physician or nutritionist orders? The problem hospitals face is that additional patient meals increase expenses without generating any additional revenues; thus, excessive meals should be minimized.

Increases in output will be positive for the organization if the additional patient days generate incremental revenue in excess of the additional expenses incurred to provide services. If the increase in patient days generates less revenue than the additional expenses or no revenue at all (unnecessarily prolonging hospitalization for case-reimbursed patients), the organization's financial performance will deteriorate. The primary question is, can managers control volume? If so, and the change improves financial performance, they should be credited; when it worsens financial performance, they should be held accountable. If volume is noncontrollable, managers should be neither praised nor blamed, but the impact of the change on the organization and future operations should be communicated to senior managers if it requires belt tightening in other areas. In terms of meals, the dietary manager cannot nor should he or she stop meals from increasing as patient days increase—three meals per day will be delivered for every patient whether the patient day was forecasted or wasn't.

It is unlikely that the total variance will be the result of a change in one factor but, generally, will arise from multiple factors. Managers

should be able to untangle the four types of variances to evaluate their effectiveness and the operation of their units. Table 11.4 allows the dietary manager to move beyond traditional variance analysis and its focus on cost per output and output quantity by furnishing the number of meals prepared and labor hours paid. When information on input and activity quantities is available, all four cost components (efficiency, intensity, price, and volume) can be calculated to produce an accurate picture of operations. Equation 11.5 shows output is *not* a factor in the calculation of the price variance; it focuses entirely on the price and number of inputs used and budgeted. Price variances focus on the cost per input rather than the cost per output, unlike Equation 11.1, which aggregated what was paid for resources with the quantity of the resources used.

$$
\begin{aligned}
\text{Price variance} &= \big((\text{Actual cost/actual input}) - (\text{Budgeted cost/budgeted input})\big) \\
&\quad * \text{actual quantity of input used} \\
&= (\$47,000/3,010 \text{ hours} - \$43,200/2,880 \text{ hours}) * 3,010 \text{ hours paid} \\
&= (\$15.61/\text{hour} - \$15.00/\text{hour}) * 3,010 \text{ hours paid} \\
&= \$0.61 \text{ unplanned cost per hour} * 3,010 \text{ hours paid} = \$1,836
\end{aligned}
\tag{11.5}
$$

The dietary department is paying $0.61 more per labor hour than budgeted. This deviation accounts for $1836, or 48.3%, of the total labor variance.

The efficiency variance should identify when inputs that can be controlled by managers are being consumed in higher or lower quantities than planned. Time for meal preparation

can increase if employees are not working effectively and/or are idle or because dietary requests, preferences, or restrictions have removed the meal from standard processes and increased preparation time. Identifying why time increased is the key issue, and variance analysis only illuminates the magnitude of the change, not the cause.

$$
\begin{aligned}
\text{Efficiency variance} &= (\text{Actual inputs/actual activity} - \text{budgeted inputs/budgeted activity}) \\
&\quad * \text{budgeted cost per input} * \text{actual activities produced} \\
&= (3,010 \text{ actual hours}/20,191 \text{ actual meals} \\
&\quad - 2,880 \text{ budgeted hours}/18,900 \text{ budgeted meals}) \\
&\quad * 43,200/2,880 \text{ budgeted cost per hour} \\
&\quad * 20,191 \text{ actual meals} \\
&= (0.1491 \text{ actual hours/actual meal} - 0.1524 \text{ budgeted hours/budgeted meal}) \\
&\quad * \$15.00 \text{ budgeted cost per hour} * 20,191 \text{ actual meals} \\
&= -0.0033 \text{ unplanned hours per meal} * \$15.00/\text{budgeted hour} \\
&\quad * 20,191 \text{ actual meals} = -\$994
\end{aligned}
\tag{11.6}
$$

The department is using less time to prepare meals (−0.0033 hours, or −0.20 minutes, or 11.88 seconds) than budgeted and is achieving higher efficiency, reducing the total labor cost by $994, or −26.2%, of the total variance.

The intensity variance identifies changes in the number of activities performed to produce an output that may or may not be in the control of managers. Additional activities may be required because work was not performed correctly the first time, for example, meals may be lost, get cold, or contain the wrong items and a second meal may be required—factors that should be controlled by managers. On the other hand, additional meals may be required because of food allergies, patient preferences (e.g., vegan), or physician ordered dietary supplements—factors that cannot be controlled by managers.

$$\text{Intensity variance} = (\text{Actual activity/actual output} - \text{budgeted activity/budgeted output})$$
$$* \text{budgeted cost per activity} * \text{actual output}$$
$$= (20{,}191 \text{ actual meals}/6{,}615 \text{ actual patient days}$$
$$- 18{,}900 \text{ budgeted meals}/6{,}300 \text{ budgeted patient days})$$
$$* \$43{,}200 \text{ budgeted expense}/18{,}900 \text{ budgeted meals}$$
$$* 6{,}615 \text{ actual patient days}$$
$$= (3.0523 \text{ actual meals/patient day} - 3.00 \text{ budgeted meals/patient day})$$
$$* \$2.2857/\text{budgeted meals} * 6{,}615 \text{ actual patient days}$$
$$= 0.0523 \text{ unplanned meals/patient day} * \$2.2857/\text{budgeted meal}$$
$$* 6{,}615 \text{ actual patient days} = \$789 \tag{11.7}$$

The unplanned increase in meals is 0.0523 per patient day, or a total of 346 unexpected meals over the month. The higher rate of activity should increase the total labor expense by $789 and accounts for 20.8% of the total labor variance. Managers will be challenged to track the reasons more time was needed per activity (need or fall in productivity) or more activities were required (need or substandard performance), but understanding these factors is essential to explaining budget variances and controlling resource use.

The formula for the volume variance when efficiency, intensity, and prices variances are calculated is identical to Equation 11.2; the volume variance still identifies the difference between budgeted and actual output and multiplies this difference by the budgeted rate per patient day.

$$\text{Volume variance} = (\text{Actual output} - \text{budgeted output}) * \text{budgeted cost per output}$$
$$= (6{,}615 \text{ actual patient days} - 6{,}300 \text{ budgeted patient days})$$
$$\times \$43{,}200/6{,}300 \text{ budgeted patient days}$$
$$= 315 \text{ unplanned patient days}$$
$$* \$6.8571 \text{ budget cost/budgeted patient day} = \$2{,}160$$

The 315 unplanned patient days continue to account for 56.8% of the total variance. The volume variance does not change, because the effects of changes in efficiency, intensity, and prices do not affect the budgeted cost per patient day. The sum of the four variances equals the total variance. The original cost variance, $1640, is only partially due to paying more for labor; it is also due to providing more meals than anticipated and was reduced by the higher efficiency achieved (**TABLE 11.6**).

Calculating four variances provides a richer and more organic insight into department operations by demonstrating why the variances arose and illuminating the extent of the manager's ability to control it. Factors under the manager's control that he or she should be held accountable for include the efficiency variance and

TABLE 11.6 Analysis of Total Labor Variance

	Actual	Budgeted	Effect on Budget Variance	% Variance (%)
Price (wage)	$15.61	$15.00	Deficit $1,836	48.3
Efficiency (meals/hour)	6.71	6.56	Surplus 994	−26.2
Intensity (meals/patient days)	3.05	3.00	Deficit 789	20.8
Volume (patient days)	6,615	6,300	Deficit 2,160	56.8
			Total = $3,791*	100.0*

*Total variance does not equal $3800, or 100.0%, because of rounding error.

some or all of the price and intensity variances. Variance analysis does not indict, try, and convict a manager of ineffectiveness or inefficiency but provides a quantitative base to undertake a qualitative analysis of budget variances. Variance analysis identifies the dollar difference between the financial plan and actual expenses and categorizes it into four areas, but it cannot pinpoint the reasons variances arose.

Price variances must be analyzed to determine what factors led to higher input prices, for example, is a higher-than-expected wage due to new hires at high wages, loss of lower-wage employees, and substitution of higher-compensated workers, overtime, temporary help, etc.? Only when the variance is analyzed from a qualitative perspective can the effectiveness of the department operations and management be determined. The key question that needs to be answered is, could the manager take effective action to prevent the higher input cost?

The second factor that should be evaluated is the efficiency variance. Efficiency in the dietary department is increasing as less time is required per meal, that is, fewer resources are consumed per activity. Is this due to better management, or does it indicate a reduction in quality? Did the manager and the employees change the production process to increase efficiency, did the mix of meals change (less special, higher preparation time meals), or were less essential duties ignored? Discovering economies in the production process is valuable, but short cuts and skimping can produce undesirable results. Did faster meal preparation lead to errors and an increase in the number of meals prepared? Changes in product specifications may be beneficial or detrimental but, ultimately, lie outside the control of managers.

Changes in intensity may or may not be controllable. The intensity factor may reflect a change in physician orders, that is, an increase in meals per patient day. On the other hand, is the uptick in meals per patient day due to meals being rejected and redone because they are incomplete, incorrect, or cold? Has the reduction in time per meal (higher efficiency) increased errors or reduced timeliness? If more meals are ordered by physicians or requested by patients, it would be inappropriate to hold the dietary manager responsible for this variance, but he or she should be accountable if the uptick in meals is due to errors or lack of timely delivery.

The final variable, patient days, is outside the control of the dietary manager and most hospital managers, so the volume variance carves out the additional expenses arising from higher output when evaluating the effectiveness of management. While increases in patient days may be uncontrollable by the dietary, nursing, or pharmacy manager, unwarranted increases in patient days must be addressed as they could have a significant negative impact on financial performance under per case and capitated reimbursement. Senior managers may have to address system issues from poor, untimely, or missed staff work to physician discharge practices that extend patient stays.

TABLE 11.7 provides the monthly variance report for the nursing unit examined in previous chapters. The variance report shows monthly (left) and year-to-date (YTD) (right) expenditures; this format allows managers to assess current and past performance, for example, staff salaries (object code 4020) are 11.8% overbudget for the year but only 6.6% for June. Did the manager take steps to reduce staff hours? Total expenses show the same pattern: YTD is 4.9% overbudget, while June is 2.6% overbudget.

Statistics are provided at the bottom of the report to guide assessment. The question, Did the manager take steps to reduce staff utilization? was asked. Statistics show that staff hours are 4.9% overbudget for the month compared to 9.9% for the year, that is, June's overage is

an improvement over past months. The statistics on output (admissions up 4.3%) and activity levels (patient days up 2.6%) indicate that some of unanticipated increase in staff hours may be due to the higher volume of patients treated. The reader should use the previously provided variances to determine how much these variance are due to changes in prices, efficiency, intensity, and volume; data is available in the Table 11.7 tab Chapter11.xlsx.

Table 11.7 provides a wealth of information for managers to assess departmental performance; it shows how far each line item varies from its budgets, provides information to determine whether variances are increasing or decreasing compared to prior months, and supplies output, activity, and input use statistics to assess the appropriateness of variances.

▶ Identifying Variances to Examine

When a manager receives his or her monthly variance report, what expenses should he or she examine? There will be dozens of expense items on the report, and it is likely that actual expenditures on the majority of object codes will differ from the budget. It is a waste of managerial effort to examine every line item where actual spending differs from the budget. Management time is a costly commodity, and managers should not expend effort calculating variances and researching the causes of variances if the benefits will not exceed their investigation cost. Management efforts should focus on expenses with large variances that can be controlled; items with small variances or those that cannot be controlled should receive a cursory review. Large, noncontrollable expenses, however, should be closely monitored to ensure they do not jeopardize the larger financial goals of the organization. What constitutes a large variance? Here are some general guidelines to focus variance analysis efforts.

TABLE 11.7 Monthly Variance Report

June 2018	June 2018	Variance	Variance (%)	Object Code	Description	YTD Actual 2018	YTD Budget 2018	Variance	Variance (%)
$31,256	$30,000	$1,256	4.2	4010	Management and clerical staff	$176,543	$180,000	($3,457)	−1.9
$196,333	$184,167	$12,166	6.6	4020	Staff salaries and wages	$1,235,642	$1,105,000	$130,642	11.8
$2,965	$3,000	−$35	−1.2	4040	Overtime	$23,833	$18,000	$5,833	32.4
$26,897	$34,000	−$7,103	−20.9	4050	Agency and temporary	$156,115	$204,000	−$47,885	−23.5
$17,637	$16,613	$1,024	6.2	4110	FICA	$109,855	$99,680	$10,175	10.2
$25,601	$25,250	$351	1.4	4120	Health insurance	$149,857	$151,500	−$1,643	−1.1
$11,528	$10,858	$669	6.2	4130	Retirement	$71,801	$65,150	$6,651	10.2
$2,667	$2,389	$278	11.6	4140	Unemployment	$15,796	$14,333	$1,463	10.2
$2,213	$2,129	$84	3.9	4210	Floor medications	$13,589	$12,775	$814	6.4
$1,016	$1,500	−$484	−32.3	4212	Medical instruments	$5,798	$9,000	−$3,202	−35.6
$859	$852	$7	0.9	4214	Bandages, gauze, etc.	$5,643	$5,110	$533	10.4
$5,269	$4,897	$372	7.6	4216	Latex gloves, gowns, etc.	$32,145	$29,383	$2,762	9.4

(Continues)

TABLE 11.7 Monthly Variance Report *(Continued)*

June 2018	June 2018	Variance	Variance (%)	Object Code	Description	YTD Actual 2018	YTD Budget 2018	Variance	Variance (%)
$458	$426	$32	7.6	4218	Sterile wipes	$2,659	$2,555	$104	4.1
$713	$767	–$54	–7.0	4250	Office supplies	$4,268	$4,599	–$331	–7.2
$102	$83	$19	22.4	4280	Cleaning supplies	$569	$500	$69	13.8
$599	$500	$99	19.8	4350	Biomed repairs/ maintenance	$3,869	$3,000	$869	29.0
$235	$200	$35	17.5	4410	Electricity	$1,156	$1,200	–$44	–3.7
$510	$480	$30	6.3	4440	Telephone	$2,645	$2,880	–$235	–8.2
$12,000	$12,000	$0	0.0	4930	Housekeeping	$72,000	$72,000	$0	0.0
$3,017	$2,975	$42	1.4	4940	Travel/professional meetings/meals	$14,523	$17,850	–$3,327	–18.6
$595	$767	–$172	–22.4	4950	Education and training	$3,688	$4,600	–$912	–19.8
$296	$276	$20	7.3	4960	Other expenses	$1,258	$1,655	–$397	–24.0
$342,766	$334,128	$8,637	2.6			$2,103,252	$2,004,769	$98,483	4.9

June 2018	June 2018	Variance	Variance (%)	Statistics	YTD Actual 2018	YTD Budget 2018	Variance	Variance (%)
108	108	0	0.0	Admissions (output)	678	650	28	4.3
531	536	(5)	−0.9	Patient days (activity)	3,295	3,213	82	2.6
920	920	0	0.0	Management and clerical hours (input)	1,040	1,040	0	0.0
8,174	7,790	384	4.9	Staff hours (input)	51,378	46,743	4,635	9.9
81	83	(2)	−2.4	Overtime hours (input)	662	497	165	33.2
672	850	(178)	−20.9	Agency hours (input)	3,903	5,100	(1,197)	−23.5

FICA, Federal Insurance Contributions Act.

Absolute Dollar Variance

A dollar threshold requires budget managers to identify and explain all variances that exceed a predetermined dollar amount, that is, all variances over $1,000 monthly (or $10,000 cumulative). A dollar-denominated monthly threshold provides an opportunity to take immediate action on problems before large losses accumulate over time. A dollar-denominated cumulative total offers the advantage of ignoring variances that may not amount to a significant amount of money or offset over time. The disadvantage is that a high-dollar threshold may green-light managers to ignore consistent budget overruns over time that will result in significant losses and should have been addressed when first observed. The primary strength of dollar thresholds is their emphasis on controlling inputs, that is, the differences between actual and budgeted expenditures must be analyzed and controlled to facilitate the larger financial goals of the organization. The primary weaknesses of absolute-dollar thresholds are the potentially large number of items to examine if the threshold is set low and the failure to consider whether the variance is high or low relative to total inputs used.

Absolute Percentage Variance

A percentage threshold requires managers to identify and explain all variances that exceed a predetermined percentage of the budget, that is, all variances that exceed 10% of the line item allocation. The primary strength of a percentage threshold is the recognition that actual inputs consumed should be proportional to the expected outlay, that is, a $1000 variance in an expense line of $2 million is trivial (0.05%), while the same variance when the budget is $2000 is significant (50% overbudget). The primary weakness of a percentage limit is it could require that a large number of low-cost items with large percentage variances be investigated. For example, given a $100 budget and 10% threshold, investigation is required

when $111 or more is spent. These variances may not be important to the operation, while a large dollar variance may not require examination. For example, a $150,000 overrun in a $2 million expense line (7.5% variance) would fall below the 10% threshold.

The AND Combination Rule

The AND combination rule requires budget managers to identify and explain all variances that exceed a predetermined percentage of the budget AND materially affect operations, that is, all variances that exceed 10% of the budget and are more than $10,000. The strength of the combination rule is that it attempts to achieve two goals simultaneously: a variance must significantly deviate from the budget (%), and the amount must be material ($). The advantage of the AND rule is that it minimizes the number of line items to review, thus conserving managerial time. On the other hand, requiring an absolute dollar and percentage of the budget threshold to be exceeded allows deviations in small budget lines to seriously overrun their budget ($8000 spent when only $2000 was budgeted means a 400% overrun but only $6000) and in large budget lines to overrun their budget by tens of thousands of dollars ($150,000, or 7.5%, in a $2,000,000 expense line) and fall below the reporting thresholds.

The OR Combination Rule

The OR combination rule requires that managers identify and explain all variances that exceed a predetermined percentage of the budget OR materially affect operations, that is, all variances that exceed 10% of the budget or are more than $10,000. The purpose is to improve budgeting processes by recognizing all large deviations from budget (%) and those that could materially affect financial performance ($). The combination rule OR would require explanations of why $8000 was spent when only $2000 was budgeted (the 400% overrun) and the dollar variance of $150,000 on a base of $2,000,000. The author recommends the OR rule because large deviations, whether as a percentage of the budget or in absolute dollars, should be understood to improve performance and ensure desired financial results are achieved.

The dollar and percentage thresholds, $1000 per month or 10% of the budget line, are given for illustrative purposes. The actual amounts employed should be determined by the financial capacity of the organization to sustain budget variation (will a $10,000 variance endanger the ability to meet payroll or pay vendors?) and the frequency, magnitude, and nature of variances (do variances offset across time?). The dollar or percentage thresholds should be lower for monthly variance reports designed for concurrent management and higher for year-end reports used for retrospective evaluation.

▶ Year-End Retrospective Evaluation

Assume 2019 has been completed. The year-end budget report, **TABLE 11.8**, shows the department overspent its budget by $121,442, or 2.9%. Should the manager be criticized or praised? The unit delivered care to 29 more patients than expected, so its expenses should be higher than the budget, but is the overrun greater or less than what should be expected, given the higher volume? The simplest calculation, dividing total budgeted expenses by total admissions ($4,202,955/1,320), indicates expenses should increase by about $3184.06 for each additional admission. Given 29 additional patients were admitted, total expenses should be approximately $92,338 higher than budgeted, so the overrun includes other factors.

Not every variance needs examination, and finance has established the following rule for determining materiality and the need to explain variances: the variance for the fiscal year must be greater than $20,000 *or* more

than 20% higher than the budget. The OR rule highlights five line items to explore: staff salaries (object code 4020), overtime (object code 4040), agency nurses (object code 4050), floor medications (object code 4210), and other expenses (object code 4960). These five object codes account for 89.6% of the total variance ($108,852/$121,442). Table 11.8 highlights the variances to be explored.

TABLE 11.9 divides the dollar variance into price, efficiency, intensity, and volume components.

The expense that accounted for 118.7% of the variances to be investigated was staff salaries and wages (object code 4020), which is unsurprising, given staff salaries constitute more than 55.0% of the total budget and actual spending. Changes in output, that is, volume variance, accounted for 56.6% of the total variance, and its impact was primarily on staff salaries and overtime. The staff salary variance arose primarily from 15.45 hours being expended per patient day, when the budget expected only 14.98 hours. The additional 0.47 hours per patient day over 6583 days of care at the budgeted hourly rate of $24.00 resulted in an additional $71,650 of labor cost. The qualitative question is, was the increase in time warranted? Adding to the staff salary overage was higher output: the 29 additional patients should increase salaries by $50,772, and higher wages, $24.00 versus a budget of $23.64, added $36,636.85. Partially offsetting this increase was a decrease in the LOS from 4.94 to 4.88 days: did the additional hours expended per day contribute to the LOS reduction and cost savings of $29,873? The reader can see the reduction in patient days did little to offset the higher expenses incurred because of lower efficiency, higher output, and higher wage.

The second major deviation was agency nurses (object code 4050), which came in $68,525 underbudget. The lower use of agency nurses may explain why staff salaries and overtime were overbudget, that is, full-time employees were utilized in place of contract workers. The budget had forecasted that 1.63 hours

TABLE 11.8 Year-End Budget Report

Object Code	Description	Actual 2019	Budget 2019	Variance	Variance (%)
4010	Management and clerical staff	$365,298	$363,679	$1,619	0.4
4020	Staff salaries and wages	$2,440,201	$2,311,015	$129,186	5.6
4040	Overtime	$78,455	$37,645	$40,810	108.4
4050	Per diem/agency nurses	$358,124	$426,649	−$68,525	−16.1
4110	FICA	$220,074	$240,287	−$20,213	−8.4
4120	Health insurance	$317,696	$317,697	−$1	0.0
4130	Retirement	$146,412	$135,718	$10,694	7.9
4140	Unemployment	$37,052	$34,551	$2,501	7.2
4210	Floor medications	$33,599	$27,237	$6,362	23.4
4212	Medical instruments	$17,654	$18,640	−$986	−5.3
4214	Bandages, gauze, etc.	$11,233	$10,583	$650	6.1
4216	Latex gloves, gowns, etc.	$59,863	$60,854	−$991	−1.6
4218	Sterile wipes	$5,366	$5,292	$74	1.4
4250	Office supplies	$9,456	$9,525	−$69	−0.7
4280	Cleaning supplies	$1,101	$1,036	$65	6.3
4350	Biomedical repairs/ maintenance	$8,542	$7,815	$727	9.3
4410	Electricity	$2,404	$2,404	$0	0.0
4440	Telephone	$5,343	$5,343	$0	0.0
4930	Housekeeping	$166,483	$147,658	$18,825	12.7
4940	Travel/professional meetings/meals	$28,633	$29,336	−$703	−2.4
4950	Education and training	$7,849	$7,450	$399	5.4
4960	Other expenses	$3,560	$2,541	$1,019	40.1
		$4,324,397	$4,202,955	$121,442	2.9

Statistics	Actual 2019	Budget 2019	Variance	Variance (%)
Output = admissions	1,349	1,320	29	2.2
Activity = patient days	6,583	6,524	59	0.9
Activity/Q = LOS	4.88	4.94	−0.06	−1.3
Staff hours (input)	101,675	97,760	3,915	4.0
Overtime hours (input)	2,179	1,039	1,140	109.8
Agency hours (input)	10,666	10,666	0	0.0
Floor medications (inputs)	13,166	11,417	1,749	15.3
Other expenses (inputs)	3,560	2,541	1,019	40.1

of agency nursing would be utilized per patient day, but only 1.36 hours were used. The lower use of agency nurses reduced spending by $72,383. There was no price variance, a favorable intensity variance, and unfavorable volume variance which had little effect on the total amount expended for agency nurses.

The last staff-related variance was overtime (object code 4040), which was $40,810 overbudget. This variance was driven by the increase in the number of overtime hours used: 2179 (0.33 per patient day) overtime hours were paid, when only 1039 (0.16) hours were planned. The increase in hours utilized increased the overtime expense by $40,976, and this overage increased by the higher number of patients treated and was slightly reduced by paying less than expected for overtime and by the decrease in the average LOS. Considering overtime and agency nurse expense simultaneously may lead one to the conclusion that the decrease in agency nurse hours was offset by the use of overtime.

The overruns in floor medications (object code 4210) and other expenses (object code 4960), although meeting the rule for review, did not contribute significantly to the total budget overrun, $6362 and $1019, and should

not command extensive manager effort. The budget variance rules specified that any expense more than 20% above its budget must be reviewed, and this required examining floor medications that were 23.4% overbudget. The variance was primarily driven by using more floor medications per patient day and a higher cost per medication. Other expenses were $1019 over the budget, but the difference amounted to 40.1%. Extensive examination of other expenses may not be worth the time because this measure captures a plethora of small items (unworthy of devoting a distinct object code to) and may not deliver any actionable information. The primary question is, will this level of expenditure be needed in future years, was it a one-time expense, or does it represent an increase in the miscellaneous costs of treating patients? The analysis demonstrates the variance was due to the higher use of other expenses per patient day.

The reader should note that the intensity variance is favorable for all expense codes because the LOS decreased and reduced the need for staff time, medications, and other expenses since patients did not stay as long as expected. The volume variance is unfavorable for all expense codes because higher

TABLE 11.9 Variance Calculations

Object Code	Description	2019 Actual	2019 Budget	Price Variance	Efficiency Variance	Intensity Variance	Volume Variance	Total Variance	Total (%)
4020	Staff salaries and wages	$2,440,201	$2,311,015	$36,637	$71,650	−$29,873	$50,772	$129,186	118.7
4040	Overtime	$78,455	$37,645	−$507	$40,976	−$487	$827	40,810	37.5
4050	Per diem/ agency nurses	$358,124	$426,649	$0	−$72,383	−$5,515	$9,373	−68,525	−63.0
4210	Floor medications	$33,599	$27,237	$2,190	$3,926	−$352	$598	$6,362	5.8
4960	Other expenses	$3,560	$2,541	$0	$996	−$33	$56	$1,019	0.9
	Total	$2,913,939	$2,805,087	$38,320	$45,164	−$36,259	$61,627	$108,852	100.0
	% Total			35.2%	41.5%	−33.3%	56.6%	100.0%	

admissions necessitate more patient days and increases in resource use.

The reader should also see that monthly and variance reports, although intimately related, are designed for two different purposes. Monthly variance reports supply managers with information to identify when excessive resource consumption is occurring and insight into its cause so that corrective action can be taken to reduce or eliminate wasteful spending in subsequent months. Year-end reports evaluate management: did managers act on the monthly reports, and were controllable budget overruns kept to a minimum?

TABLE 11.10 highlights the difference in perspective and managerial reaction to variances. Columns 2, 3, and 4 indicate three similar departments were $3000 overbudget in January. Assuming the $3000 variance is within the managers' control, manager 1 was content to let the variance run for the entire year, thus amounting to $36,000. Did manager 1 identify the source of the variance, and if so, why wasn't corrective action taken? Manager 2 received the same information but, rather than letting the variance continue, took preventive action and eliminated the variance by March. Manager 3 not only

TABLE 11.10 Management Response to Monthly Variances and the Year-End Variance

	Total Variance 1	Total Variance 2	Total Variance 3
January	$3,000	$3,000	$3,000
February	$3,000	$1,500	$1,500
March	$3,000	$0	−$450
April	$3,000	$0	−$450
May	$3,000	$0	−$450
June	$3,000	$0	−$450
July	$3,000	$0	−$450
August	$3,000	$0	−$450
September	$3,000	$0	−$450
October	$3,000	$0	−$450
November	$3,000	$0	−$450
December	$3,000	$0	−$450
Year-End Variance	$36,000	$4,500	$0

corrected the variance but also sought additional savings in the remaining months to meet the budget.

Monthly reports are not for assessment but rather supply information to managers to improve their operations. The year-end variance distinguishes management: manager 1 did nothing, manager 2 took steps to end overspending and minimize the variance, and manager 3 not only ended overspending but also took additional steps to meet the budget. Manager 3 should be evaluated higher and receive a higher salary increase than the other two managers, all other things being constant, whereas manager 1 may need remedial training, instead of a salary increase, on his or her duties as a steward of the organization's resources.

Variance analysis provides a wealth of information that is not only beneficial for management purposes but also can enhance future forecasts and budget estimates. The identification of recurring variances indicates that planning, budgeting, and/or management processes should be changed, while one-time variations suggest no action is needed.

Summary

This chapter examined the relationship between budgeting and variance analysis, explained the focus of variance analysis, discussed potential factors that produce expense variances, and provided rules to implement variance analysis. It is vital that budgeting be viewed as more than a one-time exercise in estimating future expenses. The goal of variance analysis is to improve operations, and this can only occur if budgets are used to evaluate performance and control operations.

Performance improvement requires that favorable and unfavorable variances be examined. Understanding why favorable variances arose is vital to ensuring cost savings can be continued in the future. Understanding why unfavorable variances arise is necessary to stop

budget overruns from recurring. The findings of variance analysis are also used to determine whether planning, budgeting, or management requires refinement. The use of variance analysis to tie together these three functions of an organization will improve the relationship between senior management, finance, and operating units. All three functions need a greater understanding of the goals and operations of one another, and one way of achieving this insight is by recognizing the interrelationships between desired outputs, financial plans, and operating results.

One of the major problems in large organizations is siloing—employees encased in their own areas who cannot see how their work affects the larger organization and customers. Siloing occurs when operating managers have a better understanding of what inputs (units) are required to produce output, finance understands what it costs ($) to produce the same output, but neither understands both issues. Operating managers would benefit from a better understanding of the costs of their resources, and finance would gain from a better understanding of what inputs (not simply their cost) are required to produce health services. Budgeting and variance analysis are the way to synchronize these two groups and ensure budgeting is an ongoing management tool as well as a planning and evaluation tool.

When operating managers understand the relationships between outputs, inputs, and costs, they gain fundamental insight into financial management and its relationship to their departments' operation. This insight should be used to ensure their departments receive the funding required from the budget process to fulfill operations. Managers who understand budgeting and variance analysis will have a better idea of how changes in production techniques may affect resource requirements and be better able to pinpoint production problems and reorganize departmental operations to reduce costs.

On the other side, senior management and finance who work hand-in-hand with operating managers on variance analysis will enhance their knowledge of the work of nursing, ancillary, and support departments. Nonmedical personnel generally do not understand the resource requirements necessary to produce medical services. Variance analysis using efficiency and intensity measures frames operations in an understandable way for personnel not trained in accounting and finance. Healthcare providers are probably more comfortable with quantifying their work in terms of how long it takes to deliver care and the number of activities required for a patient rather than an aggregated cost per output.

Regardless of their position in an organization, managers should be able to determine whether a variance arose from paying more or less for inputs (price variances), consuming more or less inputs to produce activities (efficiency variances), producing more or fewer activities (intensity variances), or producing more or less output (volume variances). Each variance highlights a different facet of how the operation was expected to perform and suggests different yet interrelated opportunities to improve performance.

Employing lower-priced inputs could reduce efficiency (require more units of the lower-priced resource to accomplish the same tasks) or increase the number of activities performed if work must be redone, so managers should be able to determine whether the substitution of lower-compensated inputs for higher-priced resources will be financially advantageous if productivity falls and defects increase. Similarly, if increasing the pace of work is pursued, what economic benefit should be expected if it increases the amount of work that will have to be redone? The next chapter "Ratio Analysis and Operating Indicators" examines industry benchmarks to identify whether an organization or department is paying more for resources or using more inputs than other healthcare institutions and to establish performance targets.

The cost of performing variance analysis is significant, and managers should balance the cost of variance analysis against the expected benefits. Variance analysis encompassing efficiency and intensity factors requires the collection of information on homogenous inputs and outputs that may not be currently available in healthcare organizations.

Key Terms and Concepts

Cost variance	Intensity variance	Volume variance
Efficiency variance	Price variance	

Discussion Questions

1. Explain the role of variance analysis in financial management.
2. Explain price, efficiency, intensity, and volume variances. What do they measure, and what impact does a manager have on this aspect of operations?
3. How do managers determine which variances should be investigated?
4. Discuss the difference between monthly and year-end variance analysis.

Problems

1. Given the following monthly expense report for electrocardiograms (EKGs), calculate price, efficiency, intensity, and quantity variances for each object code. Write an explanation for why expenses differ from the budget (one paragraph per expense line) and create a table similar to Table 11.4. Discuss how much of these variances the manager may be responsible for.

Object Code	Expenses	Actual	Budget	Difference	Difference (%)
4020	Staff salaries	$77,619	$75,000	$2,619	3.49
4212	Medical supplies	$11,452	$11,875	−$423	−3.56
4350	Biomedical repair/ maintenance	$6,539	$3,200	$3,339	104.34
4410	Electricity	$1,187	$1,303	−$116	−8.87
	Total	$96,797	$91,378	$5,420	5.93

Statistics		Actual	Budget	$ Difference	Difference (%)
Admissions (output)		975	1,000	−25	−2.50
Billed EKGs (activity)		1,247	1,250	−3	−0.24
Input units					
Staff salaries (hours paid)		1,186	1,250	−64	−5.12
Medical supplies (electrodes)		2,580	2,500	80	3.20
Biomedical repair/maintenance (service hours)		150	100	50	50.00
Electricity (kilowatt hours)		13,897	12,399	1,498	12.08

2. Given the following monthly expense report for the operating room (OR), calculate price, efficiency, intensity, and quantity variances for each object code. Note, management and clerical salaries are a fixed cost. Write an explanation for why expenses differ from budget (one paragraph per expense line) and create a table similar to Table 11.4. Discuss how much of these variances the manager may be responsible for.

Object Code	Expenses	Actual	Budget	$ Difference	Difference (%)
4010	Management and clerical staff	$16,975	$17,500	−$525	−3.00
4020	Staff salaries and wages	$1,340,754	$1,267,200	$73,554	5.80

4212	Medical supplies	$102,260	$95,040	$7,220	7.60
4218	Surgical instruments	$216,359	$237,600	−$21,241	−8.94
4410	Electricity	$9,622	$9,903	−$281	−2.84
	Total	$1,685,970	$1,627,243	$58,727	3.61
Statistics		**Actual**	**Budget**	**$ Difference**	**Difference (%)**
Surgeries (output)		7,863	7,920	−57	−0.72
OR minutes billed (activity)		460,944	475,200	−14,256	−3.00
Input Units					
Management salaries (hours paid)		352	352	0	0.00
Staff salaries (hours paid)		212,346	211,200	1,146	0.54
Medical supplies (surgical gowns/gloves)		48,236	47,520	716	1.51
Surgical instruments (supply carts)		11,484	11,880	−396	−3.33
Electricity (kilowatt hours)		93,877	95,040	−1,163	−1.22

OR, operating room.

3. Using Table 11.7, Chapter11.xlsx, calculate price, efficiency, intensity, and volume variances for the month of June if the variance is more than $5000 and 5% above or below the budget. Discuss significant changes between June and YTD performance, that is, which line items are moving closer or away from their budget targets?

4. Using Table 11.7, Chapter11.xlsx, calculate price, efficiency, intensity, and volume variances for YTD performance, January through June, if the variance is more than $10,000 and 10% above or below the budget. Discuss why these variances may be arising and the potential interrelationships between line items.

CHAPTER 12

Ratio Analysis and Operating Indicators

CHAPTER OBJECTIVES

1. Explain the purpose of financial ratios.
2. Calculate and interpret financial ratios.
3. Perform and interpret DuPont analysis.
4. Explain the role of operating indicators.
5. Calculate and interpret operating indicators.
6. Explain the purpose and different types of benchmarking.

▶ Introduction

Variance analysis dealt with understanding and controlling the performance of individual departments in relation to their budgets. Ratio analysis and operating indicators focus on the performance of the entire organization. One of the major weaknesses of budgeting (or human nature) is the reverence given to, self-interest pursued through, and comfort taken in past practices. How do managers who rely on the past to construct future financial plans achieve higher levels of performance?

The World Bank (1995) noted that improving the performance of state-owned enterprises requires three conditions: political desirability, political feasibility, and credibility. Political desirability arises with a change in leadership that is not tied to the past and that is willing to do things differently or with a crisis that is so severe that it makes continuation of past practice impossible. A crisis for a public organization would be the inability to secure sufficient taxes or loans to cover operating costs. Organizations, whether for-profits or nonprofits, selling their goods and services to the public cannot ignore their inability to attract customers willing to pay production costs. All three types of organizations must either increase efficiency when funds cannot be raised to cover costs or cease to exist.

In addition to an event demanding or facilitating change, political feasibility recognizes that the *status quo* confers benefits on people who will oppose reform unless their interests are satisfied.

Machiavelli (1532) noted the most dangerous activity is to implement change, as vested interests will put up a fierce defense of their privileges and potential beneficiaries will provide only lukewarm, if any, support to endeavors they believe have a low probability of success. The obvious method of neutralizing opposition and achieving political feasibility is purchasing their support or bribing them to accept change.

The last condition required for reform is management credibility. Management must have a reputation for putting its words into action and carrying the action to conclusion. Many organizations are littered with the remains of half-hearted and failed initiatives. When credibility is absent, employees see new initiatives as the latest flavor of the week to which they give lip service, while maintaining the *status quo* until the next big thing arises. The World Bank concludes that change will not be successful if *any* criterion is absent; managers pursuing reform must have a compelling reason, the ability to overcome opposition, and a reputation for follow-through.

The first step toward reaching higher performance and greater efficiency requires understanding current performance and the performance of peers. Senior managers overseeing multiple departments and responsible for ensuring departments work effectively together must take a broader view of the organization's performance—operate at the level of the master budget rather than department budgets. Second, effective managers should be capable of assessing their departments against industry performance; financial ratios provide insight into whether the organization and its subordinate operations are working above or below industry standards. Information is the key to determining when change is needed and what action should be pursued.

Financial ratios track an organization's profitability, liquidity, capital structure, and asset turnover (productivity) and are the first step toward understanding its financial health. Profitability is the measure of the effectiveness of management; first-class managers should be able to produce higher profits than peer organizations. Profitability is the culmination of effectively setting goals and managing people and physical assets. While profitability ratios provide the signposts for overall performance, turnover, liquidity, and capital structure ratios examine specific aspects of operations. The interrelationships between the various types of ratios is highlighted by DuPont analysis, which ties return on equity (ROE) to the ability of the organization to convert sales into income, assets into sales, and equity into assets. DuPont analysis provides a starting point for identifying opportunities for improvement, initiating action, and creating multiyear strategic plans.

Ratio analysis compares one financial variable to another, providing a financial view of an organization that is often poorly understood and underappreciated by nonfinancial managers. Ratio analysis assesses the relationship between income statement and balance sheet amounts to determine how resources are being used and what they are producing. Standardization of ratios allows performance to be assessed across organizations.

Operating indicators highlight how goods and services are created, that is, how care is delivered to patients, by comparing financial and operational data. Operating indicators examine operating conditions (patient mix) and performance measures (occupancy, length of stay [LOS], etc.) to explain *why* and *how* superior or substandard profits are earned; this data is often more intuitive and useful to nonfinancial managers. Superior profits should be easier to achieve if a high percentage of patients are commercially insured, while a high percentage of Medicare, Medicaid, and uninsured patients with low or no reimbursement will have an adverse effect on revenues. The challenge to managers facing a high percentage of fixed- and low-reimbursement patients is to design a care system to succeed with low revenue. Managers should ensure effective care is delivered timely, patients move through the system in the shortest possible time, resources are fully employed, and unnecessary expenses are avoided. Operating indicators drill down into financial ratios to examine performance at the level of admissions, bed utilization, labor hours, and input prices—information that can pinpoint where an organization deviates from its peers and accelerate movement toward higher performance.

▶ Ratio Analysis

The goal of ratio analysis is to understand financial statements and identify strengths and weaknesses. To the untrained, financial statements are simply a mass of numbers, that is, uninformative data. Accounting is a means to organize data to produce information and build knowledge to direct decision-making and action. One must have a basic knowledge of accounting, and data must be put into perspective to fully comprehend financial information. The magnitudes of net income to sales, sales to assets, debt to assets, etc., must be compared before any conclusion is reached on management's effectiveness.

Ratios interpret an organization's financial performance by relating income statement variables to one another and to the assets and liabilities on the balance sheet. The income statement describes the inflow and outflow of funds in a given year, while the balance sheet documents what assets are employed and how they were financed. The flow of funds largely determines whether value is created or destroyed. Ratios allow decision-makers inside and outside an organization to examine how net income relates to the tools (assets and their funding from the balance sheet) placed in the hands of managers. We expect financial performance to improve as more funds are invested in an operation; financial ratios provide a tool to assess how performance changes over time and with the size and structure of the operation.

Financial ratios indicate how an organization *is* operating and provide insight into how it *should* operate. Does a profit of $5 million indicate management is doing a good job? Before examining this question, let us ask a more intuitive question: Is a weight of 180 lb. for an adult indicative of a healthy lifestyle? Few people would jump to the conclusion that 180 lb. indicates the person is appropriately managing his or her weight. Most would ask a series of questions: What are the person's height, gender, and age? If the person is 5 feet tall, the body mass index (BMI) would be 35.1 (obese); at 7 feet, the BMI would be 17.9 (underweight). In either case, the person should take action, albeit opposite actions, to improve his or her health, life expectancy, and physical attractiveness. An individual standing 6 feet tall would have a "normal" BMI of 24.4. Another factor to consider when assessing desirable weight is an individual's muscle tone: muscle is heavier than fat, so the BMI will be higher for those with muscular bodies.

Assume a person is 5 feet tall and weighs 180 lb. with a BMI of 35.1; this person should lose weight. The goal is clear, but there are right and wrong ways of pursuing weight loss. The fastest means to lose weight would be to cut off an appendage: cutting off a leg (15%–22% of body weight) would reduce the weight by approximately 33 lb. and produce a BMI of 28.7 (overweight). Removing an appendage not only is an undesirable means to lose weight but also would further degrade health and mobility. While the example may seem flippant, this rapid weight loss approach does not differ qualitatively from managers who pursue short-term financial goals by cutting research and development funds or divesting the organization of profitable business lines. Understanding an individual's situation should indicate a combination of diet, exercise, weight loss drugs, and/or surgery to utilize to achieve a desirable weight. Similarly, improving financial performance requires managers to understand where revenues can be increased, expenses reduced, and/or changes in assets made.

The reader should see that the question of whether a $5 million profit is too high or too low cannot be answered without further information. The first question that should be asked is, what is the size of the organization? An organization's size is generally based on invested capital, assets employed, or sales. If an organization employs $500 million in equity, a $5 million profit produces a paltry 1.0% ROE. If only $10 million in equity has been invested, the organization is earning a phenomenal 50% ROE. On the basis of the average ROE (for hospitals) in 2015, 7.0%, an average organization earning $5 million should have approximately $71,429,000 in equity. Profitability varies by type of business, so whether the organization is a hospital, a physician practice, a home health agency, or other healthcare provider will determine how much the organization should earn. The third consideration is historical returns. A $5 million profit is an improvement if $2,500,000 was earned in the prior year but disappointing if $10 million was earned. A primary question is whether performance is improving or deteriorating.

A fourth consideration is how much the organization should earn. The environment in which the organization operates limits its performance. For example, hospital profits should increase with the pool of potential patients and decrease with the number of competitors. An expanding pool of patients should increase the hospital's power over the prices it charges and profitability. Pricing power is reduced by an increase in the number of organizations selling comparable services. The third major factor in health care is changes in reimbursement: provider profits move directly with changes in Medicare and Medicaid reimbursement; the more generous these payments are, the higher the profits will be. Recent trends toward lower reimbursement suggest healthcare providers may need to tighten their belts to improve their financial performance.

BOX 12.1 shows the four primary types of financial ratios: profitability, turnover, liquidity, and capital structure. **Profitability ratios** measure management effectiveness: Did management decisions and policy create wealth and value? How successful was management in converting sales into profit and/or assets into profit? **Turnover ratios** (a.k.a. activity or productivity ratios) assess the ability to

convert assets into sales and the composition of assets. **Liquidity ratios** measure the ability of the organization to meet its short-term obligations: can bills be paid as they come due? **Capital structure ratios** (a.k.a. debt or leverage ratios) assess long-term solvency: can the organization pay off its total liabilities? Capital structure ratios are also used to assess the extent of debt financing and whether organizations can handle additional debt.

TABLES 12.1 and **12.2** show actual operating results for a major U.S. hospital. The first point that leaps to attention is that regardless of the overall assessment of management, it is clear that managers initiated changes that greatly enhanced profits between 2015 and 2016. The income statement demonstrates that profit doubled in 1 year but provides little insight into the questions of why it doubled and whether it should be higher. The balance sheet shows the total assets employed decreased and liabilities increased. Ratio analysis explores how organizational performance changes over time, and can be used to compare organizational performance with industry performance.

Profit increased to $104,485,000, while total assets declined by $70,650,000, and even more notable is the decline in equity. While financial statements show the results of operations, it is clear the income statement and balance sheet do not fully explain how the organization operates or the effectiveness

---

BOX 12.1 Types of Financial Ratios

1. Liquidity: Short-term liquidity.
2. Capital structure: Long-term solvency and extent of debt financing.
3. Turnover: Ability to convert assets into sales and composition of assets.
4. Profitability: Overall measure of management effectiveness. Did management decisions create value and wealth? How successful was management in converting sales into profit and/or assets into profit?

TABLE 12.1 Oyam Hospital Income Statement		
	2015	**2016**
Operating revenue	$766,473,000	$870,598,000
Nonoperating revenue	$6,535,000	$6,519,000
Total revenue	$773,008,000	$877,117,000
Salaries and wages	$311,710,000	$317,583,000
Fringe benefits	$66,007,000	$94,759,000
Supplies	$150,957,000	$160,468,000
Rent	$10,033,000	$10,353,000
Depreciation	$32,052,000	$32,247,000
Interest	$1,363,000	$819,000
Other	$150,963,000	$156,403,000
Total expenses	$723,085,000	$772,632,000
Profit	$49,923,000	$104,485,000

of management. Ratio analysis is essential to achieving greater understanding, and the review begins by examining changes in profitability and the factors that affect profitability.

Profitability Ratios

The starting point for examining organizational performance is profitability. Profitability ratios examine how much money is earned (or value created) from operations on the basis of invested equity, assets employed, and sales. Profitability ratios are the net results of management decision-making and direct indicators of the ability of managers to achieve the goals of the organization.

■ **ROE = Profit/Equity** (or fund balance; numerator from the income statement and denominator from the balance sheet)

The ROE assesses management's ability to generate wealth for the organization's owners. Managers should work to maximize the ROE, that is, the higher the ratio, the better.

2015 $49,923,000/$487,322,000 = 10.2%

2016 $104,485,000/$391,916,000 = 26.7%

Benchmark (2015): 7.0%

TABLE 12.2 Oyam Hospital Balance Sheet

	2015	2016
Cash	$25,435,000	$25,270,000
Accounts receivable	$181,767,000	$161,841,000
Other current assets	$162,936,000	$142,851,000
Fixed assets	$495,057,000	$444,822,000
Total assets	$708,834,000	$638,184,000
Current liabilities	$28,638,000	$32,344,000
Current portion long-term debt	$6,430,000	$7,130,0000
Long-term debt	$186,444,000	$206,794,000
Total liabilities	$221,512,000	$246,268,000
Equity	$487,322,000	$391,916,000

The ROE in 2015 indicates that Oyam is earning 26.7 cents for every $1.00 of equity investment. The reader should note that benchmarks are often 2 or more years out of date, and obtaining contemporary data is an obstacle most organizations face in **benchmarking**, that is, comparing an organization's processes and outcomes against those of other organizations. Relying on Linnaeus' observation that "nature does not leap," older benchmarks can still be used to assess current performance. Accordingly, Oyam's management seems capable of producing higher-than-industry returns for its owners (more precisely, on its fund balance since this is a nonprofit organization) and substantially increasing profit over the prior year. While superior performance relative to the industry and past performance is desirable, further analysis is needed to understand how this return was achieved.

■ **Return on assets (ROA) = Profit/Total assets** (numerator from the income

statement and denominator from the balance sheet)

The ROA assesses management's ability to convert assets into profit (wealth). The ROA assesses the use of all assets employed by the organization, whether provided by equity holders or obtained through debt. The ROA is used to determine whether the organization has over- or underinvested in assets; like the ROE, managers should attempt to maximize the ROA, that is, produce the maximum return possible from available assets.

2015 $49,923,000/$708,834,000 = 7.0%

2016 $104,485,000/$638,184,000 = 16.4%

Benchmark (2015): 3.7%

The ROA in 2016 indicates 16.4 cents is earned for every $1.00 of assets employed.

Unlike the ROE, which can be enhanced by debt financing, the ROA is a superior measure of whether the organization effectively uses its assets or employs the "correct" level of assets. Oyam's higher ROA in 2016 was driven by the increase in profit and reduction in assets.

- **Total margin = Profit/Total revenue** (both from the income statement)

    The total margin measures the ability to generate profit (wealth) from any source (operations, nonoperating income, etc.). The total margin primarily focuses on the organization's ability to convert sales into profit. Managers maximize the return from each dollar of sales by setting appropriate prices and holding down costs.

    2015 $49,923,000/$773,473,000 = 6.5%

    2016 $104,485,000/$877,117,000 = 11.9%

    Benchmark (2015): 4.5%

    The total margin in 2016 indicates Oyam generates 11.9 cents in profit for every $1.00 in sales. Oyam's improvement between 2015 and 2016 appears to be driven by its higher operating margin: total revenue increased by $104 million, while profit increased by $54 million. The $54 million in additional profit was largely the result of controlling expenses rather than increasing sales.

- **Operating margin = Net operating income/Net operating revenue** (both from the income statement)

    The operating margin measures the ability to convert sales into profit (wealth): unlike the total margin, the operating margin focuses on the primary business of the organization and the managers' ability to manage core operations. The goal of managers should be maximization of the operating margin.

    Benchmarks (2015): 3.76%

- **Nonoperating gain = Nonoperating gain/Total revenue** (both from the income statement)

    Nonoperating gain shows the amount of income generated from nonoperating activities. A lower nonoperating ratio may be better as the organization should derive the majority of its income from its core business, that is, it should be competent in its major field of activity to produce sufficient income and should not have to rely on nonoperating sources (especially if these funds are unstable) to sustain itself. On the other hand, organizations with large endowments that provide a stable stream of income are in an enviable situation, where they can invest in less desirable or money-losing activities without jeopardizing their viability.

FIGURE 12.1 provides a visualization of the changes in the three major profitability ratios from 2015 through 2018. The ROE, ROA, and total margin increased sharply in 2016 and have seen modest declines in the subsequent 2 years. The changes in 2016 could be management, programming, the economy, or other factors. Another useful visualization (**FIGURE 12.2**) tracks organizational profitability against industry or peer group averages to determine whether the organization followed industry trends.

Figure 12.2 tracks the ROA against the industry average, and the 25th percentile, industry performance, was projected by the author (since data is not available for performance after 2015). In

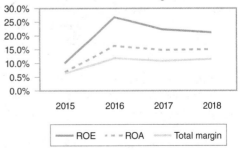

FIGURE 12.1 Profitability Trends

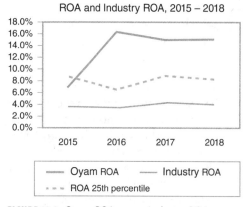

FIGURE 12.2 Oyam ROA versus Industry ROA

2015, Oyam was above the industry average but below the top 25% of hospitals; 2016 saw industry profitability decline, while Oyam improved. Since 2016, Oyam's ROA has been 70%–80% higher than the performance of the top 25th percentile. This type of performance speaks volumes about management's performance, liquidity, capital structure, and turnover ratios, as well as operating indicators, may shed light on the major factors that propelled the leap in profitability from 2015 and the continuing above-average returns.

Turnover Ratios

Turnover (or asset efficiency) ratios assess the productivity of assets and the balance between assets. Does the organization have too many assets producing too little revenue? Turnover ratios assess whether management was wise in accumulating assets and its ability to keep assets fully employed. Turnover ratios are a prime example of combining income statement information (flow of funds) with balance sheet information (stock of funds)—assets are acquired to generate revenue.

■ **Total asset turnover = Total revenue/ Total assets** (numerator from the income statement and denominator from the balance sheet)

Total asset turnover shows how many dollars of revenue each dollar of assets

produces in a year. The goal is to maximize revenue per dollar of asset. Two complications that distort comparisons of turnover ratios across organizations are asset age and depreciation methods used. Organizations employing assets with low book values due to age or use of accelerated depreciation methods will appear to have more productive assets than organizations with newer and/ or less depreciated equipment and buildings.

2015 $773,008,000/$708,834,000 = 1.09

2016 $877,117,000/$638,184,000 = 1.37

Benchmark (2015): 0.99

In 2015, Oyam's total asset turnover was higher than the industry average: every dollar of assets produced $1.09 in revenue. Depending on higher revenue and lower assets, Oyam's assets were 38.4% more productive than the industry average.

■ **Fixed asset turnover = Total revenue/ Fixed assets** (numerator from the income statement and denominator from the balance sheet)

Fixed asset turnover measures how many dollars of revenue each dollar of fixed assets produces in a year. Regardless of what the total asset turnover reports, the composition of assets should be analyzed to ensure an excess of current assets are not offset by a deficiency in fixed assets or vice versa. Managers should attempt to maximize revenue from fixed assets. Given the life span of fixed assets, the comparison problems created by asset age and depreciation methods may be greater than seen in the total asset turnover ratio.

2015 $773,008,000/$495,057,000 = 1.56

2016 $877,117,000/$444,822,000 = 1.97

Benchmark (2015): 2.54

Oyam's fixed assets are less productive than the industry average: $1.97 in revenue for every $1.00 of fixed assets. But 2016 was a distinct improvement over 2015, when only $1.56 in revenue was generated by each $1.00 of fixed assets. The 2016 improvement was driven by higher revenue and a reduction in fixed assets.

- **Current asset turnover = Total revenue/ Current assets** (numerator from the income statement and denominator from the balance sheet)

   Current asset turnover reports how many dollars of revenue are generated for every dollar invested in current assets. Given the low return typically earned on current assets, these assets can be characterized as low-risk and high-turnover assets. Managers should attempt to maintain current assets at the minimum level required to support operations.

2015 $773,008,000/$213,777,000 = 3.62

2016 $877,117,000/$193,362,000 = 4.54

Benchmark (2015): 3.72

Oyam has shifted from underperforming compared to the industry in 2015 to overperforming in 2016 primarily by reducing days in accounts receivable (AR). In 2016, Oyam produced $4.54 in revenue for every $1.00 of current assets.

The fixed and current asset turnover ratios allow managers to investigate where they may have a problem if total asset turnover is not as productive as desired; that is, has the organization overinvested in buildings and equipment (fixed) or cash, AR, and/or inventories (current)? Examining the three turnover ratios suggests that further improvement will require Oyam to reduce its investment in fixed assets if revenue is constant or increase the amount of revenue generated from existing fixed assets. Turnover ratios are good measures of managerial performance and help assess whether managers are requesting and investing in underutilized assets.

Liquidity Ratios

It is obvious from the increase in profitability and the comparison with other hospitals that Oyam's management is highly effective, but what insight can other organizations draw from Oyam's performance? The next step in the analysis examines how Oyam has generated high profits by managing its short-term assets and liabilities. Liquidity ratios are designed to assess an organization's ability to meet its short-term debt obligations.

- **Current ratio = Current assets/Current liabilities** (both numerator and denominator from the balance sheet)

   The current ratio measures the ability to meet short-term obligations with current assets. Current assets can be converted to cash within 12 months, and current liabilities should be paid (cash outflows) within 12 months. The primary question is, does the organization have sufficient cash to pay its short-term obligations? A ratio of 1.00 (current assets = current liabilities) implies the organization has just enough funds to pay off its current obligations. The higher the current ratio, the larger the amount by which current assets exceed current liabilities, the more likely the organization will be able to meet its obligations on time.

2015 $213,777,000/$28,638,000 = 7.45

2016 $193,362,000/$32,344,000 = 5.98

Benchmark (2015): 2.18

In 2015, Oyam had $7.46 in current assets for every dollar of current liabilities—payment should not be a problem. In 2016, Oyam reduced its current assets by $20,415,000 and increased its current liabilities by $3,706,000; the current ratio fell to 5.98 but remains well above the industry average.

- **Acid (or quick) ratio = (Cash + Marketable securities + AR)/Current liabilities** (all amounts from the balance sheet)

The acid ratio also measures the ability of an organization to meet its short-term obligations. Use of the current ratio is criticized because certain types of current assets (e.g., inventory and prepaid expenses) are not well suited to pay current liabilities. The acid ratio recognizes that some current assets cannot be quickly converted to cash and rectifies this problem by using only highly liquid current assets, that is, cash and marketable securities, which can be immediately converted at full value. As we will see, collecting the full value of AR takes roughly 50 days. A higher ratio, having more liquid assets in the numerator to repay current liabilities, is better.

2015   ($25,435,000 + $181,767,000)/
        $28,638,000 = 6.58

2016   ($25,270,000 + $161,841,000)/
        $32,344,000 = 5.20

In 2016, Oyam had $5.20 in readily convertible current assets for every $1.00 in current liabilities, down from 2015 but more than adequate to meet its obligations.

- **Cash on hand = (Cash + Marketable securities)/((Annual expenses − Depreciation)/365)** (numerator from the balance sheet and denominator from the income statement)
    Cash on hand assesses an organization's ability to meet daily expenses with currently available liquid assets. The numerator includes only highly liquid assets (those can that be converted to full value immediately), and the denominator calculates average daily cash expenses (how much money flows out of the organization daily). Depreciation is an accounting entry and does not require cash outlay, so it is subtracted from the total annual expense. One could think of cash on hand as answering the question: If cash inflows stopped today, how many days could the organization pay its bills (meet its daily cash obligations) before its

liquid assets are exhausted? An organization has less risk as cash on hand increases.

2015 $25,435,000/(($723,085,227 −
        32,052,026)/365) = 13.4 days

2016 $25,270,000/(($772,632,296 −
        32,247,496)/365) = 12.3 days

Benchmark (2015): 25.8 days

In 2016, Oyam could pay its cash expenses for 12.3 days if no additional money flowed into the organization, which was roughly half the time of other hospitals. In light of its profitability, it is clear that Oyam is deliberately minimizing highly liquid assets in favor of higher-return, lower-liquidity assets.

- **Days in AR = Accounts Receivable/ (Annual revenue/365)** (numerator from the balance sheet and denominator from the income statement)
    Days in AR shows the ability to convert sales into cash, that is, what is the time lag between production of a good or service and receipt of payment for this work? This ratio measures how many days of revenue (an asset) are tied up in AR i.e. total uncollected revenue. The denominator is the calculation of average daily revenue. Management should strive to minimize days in AR by collecting payment at the time of service, ensuring charges accumulated and physician attestations are promptly completed and claims are submitted to the correct payer without error.

2015 $181,766,929/($773,008,357/365) =
        85.8 days

2016 $161,841,233/($877,116,629/365) =
        67.4 days

Benchmark (2015): 47.3 days

In 2015, Oyam waited 85.8 days to collect revenue for the services it provided. The problem is AR is a non-interest-bearing asset; the funds tied up in AR could be earning interest income in a bank or be reinvested in the operation to generate sales and income. Funds tied up in AR represent an opportunity cost, while the cost for hospitals with sufficient funds to meet their obligations may only be foregone interest; liquidity-constrained organizations may have to borrow funds to pay bills and pay interest on these loans. The days in AR ratio is primarily a measurement of the effectiveness of receivables management: is management ensuring patient accounts are correctly and timely billed and collected? In 2016, Oyam had substantially improved its receivables management by reducing the total amount of receivables by $20,000,000 (−11%), while increasing revenue per day by $285,000 (+13%). Oyam's investment in AR is still high in light of industry performance, and reducing days in AR to the industry average would free up roughly $33,600,000 for reinvestment.

A problem that arises in comparing AR is, what are AR and daily revenue? Is AR gross (what is billed to patients) or net (what is expected to be collected)? If AR is recorded on a net basis, average daily revenue should be net and vice versa, but when do organizations write off contractual allowances? Is it at the time of billing or payment? And when are bad debts written off, that is, removed from AR? Organizations that remove questionable accounts quickly, eliminating accounts 90 days past due, will have a lower days in AR ratio than organizations that work accounts longer. Differences in accounting policy, primarily when contractual adjustments, charity, and bad debt are written off, can cloud comparisons between organizations.

- ■ **Average payment period = Current liabilities/((Annual expense − Depreciation)/365)** (numerator from the balance sheet and denominator from the income statement)

    The average payment period shows how quickly short-term liabilities are paid and measures how many days of

expense are unpaid. The denominator is average daily cash expense minus depreciation that does not require a cash outlay. Faster payment demonstrates the ability of an organization to meet its short-term obligation (as well as taking advantage of trade discounts), but substantial funds in current liabilities, particularly accounts payable, can be viewed as taking advantage of interest-free loans.

| 2015 | $28,637,701/(($723,085,227 − 32,052,026)/365) = 15.1 days |
| 2016 | $32,343,983/(($772,632,296 − 32,247,496)/365) = 15.9 days |

Benchmark (2015): 54.1 days

In 2015, Oyam had only 15.1 days of average daily expense unpaid in current liabilities, well below the industry average of 54.1 days. Interpreting a high (or low) average payment period requires understanding why the ratio is high (or low); if current liabilities are largely interest-free loans and the organization has the resources necessary to pay them off, a high payment period is good. It is better to have cash sitting in your bank account, drawing interest, than with your suppliers. The determination of whether to pay bills promptly or delay payment should consider whether and how much of a prompt payment discount the organization could receive. A high average payment period could mean suppliers offer no incentive for prompt payment or the organization lacks the funds to quickly pay its obligations. The average payment period can also be used to measure the effectiveness of management over its disbursement function: are the payment approval processes and check-writing function well run?

Capital Structure Ratios

Capital structure ratios assess how assets are financed and an organization's ability to meet its long-term debt obligations. These ratios are used by creditors to assess the safety of their loans and whether they should lend additional funds. Capital structure ratios gauge creditor power over an organization, as overreliance on debt confers control to outside parties. A key responsibility of managers is to minimize the total cost of capital by balancing lower-cost debt and higher-cost equity. Managers have an incentive to substitute debt for equity in the organization's capital to increase returns to its owners. Overuse of debt, that is, excessive leverage, however, increases financial risk. More debt increases interest expense and may reduce an organization's ability to make interest and principal payments, especially during a business downturn accompanied by falling revenue. We should be circumspect when evaluating capital structure ratios, as high use of debt confers advantages and disadvantages.

Conservative managers may choose to rely on equity rather than debt to reduce total organizational risk, yet higher use of equity reduces the ROE (ROE↓ = Profit/Equity↑). On the other hand, some managers may choose to aggressively leverage the organization to minimize equity financing and maximize the ROE. The interpretation of whether leveraging is positive or negative must be couched in why debt is being used: if it is due to the inability to raise funds internally (retained earnings), this is bad. If the operation is earning high profits, has large cash reserves, and can meet debt obligations, increasing the use of debt is a prudent way to maximize returns to the organization's owners. Industries with stable demand, like health care and utilities, typically rely more heavily on debt than industries with unstable revenues.

- **Equity financing ratio = Equity (or fund balance)/Total assets** (both numerator and denominator from the balance sheet)

The equity financing ratio shows the proportion of total assets financed by the organization's owners. An organization faces less risk, that is, it does not have to pay interest to others for the use of funds

to acquire assets, when it finances its own assets. A higher equity financing ratio lowers financial risk and is desirable to risk-averse investors. Of course, aggressive use of debt financing is desirable if managers can borrow funds and invest them at a rate higher than the interest rate they pay. A higher equity financing ratio indicates less risk, while lower ratios and higher risk may increase the ROE, 1.0 minus the equity financing ratio provides the percentage of the organization's assets financed by creditors.

| 2015 | $487,322,000/$708,834,000 = 68.7% |
| 2016 | $391,915,642/$638,184,000 = 61.4% |

Benchmark (2015): 55.2%

In 2015, Oyam internally financed 68.7 cents of every $1.00 of assets and was significantly higher than the industry average of 55.2 cents. In 2016, Oyam reduced total assets by $70 million and equity by $96 million (transferred to related organizations), reducing the percentage of total assets financed by equity by 7.3%. The 2016 equity financing ratio is still higher than the industry average, where 55.2% of assets are internally financed. Oyam appears to be choosing a more conservative method of financing its assets than the average hospital.

- **Equity multiplier** is the inverse of the equity financing ratio, that is, it measures the total amount of assets supported by equity investment and is used in the DuPont analysis formula.

| 2015 | 1/0.687 = $708,834,000/$487,322,000 = 1.45 |
| 2016 | 1/0.614 = $638,184,000/$391,915,642 = 1.63 |

Benchmark (2015): 1.00/0.552 = 1.81

In 2016, every $1.00 of equity in Oyam supports $1.63 in assets; Oyam's ample net income relative to the industry average allows it to fund its investments through retained earnings, and its low use of debt guarantees access to debt at favorable rates should it pursue funding through banks or bond markets.

- **Long-term debt to equity** = **Long-term debt/Equity** (or fund balance) (both numerator and denominator from the balance sheet)

  Long-term debt to equity identifies the percentage of assets permanently financed by debt and ignores short-term liabilities.

2015 $192,874,000/$487,322,000 = 39.6%

2016 $213,924,000/$391,916,000 = 54.6%

Benchmark (2015): 28.2%

The long-term-debt-to-equity ratio indicates the ability of an organization to repay long-term debt, that is, equity provides a cushion to protect debt holders, and the greater the equity, the lower the risk to creditors. The same changes seen in the equity financing ratio are seen in the long-term-debt-to-equity ratio; equity has been reduced, but Oyam still has $1.83 (1/0.546) in equity for every dollar of long-term debt owed, although this is down from $2.53 in 2015.

- **Times interest earned** = **(Profit (Loss) + Interest expense)/Interest expense** (both numerator and denominator from the income statement)

  Times interest earned identifies the ability of an organization to pay its annual interest expense (the cost of borrowing funds) from current earnings. The numerator adds net income (did the organization earn a profit or suffer a loss?) to its interest expense. If the organization earns neither a profit nor a loss, the ratio is 1.00 and the interest expense can be paid from current revenues. If the organization earns a profit, the ratio will be greater than 1.00, that is, the organization has more than enough resources to pay its interest expense. If it is losing money, the ratio will be less than 1.00, that is, operating results are insufficient to pay interest cost, and the interest expense must be met by drawing down assets or increasing debt. Managers maximizing profits will be simultaneously increasing the times interest earned ratio.

2015   ($49,923,000 + $1,363,000)/ $1,363,000 = 37.63

2016   ($104,485,000 + $819,000)/ $819,000 = 128.56

Benchmark (2015): 4.24

Oyam's low use of debt combined with a low interest rate on debt and large profits has resulted in an extremely high times interest earned ratio. In the prior year, the doubling of net income combined with a 40% reduction in interest expense drove an already high ratio to an astronomical level of having $128.56 in resources to pay every dollar of interest expense (despite a $19 million increase in long-term debt).

- **Debt service coverage** = **(Profit (Loss) + Interest expense + Depreciation)/ (Interest expense + Principal)** (all amounts from the income statement)

  The limitation of the times interest earned ratio is that organizations are responsible for paying interest and principal on debts, and creditors want to know whether both obligations can be met. Debt service coverage adds depreciation (a noncash expense that can be used to pay the principal) to the numerator and the principal to the denominator (an additional cash outflow). A high debt service coverage ratio shows the organization can pay all cash flows associated with the use of debt; a higher ratio demonstrates a greater ability to meet the total outflows associated with the use of debt.

2015	($49,923,000 + $1,363,000 + $32,052,000)/ ($1,363,000 + $6,430,000) = 10.69
2016	($104,485,000 + $819,000 + $32,247,000)/ ($819,000 + $7,130,000) = 17.30

The debt service coverage reinforces the information provided by the times interest earned ratio. In 2016, Oyam had $17.30 of resources to pay each $1.00 of interest and principal payments due.

- **Cash flow to debt = (Profit + Depreciation)/(Current liabilities + Long-term debt)** (numerator from the income statement and denominator from the balance sheet)

    The cash-flow-to-debt ratio reports an organization's ability to liquidate its liabilities (rather than meet annual debt service). When the ratio is 1.0, the organization could discharge all of its obligations in a single year: profit plus depreciation equals total liabilities. A higher cash-flow-to-debt ratio signals a stronger organization.

2015	($49,923,000 + $32,052,000)/ ($28,638,000 + $192,874,000) = 0.37
2016	($104,485,000 + $32,247,000)/ ($32,344,000 + $213,924,000) = 0.56

In 2016, Oyam could pay 56% of the sum of current and long-term obligations by committing its current profit and depreciation expense; at this rate, Oyam could be debt free in 1.78 years (1.0/0.56). On the other hand, the average hospital needs 22.4 years to extinguish its debt.

- **Capital expense = (Interest expense + Depreciation + Amortization)/Total expense** (all amounts from the income statement)

Capital expense assesses how much of the total expense the organization devotes to using funds.

2015	($1,363,000 + $32,052,000)/ $723,085,000 = 4.6%
2016	($819,000 + $32,247,000)/ $772,632,000 = 4.3%

Benchmark (2015): 6.0%

The capital expense ratio shows Oyam may have a competitive advantage over other hospitals due to its ability to hold down financing costs in its cost structure. In 2016, the average hospital's total expense was 1.7% higher than Oyam's, simply to finance assets. **TABLE 12.3** summarizes the ratios in a concise format where the reader can quickly assess the level of performance and the change from 1 year to the next.

One of the important things to remember about ratios is they are **fractions**. When managers are confronted by a ratio that is too high or too low, there are two ways of improving performance, change the numerator or change the denominator. When the current asset turnover ratio (total revenue/current assets) is too low, managers should increase total revenue, reduce current assets, or do both to improve performance. The second solution, reducing current assets, requires understanding the composition of these assets; reducing current investments if they earn more than the organization's ROA may not be desirable, but reducing non-interest-bearing assets like AR and/or excess inventory is desirable.

Like with all financial information, when using ratios, it is wise to be alert to ways in which the information can be skewed. Managers can manipulate or window-dress information by postponing maintenance (↓expense) and investment (↓capital outlays and depreciation). These actions increase short-run profitability but can have adverse effects on future competitiveness (Weston & Brigham, 1978, p. 69).

TABLE 12.3 Ratio Analysis		
Profitability	**2015**	**2016**
ROE	10.24%	26.66%
ROA	7.04%	16.37%
Total margin	6.46%	11.91%
Liquidity		
Current	7.46	5.98
Acid	7.24	5.79
Cash on hand	13.43	12.46
Days in AR	85.83	67.35
Average payment period	15.13	15.95
Capital structure		
Equity financing	68.75%	61.41%
Times interest earned	37.63	128.58
Debt service coverage	10.69	17.30
Capital expense	4.62%	4.28%
Turnover		
Total asset	1.09	1.37
Fixed asset	1.56	1.97
Current asset	3.62	4.54

Ratio analysis, like variance analysis, does not determine why things change; it only identifies how things have changed. It is up to managers and analysts to determine what changes should be investigated, why they occurred, and what action can or should be taken.

A final caution is that comparisons should be tentative, changes in accounting, location, and industry have large effects on financial performance so users of ratios should be confident that comparisons across organizations are appropriate: do both organizations measure the same economic entities the same way? Accounting provides multiple ways to measure and report financial transactions; one should be sure that consistent reporting is in place when making comparisons across time or organizations.

DuPont Analysis

DuPont analysis is a shorthand model capturing three critical elements of an organization's operation to illuminate how wealth is produced from equity. DuPont analysis focuses

on the ROE: the product of total margin, total asset turnover, and equity multiplier.

$$
\text{ROE} = \text{Total margin} * \text{total asset turnover} * \text{equity multiplier} \quad (12.1)
$$

$$
\text{ROE} = \frac{\text{Profit}}{\text{Total revenue}} * \frac{\text{Total revenue}}{\text{Total assets}} * \frac{\text{Total assets}}{\text{Total equity}}
$$

Assume an industry averages 7.2% ROE; this financial outcome could be produced by the following industry averages for total margin, total asset turnover, and equity multiplier:

Industry average	=	7.2%	=	4.0%	*	1.20	*	1.50
		7.2%	=	$\dfrac{\$3,600,000}{\$90,000,000}$	*	$\dfrac{\$90,000,000}{\$75,000,000}$	*	$\dfrac{\$75,000,000}{\$50,000,000}$

DuPont analysis shows that 7.2 cents is earned for every $1.00 of equity. Every dollar of equity supports $1.50 in assets, every $1.00 of assets produces $1.20 in revenue, and every $1.00 of sales generates 4.0 cents in profit. Assume an organization experiences difficulty in turning revenue into profit due to excessive expenses that drive its total margin to 2.0%; the ROE would fall to 3.6%, and the necessary action would be to raise prices and/or reduce expenses.

ROE = 3.6% = **2.0%** * 1.20 * 1.50

If an organization overinvests in assets, resulting in its total asset turnover being two-thirds the industry average, its ROE would fall to 4.8%, and the necessary action would be to reduce assets or make existing assets produce more revenue.

ROE = 4.8% = 4.0% * **0.80** * 1.50

If an organization is underleveraged, that is, each dollar of equity supports $1.20 in assets (versus $1.50 in the industry), the ROE would fall to 5.8%, and the necessary action would be to increase debt-financed assets or reduce equity.

ROE = 5.8% = 4.0% * 1.20 * **1.20**

If the organization underperforms the industry on every measure, its ROE would be only 1.9%, or every dollar of equity would earn 26.3% of the return received in an average organization.

ROE = 1.9% = 2.0% * 0.80 * 1.20

Comparing Oyam's and the industry's performance using DuPont analysis highlights why Oyam is so successful.

ROE = Total margin * Total asset turnover * Equity multiplier	
Oyam (2015)	10.2% = 6.5% * 1.09 * 1.45
Oyam (2016)	26.7% = 11.9% * 1.37 * 1.63
Benchmark (2015)	7.0% = 4.4% * 0.99 * 1.60 note: 1.60 does not tie to the equity multiplier reported on page 356

DuPont analysis shows Oyam's strength is its total margin; in 2015, its total margin was

47.7% above the benchmark, and in 2016, it improved further. Oyam's assets were also more productive than the industry average. Reducing the ROE is Oyam's conservative funding of assets; managers are using less debt than other hospitals. In 2015, Oyam funded significantly less assets for every dollar of equity; however, it moved closer to the industry average in 2016.

DuPont analysis highlights the remarkable improvement in Oyam's financial performance: the ROE more than doubled between 2015 and 2016, and improvement crossed all areas. First, Oyam's ability to turn a dollar of sales into profit increased by 83%: total revenues increased by $104 million, while total expenses only increased by $50 million. Second, total asset turnover increased by 26.5%, or every dollar of assets generated more revenue. Finally, the organization is more highly leveraged: In 2015, every dollar of equity supported $1.45 investment into assets; in 2016, every dollar of equity supported $1.63 of assets. Oyam has improved its ability to translate sales into profit, increased the productivity of assets, and reduced its reliance on equity financing. In 2015, the ROE of half of all hospitals was less than 7.0%, and 75% had an ROE less than 13.9%; Oyam's financial performance places it in the upper echelon of all hospitals.

▶ Operating Indicators

Hospitals and other firms are governed by economies and diseconomies of scale, that is, organizations of a certain size are capable of performing efficiently, while larger and smaller organizations have higher costs. The budget should operate similar to the vital signs in a human, temperature at 98.6°F, heart rate 70 beats per minute, and blood pressure 120/80 mmHg, to determine whether the operation is functioning as it should. Is the operation in control, is it running too hot or too cold, is it exerting too much or too little energy, and is there too much stress or not enough urgency?

When assessing vital signs, it is obvious that extremely young or old persons will deviate from the above measures, so the question is, how much variation from desired performance should be accepted on the basis of the characteristics of the individual, and when should corrective action be taken? This is where benchmarking comes into play; it is inappropriate to compare the vital signs of a 30-year-old with those of a person in his or her 70s or compare the financial performance of a 500-bed hospital to a 100- or 1200-bed institution or compare a sole practitioner physician office with a multiphysician/specialty practice.

The *2017 Almanac of Hospital Financial and Operating Indicators* (Optum360°, 2016) provides trends and benchmarks for hospitals at the 25th, 50th, and 75th percentiles for various metrics. The almanac provides benchmarks by geographic region (Northeast, South, Near West, East North Central, and Far West), total revenues (<$10, $10–25, $25–60, $60–100, $100–150, and >$150 million), urban or rural location, bed size (<100, 100–199, 200–299, 300–399, 400–499, and >500 beds), teaching status, system affiliation, bond rating, state (AA+, A+, A, A−, BBB, and below), critical access by region, case mix index (CMI) by quartile, wage index by quartile, operating margin by quartile, inpatient percentage by quartile, ownership (profit, nonprofit, government), quality by quartile, and specialty (psychology, rehabilitation, pediatric). These breakdowns allow managers to select a peer group similar to their hospital to enhance the validity of comparisons; a community hospital with 250 beds in the South can be compared with similar hospitals rather than an average including teaching hospitals and all beds sizes across the United States.

Operating indicators drill down into operations to identify why financial performance is what it is. Profitability ratios may indicate an organization's profit is too little for the amount of sales generated, assets employed, and/or funds invested but provide little insight into why net income is low. Operating indicators attempt to determine where the deficiency arises (is it in the inpatient area, outpatient area, or both areas?) by examining price, volume, LOS, intensity of service, efficiency, and unit cost measures to identify areas where improvements can be made. Operating indicators, unlike financial ratios, often examine the relationship between financial variables and operational measures such as inputs used, activities performed, and outputs produced.

Profitability Indicators

The goal of profitability indicators is to identify how inpatient and outpatient services contribute to net income, the impact of the cost of living and the needs of patients served on the profit, and where profit is earned (or lost). Averages and the 25th and 75th percentile metrics for 2015 are provided to allow the reader to determine whether an organization is in the top or the bottom half in performance and to assess the difference in performance between the top 25% and the bottom 25%.

- Profit per discharge = (Inpatient net revenue − Inpatient operating expenses)/ Total discharges = −$27; range: −$716 (25th) to $761 (75th)

- CMI- and wage-adjusted profit per discharge = (Inpatient net revenue − Inpatient operating expenses)/(Total discharges * All patient CMI * Wage index) = $41; range: −$364 (25th) to $477 (75th)

- Profit per outpatient visit = (Outpatient net revenue − Outpatient operating expenses)/Total visits = Not available

First, profit indicators should be used to determine whether earnings are less than desired in inpatient care, outpatient care, or both types of care. The profit per adjusted discharge indicator introduces the CMI into the denominator to assess the impact of changes in case severity on the profit. In 2015, the average hospital lost a small amount of money on inpatient care but profited when the CMI and

the wage index were considered. The adjusted profit per discharge introduces the wage index to recognize the impact on profit due to higher or lower market-driven salaries. These adjustments should reduce the profit or loss per discharge due to inflation of the denominator. The marginal profit earned as the CMI increases may be the result of the higher reimbursement received as the diagnosis-related drug (DRG) weight increases, the ability of hospitals to better manage difficult cases, or both. Future indicators will use the CMI and the wage index to increase the comparability of the LOS, unit cost, and other measures between hospitals serving patients with different needs for care.

The benchmarks suggest the average hospital lost money on inpatient care but profited from outpatient care since the average hospital had a positive ROA and ROE in 2015. These indicators are obviously at a high level but identify why managers should focus on improving inpatient care to improve their financial results. The reader should see whether profit per discharge or outpatient visit was calculated by medical service line or payer; it would provide precise information that could be used to set future market plans and improve operations.

Price Indicators

While the profit indicators show where hospitals are earning or losing money, price indicators explore whether inpatient and outpatient prices are too high or too low, what the impact of the inpatient/outpatient service mix and payer mix is, and how much revenue is written off as contractual discounts.

- Gross price per inpatient discharge = Gross inpatient revenues/Total discharges = $26,932; range: $17,410 (25th) to $45,196 (75th)

- CMI- and wage-adjusted gross price per discharge = Gross inpatient revenues/ (Total discharges * All patient CMI * Wage index) = $22,038; range: $17,902 (25th) to $31,813 (75th)

– Net price per inpatient discharge = Net inpatient revenues/Total discharges = $10,154; range: $7,553 (25th) to $14,511 (75th)

– CMI- and wage-adjusted net price per discharge = Net inpatient revenues/(Total discharges * All patient CMI * Wage index) = $6,688; range: $5,752 (25th) to $7,827 (75th)

– Gross price per ambulatory payment classification (APC) = Gross APC revenues /Total APCs = $669; range: $430 (25th) to $1,075 (75th)

– Wage adjusted gross price per APC = Gross APC revenues/(Total APCs * Wage index) = $882; range: $586 (25th) to $1,292 (75th)

– Medicare payment percentage = (Medicare discharges/Total discharges) * 100 = 40.3%; range: 30.0% (25th) to 52.9% (75th)

– Deductible ratio = (Contractual allowance/Total gross revenue) * 100 = 62.7%; range: 48.8% (25th) to 72.0% (75th)

– Inpatient revenue percentage = Net inpatient revenue/Total net revenue * 100 = 45.8%; range: 30.5% (25th) to 64.1% (75th)

– Outpatient revenue percentage = net outpatient revenue/total net revenue * 100 = 58.4%; range: 44.2% (25th) to 71.5% (75th)

– Nonoperating revenue percentage = Nonoperating revenue/Total net revenue * 100 = 0.02%; range: 0.00% (25th) to 0.39% (75th)

Price indicators should be used to determine whether prices should be raised or lowered and what bargaining position to take with managed care payers. Does a hospital charge less than its peers, and could it successfully raise prices? The price indicators highlight a common misconception in health care: hospitals do not receive what they bill to patients. CMI and APC adjustments factor in the difference in the intensity of care provided to inpatients and outpatients to facilitate price comparisons across organizations. Patients and providers do not understand this fact; the contractual allowance percentage, the difference between the gross and net price per discharge, demonstrates the average hospital receives only 37.3 cents for every $1.00 billed. Hospital managers and employees should understand revenue constraints and that they must hold costs below what third parties are willing to pay for treatment.

Inpatient Occupancy and Length-of-Stay Indicators

Inpatient occupancy and LOS indicators identify the utilization of inpatient beds and report the time between admission and discharge. These indicators evaluate past investment decisions and current treatment practice.

– Hospital occupancy = (Patient days/ (Licensed beds * 365)) = 49.5%; range: 32.7% (25th) to 65.0% (75th)

– Hospital discharges per bed = Total discharges/Licensed beds = 33.0 discharges; range: 17.4 discharges (25th) to 47.5 discharges (75th)

– Average LOS = Total patient days/Total inpatient discharges = 4.5 days; range: 3.8 days (25th) to 6.7 days (75th)

– CMI-adjusted LOS = Total patient days/ (Total inpatient discharges * All patient CMI) = 2.70 days; range: 2.4 days (25th) to 3.0 days (75th)

– Adjusted LOS, Medicare = Medicare patient days/(Total Medicare discharges * Medicare CMI) = 3.1 days; range: 2.7 days (25th) to 3.1 days (75th)

The occupancy and LOS indicators assess how inpatient assets are utilized and what the duration of inpatient stays is. The cost per inpatient bed is estimated to be over $1 million per bed, so having 50.5% of beds unoccupied imposes a large fixed cost on hospitals. While current managers cannot undo past investment decisions, they should be accountable for how fixed resources are utilized. Increasing the LOS is one way of increasing occupancy rates, but managers must also understand that a higher LOS may not produce additional revenue under fixed reimbursement systems and could lower net income.

Occupancy and LOS indicators gathered at the organizational level are the starting point for examining performance at the nursing unit, physician, or program level. Programming decisions and improvement initiatives should be based on identifying outliers and taking appropriate action: Should low-occupancy programs be promoted to increase volume and efficiency, scaled back, or shuttered? How should high-LOS nursing units, physicians, and/or programs be handled?

Intensity-of-Service Indicators

Intensity-of-care indicators focus on the cost per discharge and how costs vary with the needs of the patients served. While cost information is imprecise in health care, especially when applied to individual procedures or patients, it remains one of the most available and commonly used measures to evaluate the level of resources consumed by an admission or outpatient visit.

– Cost per discharge = Inpatient operating expenses/Total inpatient discharges = $10,162; range: $7,627 (25th) to $14,503 (75th)

– Adjusted cost per discharge = Inpatient operating expenses/(Total inpatient discharges * Wage index * All patient CMI) = $6,609; range: $5,595 (25th) to $7,835 (75th)

– Cost per APC service = APC operating expenses/Total APCs = $185; range: $145 (25th) to $250 (75th)

– Cost per APC service weight-adjusted = APC operating expenses/(Total APCs * Wage index) = $71; range: $53 (25th) to $104 (75th)

The intensity indicators allow managers to compare their average costs per discharge or outpatient visit against their peers' to determine whether their inpatient and outpatient costs differ substantially from other institutions. Like occupancy and LOS indicators, improving performance will require information by unit or program to identify and correct outliers.

Efficiency Indicators

Efficiency indicators examine the productivity of labor: does the hospital employ too many or too few people, depending on the quantity and level of care they provide? Efficiency indicators use the concept of **full-time equivalent (FTE)** to account for the use of part-time personnel; the FTE indicates 2080 hours paid, whether it is one employee paid for 40 hours per week across 52 weeks or two people working 20 hours per week over 52 weeks.

– FTE per occupied bed = Inpatient FTEs/(Total patient days/365 (average daily census)) = 4.66 FTEs; range: 3.68 FTEs (25th) to 5.90 FTEs (75th)

– CMI-adjusted FTE per occupied bed = Inpatient FTEs/(Average daily census * All patient CMI) = 3.30 FTEs; range: 2.75 FTEs (25th) to 4.05 FTEs (75th)

– Staff hours per discharge = (Inpatient FTE * 2080)/Inpatient discharges = 131.1 hours; range: 101.0 hours (25th) to 194.3 hours (75th)

– CMI-adjusted staff hours per discharge = (Inpatient FTE * 2080)/(Inpatient discharges * All patient CMI) = 75.2 hours; range: 62.9 hours (25th) to 92.8 hours (75th)

– Outpatient person-hours/visit = (Outpatient FTE * 2080)/Visits = Not available

If intensity indicators conclude the cost per admission or outpatient visit is too high, efficiency indicators should be used to determine whether the hospital is using too much labor for the services provided: does the hospital use more or less than the 4.66 FTEs per occupied bed used by the average hospital? One difficulty using these indicators is the allocation of personnel between inpatient and outpatient services; ancillary personnel provide services to inpatients and outpatients, and many organizations have difficulty in determining how much time is spent in each area. To improve labor scheduling, efficiency indicators need to identify personnel use at the department level.

Unit (Input) Cost Indicators

If profits are too low, a major reason may be costs are too high. The efficiency indicators explored whether the hospital utilized too many workers, but costs could also be higher than comparable hospitals due to wages. Unit cost indicators examine input prices and costs per discharge by major expense to determine which factors, wages or capital, explain excessive costs. Managers would also need to explore how fringe benefits, supplies, and malpractice insurance affect costs.

- Salary per FTE = Total salary + Wages/Total FTE = $59,380; minimum, $50,276, Alabama; maximum, $77,081, Oregon
- Wage-adjusted salary per FTE = Total salary + Wages/(FTE * Wage index) = $65,432; minimum, $56,857, Massachusetts; maximum, $75,616, Maine
- Salaries and wages as % of total operating expenses = 41.0%; range: 35.5% (25th) to 45.6% (75th)
- Capital cost per discharge = (Inpatient interest + Depreciation)/Discharges = $513; range: $324 (25th) to $770 (75th)
- Depreciation as % of total operating expenses = 4.9%; range: 3.7% (25th) to 6.2% (75th)

- CMI- and wage-adjusted capital cost per discharge = (Inpatient interest + Depreciation)/(Discharges * All patient CMI * Wage index) = $352; range: $257 (25th) to $476 (75th)
- Salaries per discharge = Inpatient salaries/Discharges = $3,849; minimum, $2,598, Louisiana; maximum, $7,401, Alaska
- CMI- and wage-adjusted salaries per discharge = Inpatient salaries/(Discharges * All patient CMI * Wage index) = $2,382; minimum, $1,994, Utah; maximum, $3,250

If the cost per discharge is higher than average, unit cost indicators should be used to identify where major deviations arise between the institution and industry standards. Even if a hospital's cost per discharge is equivalent to the industry average, these indicators can be used to identify cost-saving opportunities in labor and capital expenses. Instead of the 25th and 75th percentiles, wage indicators provide the minimum and maximum expenses to highlight how costs differ across the country.

FIGURE 12.3 highlights the role operating indicators can play in identifying improvement opportunities. Profitability, at the top of the diagram, identifies whether profits in inpatient and outpatient services meet expectations. If profits are less than desired, the deficiency must arise from inadequate revenues or excessive expenses. The revenue indicators examine whether the deficiency arises from low inpatient or outpatient prices, excessive contractual discounts to third-party payers, the payer mix, and/or the service (inpatient and outpatient) mix. The other cause of low profits is excessive expenses; the expense indicators track utilization of fixed resources, efficiency of variable resources, and unit (input) costs.

Given the operating indicators reported, low profits are the result of losses on inpatient care. Given extensive fixed reimbursement systems, it is unlikely a hospital could successfully raise prices. Price increases would widen the

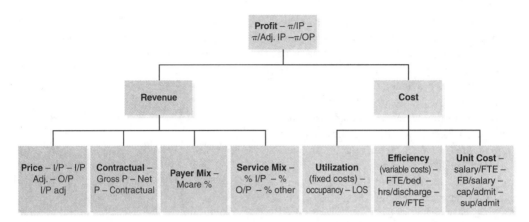

FIGURE 12.3 Operating Indicators

gap between gross charges and net payments and increase the contractual adjustment. Revenue-improving action may be limited to targeting payers with higher reimbursement or growing outpatient care, given its positive returns.

Actions to reduce expenses may include increasing occupancy to spread fixed costs over a larger patient base and generate more revenue. One means to improve occupancy is to increase the LOS, but given Medicare provides 40.3% of all discharges, this would increase expenses without increasing revenue for a large percentage of patients. Reducing variable expenses should be considered; reducing staff hours per bed should have an immediate and positive impact on profitability. The third approach examines input consumed: is the organization paying too much for labor, are wages or fringe benefits too generous, and are supply, capital, and malpractice costs per discharge too high?

Determining whether an institution is earning less than it should using ratio analysis is the launch pad for exploring whether revenues are inadequate or expenditures for inputs are excessive. Operating indicators provide specific data to pinpoint areas where and why revenues are lower or costs are higher than peer institutions so that managers can improve

their departments and the net income of the organization.

▶ Benchmarking

Benchmarking seeks to provide managers with valid measures of comparison to determine whether departmental or organizational performance is superior or substandard and whether it is improving, deteriorating, or remaining stable. The ratios and operating indicators examined were based on industry standards, but there are other sources of information managers may use to encourage performance improvement. The main point is the source and accuracy of the data may be less important than if the information propels positive action.

Benchmarking is commonly seen as a process of comparing an organization's processes and outcomes against those of other organizations. Benchmarking is a shorthand and ongoing method of improvement that does not require organizations to discover better ways of doing things or reinvent practices used by others. Camp and Detoro state that benchmarking "ensures the best practices are uncovered, adopted and implemented" (Juran & Godfrey, 1999). A *best practice* is defined as a method or technique that consistently shows superior results to those achieved through other means (BusinessDictionary, 2011).

Benchmarking can also be performed internally, where targets can be based on the performance achieved by other departments or the historical performance of a single department. The goal, whether internal or external targets are used, is to determine how an organization or department is performing and identify areas where improvements can be made. If an external benchmark is used, the initial target could be to achieve the average performance of the industry. Once an organization achieves average industry performance, managers should set their sights on reaching the performance of organizations deemed best-in-class. One of the advantages of benchmarking is the establishment of credible improvement goals. Employee awareness that superior performance has been achieved in other places or by rivals should encourage improvement.

BOX 12.2 describes four major types of benchmarks. The type of benchmarking pursued will be determined by the organization's goals and the availability of information. Internal benchmarking is the fastest and easiest to undertake as the organization controls the information. Internal benchmarking could entail comparing the current performance of a process to history or the performance of one department to a similar department. The LOS, hours per discharge, or unit costs of one surgical nursing unit could be compared to historical rates or the performance of similar units in the same period.

Industry benchmarking involves comparing the organization's performance against the industry average or best-in-class performance. The complication in implementing industry benchmarking is locating data: is industry data available through trade associations or in published reports? Current performance should dictate the benchmark target. Organizations lower than the industry average should first target the mean; organizations higher than the industry average should strive for the upper quartile or the performance of industry leaders.

Competitive benchmarking seeks to meet or exceed the performance of rival organizations, that is, organizations pursuing the same customers. The obvious problem in implementing competitive benchmarking is that rivals do not share information. Knowledge of a rival's superior performance could dilute the rival's competitive advantage, and knowledge of your own superior performance could provide the basis for an effective marketing campaign. The goal of every organization should be to provide superior value to its customers than the competition.

The final type of benchmarking is functional; this requires the organization to identify a recognized leader in the performance of a process. An advantage of functional benchmarking is that the recognized leader may not be in the same industry and may be willing to share its methods. For example, hospitals have multiple different functions such as room scheduling, guest relations, and food service. The best performers in these functions may be found in the hospitality industry, and hotels and restaurants may be willing to share their expertise with healthcare organizations.

The Benchmarking Process

The first step in the benchmarking process is to determine what to benchmark. Managers should understand what patients, physicians,

---

BOX 12.2 Types of Benchmarking

1. Internal or historical
2. Industry average or best-in-class performance
3. Competitive
4. Functional

and third-party payers want, and these wants encompass both financial and nonfinancial components. Financial performance may be lower than desired because of the organization's inability to meet patient or physician expectations or third-party payers' demand for cost-effective care. The benchmark targets must be important (relevant) to customers if benchmarking is going to be impactful. Processes or outputs to be benchmarked may be selected on the basis of the frequency of complaints, a high number or rate of defects, or high cost.

The second step is to identify a benchmark the organization will strive for. What should be the goals or targets the organization will attempt to achieve? External benchmarks may be used when the goal is to achieve a competitive advantage over rivals operating in the same market or to achieve better-than-average performance or best-in-class performance.

The third step is to determine how targets will be achieved. Assume an organization seeks to be the lowest-cost provider in its market. The recognition that its total cost per adjusted discharge is higher than other hospitals should encourage change and raise questions as to how costs can be lowered. Rivals will not be willing to share trade secrets that could decrease their competitiveness; however, managers may be able to find providers in another geographic region who are willing to share information. The probability of information exchange will be increased if the information-seeking organization offers an opportunity for collaborative benchmarking (a fifth type of benchmarking). Collaborative benchmarking involves a two-way flow of information, where each organization is recognized as having superior performance in a given area and both organizations can learn from each other. Collaborative benchmarking provides the potential for partnership and mutual gain.

Lean Six Sigma offers three approaches to analyzing and optimizing processes: value stream map, product process flow, and operator full-work analysis. Value stream mapping documents the major activities in a process,

with an eye toward improving work and eliminating redundant or non-value-adding steps. Product process flow follows the product (the patient) to determine where value is added or lost because of unnecessary delays. Similarly, operator full-work analysis documents how workers use time, whether they are engaged in activities that please customers (necessary but non-value-adding activities), or whether they are idle. The three foci, process, product, and labor, all aim to increase customer satisfaction and reduce waste. Both ends must be realized for a hospital to be successful as the lowest-cost provider (**BOX 12.3**).

Functional benchmarking is used to identify a best-in-class performer from inside or outside the industry. Identifying a best-in-class performer from outside one's industry does not raise competitive concerns and may increase the probability that the best-in-class performer will share information. A prime example of functional benchmarking was the recognition that LL Bean had a world-class order-processing system. LL Bean's reputation led companies like Xerox and Chrysler to study and adopt its order-filling process (Heizer & Render, 1996). The focus of functional benchmarking is not what is produced but rather how operations are run; thus manufacturers of copiers and automobiles could learn how to improve their order-filling processes from a retail firm specializing in clothing and outdoor equipment.

The final step is organizing resources to achieve targets. Leadership is essential to ensure staff is motivated toward achieving the targets and monitoring systems are in place to assess and communicate performance to

---

BOX 12.3 Benchmarking Steps

1. Determine the area of concern (complaints, defects, cost, etc.).
2. Identify and set performance targets.
3. Determine how to achieve targets.
4. Organize resources and motivate staff to achieve or exceed targets.

employees. Change will be unsuccessful if management lacks credibility, if performance and outcomes are not measured, and/or if performance is not tied to compensation.

There are four essential prerequisites to benchmarking. The first is an organization must be committed to the process and carry it through to its conclusion (Goetsch & Davis, 2010). Senior management should understand the benefits of benchmarking, be committed to the process, and be actively involved to demonstrate to employees why benchmarking should be embraced by everyone in the organization. If senior managers announce a benchmarking program and delegate responsibility to lower-level employees, the message subordinate employees will receive is that benchmarking is not important to senior staff, and they will subsequently assign it a low priority.

Second, benchmarking programs must be consistent with the organizational vision and its strategic objectives. The first step in the benchmarking process requires that employees understand their customers; in health care, this requires providers to recognize what attracts patients, physicians, or insurers. Benchmarking should identify and track patient-valued activities and their costs. If benchmarking compares product or service attributes that patients place little or no value upon, the program will not enhance organization performance and will simply add another bureaucratic record-keeping task.

The third prerequisite is the organization must be open: managers and employees should avoid the "not invented here" mentality. Employees should not think so highly of themselves and their work that they fail to recognize they can learn from others, including organizations they may consider inferior. The second element of openness is a willingness to change. Recognizing that improvement can be made is only the first step; managers must develop a culture willing to accept the risks that accompany learning new ways of doing things and changing work processes.

The final prerequisite is that managers and employees must understand current processes,

products and services, support services, and customer desires. Implementing change when one is unfamiliar with current practices is a random process with an equal probability of improving or reducing outcomes. Benchmarking identifies a goal, but the third step of the process, determining how to achieve targets, requires clear ends and means thinking. What are the opportunities in the current processes to increase revenue and/or reduce costs, and what changes can be introduced to capture these opportunities?

The primary goal of benchmarking is self-assessment: is the organization performing effectively and efficiently? System effectiveness is measured by outcome: does a good or service satisfy the need or desire it was created for? Efficiency concerns output: did expended resources produce the maximum amount of goods or services? Successful organizations must be effective and efficient; organizations that fail on either measure will lose customers to higher-performing providers. The first question benchmarking should answer is, are the desired results being achieved? If the desired results are being achieved, the second question is, are the results being produced at the lowest-possible cost? A successful provider must not only produce what patients want but also produce the desired goods and services at prices patients and third-party payers are willing to pay.

The absence of any prerequisite, senior management commitment, openness, the selection of benchmarks that enhance an organization's competitiveness, or an understanding of current processes and products, will doom a benchmarking project. **BOX 12.4** details these and other obstacles that frequently undermine benchmarking programs. The first obstacle is a lack of senior management support: if senior management does not devote itself to the program, lower-level employees will do the same. Deming (1982, p. 21) reports the response sent to a vice president wanting to observe the quality program at Nashua Corporation: " . . . and if you can't come, send nobody." The point is clear: either quality improvement is worth devoting senior staff time to, or it should not

BOX 12.4 Obstacles to Benchmarking

1. Insufficient senior management support
2. Organizational culture and the illusion of uniqueness
3. Poorly chosen or defined objectives
4. Lack of employee buy-in
5. Poor team composition
6. Overemphasis on processes rather than goals
7. Too high or too low benchmark objectives
8. Too little or too much time provided for implementation
9. Lack of data
10. Insufficient resources
11. Physician and stakeholder opposition

be undertaken. Expectations are set at the top of the organization, and when senior managers demonstrate an initiative is not worth their time, lower-level behavior follows their example.

The second obstacle is cultural: are employees excessively internally focused and have illusions of uniqueness? An excessive internal focus is the opposite of openness: organizations that see themselves or their processes as unique cannot imagine they can learn from others. The "not invented here" attitude dismisses the effectiveness of other organizations' processes and/or ability of these processes to be applied to the organization's problems.

In one case, a hospital's admissions department believed its admissions process was so unique that it could not use existing software but had to create its own system. Not only was the admissions process similar to the 5000+ other hospitals in the country, the process also shared characteristics with the check-in function of the hotel industry. If the admissions staff could have seen beyond themselves, they would have learned other organizations' admissions and check-in processes moved patients and guests to their rooms in significantly less time and with less error.

To address employee resistance to adopting methods developed by other organizations, Camp and Detoro (Juran & Godfrey, 1999) emphasize that benchmarking is not simply the blind copying of processes of other organizations. Benchmarking requires recognizing the superior results of other organizations and the ability to creatively adapt another organization's processes to one's operations. Those who believe their uniqueness will be lost by using processes developed outside their organization miss the point of making comparisons. The point is to improve activities where others demonstrate superior performance, while retaining those aspects of operations that have delivered superior outcomes.

The third obstacle is a poorly defined and/or communicated benchmarking objective. Often the benchmark goal is too broadly defined; poor goals include increasing profit or improving quality. While these goals summarize what managers want, their broadness fails to provide direction or motivation. Superior goals provide clear direction to employees and address issues important to patients and employees. Superior benchmark targets would be reducing hours per admission by four hours or reducing the cost per admission by $500. Beyond establishing a worthwhile goal, employees need to understand why the goal was selected and how the organization (and they) will benefit if the target is achieved.

The fourth obstacle is related to the first three obstacles: lack of employee buy-in. Lack of buy-in may arise from poorly defined objectives or targets that are not accepted or internalized by employees. Profitability objectives regularly fail to motivate healthcare workers who see their jobs as improving patient health, so benchmarks must be formulated to appeal to the interests of employees. If employees see the process as adding another unproductive task to their workload without a corresponding reduction in other tasks or the addition of resources, they will be unlikely to embrace the improvement initiative. Employee commitment will parallel the dedication exhibited by senior management, and if senior managers are detached from the process and satisfied with the current performance, this attitude will permeate all levels of the organization.

The fifth problem is poor team composition. The benchmark team must include members who understand medical processes, patient needs and desires, and benchmark goals and processes and have the authority to institute change. A mix of talent is essential to ensure benchmarks are properly chosen, operations are examined from medical and process perspectives, and necessary actions are taken.

Another common problem in many organizations is the means become more important than the ends, the outcome sought. In benchmarking, this tendency manifests itself by an overemphasis on data collection rather than process improvement. Managers and employees who lose sight of the goal of improving operations end up creating and filing reports but are unable to use the benchmark data to focus on areas of opportunity. Creating a benchmark report will have no impact if it is not used to evaluate processes, drill down to discover the source of performance gaps, and identify ways of enhancing operations.

The seventh obstacle is the specific benchmark targets may be set too high or too low. Setting a target too high may demoralize staff if the objective cannot be reached. An example of oversetting goals may be the use of benchmarks achieved by a teaching hospital for a community hospital. Differences in the structure and patient mix of hospitals may preclude one institution from meeting the performance of another. Objectives can also be set too low and provide no challenge to employees and require no change. If the target is set at the industry average, 50% of hospitals will have already met or exceeded the goal without taking any action. Benchmarks should set targets that require improvement and are challenging and obtainable.

The eighth obstacle arises from how benchmarking is implemented and when results are expected. Given the magnitude of the improvement sought, managers should not expect rapid results. When employees believe the demands for rapid improvement are too much, too soon they will be demoralized and discouraged. On the other hand, an overly long implementation may telegraph a lack of urgency and encourage the belief that other matters should take precedence, resulting in no action. Managers walk a fine line between pushing too far too fast and allowing workers to determine when and what is undertaken. Managers should set goals of slow and steady progress toward a target and continually communicate achievements to workers.

Obstacles that are more apparent in health care than other organizations include a lack of information, insufficient resources to run a benchmarking program, and stakeholder opposition. Health care is data rich and information poor. The primary problem facing health care is a lack of integration of information systems within organizations and the fragmentation of care between providers. Healthcare organizations frequently employ different information systems for different tasks, hindering the ability to derive benchmarks. Providers often have different registration, medical record, clinical, inventory, payroll, billing, and accounting systems that do not talk to each other. Nonintegrated systems complicate work for employees who must use information across platforms. Between providers, there is the problem of different and incompatible systems, making it impossible to compile a comprehensive record of patient care.

Benchmarking must overcome the perception and values of healthcare professionals; there is widespread perception that health care is understaffed and workers are being asked to do more. Healthcare professionals value delivering patient care above other tasks, and benchmarking programs are often seen as another, dispensable bureaucratic task. Benchmarking should not require extensive data collection by line workers and should emphasize how it can improve care to their patients. Likewise, the support of physicians is essential to successfully implementing benchmarking. Physicians are the primary decision-makers in health care, so benchmarking must be seen as a way to improve healthcare processes and patient outcomes.

While obstacles have doomed many a benchmarking program, Camp (1989) offers an engaging set of reasons employees should embrace benchmarking. Camp makes it evident that internally focused organizations that refuse to utilize the benefits of benchmarking will make decisions on a severely restricted set of information. Internally focused organizations will often fail to identify critical pieces of information, and their decisions regarding customer desires, goals, and processes will often be suboptimal. In three critical areas (identifying customer wants, establishing goals, and measuring performance), internally focused organizations will be operating blind. Benchmarking forces an organization to look beyond itself and observe how other organizations are meeting customer demands, what goals they pursue, and what the productivity of their workforce is.

Camp (1989) presents a compelling case for moving beyond an organization's comfort zone to challenge employees to think about what they are attempting to achieve and how they perform their work. The goal of an externally focused, benchmarking organization is to identify and implement best practices. Only by focusing on objective data can an organization ensure it is providing customers with what they want (versus what employees think they want) and operating efficiently and effectively. Benchmarking is a data-driven approach to process improvement that relies on identifying processes and outcomes where others have demonstrated higher performance. Benchmarks provide stark examples that processes can be improved and models for the types of changes that can be implemented to improve output and increase competitiveness.

One of the chief benefits of benchmarking is it signals managers are beginning to explicitly examine what the organization does and what it achieves. Rather than accepting the *status quo*, benchmarking highlights the possibilities for improvement and establishes expectations and goals. When goals are based on the results achieved by other organizations, especially outcomes achieved by rivals, they can provide a strong motivation for change.

Industries and rivals do not stand still, so benchmarking is not a one-time review of operations but a continuous process. This assessment should be directed toward identifying changes in performance as well as shifts in what measures are being tracked. **FIGURE 12.4** demonstrates two of the potential benefits of benchmarking, identifying performance gaps and communicating goals and progress.

Benchmarking facilitates improvement in three ways. Improvement first arises from recognizing the gap between organizational performance (the solid line in Figure 12.4)

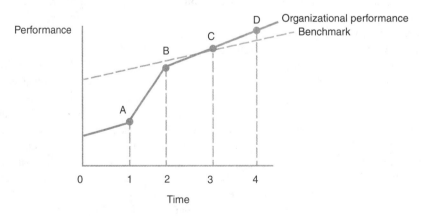

FIGURE 12.4 Improving Performance Through Benchmarking

and the benchmark, industry average or best-in-class performance (the dashed line). While the organization's and the benchmark's performances are assumed to be improving (organizations that stand still will fall behind their improving competitors), the recognition of a gap between the organization and the benchmark should lead to the adoption of new processes and dramatic improvement, that is, capturing low-hanging fruit.

Between time 0 and time 1, the organization is unaware it has inferior performance, and recognition of the large gap at time 1 (point A) leads it to adopt new methods. Stage 2 documents the implementation of new methods that produce rapid improvement from point A to B. After new methods are adopted, they must be refined to capture their full potential; the movement from point B to C documents the gradual refinement until the industry average is reached. The third stage, time 3 to 4, arises from the desire of employees to push beyond the industry average toward best-in-class performance. Once the organization reaches best-in-class performance, point D, employees will not have any model to follow and must rely on continuous quality improvement (CQI) or the plan-do-check act (PDCA) cycle to propel further improvement.

Benchmarking is most effective when it is initiated and operated by the employees closest to the process who have the greatest understanding of patient needs and desires and how work is performed. These employees will need assistance from quality improvement and finance personnel to identify performance targets and implement change. The goal is to establish a system of self-management where employees know desired goals, monitor their performance, and initiate changes when they see fit.

Summary

Ratio analysis and operating indicators explore financial analysis at the organizational and operational levels. Profitability ratios examine net income from the perspective of the amount of equity invested, investment in assets, and sales required to produce operating results. Turnover ratios assess the productivity of assets, while liquidity and capital structure ratios examine the short-term and long-term ability to manage debt. Profitability ratios ultimately assess the ability of management to make decisions and take action that increases the value of the organization.

DuPont analysis provides a single-shot picture of financial performance from the owners' perspective that the purpose of the organization is to generate the maximum-possible ROE. The ROE is a function of the managers' ability to convert a dollar of sales into profit (total margin), maximize the amount of sales from assets employed (total asset turnover), and optimize the amount of assets financed by equity (equity multiplier). The results of ratio and DuPont analyses are often compared against industry averages to assess how an organization measures up with similar organizations. The ROE may compare favorably or unfavorably with other organizations, but in either case, managers should recognize where improvements can be made or cost-saving opportunities lie.

Improvements to financial performance are rarely made at the organizational level but, rather, require identifying opportunities in departments. Information at the organizational level, financial statements, may suggest revenues are too low and/or expenses are too high, but they cannot identify why inflows are low or outflows are high. The first step toward identifying why and what to do is calculating operating indicators at the organizational and departmental levels; on the revenue side, this includes profitability, price, contractual adjustments, payer mix, and service mix, and on the expense side, this includes utilization, efficiency, and intensity indicators. Operating indicators tie financial performance to inputs used, activities performed, and outputs produced to more precisely identify where improvements can be made.

Benchmarking often provides the final encouragement to initiate action based on the insights provided by operating indicators: which departments and what specific aspects of their operation offer the greatest opportunity for improvement? Given prices, payer mixes, and operating expenses vary by department and program, what prices are set too low, where are unfavorable patient mixes reducing revenues, which production processes can be improved, and what adjustments should be made? Translating the insights of financial ratios and operating indicators to operational changes requires understanding what each department does and the resources it consumes; improvement cannot be made without information on current outcomes and knowledge of what can be achieved. The focus of ratios and operating indicators on outcomes and processes complements budgeting and provides essential inputs for setting priorities.

Key Terms and Concepts

Benchmarking	Full-time equivalent (FTE)	Profitability ratios
Capital structure ratio	Liquidity ratios	Ratio analysis
DuPont analysis	Operating indicators	Turnover ratios

Discussion Questions

1. Explain the purpose of financial ratios.
2. Discuss the various components of the DuPont analysis formula and how it provides an overview of financial operations.
3. What issues should an analyst consider when using financial ratios for comparing organizations?
4. Explain the role of and calculate and interpret operating indicators.
5. Explain the purpose and different types of benchmarking.

Problems

1. Problems 1 through 4 reference the balance sheet and income statement of Tanvon Health System, available as a Microsoft Excel file in Chapter12.xlsx, Problem 12.1 tab. Calculate the following ratios:

	2017	2018
Current ratio	_____	_____
Days cash on hand	_____	_____
Days in AR	_____	_____
Debt ratio	_____	_____
Debt to equity	_____	_____
Times interest earned	_____	_____

Cash flow coverage	_____	_____
Total asset turnover	_____	_____
Current asset turnover	_____	_____
Fixed asset turnover	_____	_____
Total margin	_____	_____
Return on equity	_____	_____

2. Explain for the following ratios the calculated results, whether the financial performance improved or deteriorated, and why the ratio increased or decreased:
   A. Days cash on hand
   B. Times interest earned
   C. Total asset turnover
   D. ROE

3. Prepare a DuPont analysis of the organization and discuss the change in the ROE.

4. Comment on the change in the financial condition of this organization on the basis of your analysis and provide any specific operating recommendations, as needed, to improve financial performance.

Income Statement—Tanvon Health System

	2017	2018
Operating revenue	$511,256,300	$568,318,572
Nonoperating revenue	$68,246,711	$89,297,336
Total revenue	$579,503,011	$657,615,908
Expenses		
Salaries and wages	$222,614,230	$234,705,059
Fringe benefits	$48,064,237	$59,474,808
Supplies	$37,871,064	$38,504,945
Lease	$40,419,807	$39,043,322
Information technology	$18,188,560	$19,802,431

(continues)

Income Statement—Tanvon Health System		*(continued)*
Expenses		
Depreciation	$51,297,583	$58,480,314
Interest	$24,587,633	$25,927,328
Other	$132,302,939	$151,747,507
Total expenses	$575,346,053	$627,685,714
Profit	$4,156,958	$29,930,194
Balance Sheet—Tanvon Health System		
Cash	$489,205,269	$454,025,775
Accounts receivable	$58,162,040	$50,136,237
Inventory	$14,809,503	$16,139,581
Property, plant, and equipment	$657,564,480	$715,810,262
Investments	$224,569,789	$245,903,919
Total assets	$1,444,311,081	$1,482,015,774
Accounts payable	$382,108,428	$384,026,716
Long-term debt	$739,310,809	$745,167,020
Total liabilities	$1,121,419,237	$1,129,193,736
Equity	$322,891,844	$352,822,038

5. Problems 5 through 8 reference the balance sheet and income statement of Oyam Hospital. Operating results have been added for 2017 and 2018, available as an Excel file in Chapter12.xlsx, Problem 12.5 tab. Extend the text analysis from 2016 through 2018 and calculate the following ratios:

	2017	2018
Current ratio	_____	_____
Acid ratio	_____	_____
Days cash on hand	_____	_____
Days in AR	_____	_____
Average payment period	_____	_____
Equity multiplier	_____	_____
Times interest earned	_____	_____
Debt service coverage	_____	_____
Total asset turnover	_____	_____
Current asset turnover	_____	_____
Fixed asset turnover	_____	_____
Total margin	_____	_____
Return on equity	_____	_____
Return on assets	_____	_____

6. Create run charts showing the change in the following ratios from 2015 through 2018. Did financial performance improve or deteriorate?
   A. Total margin
   B. Days in AR
   C. Equity multiplier
   D. Fixed asset turnover

7. Prepare a DuPont analysis of the organization and discuss the change in the ROE.

8. Comment on the change in the financial condition of this organization on the basis of your analysis and provide any specific operating recommendations, as needed, to improve financial performance.

Income Statement	2015	2016	2017	2018
Operating revenue	$766,473,000	$870,598,000	$888,568,000	$933,495,000
Nonoperating revenue	$6,535,000	$6,519,000	$9,285,000	$9,580,000
Total revenue	$773,008,000	$877,117,000	$897,853,000	$943,075,000
Salaries and wages	$311,710,000	$317,583,000	$300,747,000	$320,383,000
Fringe benefits	$66,007,000	$94,759,000	$113,730,000	$108,644,000
Supplies	$150,957,000	$160,468,000	$155,852,000	$163,880,316
Rent	$10,033,000	$10,353,000	$14,720,029	$9,180,000
Depreciation	$32,052,000	$32,247,000	$32,178,000	$32,251,000
Interest	$1,363,000	$819,000	$52,288	$0
Other	$150,963,000	$156,403,000	$183,149,683	$200,358,684
Total expenses	$723,085,000	$772,632,000	$800,429,000	$834,697,000
Profit	$49,923,000	$104,485,000	$97,424,000	$108,378,000
Balance Sheet				
Cash	$25,435,000	$25,270,000	$23,674,000	$25,560,000
Accounts receivable	$181,767,000	$161,841,000	$261,045,000	$226,858,000
Other current assets	$6,575,000	$6,251,000	$6,899,000	$7,181,000
Fixed assets	$495,057,000	$444,822,000	$357,980,000	$457,896,000
Total assets	$708,834,000	$638,184,000	$649,598,000	$717,495,000
Current liabilities	$28,638,000	$32,344,000	$48,098,000	$55,718,000
Current portion of long-term debt	$6,430,000	$7,130,000	$5,456,000	$5,174,000
Long-term debt	$186,444,000	$206,794,000	$158,213,000	$150,044,000
Total liabilities	$221,512,000	$246,268,000	$211,767,000	$210,936,000
Equity	$487,322,000	$391,916,000	$437,831,000	$506,559,000

References

BusinessDictionary. (2011). *Best practice.* Retrieved August 15, 2011, from http://www.businessdictionary .com/definition/best-practice.html

Camp, R. C. (1989). *Benchmarking: The search for industry best practices that lead to superior performance.* Milwaukee, WI: Quality Press.

Deming, W. E. (1982). *Out of the crisis.* Cambridge, MA: Massachusetts Institute of Technology.

Goetsch, D. L., & Davis, S. B. (2010). *Quality management for organizational excellence* (6th ed.). Upper Saddle River, NJ: Pearson Prentice Hall.

Hezier, J., & Render, B. (1996). *Production and operations management* (4th ed.). Upper Saddle River, NJ: Prentice Hall.

Juran, J. M., & Godfrey, A. B. (1999). *Juran's quality handbook* (5th ed.). New York, NY: McGraw-Hill.

Machiavelli, N. (1532). *The prince.* New York, NY: New American Library.

Optum360°. (2016). 2017 *Almanac of hospital financial and operating indicators.* Salt Lake City, UT: Author.

Weston, J. F., & Brigham, E. F. (1978). *Managerial finance* (6th ed.). Hinsdale, IL: Dryden Press.

World Bank. (1995). *Bureaucrats in business.* New York, NY: Oxford University Press.

CHAPTER 13

Capital Budgeting

CHAPTER OBJECTIVES

1. Calculate the time value of money.
2. Explain the steps in building a capital budget.
3. Construct a capital budget.
4. Explain the strengths and weaknesses of capital budgeting.
5. Explain the roles of sensitivity analysis and postexpenditure review in the capital budgeting process.

▶ Introduction

Capital budgeting explores how investments on inputs providing services over a multiyear horizon should be examined versus the 1-year focus of operating budgets in previous chapters. Capital investments are defined by their differences from operating expenditures: they are high-cost, typically multimillion-dollar expenditures and infrequent purchases with long life spans. The use and cost of operating expenses like labor and supplies can be varied rapidly to match resource use with output. When a higher demand for output arises, managers can hire additional workers and/or use overtime and requisition more materials from suppliers. When demand falls, hours can be reduced and supply purchases postponed or cancelled. Complex equipment and facilities,

unlike labor and materials that can be varied on a daily basis, can take months and years to put online and take out of service.

What investors, lenders, and/or taxpayers want to know is whether the benefits of capital investment typically measured as a stream of future net revenues will be greater than, equal to, or less than its cost. Money is expended today for a stream of future, uncertain earnings, so capital investments should be closely scrutinized because of their high cost, the lack of experience managers have with these decisions (versus routine hiring and purchase of supplies decisions), and the difficulty in correcting poor decisions. If a hospital overinvests in capital, constructs too many beds, or doesn't uses its full capacity, the hospital is saddled with acquisition costs (interest, depreciation) and operating expenses (security, maintenance, utilities, etc.) and average total costs (ATCs) are higher than necessary. Once assets are acquired, reselling excess capacity may produce steep losses, if a buyer can be found, due to the limited usability of health-care equipment and facilities. If too few beds or equipment are in place, the hospital may be unable to expand or provide required care and lose patients to other providers (or have to purchase or lease additional capacity at exorbitant prices). Neither losing patients nor incurring higher-than-necessary costs is desirable.

Mikesell (1995, pp. 225–226) recognizes that different types of investments should receive different levels of scrutiny. The key factors in capital budgeting decisions are output, output prices (and revenue), and expenses, and their variability is directly related to the type of investments being considered (**BOX 13.1**). Mandatory investments to comply with health and safety regulations (meet the standard or shut your doors) do not require the same level of review as discretionary investments like replacing existing equipment, expanding existing services, or adding new services. Mandatory investments are not isolated go/no-go decisions—they must be undertaken to continue operations. Managers should know current output, output prices and revenues, and expenses, know how they have changed over time, and be reasonably able to project these variables into the future (in the absence of dramatic industry change). The key question is, should operations be continued? Marginal analysis is not needed; are total revenues greater than total expenses? The key decision for mandatory expenditures is how the mandate will be met, what the capacity and functionality of the investment are, and how they affect its cost.

The second type of capital investment is discretionary replacement of existing capacity; in this case, the question is not whether operations should be continued but at what level. Again, managers should know current output, output prices and revenues, and expenses, know how they have changed over time, and be able to project these variables into the future with some degree of accuracy. Given what was a fixed cost has now become a variable cost, that is, no sunk costs, managers can assess current services and determine whether they should be continued at current levels, expanded, or contracted. Unlike all-or-nothing mandatory investments, marginal analysis may be desirable, for example, if capacity is expanded by 10%, what will be the change in marginal revenue and expenses?

The risk associated with replacement should be minimal in the absence of dramatic industry change. The purchase/do-not-purchase decision is straightforward: Is the service worth continuing at its current scale? Do revenues exceed costs, or is there a compelling community need that may go unmet if operations are reduced or halted? In the absence of an altering scale, the key decision is between higher- and lower-cost methods for continuing current output.

Decisions to expand services are riskier. While managers are knowledgeable about existing operations, there are numerous unknowns associated with expanding a business: Can additional output be sold at existing prices? How much unmet need or desire for the good or service is there? Will prices have to be reduced to sell more, and if so, by how much? How will competitors respond to attempts to increase market share? How will labor markets and suppliers respond to a higher demand for inputs?

Investments to expand operations require more analysis to determine how much additional

---

BOX 13.1 Types of Capital Investments Ranked from Least to Most Scrutiny (Risk)

1. Mandatory
2. Discretionary replacement of existing capacity
3. Discretionary expansion of existing products, services, or markets
4. Discretionary expansion into new products, services, or markets

capacity should be added. Given the uncertainty over future demand, sensitivity analysis should be performed to determine how far below projections demand can fall, prices decline, or costs rise before expansion is undesirable. Marginal analysis is essential; in the absence of nonfinancial goals, marginal revenue should be greater than marginal cost to warrant expansion.

Expansions into new product areas involve the greatest risk because managers may lack knowledge of the good or service, customers, competitors, regulations, etc. These types of investments are subject to the normal variability expected in forecasting output, but they also carry the risk that the initial projection may be wildly inaccurate (like scratch budgeting) because of the organization's lack of expertise in the area. The analysis should recognize and quantify the greater uncertainty of the expected cash flow to determine whether the investment should be undertaken. Approximately 56% of new businesses fail within 4 years, providing insight into the risk organizations face introducing new products or entering new markets.

One of the key features of capital budgeting, especially in the public sector, is a tendency to overestimate the benefits of an expenditure and underestimate costs. Reports of construction costs for public projects running two or three times their original estimates seem to be daily news stories. The F35A joint strike fighter originally was slated to cost $49 million; current estimates after a highly publicized cost drop are $85 million (Popular Mechanics, 2017). When cost estimates are dramatically understated, the question that should be asked since the project cannot generate the return originally promised is, what return will be made? Unfortunately, this question is not routinely asked, and managers seeking to expand their budgets use the foot-in-the-door strategy to acquire additional resources, believing funding will not be reduced even if the investment does not perform as promised. Inertia regularly triumphs, and incrementalism ensures the resources necessary to operate the investment receive annual inflation increases.

The job of capital budgeting is to ensure large, one-time expenditures receive a thorough review and resources flow to their highest-value uses. Capital expenditures made to expand output or enter new areas are strategic decisions that may determine an organization's future and warrant extensive analysis. The estimates of output, revenues, and expenses calculated prior to the expenditure of funds have often constituted the bulk of capital budgeting work, that is, justify the expenditure and get it approved. Like operating budgets, the true value of capital budgeting is based on how well plans are met. Improving the effectiveness of capital budgeting requires postexpenditure analysis. Were the output, revenue, and cost projections accurate, which managers proposed investments that met or exceeded expected performance, and how can the capital budgeting process be improved by learning from past mistakes?

▶ Time Value of Money

One of the biggest differences between an operating budget and a capital budget is time. Operating expenditures are made and revenues are received within a single year, and we are not concerned with differences in purchasing power—a dollar is a dollar. One dollar of revenue (received in December, or the twelfth month of the fiscal year) is roughly equal to a dollar paid out in wages (in January, or the first month of the year) in the absence of hyperinflation. Capital investments provide service and produce revenues over an extended period, 10 or 20 years, so a dollar paid to purchase buildings or equipment in 2018 is worth considerably more than a dollar of revenue received in 2028. The difference in the purchasing power of a dollar expended today and money received in the future is determined by when revenues are received, the number of years in the future, and interest rates. The major differences between capital and operating budgets are the greater unpredictability of future events: predicting events over a multi-year horizon is considerably harder than predicting what will occur in the upcoming year and the declining purchasing power of money, that is, the value of future revenues adds another element of risk.

Making astute investment decisions across time, whether assessing whether money spent today will generate a sufficient return to justify the outlay of funds or how much money will have to be set aside to satisfy a future obligation or goal, requires discounting future cash inflows and compounding current investments. **TABLE 13.1** shows the decline in the purchasing power of the dollar from 2000 to 2016.

The **consumer price index (CPI)**, the average price change seen for a market basket of goods and services purchased by an urban consumer, currently uses 2010 as the base year for establishing when $1.00 purchased $1.00 of goods and services. In 2016, $1.00 could purchase only 90.9¢ of goods and services, as measured in the 2010 purchasing power. Carrying the comparison back to 2000, one would need $1.10 in 2016 to purchase the same amount of goods and services that could be purchased for 79¢ in 2000; in 16 years, the dollar has lost 28.3% of its purchasing power. The value of a single good or service or a set of goods and services measured in current dollars is called its **nominal value,** while the value of a single good or service or a set of goods and services measured in constant dollars, no change in purchasing power, is called its **real value**.

Examining the gross domestic product (GDP) highlights the dramatic difference price increases have on our perception of economic vitality. In 2016 and 2000, the nominal GDP was $18,569B and $11,226B, respectively, and it appears the economy increased by 65.4% ($18,569B/$11,226B), but this comparison ignores the fact that a dollar in 2016 buys fewer goods and services than a dollar in 2000. In terms of the purchasing power, $18,569B in 2016 would only purchase

$13,323.8B, depending on changes in the CPI ($18,569B * 0.79/1.101). The increase in the amount of additional goods and services that were consumed between 2000 and 2016 is 18.7% ($13,323.8B/$11,226B). As consumers, we should not be concerned with nominal prices but rather the amount of real goods and services we can consume.

Time-value-of-money mathematics is the method of comparing monetary magnitudes across time. The present value (PV) (discounting) provides the value today of money received in the future, for example, how much should be paid today for a dollar received 10 years in the future? The future value (FV) (compounding) estimates what the money invested today will grow to in the future, for example, if $1.00 is invested today, what will it be worth 10 years from now? Capital investment requires the expenditure of funds today to receive future cash payments. The primary question is, will the benefits received in the future be greater than the benefit foregone today? PV comparisons must be used to answer this question when the value of a dollar received in the future is less than the value of a dollar today.

The first step in determining the value of future cash flows is to identify the price of using (borrowing) money, that is, the **discount rate**. The three components of the discount rate are (1) **inflation**, a general increase in wages and prices; (2) risk; and (3) deferred gratification. Given the prices of most goods and services are increasing (or the purchasing power of the dollar is decreasing), if money is invested today, the amount received in the future (principal plus interest) to allow the lender (investor) to purchase the same market basket of goods that could be purchased with the funds today must increase. The amount of money received by a lender in the future should have at least the same purchasing power as the money expended today on the investment. For example, if a good is sold for $1.00 in 2000, the same good may sell for $1.39 in 2016 as the purchasing power of the

TABLE 13.1 Purchasing Power of the Dollar, 2000–2016

Year	CPI	Needed to Purchase $1.00 in 2000	Loss of Purchasing Power (%)
2000-01-01	0.790	$1.00	0.0
2001-01-01	0.812	$1.03	2.7
2002-01-01	0.825	$1.04	4.3
2003-01-01	0.844	$1.07	6.4
2004-01-01	0.866	$1.10	8.8
2005-01-01	0.896	$1.13	11.8
2006-01-01	0.925	$1.17	14.6
2007-01-01	0.951	$1.20	17.0
2008-01-01	0.987	$1.25	20.0
2009-01-01	0.984	$1.25	19.7
2010-01-01	1.000	$1.27	21.0
2011-01-01	1.032	$1.31	23.4
2012-01-01	1.053	$1.33	25.0
2013-01-01	1.068	$1.35	26.1
2014-01-01	1.086	$1.37	27.3
2015-01-01	1.087	$1.38	27.4
2016-01-01	1.101	$1.39	28.3

Federal Reserve Economic Data (2017).

dollar decreased by 28.3%. If a lender invested $1 million in 2000 and received a single lump-sum payment in 2016, he or she would have to receive $1,393,820 to purchase the same amount of goods and services as the $1 million would have purchased in 2000.

Second, the interest rate must cover the possibility of default: not all debts are repaid.

Lenders should consider the possibility that loans will not be repaid, as well as the lower purchasing power of money. Charge-off rates are the value of loans removed from the books of banks. In the fourth quarter of 2016, commercial banks removed 0.51% of total loans as uncollectible versus 3.14% in the fourth quarter of 2009 (Board of Governors of the Federal Reserve System, 2017). Loan underwriting assesses the risk of default and offers low interest rates to individuals or organizations with good credit histories and charges high rates to those with poorer histories and less likely to repay loans.

Third, individuals prefer satisfaction today versus in the future (time preference or present bias), so the future stream of benefits must provide lenders with something above inflation and indemnification of default. The interest rate must not only allow lenders to purchase the same amount of goods and services as they could consume today, it must also compensate them for postponing the benefits they could have received from consuming those goods and services today. Assume an individual has $200,000, which could purchase a home. However, rather than purchasing the home, the $200,000 is invested in bonds, or the stock market, for 5 years. If home prices increase 2% annually, the individual will need $220,816 to purchase a comparable house in 5 years, but the return on investment (ROI) should be greater than $220,816 to compensate the investor for the time he or she could have enjoyed living in the home.

The rate of time preference, the willingness to give up current consumption for future consumption, varies by individual. Individuals with low time preference are willing to forego consumption today for slightly more consumption in the future and would settle for an interest rate slightly above the expected inflation rate. Individuals with high time preference want to consume now and must be coaxed into saving (foregoing current consumption) by the prospect of significantly higher consumption in the future; these individuals demand higher interest rates for the use of their funds. Some believe older people have lower time preference, given they have accumulated goods, and thus their demand for consumption is lower than younger people; on the other hand, given their shorter life expectancies, older people may want to consume now rather than bet on an uncertain future. The value of $1.00 received 20 years in the future should be significantly different for a 50- and a 70-year-old.

The **Fisher equation** holds that the nominal interest rate (i) equals the expected inflation rate (π^e) plus the real interest rate (i_r). The real interest or time preference rate (the increase in resources a lender can consume) is believed to be roughly 2.0%. If expected inflation is 3.0%, the nominal interest rate should be 5.0%; if inflation is expected to increase to 5.0%, then interest rates should increase to 7.0%. Equation 13.1 calculates how much a sum of money received in the future is worth today, that is, its PV.

$$PV = \frac{FV}{(1+i)^n}, \qquad (13.1)$$

where PV is the value today of a benefit received in the future, FV is the amount of money received in the future, i is the nominal interest (discount) rate, and n is the number of years in the future.

TABLE 13.2 and **FIGURE 13.1** show the decrease in the value of a dollar on the basis of the discount rate and year received. PVs can be calculated using Microsoft Excel's PV function, $=$**PV(i,n,pmt, $-$FV,type)**. The first and second arguments (**i** and **n**) are the discount rate and the number of years in the future payment is received, respectively. The third argument (**pmt**) is for a series of payments, to be discussed in the annuity section. The fourth argument ($-$**FV**) is the amount of money to be received in the future (the author used a negative sign to produce a positive PV). The fifth argument (**type**) indicates when the payment is received: 0 or blank indicates receipt at the end of year, while 1 indicates payment

TABLE 13.2 Present Value of a Single Sum

Discount Rate =	0%	2%	5%	10%	20%
Year					
0	$1.00	$1.00	$1.00	$1.00	$1.00
1	$1.00	$0.98	$0.95	$0.91	$0.83
2	$1.00	$0.96	$0.91	$0.83	$0.69
3	$1.00	$0.94	$0.86	$0.75	$0.58
4	$1.00	$0.92	$0.82	$0.68	$0.48
5	$1.00	$0.91	$0.78	$0.62	$0.40

is received on the first day of the year. Calculating the PV of $1.00 received in 5 years in the future with a discount rate of 10% gives $=PV(0.10, 5,, -1) = \$0.62$.

Table 13.2 and Figure 13.1 highlight two important characteristics about discounting. The first is that future cash flows are more valuable when the discount rate is low. When the discount rate is 1.0%, a dollar will purchase 99¢ of goods and services at the end of the first year; the same dollar would only purchase 83¢ in goods and services if the discount rate is 20%, that is, money loses value faster as the discount rate increases. At a discount rate of 1.0%, lenders must receive at least $1.01(1/0.99) at the end of the year to induce them to save; if the discount rate is 20%, they must receive $1.20(1/0.83) to equal the purchasing power they had at the beginning of the year.

Second, cash is more valuable the sooner it is received. The value of future cash flows diminishes as the period of time increases before the cash is received. At the end of the first year, with a discount rate of 1.0%, $1.00 purchases 99¢ of goods and services; at the end of 5 years, the dollar is worth only 95¢. Whereas the promise of $1.01 would entice lenders to loan $1.00 for 1 year, $1.051 must be promised to elicit a 5-year loan. A borrower would have to offer $2.488 to potential lenders to obtain a 5-year loan when the discount rate is 20%. The use of PV includes calculating the desirability of stock and bond investments and pension returns.

FV (compounding) is the flip side of PV (discounting): it asks the question, if funds are invested today, what will its nominal value be in

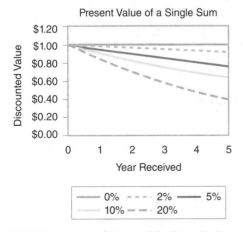

FIGURE 13.1 Impact of Time and the Discount Rate on the Present Value of a Single Sum

the future? Equation 13.2 calculates how much a sum of money invested today (PV) will grow to the future, given the discount rate (i) and the number of years the money is invested (n).

$$FV = PV * (1+i)^n \qquad (13.2)$$

TABLE 13.3 and **FIGURE 13.2** show the increase in the nominal value of an investment on the basis of the discount rate and the number of years invested. FVs can be calculated using Excel's FV function, =**FV(i,n,pmt,** −**PV,type)**. −PV indicates the amount invested at the end of the year when the fifth argument (**type**) is blank or 0. Calculating the FV of $1.00 received in 5 years in the future with a discount rate of 10% gives =FV(0.10,5,,−1.00) = $1.61.

Table 13.3 and Figure 13.2 highlight the two main factors in compounding, first, amounts invested today will be worth more in the future the longer the period of time the funds are invested and second, their value increases with the discount rate. At a discount rate of 5.0%, $1.00 grows to $1.05 after 1 year and $1.276 after 5 years. The impact of compounding is seen in the fact that 5¢ is not earned every year (5.0% of $1.00) but that interest is earned on prior interest earned: in the fifth year, 6.1¢ is earned (5.0% of $1.216). At higher discount rates, compounding works in a similar fashion: at 20%, the accumulated value of $1.00 would grow to $2.07 after 4 years, and 20% interest on the balance would generate an additional increase of 41.5¢ in year 5. The use of FV includes calculating growth in investments invested at fixed interest rates or historical growth rates, for example, stock markets.

Present Value of an Annuity

While PV and FV analyses of a single amount highlight the two critical factors in the time value of money, discount rate and duration, most financial transactions involve a series of future payments. **Annuities** are special cases where future payments or investments are equal. Capital expenditures or the purchase of bonds may provide (or be assumed to create) a series of equal payments, and thus investors examine the PV of the stream of cash flows to determine whether the investment is worthwhile. People setting aside funds

TABLE 13.3 Future Value of a Single Amount					
Discount Rate	**1%**	**2%**	**5%**	**10%**	**20%**
Year					
0	$1.00	$1.00	$1.00	$1.00	$1.00
1	$1.01	$1.02	$1.05	$1.10	$1.20
2	$1.02	$1.04	$1.10	$1.21	$1.44
3	$1.03	$1.06	$1.16	$1.33	$1.73
4	$1.04	$1.08	$1.22	$1.46	$2.07
5	$1.05	$1.10	$1.28	$1.61	$2.49

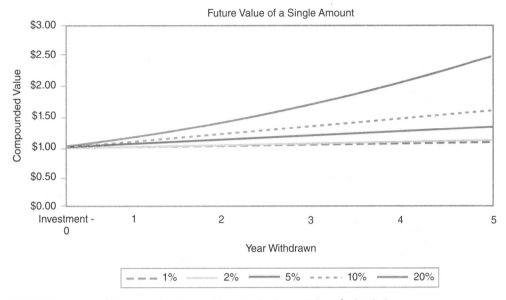

FIGURE 13.2 Impact of Time and the Discount Rate on the Future Value of a Single Sum

for retirement, investing a portion of income during an individual's working life (FV) to fund a series of payments from retirement till death (PV), want to know whether they will have a sufficient nest egg to support them in their expected lifestyle. Savers want to know if they save a certain amount of income each year, how much they will accumulate for retirement, that is, the FV of a series of equal contributions.

A second consideration when dealing with annuities is, when are payments received? An **ordinary annuity** is a series of payments paid or received at the end of the year, while an **annuity due** calculates the value of the cash flow, assuming payments are paid or received on the first day of the year. The difference between an ordinary annuity and an annuity due is 1 year of interest; in a PV of an annuity due, when payment is received at the start of the first year, no purchasing power is lost on the first payment and hence no discounting is required. In an ordinary annuity, payment is received at the end of the year and thus 1 year of purchasing power is lost.

The formula for the PV of an annuity is

$$PV = FV * \frac{\left(1 - 1/(1+i)^n\right)}{i}. \qquad (13.3)$$

Present Value of an Annuity

Assume an investor has an opportunity to receive $100 per year for 5 years at the end of each year. If the discount rate is 0.0%, he or she would be willing to pay $500, given a discount rate of 2.0%, the maximum the investor should pay is $471.35. **TABLE 13.4** shows the PV factor for each year and illustrates that an annuity is simply the sum of the PVs of the individual cash flows. Table 13.4 also shows that the maximum payment for five payments of $100 over 5 years falls to $379.08 when the discount rate is 10.0%. The PV of an annuity can be calculated using Excel's PV function, $=\textbf{PV(i,n,pmt, }-\textbf{FV,type})$. Unlike the single payment received where the cash flow was entered into the fourth argument, $=\textbf{PV(}\textit{i,n,}\textbf{, }-\textbf{FV)}$, a series is indicated in the third argument, **pmt**. Calculating the PV of $100.00 received every year for 5 years with a

TABLE 13.4 Present Value of an Annuity

Year	Nominal Payment	Present Value Factor (2%)	Value of Each Payment	Total Value @ 2%	Total Value @ 5% (5%)	Total Value @ 10% (10%)	Total Nominal
0	$0.00	1.0000	$0.00	$0.00	$0.00	$0.00	$0.00
1	$100.00	0.9804	$98.04	$98.04	$95.24	$90.91	$100.00
2	$100.00	0.9612	$96.12	$194.16	$185.94	$173.55	$200.00
3	$100.00	0.9423	$94.23	$288.39	$272.32	$248.69	$300.00
4	$100.00	0.9238	$92.38	$380.77	$354.60	$316.99	$400.00
5	$100.00	0.9057	$90.57	$471.35	$432.95	$379.08	$500.00
	$500.00		$471.35				

discount rate of 10% gives $=PV(0.10,5,-100)=$ $379.08.

FIGURE 13.3 graphically demonstrates the impact of the discount rate and the length of time to receive payments on the maximum value of an annuity. **TABLE 13.5** demonstrates the impact of payments received at the beginning of the year (an ordinary annuity) versus year-end payments (an annuity due). When the discount

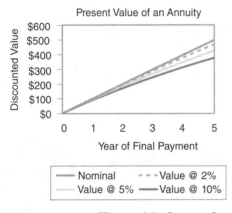

FIGURE 13.3 Impact of Time and the Discount Rate on the Present Value of an Annuity

rate is 10.0% and payments are received on the first day of the year, investors would be willing to pay up to $416.99 for the stream of payments, that is, $500. If payments are received at the end of the year, the value of the cash flow declines, and an investor would be willing to pay a maximum of $379.08; the $37.91 difference is the loss of one additional year on the payments received at the end of the year.

Table 13.5 and **FIGURE 13.4** display how much investors would be willing to pay to receive $100 per year on the basis of how many payments are received and when payments are received when the discount rate is 10.0%.

Future Value of an Annuity

Assume a recent college graduate decides to set aside $1000 per year for retirement. How much will this series of payments be worth in 40 years? Again, the question is, what is the discount rate (or how much interest will be earned on contribution) and when is the contribution made? The FV increases as the discount rate increases and the earlier contributions are

TABLE 13.5 Present Value of an Ordinary Annuity and an Annuity Due

Year	Payment	Value of Each Payment	Ordinary Annuity	Annuity Due	Nominal
0	$0.00	$0.00	$0.00	$0.00	$0.00
1	$100.00	$90.91	$90.91	$100.00	$100.00
2	$100.00	$82.64	$173.55	$190.91	$200.00
3	$100.00	$75.13	$248.69	$273.55	$300.00
4	$100.00	$68.30	$316.99	$348.69	$400.00
5	$100.00	$62.09	$379.08	$416.99	$500.00
		$379.08			

Present Value of Ordinary Annuity and Annuity Due

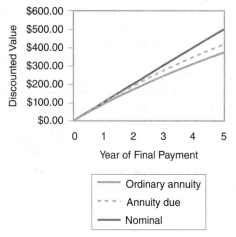

FIGURE 13.4 Impact of Time on the Present Value of an Ordinary Annuity and an Annuity Due

made. If the contribution is made on the first day of the year, the first payment will accrue 40 years of interest, the second 39 years, and so on. If contributions are made on the last day of the year, the first $1000 will only accumulate 39 years of interest, and each subsequent contribution will also receive 1 less year of interest.

Equation 13.4 calculates the FV of an annuity, and **TABLE 13.6** and **FIGURE 13.5** show how much a series of $1000 payments will be worth on the basis of the interest rate and the number of years invested if contributions are made at the beginning or the end of the year.

$$FV = PV * \frac{\left((1+i)^n - 1\right)}{i} \quad (13.4)$$

TABLE 13.6 Future Value of an Annuity

Interest Rate =		4%	8%	0%
Year	Contribution	Ordinary Annuity	Ordinary Annuity	Nominal
0	$0.00	$0.00	$0.00	$0.00
5	$1,000.00	$5,416.32	$5,866.60	$5,000.00
10	$1,000.00	$12,006.11	$14,486.56	$10,000.00
15	$1,000.00	$20,023.59	$27,152.11	$15,000.00
20	$1,000.00	$29,778.08	$45,761.96	$20,000.00
25	$1,000.00	$41,645.91	$73,105.94	$25,000.00
30	$1,000.00	$56,084.94	$113,283.21	$30,000.00
35	$1,000.00	$73,652.22	$172,316.80	$35,000.00
40	$1,000.00	$95,025.52	$259,056.52	$40,000.00
Excel formulas:				
= FV(0.05,40,−1000,,0)		$95,025.52		
= FV(0.08,40,−1000,,0)		$259,056.52		

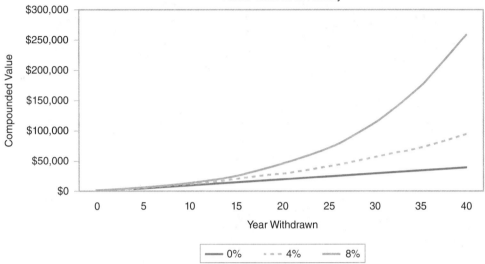

FIGURE 13.5 Impact of Time and the Discount Rate on the Future Value of an Ordinary Annuity

Figure 13.5 dramatically demonstrates the power of compounding; at a 0.0% discount rate, the investor has $40,000 at the end of 40 years, and when the discount rate is 4.0%, the investor will more than double his or her nest egg to $95,025. More remarkably, if the investor selects a riskier investment offering 8.0%, he or she can almost triple the nest egg to $259,057. **TABLE 13.7** and **FIGURE 13.6** demonstrate the impact of first-of-the-year contributions versus waiting until year-end.

Table 13.7 and Figure 13.6 show a $1000 annual contribution invested for 40 years at 8.0% will grow to $259,057 if the contribution is made at the end of each year and $279,781 when payments are made at the start of the year. While contributions made at the start of the year produce an additional $20,725 in interest, both increase the nominal contributions by more than sixfold.

Unequal Cash Flows

It is unlikely that individuals or organizations will be able to make equal contributions or receive equal payments each year. Most

pensions, 401(k) plans, and social security entail contributions based on an individual's income, and pension contributions increase with income. Similarly, social security and some pension benefits are tied to the cost of living and increase annually, which do not meet the criterion of an annuity.

If payments or contributions are not equal, an analyst will have to calculate the value for the payment made or received each year. The following example assumes an organization is evaluating the PV of an investment in a program that produces revenue over 10 years. Revenue is expected to be 50% of an established program in the first year as the patient base is built and increase to capacity in year 2; subsequent years' revenues are expected to increase by 5.0% due to price increases. In year 10, an additional $1 million is expected from the sale of program assets, that is, **salvage value**.

TABLE 13.8 shows the expected cash flows in column 2, the PV factor based on a discount rate of 6.0%, $1/(1 + i)^n$, in column 3, and the PV of the cash flow (PVCF) in column 4 (cash flow * PV factor).

TABLE 13.7 Future Value of an Ordinary Annuity and an Annuity Due				
Interest Rate =	8%			
Year	**Contribution**	**Ordinary Annuity**	**Annuity Due**	**Nominal**
0	$0.00	$0.00	$1,000.00	$0.00
5	$1,000.00	$5,866.60	$6,335.93	$5,000.00
10	$1,000.00	$14,486.56	$15,645.49	$10,000.00
15	$1,000.00	$27,152.11	$29,324.28	$15,000.00
20	$1,000.00	$45,761.96	$49,422.92	$20,000.00
25	$1,000.00	$73,105.94	$78,954.42	$25,000.00
30	$1,000.00	$113,283.21	$122,345.87	$30,000.00
35	$1,000.00	$172,316.80	$186,102.15	$35,000.00
40	$1,000.00	$259,056.52	$279,781.04	$40,000.00
Excel formulas:				
= FV(0.08,40,−1000,,0)		$259,056.52		
= FV(0.08,40,−1000,,1)		$279,781.04		

Table 13.8 demonstrates the impact of the timing of revenues on the expected value of a project; when individual-year revenues are discounted, the total is significantly less than assuming equal cash flows are received. The annuity calculation using an average annual cash flow of $1,252,656 values the cash flow stream at $9,219,660, while calculation matching the expected cash receipts in each period values the stream of payments at $8,744,358—a difference of $475,302, or 3.5%. This result is expected as the low yearly revenues, years 1 and 2, are worth 94% and 89%, respectively, of their nominal value, while high, out-year revenues, years 9 and 10, are worth less than 60% of their nominal value. The PV of unequal cash flows can be calculated in Excel using $=$**NPV(i,cf$_1$,cf$_2$...cf$_n$)**, that is, $=$NPV(0.06, 500,000, 1,000,000,...2477455) = $8,744,358. The reader should note this function discounts the first-year cash flow, assuming it is received on the last day of the year.

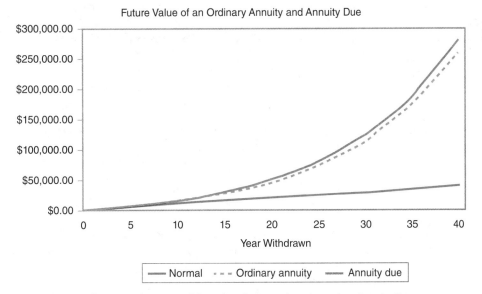

FIGURE 13.6 Impact of Time on the Future Value of an Ordinary Annuity and an Annuity Due

Year	Cash Flow	PV Factor	PVCF
TABLE 13.8 Unequal Cash Flows			
1	$500,000	0.9434	$471,698
2	$1,000,000	0.8900	$889,996
3	$1,050,000	0.8396	$881,600
4	$1,102,500	0.7921	$873,283
5	$1,157,625	0.7473	$865,045
6	$1,215,506	0.7050	$856,884
7	$1,276,282	0.6651	$848,800
8	$1,340,096	0.6274	$840,793
9	$1,407,100	0.5919	$832,861
10	$2,477,455	0.5584	$1,383,398
Average	$1,252,656		$8,744,358
=PV(0.06,10, −1252656)			$9,219,660
Difference			$475,302

SIDEBAR Lotteries: Taxes on the Mathematically Challenged

Lotteries provide a practical, if improbable, example of time value analysis. First, the author does not suggest anyone play a lottery ever; when lotteries are introduced in class, the title of the topic is "Why No One Should Play the Lottery." The primary reason no one should play is it is not a fair gamble: $1.00 wagered does not produce an expected return of $1.00, and as you will see, the only people who should purchase lottery tickets are those who enjoy losing money.

The Powerball prize is enticing; who would not want to win $40,000,000 paid in $1,333,333 installments over 30 years, i.e., the prize on December 19, 2016? However, having reached this point in the text, we know $1,333,333 received over 30 years is *not* worth $40,000,000 in today's purchasing power. The lottery knows this as well and offers winners a lump-sum payment of $23,700,000, or 59.25% of the announced jackpot. The decision whether to take the installments or the lump sum requires the use of PV. First, the winner must determine what the discount rate is; we will assume discount rates of 4.0% and 5.0%.

At 5.0%, the value of 30 payments of $1,333,333 is worth $21,521,431 (assuming an annuity due), and the winner should elect for the lump-sum payment. At 4.0%, the stream of payments is worth $23,978,286, and the 30 installments should be selected.

Of course, none of this explains why no one should play the lottery; understanding this point requires us to determine what the jackpot should amount to in order to be a fair gamble. The odds of winning the jackpot are 1 in 292,201,338, and the bet is $2.00. The simple mathematics is as follows:

$$\text{Bet}: \$2.00 > 8.11 \cent (\$23,700,000 * 1/292,201,338), \text{expected payout}$$

The undesirability of losing $1.92 for every $2.00 wagered should be clear, but the expected payout *overstates* what winners receive. Players use after-tax earnings to purchase tickets, and their winnings are taxable. The maximum U.S. tax rate is 39.6% for income over $415,051 for a single taxpayer and $466,951 for a couple, assuming an average state income tax rate of 5.0% (if you win, you should consider moving to a state without income tax; Alaska leaps to mind). The after-tax loss is thus larger than calculated:

$$\text{Bet}: \$2.00 > 4.49\cent (8.11\cent * (1.00 - 0.396 - 0.05)), \text{after-tax payout}$$

How much should the jackpot amount to in order to be a fair gamble?

The answer is $1,780,385,614. When the jackpot reaches this level, you could purchase every ticket combination and be assured of winning; however, you would only receive your investment back:

$$\text{Bet}: \$2.00 = \$6.09 (\$1,780,385,614 * 1/292,201,338), \text{odds of winning}$$

$$= \$3.61 (\$6.09 * 0.5925), \text{lump-sum payment or present value of winnings}$$

$$= \$2.00 (\$3.61 * (1 - 0.396 + 0.05)), \text{after-tax payout}$$

Of course, to get your bet back, you must make the strong assumption that only one player matches all the jackpot numbers. The author would rather toss $2.00 out the car window, knowing that the satisfaction of someone's finding the money would be greater than the dissatisfaction of wagering $2.00 to win 4.49¢.

Practical Considerations

Having examined the theoretical factors of the time value of money, it is time to examine how capital investment analyses should be structured. The first issue is determining the discount rate to use, or the cost of capital/capital hurdle rate. Organizations have choices in their source of funds: they can use debt, equity, or a combination of debt and equity. The use of equity funding is more expensive than debt financing because of the fact that equity holders are residual claimants (the last to be paid) in the event of default and assume greater risk.

Selecting a Discount Rate

The equity discount rate is the return on equity (ROE). In Table 12.4, the ROE for Oyam in 2015 was 10.24% ($49,923,000 earned on $487,322,000 of equity). Stockholders in publicly traded corporations calculate the discount rate as the dividend yield plus the expected increase in stock price. For example, a stock selling for $40.00 with a $1.00 dividend that is expected to sell for $44.00 in 1 year would have a discount rate of 12.5%, $1.00/$40.00 + ($44.00 − $40.00)/$40.00 = 2.5% + 10.0%. When discount rates increase, investment decreases as it is more difficult to identify projects that earn more than the discount rate.

Assume a desired project cannot meet the equity discount rate; to make it more financially enticing, a discount rate based on lower cost, debt financing, could be used. One way of determining the debt financing rate would be to use the current interest rate available through banks or bond markets; current interest rates on 30-year treasury bonds are 2.95% (Yahoo, 2017). A second method uses the average cost of debt. The chapter "Ratio Analysis and Operating Indicators" shows Oyam paid $1,363,000 in interest on $221,512,000 of debt in 2015, or an interest rate of 0.6%. The use of a discount rate under 1.0% will expand the field of desirable projects greatly; future borrowing,

however, is unlikely to obtain an interest rate at 0.6%, so current interest rates should be used.

A midpoint between the use of the equity discount rate and the interest rate on debt is the use of the weighted average cost of capital (WACC). The WACC calculates the discount rate on the basis of the cost of equity and debt and the percentage of assets financed by each means.

$$\text{WACC} = w_e * c_e + \left(1 - w_e\right) * d_e, \quad (13.5)$$

where w_e is the percentage of equity in the capital structure (equity/total assets), c_e is the cost of equity (ROE), $(1 - w_e)$ is the percentage debt in the capital structure (total liabilities/total assets), and d_e is the cost of debt (current or average interest rate).

$$\text{For Oyam, WACC} = 68.75\% * 10.24\% \\ + \left(100\% - 68.75\%\right) \\ * 0.6\% = 7.23\%.$$

The WACC is higher than the return on assets (ROA) as the ROA is profit/total assets and the WACC is (profit + interest expense) / total assets.

The project cost of capital is a fourth approach that analyzes the riskiness of the individual investment rather than using an organizationally determined discount rate. Are the revenues and expenses from the project expected to be more or less variable than the overall organization? If net revenue is expected to be more variable than the overall organization, the discount rate should be increased. For example, if the variability of project net income is expected to be 20% greater than the total organization, the discount rate could be raised to 8.68% (1.20 * 7.23%). Similarly, if revenues are guaranteed and expenses are locked in, the variability of project net income may be less than the overall organization and the discount rate can be reduced. If the variability of project net income is expected to be 20% less than the overall organization, then the discount rate could be reduced to

5.78% (0.80 * 7.23%). A second way of calculating a project-specific discount rate would use the actual mix of financing expected. If the project is expected to be 20% equity and 80% debt-financed (assuming current interest rates on debt are 5.0%), then the discount rate would be 6.05% ([0.20 * 10.24%] + [0.80 * 5.0%]).

Selecting an Evaluation Measure to Compare Projects

The selection of a higher or lower discount rate reduces or increases the economic desirability of a project; a second factor that affects the probability that a project will be pursued is the evaluation measure used to rank projects. There are four frequently used evaluation measures: net present value (NPV), payback period, benefit–cost ratio (BCR), and internal rate of return (IRR). The NPV ranks projects on the basis of their total discounted net cash flow from the highest amount to the lowest. The payback period identifies how many years of revenue are needed to recoup investment and ranks projects from the shortest recovery period to the longest. The BCR calculates the return earned per dollar of investment, and the IRR calculates the discount rate that equates discounted cash inflows and outflows; both rank projects from the highest to the lowest percentage returns.

In situations in which an organization has more funds available than projects, the use of a ranking method is academic; all projects that surpass the discount rate can be pursued. In capital-rationing situations, where organizations have requests for funds that exceed available funding, the choice of an evaluation measure can alter the order in which projects are pursued.

The NPV is built on the time value of money and recognizes that an investment must generate revenues greater than the cost of the investment. The NPV discounts and totals the cash inflows received each year (PVCF) and subtracts the PV of the investment (−PV investment), producing the net

profit or loss resulting from pursuing a project. Equation 13.6 assumes the investment is made in year 0 and does not discount the initial cash outflow. If additional cash outflows occur after year 0, they should be discounted.

$$NPV = \frac{CF_1}{(1+i)^1} + \frac{CF_2}{(1+i)^2} + \cdots \frac{CF_n}{(1+i)^n} - Investment_0 \qquad (13.6)$$

The decision rule to determine whether a project should be pursued is that if $NPV \geq 0$, invest; if $NPV < 0$, do not invest. If $NPV = 0$, the project is producing sufficient revenue to cover the investment; if $NPV > 0$, the project produces more revenue than the investment and the organization will be better off if the project is pursued. If $NPV < 0$, the organization will have less funds available and be less capable if the project is undertaken.

Under capital rationing or mutual exclusivity of projects, the decision rule is invest in the highest-NPV project(s), those that produce the largest net cash inflows, until investment funds are exhausted. The chief problem with the NPV is it does not consider the size of the investment, that is, its focus on total net dollar return produces an inherent bias towards large projects that should produce larger revenues than smaller projects. **TABLE 13.9** compares two projects: project A requires an investment of $500,000 in year 0, and project B $360,000; both produce revenues over 5 years.

Project A can be analyzed as an annuity **=PV($i,n,$-cf)-investment**, while the uneven cash flows generated by project B require the use of **=NPV(i,cf$_1$,cf$_2$...cf$_n$)**; this function discounts the year 0 investment (cf$_1$), and subsequently the first year of cash inflows (cf$_2$) is discounted 2 years. If no discount is wanted for the initial cash outflow, the analyst can enter **=NPV(rate,cf$_1$,cf$_2$... cf$_n$)-investment$_0$**. In this example, the NPV prefers project A over project B due to the higher level of discounted cash generated.

The payback period is the second and least complicated evaluation measure in that it does not discount future cash flows and only

TABLE 13.9 NPV Comparison of Projects A and B

	PVCF	Investment	NPV
$NPV_A =$	$649,422	−$500,000	= $149,422[a]
$NPV_B =$	$460,786	−$360,000	= $100,786

[a] Project selected based on NPV.

TABLE 13.10 Payback Period Comparison of Projects A and B

	Investment	Cash Inflow	Payback
$Payback_A =$	$500,000	/$150,000	=3.33 years
	$500,000	−$150,000 − 150,000 − 150,000 − (0.33 * 150,000) = 0	
		Year 1 + Year 2 + Year 3 + 0.33 * Year 4 = 3.33	
$Payback_B =$	$360,000	−$150,000 − 130,000 − 0.73 * 110,000 = 0	
		Year 1 + Year 2 + 0.73 * Year 3 = 2.73[a]	

[a] Project selected based on payback period.

focuses on how many years of cash inflow are needed to recoup the year 0 investment. The payback period is

$$\text{Payback period}(\text{years}) = \frac{\text{Investment (outflow)}}{\text{Average cash inflow}},$$

(13.7)

or

in the case of uneven cash flows

$$\text{Payback period} = \text{Investment} - cf_1 - cf_2$$
$$\dots cf_n \text{ until cash outflow} = \text{inflow.}$$

Managers may arbitrarily set a maximum number of years as the decision rule to determine acceptable projects, for example, investments with a payback period of 5 years or less. When investment funds are limited and not all projects can be financed, invest in the projects with the shortest payback periods until funds are exhausted. Revisiting projects A and B, **TABLE 13.10**, shows project B recoups its investment 0.6 years faster than project A and is more desirable when the payback period is the evaluation measure.

The first problem associated with the payback period is it ignores the time value of money. If project A only produced $150,000 each year for 3 years and $50,000 in year 4, it would not repay the initial investment because of the lower purchasing power of money received in years 1–4 relative to when funds were expended in year 0. Second, it ignores postpayback cash flows, that is, inflows received after 2.73 or 3.33 are ignored by the analysis; the higher these postrecoupment cash inflows are and the longer they continue, the more the desirability of the investment increases.

The NPV and payback period have created a quandary: the NPV favors project A, while the payback period favors project B. The BCR remedies the problems associated with each by incorporating the size of the investment (ignored by the NPV after the investment is recovered) and discounting future cash flows (ignored by the payback period), **TABLE 13.11**. The BCR determines the rate of return earned per dollar of investment. The formula is

$$BCR = \frac{\Sigma(PVCF)}{PV \text{ investment}}. \quad (13.8)$$

The BCR decision rule is to invest if BCR ≥ 1.0, that is, every dollar invested returns at least an equal amount of purchasing power. Project A generates $1.30 for every dollar invested, while project B generates $1.28 per dollar, and thus A is more desirable than B. When projects are mutually exclusive or the organization must ration its capital, the highest BCRs should be selected until funds are exhausted.

The IRR calculates the discount rate that equates the PVs of the net cash inflows (revenues) with the PV of the outflow (the investment).

$$IRR = \frac{\Sigma CF}{(1+i)^t} - Investment_0 = 0 \quad (13.9)$$

The manual calculation of the IRR is cumbersome, but Excel provides a function that avoids this problem, $= \mathbf{IRR(cf_1, cf_2, \ldots cf_n)}$. The IRR decision rule is to invest in all IRRs that exceed the discount rate or, if investment funds are limited, invest in the highest-IRR projects until funds are exhausted. The IRR function reports that project A is expected to earn 15.2% per year on its investment, while project B earns 16.6%, and thus B is more desirable than A, **TABLE 13.12**.

The four evaluation measures rank projects differently on the basis of the size of the investment and the timing of cash flows. These differences become significant mainly when two or more projects serve a single end or where requests for funds exceed the availability of funds. **TABLE 13.13** and **FIGURE 13.7** highlight a capital-rationing situation with seven potential investments, $7 million in available funds and a discount of 6.0% that compares projects using the IRR.

On the basis of IRRs, project C should be invested in first, followed by projects F, E, A, and D. Projects G and B should not be pursued, even if money is available (in the absence of a compelling nonfinancial reason). The capital budget is $7 million and eliminates project D from pursuit in the current year despite the fact that it earns more than the discount rate (6.05% > 6.0%).

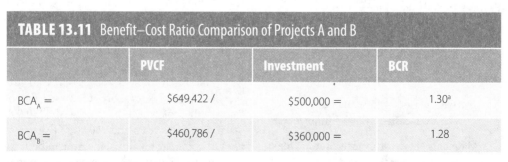

TABLE 13.11 Benefit–Cost Ratio Comparison of Projects A and B			
	PVCF	**Investment**	**BCR**
$BCA_A =$	$649,422 /	$500,000 =	1.30[a]
$BCA_B =$	$460,786 /	$360,000 =	1.28

[a] Project selected based on BCR.

TABLE 13.12 Comparison of Project Evaluation Measures

Year	Project A	Project B	PV Factor	PVCF Project B
0	−$500,000	−$360,000	1.0000	−360,000
1	$150,000	$150,000	0.9524	142,857
2	$150,000	$130,000	0.9070	117,914
3	$150,000	$110,000	0.8638	95,022
4	$150,000	$80,000	0.8227	65,816
5	$150,000	$50,000	0.7835	39,176
	$750,000	$520,000		$100,786
NPV	$149,422	$100,786		
Payback	3.33	2.73		
BCA	0.30	0.28		
IRR	15.24%	16.62%		

▶ Capital Budgeting

The analysis to evaluate an investment should be proportionate to the flexibility of making the investment. Essential or mandatory investments require less scrutiny than discretionary investments. Mandatory investments are required by the government or an accrediting body to remain in business. Mandatory investments include health and safety, the Environmental Protection Agency (EPA), etc. The primary question is not whether the expenditure will be made but rather the size of the expenditure: what is the least expensive way of meeting the standard versus what additional benefits can be derived from increasing the size of the expenditure, for example, longer life span and higher performance.

Discretionary investments, assuming the same level of output is desired, require a lower level of scrutiny, but since an organization has a choice to reinvest or do something else, the desirability of the investment should be examined. Replacement of capital decisions does not involve great risk as output quantity as well as current output prices and resource costs are known. The questions to be determined for reinvestment are, will the investment lower (or increase) costs, and will it increase quality or lower risk? Over time, investment costs are expected to increase, new equipment and buildings may become more expensive, but the ATC can increase, decrease, or remain unchanged. Newer technology and facilities may reduce the ATC, improve product quality, and/or provide higher safety. If the ATC increases, the questions that should be asked are whether consumers are willing to pay more for the product and, if so, how much can output prices be increased.

TABLE 13.13 Capital Rationing

Discount Rate =	6.0%						
Available Funds =	$7,000,000						
Project							
Year	A	B	C	D	E	F	G
0 (Investment)	−$1,000,000	−$2,000,000	−$750,000	−$1,250,000	−$750,000	−$4,500,000	−$1,650,000
1 (Cash inflow)	$175,000	$450,000	$200,000	$195,000	$150,000	$700,000	$450,000
2	$175,000	$400,000	$200,000	$205,000	$175,000	$735,000	$450,000
3	$175,000	$350,000	$200,000	$215,000	$200,000	$772,000	$450,000
4	$175,000	$300,000	$200,000	$226,000	$225,000	$811,000	$450,000
5	$175,000	$250,000	$200,000	$237,000	$250,000	$852,000	
6	$175,000	$400,000		$249,000		$895,000	
7	$175,000			$261,000		$940,000	
8	$175,000					$1,455,000	
IRR	8.15%	2.22%	10.42%	6.05%	9.53%	10.40%	3.57%

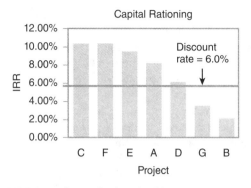

FIGURE 13.7 Project Ranking by IRR

Investments that increase capacity enabling greater output of existing products and services or entry into new geographic markets or product lines carry higher risk. Can more products be pushed into existing markets? Will new markets be as receptive as existing markets? New markets or product lines carry higher risk than current markets, given quantity, output prices, expenses, and competition are less familiar. Knowledge of current markets may be useful for entering new markets, while expansion into new products or services may place the organization in unknown territory. In addition, managers may fail to understand the capital investment necessary to enter new markets or product lines. In higher-risk situations, multiple scenarios (the best case, the most likely one, and the worst case) should be examined.

Capital budgets, like operating budgets, are a means to organize information to reduce financial risk. The capital budgeting process attempts to determine whether a large investment will generate more revenue than its cost. The key factors are the capital investment or initial cash outflow and the future net cash inflows (future revenues – expenses). If current resources are allocated to the project, their costs should be recognized. A hospital may have unused space that can be used to support a project; neither is its cost zero, nor is

its acquisition (or historical) cost, the relevant cost is its current market value.

If unused space is attributed a cost of zero, it understates the cost of a project and fails to recognize the revenue that could be generated if the space was used for another purpose, leased, or sold to others. Similarly, if a building is purchased for $2 million and the cost of capital is 6.0%, recognizing an annual cost of $120,000 will overstate expenses if the organization cannot obtain this rent on the open market. Sunk costs are irrelevant in capital budgeting; only opportunity costs matter, so "owned" assets should be included at their current market value rather than historical cost.

The Capital Budgeting Process

Capital budgeting is a seven-step, often iterative process (**BOX 13.2**). The first step is to determine the goal: is the objective to maximize financial returns, meet a particular need, or both? A goal to maximize profit by investing available funds in the most advantageous ways would create a more wide-ranging search for alternatives than a goal of meeting mandates

---

BOX 13.2 The Capital Budgeting Process

1. Identify the desired goal and alternatives.
2. Estimate output, output prices, and revenues, including when cash will be received.
3. Identify the type and quantity of resources needed, input prices, and when expenses will be paid.
4. Select a discount rate and calculate the PV of future cash flows.
5. Select an evaluation measure to assess cash flows.
6. Conduct sensitivity analysis.
7. Make recommendations.

or replacing existing equipment. Assume the chosen goal is to maximize the ROI; the three most important variables affecting the ROI are units sold, the price of the outputs, and production cost.

$$\text{ROI} = f(\text{output quantity (sales)},$$
$$\text{output prices, operating expenses)}$$

$$(13.10)$$

Once again, we are faced with the task of estimating future events and must recognize the uncertainty surrounding these estimates. Obviously, demand, competition, production technology, and input prices may experience radical shifts, which may neither be seen nor be foreseeable. The degree of risk inherent in the estimates varies with the type of investment under consideration, with the least risk being replacement decisions and the greatest risk lying with investments in new markets. Steps 2 and 3 attempt to define the critical variables that affect the benefits from and costs associated with the investment.

Step 2 begins the process of specifying the expected benefits of an investment. What value will the investment bring to the organization? Will output change? If so, by how much? How much revenue will the output generate? If revenue is generated, when will it be received? Capital budgeting is often an iterative process, where output and revenue forecasts, expense projections, and discounts rates are modified if potential investments fail to generate sufficient returns.

The demand for healthcare services is expected to be affected by their price; the income of patients; the number, age, and medical status of the population; insurance coverage or lack thereof; and the number of competitors. Obviously, price and insurance status assume that medical services are being sold, and the law of demand states that as the price of a good or service increases, fewer units will be sold. Similarly, an increase in insurance coverage that insures more individuals, covers a greater range of health conditions, and/or reduces deductibles or copayments will increase demand for healthcare goods and services. Besides price and insurance coverage, an increase in the patients' income should increase their use of health services. A proxy measure for income is the economy and its rate of growth. Beyond the obvious impact on consumer income, economic growth also affects government revenues and determines the generousness of Medicare and Medicaid reimbursement.

$$\text{Demand } (Q) = f \begin{pmatrix} \text{price,} & \text{insurance,} & \text{economy,} & \text{population,} \\ \text{(--)} & \text{(+)} & \text{(+)} & \text{(+)} \\ \text{median age,} & \text{medical status,} & \text{competition\ldots} \\ \text{(+)} & \text{(--)} & \text{(--)} \end{pmatrix} \qquad (13.11)$$

The demand for healthcare goods and services is expected to increase with the size of the population, the age of the population, and its health status. The final demand determinant is the number of competitors providing the service; an increase in competitors should reduce the market share for every individual provider as patients are spread between them. Equation 13.11 encapsulates these relationships and shows the expected change in demand. The capital budget analyst needs to quantify these variables to the extent possible to reduce the uncertainty surrounding output forecasts.

The second element to calculating revenue, assuming the good or service is sold, is the price. Price for the majority of patients may be set by third party payers, so government policy toward reimbursement will have a major impact on reimbursement levels; as noted, reimbursement should be higher when government revenues are high. The second, related factor is who insures the patients or the organization's patient mix. Equation 13.12 assumes reimbursement rates will be lower for patients covered by Medicare, Medicaid, and managed care payers and the uninsured and higher for commercial insurers. Average prices (or reimbursement) should be higher for providers with high percentages of commercial patients and lower percentages of Medicare, Medicaid, managed care, and uninsured patients.

$$\text{Price } (P) = f \begin{pmatrix} Q, \underset{(-)}{\text{government policy}}, \underset{(+/-)}{\text{Medicare}}, \underset{(-)}{\text{Medicaid}}, \underset{(-)}{\text{commercial}}, \\ \underset{(-)}{\text{managed care}}, \underset{(-)}{\text{competition}}, \underset{(+)}{\text{negotiation power}} \end{pmatrix} \quad (13.12)$$

Competition not only affects the number of patients a provider may serve but also prices. An increase in providers should hold down prices as patients or their insurers shop for lower rates. The final determinant of price is their negotiating power; if the provider is the sole supplier of a good or service, this enhances the provider's ability to negotiate high reimbursement rates. However, negotiating power is also enhanced by reputation, quality and outcomes, location, and other factors. The product of output (Q) and price (P) is revenue, and the ROI is determined by the difference between revenue and expense.

Step 3 quantifies the operating expenses expected to be needed, in conjunction with the investment to produce goods or services. Like operating budgets, the manager needs to identify labor, supplies, utilities, and other expenses to support the investment and when these expenses will be incurred. Operating expenses, Equation 13.13, vary on the basis of the location of the provider; in high-cost areas, wages (as recognized in the diagnosis-related group [DRG] system by the wage index), supplies, and utilities will be higher.

$$\text{Operating cost } (ATC) = f \begin{pmatrix} \underset{(+)}{\text{labor}}, \underset{(+)}{\text{supplies}}, \underset{(+)}{\text{utilities}}, \underset{(-)}{\text{output}}, \underset{(+)}{\text{competition}} \ldots \end{pmatrix} \quad (13.13)$$

The average cost per unit should decrease as output increases because of spreading of fixed costs, but the analyst should recognize when further increases in output will require additional fixed resources or produce congestion leading to higher costs. Competition for inputs should also increase the ATC. Steps 2 and 3 provide estimates for the three largest unknowns: quantity of output, output price, and input costs. While none of these variables can be determined exactly, the analyst can develop estimates based on the normal (or Poisson) distribution to quantify risk.

Step 4 requires the analyst to identify a discount rate to use to obtain the PV of future cash flows; as stated previously, the rate could be based on how the investment is be funded, equity, debt, or the weighted average, or project risk. Once the discount rate is identified, future cash flows are reduced to current purchasing power.

Step 5 determines how benefits and costs will be compared. The analyst must determine which evaluation or ranking measure(s) to use. The evaluation measure(s) is/are then applied to the forecasted and discounted cash flows. The output of step 5 is either a go/no-go decision if a single project is being evaluated or a list ranking multiple projects from most desirable to least desirable. After the initial IRRs, NPVs, BCRs, or payback periods are calculated, it is common for the estimated quantities, output prices, and expenses to be adjusted to tweak the analysis.

TABLE 13.14 shows the results of steps 2–5; key assumptions are displayed at the top;

TABLE 13.14 Capital Budgeting Worksheet

All dollar amounts in thousands (000)

Discount rate:	6%
Inflation, output price:	2%
Inflation, expenses:	3%
Growth rate of demand:	2%

Year	0	1	2	3	4	5
Investment	−$1000.00	$0.0	$0.0	$0.0	$0.0	$0.0
Price	0.0	$1.00	$1.020	$1.040	$1.061	$1.082
Quantity	0.0	400.0	408.0	416.2	424.5	433.0
Revenue	$0.0	$400.00	$416.20	$433.00	$450.50	$468.70
Expenses						
Salaries	$0.0	$100.00	$103.00	$106.10	$109.30	$112.60

Supplies	0.0	60.0	61.8	63.7	65.6	67.5
Utilities	0.0	10.0	10.3	10.6	10.9	11.3
Total expense	$0.0	$170.00	$175.10	$180.40	$185.80	$191.30
Net cash flow	−$1000.00	$230.00	$241.10	$252.60	$264.70	$277.30
PV factor	1.0000	0.9434	0.8900	0.8396	0.7921	0.7473
PVCF	−$1000.00	$217.00	$214.50	$212.10	$209.70	$207.20

Evaluation Measures

Payback	3.95	= −D53/(AVERAGE (E65:I65))
NPV	$60.50	= NPV(B6,C24:G24)
BCR	1.06	= NPV(B6,C24:G24)/Investment
IRR	8.2%	= IRR(B24:G24)

output quantities, prices, and expenses and the resulting cash flow are shown in the middle; and evaluation methods are included at the bottom. The project is a go as the IRR, BCR, and NPV exceed the discount rate and the payback period is less than 4 years.

Sensitivity analysis, step 6, examines the robustness of the results: how much will the ROI change when key variables change? In Table 13.14, project A is expected to earn an IRR of 8.15%, well above the 6.0% cost of capital. Sensitivity analysis asks how much output or revenue projections can be overstated or expenses understated before the IRR falls below 6.0%. Will an adequate return be produced if output comes in at 90% of expectations, 80%, and so on? The more resilient financial results are to changes in output, output prices, and expenses, the less risky is the investment. Projects that can sustain a 20% overstatement of output and still produce an IRR greater than the cost of capital are more desirable than projects that are unable to sustain a 10% overstatement.

Sensitivity analysis typically alters each of the key variables to determine when a project moves from desirable to undesirable.

The key problems with sensitivity analysis are correlation between variables and nonlinearity. Correlation between variables recognizes that variables are not independent. For example, price and quantity are correlated: increases in price reduce the quantity sold—the law of demand. The presence of correlation weakens the validity of altering one variable, while assuming no change in other variables to assess the impact on the bottom line. The second problem is nonlinearity: not only are quantity and expenses correlated, but changes in quantity may also result in more than or less than proportionate changes in expenses. In the presence of economies of scale, a 10% increase in output may not increase expenses by 10%; when diseconomies of scale are present, increases in output produce disproportionately larger increases in expenses.

Sensitivity analysis is easily performed in Excel, **FIGURE 13.8**. The analyst selects **Data**

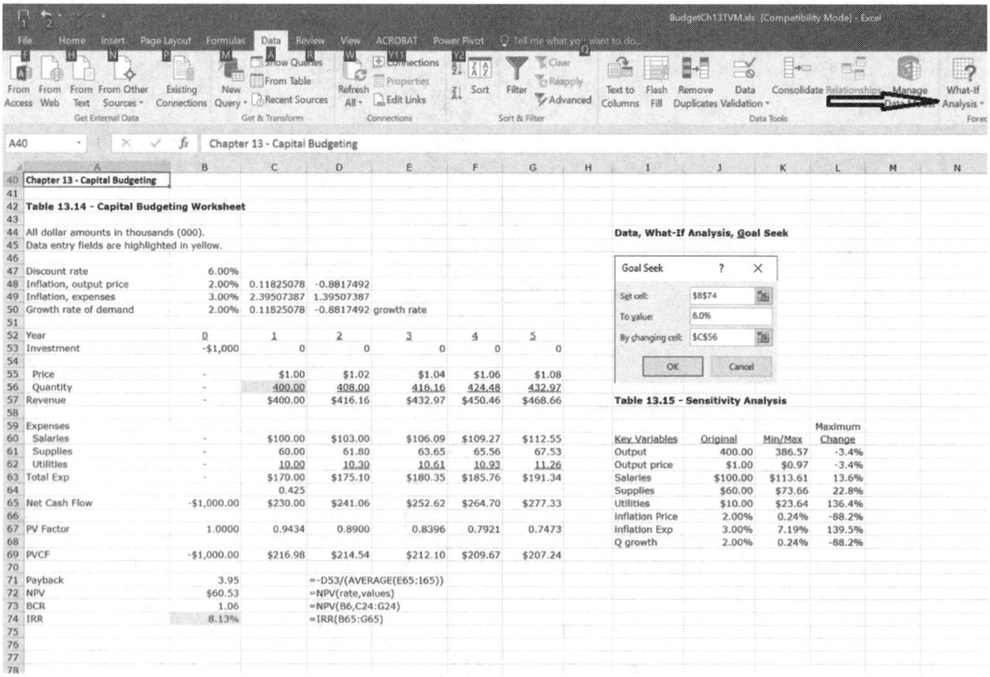

FIGURE 13.8 Goal Seek Screenshot

from the main menu, **What-If Analysis**, and then **Goal Seek**. Goal Seek requires the analyst to specify the target variable, the minimum acceptable value, and a variable to minimize or maximize that would still provide the desired outcome. For example, how much can quantity fall below 400, the specified value in the capital budget analysis, before the IRR (the target variable) falls below 6.0% (the minimum acceptable value)?

Goal Seek calculates that the output quantity can fall to 386.6 units, or 3.4%, before the IRR, currently 8.1%, falls below the 6.0% discount rate. **TABLE 13.15** displays the maximum percentage change in each of the key variables before the IRR falls below 6.0%.

Assessing Table 13.15 shows that the key factors are output and output prices. The question for managers is, how confident are they that output will not fall below 386.6 units or price will not fall below $966? Neither variable can fall more than 3.4% below the expected amount before the IRR falls below 6.0%. The other sensitive variable is salary expense; salaries cannot

increase more than 13.6% before the IRR falls below the minimum desired value. Changes in other variables, supplies, utilities, inflation rates, and output growth rate, can sustain large changes before the project's financial performance falls below the discount rate, and the magnitude of these changes reduces the likelihood that they will occur.

Capital Budgeting for a For-Profit

If the organization in Table 13.14 is a for-profit hospital, the capital budgeting analysis is altered to recognize the impact of depreciation on taxes. In the original analysis, depreciation was ignored as the cost of the investment was recognized when purchased (year 0); since for-profits must pay tax and investment costs are depreciated over time, the analysis must recognize tax benefits. In this example, the investment is depreciated over 5 years, reducing taxable income by $200 each year and saving the organization $80 in taxes if the tax rate is 40% (**TABLE 13.16**).

TABLE 13.15 Sensitivity Analysis

Key Variables	Original	Min./Max.	Maximum Change (%)
Output	400.00	386.57	−3.4
Output price	$1.00	$0.97	−3.4
Salaries	$100.00	$113.61	13.6
Supplies	$60.00	$73.66	22.8
Utilities	$10.00	$23.64	136.4
Inflation price	2.00%	0.24%	−88.2
Inflation expense	3.00%	7.19%	139.5
Q growth	2.00%	0.24%	−88.2

TABLE 13.16 Capital Budgeting Worksheet for a For-Profit

Discount rate	6%					
Inflation, output price	2%					
Inflation, expenses	3%					
Growth rate of demand	2%					
Tax rate	40%					

Year	0	1	2	3	4	5
Investment	−$1000.00	$0.0	$0.0	$0.0	$0.0	$0.0
Price	$0.0	$1.000	$1.020	$1.040	$1.061	$1.082
Quantity	0.0	400.0	408.0	416.2	424.5	433.0
Revenue	$0.0	$400.00	$416.20	$433.00	$450.50	$468.70
Expenses						
Salaries	$0.0	$100.00	$103.00	$106.10	$109.30	$112.60
Supplies	0.0	60.0	61.8	63.7	65.6	67.5
Utilities	0.0	10.0	10.2	10.4	10.6	10.8
Depreciation	0.0	200.0	200.0	200.0	200.0	200.0
Total expense	$0.0	$370.00	$375.00	$380.10	$385.40	$390.90
Profit		$30.00	$41.20	$52.80	$65.00	$77.80
−Tax		$12.00	$16.50	$21.10	$26.00	$31.10
After-tax profit		$18.00	$24.70	$31.70	$39.00	$46.70
+Depreciation		$200.00	$200.00	$200.00	$200.00	$200.00
Net cash flow	−$1000.00	$218.00	$224.70	$231.70	$239.00	$246.70

PV factor		1.0000	0.9434	0.8900	0.8396	0.7921	0.7473
PVCF		−$1000.00	$205.70	$200.00	$194.50	$189.30	$184.30
Payback		4.31					
NPV		−$26.20					
BCR		0.97					
IRR		5.1%					

Depreciation does not result in any cash flowing out of the organization, so depreciation is added to after-tax income to obtain cash flow. The financial performance of the for-profit is lower than a comparable nonprofit as $106.7 is taxed away. The IRR is 5.1% for the for-profit, while a comparable nonprofit would earn 8.1%. The reader should also see that the NPV is negative and the BCR is less than 1.0, indicating the investment should not be undertaken—these results are based on the use of a 6.0% discount rate. A for-profit should use the after-tax discount rate as the hurdle rate, that is, if a for-profit earns 6.0% pretax, it would only net 3.6% after tax, so this investment may still be a desirable investment.

Incorporation of Capital Budgeting Results into the Operating Budget

When expanded or new services are contemplated that require additional resources, the new resources must be added to current expenses to ensure the operating budget expense estimates are as accurate as possible for the coming year. Previous chapters emphasized expenses were estimated assuming operations remained relatively constant, and increases were calculated for higher prices of resources as well as any incremental volume growth, capital budgeting often is the first step in a quantum shift in operations.

Opening a new practice site shifts an organization away from the incremental growth in output it has historically experienced and may result in large increases in output, revenue, and expenses. A second consideration in opening new sites is the possible cannibalization of existing practice sites; patients who have travel long distances for care may be willing to change to a closer site within the provider's organization, so one or more existing sites may see a decline in patient volume. Any jump in output and revenue should require similar increases in labor, supplies, and utilities above prior growth rates. On the other hand, if investments are made in cost-reducing technologies, the predicted increase in expenses should be lower than historical growth rates.

▶ Postexpenditure Review

While the primary job of capital budgeting is to determine whether a high-cost resource should be purchased, the capital budgeting process should be structured to recognize its weaknesses and improve future analyses. Like operating budgets, the usefulness of capital budgets is not determined by the initial estimates but by whether the estimates are accurate and used to manage operations. Given the infrequent nature of capital purchases, it is tempting to approach capital budgeting as a one-and-done process: prepare the capital budgeting proposal, submit it, and, if approved, purchase.

Capital budgeting requires a review process similar to the variance analysis performed with operating budgets where the accuracy of estimates and management effectiveness can be evaluated. Given the multiyear time frame of capital budget requests, annual reviews of actual and realized output, output prices, and expenses (prices and efficiency standards) should be undertaken to determine whether the expected return was achieved. The goal of postexpenditure review is to identify managers who produce the best and worst forecasts, discover how and why forecasts differed from what actually occurred, and improve future forecasts.

Inaccurate forecasts may indicate the need for financial training; many managers graduate into management from nonfinancial fields and have little, if any, financial training. Organizations often supply their managers with little more than the required forms that must be submitted for capital requests. On the other hand, financially savvy managers wanting to expand their budgets use the overestimation of needs, foot-in-the-door, bandwagon, or other strategies to acquire more funds and systematically overestimate output and revenue, while underestimating expenses. Tracking the performance of capital budget requests is essential to determining the type of bias contained in estimates and implementing effective training and oversight to reduce forecast error.

The key question is, did a project produce the expected result? Education may be able to improve the forecasts of naive managers, but savvy managers may continue to intentionally produce faulty forecasts. Tracking performance could enable organizations to reward or punish managers for their estimates: Managers whose forecasts are on target may be allowed to use the average cost of capital when discounting future cash flows, while managers who consistently overestimate quantity and output prices and/or underestimate expenses should be forced to use a higher capital hurdle rate.

TABLE 13.17 examines the current-year and cumulative performance for the investment analyzed in Table 13.14. That analysis indicated the organization could expect an IRR of 8.1%, based on the first 3 years of operation the IRR appears to be only 4.9%. Since this is below expectations as well as below the minimum threshold of 6.0% further analysis is needed.

Analyzing performance shows current reimbursement, which may be uncontrollable, is lower than expected and utilization is slightly behind the forecast. As a result of unfavorable variances in reimbursement and utilization, revenue is 8.2% below target. The variation in expenses may be of greater concern. Even though it is running only 4.9% overbudget and accounts for only 27.7% of the total variance, this may be the most controllable variable, and additional analysis is needed to determine which expenses are overbudget and why.

Comparing current to cumulative results provides additional insight into trends and managerial effectiveness. Reimbursement is getting worse over the life of the project; price is only 2.5% below forecast overall but is 5.4% underbudget in the current year. Utilization in the current period continues to fall behind target: overall it is 1.5% below target, but in the last year, it has fallen to 2.7% below target. Both of these trends have had an adverse impact on revenue: for the 3-year period, it is only 1.0% lower than planned, while the gap in the current period is 8.4%. On a positive note, expenses for the 3-year period were running 9.8% overbudget, and currently expenses are 4.9% overbudget. While the trend is positive, the manager should also consider the relationship between output and expenses: The current-year output is 2.5% below forecast, and expenses are 4.9% above forecast; over 3 years, output is only 1.5% below forecast, but expenses are 9.8% over. This trend suggests the cost per unit is heading down.

TABLE 13.17 Postexpenditure Review

	Year 3 Actual	Year 3 Budget	Difference	Difference (%)
Price	$0.985	$1.040	−$0.06	−5.4
Quantity	405	416.2	−11.16	−2.7
Revenue	$398.925	$432.973	−$34.05	−8.2
Expense	$188.900	$180.353	$8.55	4.9
Cash flow	$210.025	$252.620	−$42.59	−17.7

	3 Year Actual	3 Year Cumulative	Difference	Difference (%)
Price	$0.995	$1.020	−$0.03	−2.5
Quantity	1243.0	1224.2	−18.36	−1.5
Revenue	$1236.325	$1248.81	−$12.48	−1.0
Expense	$576.947	$525.453	$51.49	9.8
Cash flow	$659.378	$723.680	−$64.30	−8.9

While costs are improving, the reduction in revenue is lowering cash flow. The current-year cash flow is off 17.7%; for the 3-year period, it was only 8.9% below forecast. Management needs to take swift and dramatic action to improve operating performance in the last 2 years of the investment to move actual results toward those expected in the original analysis.

Gapenski (2012) provides four goals for postexpenditure review. The first is to assess risk and credibility, that is, which managers produce the best estimates? The second goal is to improve future forecasts. Improving future forecasts requires the direction of error be recognized. If consistent errors are made, that is, overestimating revenues and/or underestimating expenses, adjustments can be made to increase the accuracy of future forecasts. Third,

operating and capital budgets provide an operations guide, so when projections are not met, the reasons need to be determined. Managers should also feel the pressure to meet their budgets. Lastly, postexpenditure review and the knowledge that managers will be held to their estimates should reduce losses by reducing nonprofitable investments or by making managers work harder to realize the expected income.

▶ Nonfinancial Capital Budgeting Criteria

To this point, the decision to invest or forego investment has been discussed purely in financial terms: does the project produce an adequate monetary return to justify its pursuit? While this may be the primary criteria for for-profit organizations in other industries, healthcare organizations regardless of ownership often recognize other factors that influence their investment decisions. Issues of community need, patient outcomes/quality improvement, physician demands, public image, staying abreast of technological development, etc., are often weighed with financial performance to decide what projects should be pursued.

Assume an organization bases 50% of the capital investment decision on financial performance, 25% on quality (will the expenditure improve patient outcomes, that is, life expectancy?), and 25% on community need (how many other providers offer the service within 50 miles?). **TABLE 13.18** demonstrates how these variables are measured and ranked; the highest-scoring projects are funded first.

Consider three potential investments in a capital-rationing situation where only two projects can be pursued. Project A is expected to produce a return in excess of the organization's ROA, but more than two providers already provide the service, and it is not expected to improve patient outcomes. Project B appears certain to lose money but will provide a service not currently available in the area and greatly improve patient outcomes. Project C is expected to produce an equivalent return to the organization's ROA by providing a readily available service and will not change patient outcomes. The financial decision would be to fund A and C and forego B. **TABLE 13.19** reassesses the decision using community need and patient outcome considerations.

TABLE 13.18 Factor Weights and Ranking

Factor Rank	1	2	3	4
Finance (50%)	ROI < 0	ROI < ROA	ROI = ROA	ROI > ROA
Community need (25%)	>2 providers/ 1000	>1–2/1000	>0–1/1000	0
Patient outcomes (25%)	No change or worsens	1–12 months	1–3 years	3 years or more

TABLE 13.19 Project-Scoring Matrix

Project	Finance (50%)	Community Need (25%)	Patient Outcomes (25%)	Score
A	4 (4 * 0.50 = 2.00)	1 (1 * 0.25 = 0.25)	2 (2 * 0.25 = 0.50)	2.75
B	1 (1 * 0.50 = 0.50)	4 (4 * 0.25 = 1.00)	4 (4 * 0.25 = 1.00)	2.50
C	3 (3 * 0.50 = 1.50)	1 (1 * 0.25 = 0.25)	2 (2 * 0.25 = 0.50)	2.25

When nonfinancial criteria are incorporated into the capital investment decision, project B is selected over project C, that is, the organization's managers place the importance of providing a money-losing service not presently available in the area, B, over the possibility of obtaining an average ROA from C.

It is perfectly acceptable to choose to lose money to support a higher goal, but financial prudence dictates that the size of the loss be understood, minimized to the extent possible, and offset. It would be irrational to supply a service that imposes a large loss on an organization that would endanger its survival, so managers should have a plan to accommodate the loss and maintain operations.

Summary

This chapter shifts away from financial issues that are a daily part of managers' lives toward decisions that arise sporadically. Capital investments are made infrequently and commit large amounts of money over multiple years. Due to the magnitude of resources involved and the rarity of making these commitments, capital expenditures are handled separately from operating budgets to ensure a thorough review is performed and scarce resources are allocated to their best uses.

The first major departure from operating budgets is revenues are received over many years and analysts must recognize the time value of money. Money received in the future is worth less than money today, so equitable measurement of investment cost and revenues requires that future cash flows be discounted to their PV. The first step in calculating the time value of money is to identify the discount rate, which determines how much future cash flows will be reduced to account for inflation, default risk, and postponed consumption. The second step is to identify the evaluation measure(s) to be used to judge investments.

The capital budgeting process involves up to seven steps, starting with identification of the goal and ending with the purchase decision. Between the identification of the objective and the purchase decision, managers must quantify output, output prices, and expenses; select a discount rate and evaluation measure; and, in some cases, determine how the expected results will change, given changes in key variables. A capital budgeting worksheet was provided to guide managers in developing their own capital budgeting templates for the specific needs of their projects and organizations. The use of Excel's What-If Analysis was demonstrated to identify how far key variables can vary from their forecasted values before insufficient financial results arise.

The value of capital budgeting, like all things, should be measured by how well it improves operations, and this requires that capital budget requests be integrated into the work of departments. After capital projects are approved and put into service, their performance should be assessed to facilitate midcourse correction if projections are not meeting expectations, and steps should be taken to improve the accuracy of future capital budget requests. No organization is operated solely on financial criteria, so capital budgeting processes should include mechanisms to incorporate other criteria into the evaluation process and ensure funds are allocated to the ends that maximize the value of the organization.

Key Terms and Concepts

Annuity	Future value (FV)	Present value (PV)
Annuity due	(compounding)	(discounting)
Consumer price index (CPI)	Inflation	Ordinary annuity
Fisher equation	Nominal value	Real value

Discussion Questions

1. Explain the difference between PV and FV.
2. Explain the impact of the length of time in which payments are received and the discount rate on the PV of a stream of payments.
3. Explain the difference between the NPV, payback period, BCR, and IRR.
4. What factors have the largest impact on the rate of return of capital investments, and what variables are these factors subsequently determined by?
5. Discuss the goals of postexpenditure review.

Problems

1. Calculate the PV of the following cash flows:
   A. What is $10,000 received 5 years in the future worth today if the discount rate is 4%?
   B. What is $10,000 received 10 years in the future worth today if the discount rate is 4%?
   C. What is $10,000 received 5 years in the future worth today if the discount rate is 8%?
   D. What is $10,000 received 10 years in the future worth today if the discount rate is 8%?
   E. What is an annuity of $10,000 received on the first of every year for 5 years worth today if the discount rate is 4%?
   F. What is an annuity of $10,000 received at the end of every year for 5 years worth today if the discount rate is 4%?
   G. What is an annuity of $10,000 received on the first of every year for 5 years worth today if the discount rate is 8%?
   H. What is an annuity of $10,000 received at the end of every year for 5 years worth today if the discount rate is 8%?
   I. What is a series of payments of $70,000, $60,000, $50,000, $40,000, and $30,000 received on the first of every year for 5 years worth today if the discount rate is 8%?
   J. What is a series of payments of $30,000, $40,000, $50,000, $60,000, and $70,000 received at the end of every year for 5 years worth today if the discount rate is 8%?

2. Calculate the FV of the following cash flows:
   A. If you invest $10,000 today at 4%, how much money will you have in 5 years?
   B. If you invest $10,000 today at 4%, how much money will you have in 10 years?
   C. If you invest $10,000 today at 8%, how much money will you have in 5 years?
   D. If you invest $10,000 today at 8%, how much money will you have in 10 years?
   E. If you invest $10,000 on the first of every year for 5 years at 4%, how much money will you have in 5 years?
   F. If you invest $10,000 on the last day of each year for 5 years at 4%, how much money will you have in 5 years?
   G. If you invest $10,000 on the first of every year for 10 years at 8%, how much money will you have in 10 years?
   H. If you invest $10,000 on the last day of each year for 10 years at 8%, how much money will you have in 10 years?

I. If you invest $70,000, $60,000, $50,000, $40,000, and $30,000 on the first day of the every year for 5 years, how much money will you have in 5 years if the interest rate is 8%?

J. If you invest $30,000, $40,000, $50,000, $60,000, and $70,000 on the first day of every year for 5 years, how much money will you have in 5 years if the interest rate is 8%?

3. A hospital is considering the purchase of a piece of medical equipment that costs $1,500,000 and has a useful life of 5 years and no salvage value at the end of its useful life. The equipment generates revenues of $650,000 per year and operating expenses of $300,000. Calculate the NPV, payback, BCR, and IRR. Should the equipment be purchased if the discount rate is 6% or 10%?

	Revenue	Expense
Year 0	–	$1,500,000 (investment)
Year 1	$650,000	$300,000
Year 2	$650,000	$300,000
Year 3	$650,000	$300,000
Year 4	$650,000	$300,000
Year 5	$650,000	$300,000

4. A hospital is considering the purchase of a piece of medical equipment that costs $1,500,000 and has a useful life of 5 years and a salvage value of $250,000 at the end year 5. The equipment generates revenues of $450,000 per year and

operating expenses of $200,000. Calculate the NPV, payback, BCR, and IRR. Should the equipment be purchased if the discount rate is 6% or 10%?

	Revenue	Expense
Year 0	–	$1,500,000 (investment)
Year 1	$450,000	$200,000
Year 2	$450,000	$200,000
Year 3	$450,000	$200,000
Year 4	$450,000	$200,000
Year 5	$450,000	$200,000

5. Assume revenues decrease and expenses increase with the age of the machine, as given in the table here, and it can be sold for $200,000 at the end of year 5. Calculate the NPV, payback, BCR, and IRR. Should the equipment be purchased if the discount rate is 6% or 10%?

	Revenue	Expense
Year 0	–	$1,500,000 (investment)
Year 1	$850,000	$200,000
Year 2	$750,000	$250,000
Year 3	$650,000	$300,000
Year 4	$550,000	$350,000
Year 5	$450,000	$400,000

References

Board of Governors of the Federal Reserve System. (2017). *Charge-off and delinquency rates on loans and leases at commercial banks*. Retrieved June 8, 2017, from https://www.federalreserve.gov/releases/chargeoff/chgallnsa.htm

Federal Reserve Economic Data. (2017). *Economic research*. Retrieved June 8, 2017, from https://fred.stlouisfed.org/series/CPALTT01USA661S.

Gapenski, L. C. (2012). *Healthcare finance* (5th ed.). Chicago, IL: Health Administration Press.

Mikesell, J. (1995). *Fiscal administration* (4th ed.). Belmont, CA: Wadsworth Publishing Company.

Popular Mechanics. (2017). *The F-35 is about to get a lot cheaper. Sort of*. Retrieved June 8, 2017, from http://www.popularmechanics.com/military/weapons/a21776/f-35-cheaper

Yahoo. (2017). *US Treasury Bond Rates*. Retrieved from https://finance.yahoo.com/bonds?.tsrc=globe?date=20120821

CHAPTER 14

Cost–Benefit Analysis, Cost-Effectiveness Analysis, and Program Evaluation

CHAPTER OBJECTIVES

1. Explain the purpose of cost–benefit analysis, cost-effectiveness analysis, and program evaluation.
2. Perform a cost–benefit analysis.
3. Perform a cost-effectiveness analysis.
4. Explain the steps in program evaluation and how it differs from cost–benefit and cost-effectiveness analyses.

▶ Introduction

I s an ounce of prevention worth a pound of cure? It is an article of faith to many, but an ounce or many ounces of one material may be more expensive than a pound of another material. An ounce of gold, \$1137.80, is significantly more expensive than a pound of silver, \$256.80 = \$16.05 * 16 (prices as of 12/21/16). The first question that should be asked is, what resources are needed to produce an ounce of prevention and a pound of cure? A second consideration is the total number of people and the number

at risk, that is, how many ounces of prevention and pounds of cure are needed? Assuming prevention and cure cost the same on a per ounce basis, it is easy to see that if less than 1 person in 16 will contract a disease, providing a pound of cure to the people who become sick is cheaper than providing an ounce of prevention to 16 people. If more than 1 person in 16 will contact a disease, prevention is cheaper; if 2 people in 16 will become ill, it will be twice as expensive to treat 2 patients than to inoculate 16. A third consideration is whether prevention is 100% effective, what level of false negatives and false positives screening tests produce, whether there are any negative side effects, and what additional costs faulty findings and side effects impose.

This chapter explores methodologies for organizing information to support decision-making and process improvement. **Cost–benefit analysis (CBA)** is used to determine whether activities should be performed, for example, when is prevention cheaper than cure? CBA is used to determine whether investments should be undertaken and whether existing operations should be continued, while capital budgeting assesses future investments. CBA is a means to clarify goals, identify available methods to achieve goals, determine who receives the benefits and pays the costs of programs, and recognize the incentives and/or disincentives a program may have on affected parties and how secondary or unintended effects will affect the desired goal. CBA is a tool to identify programs that should be undertaken or expanded (and the order in which they should be pursued), processes to alter, and programs to scale back or eliminate. CBA is not simply about dividing up a budget but should be used to determine the size of the budget.

CBA compares the benefits and costs of an activity, measured in dollars, to determine whether it creates or destroys value. Value is created when benefits exceed costs, and a forceful argument can be made that expanding the activity and budget is warranted. When costs exceed benefits, the activity reduces value and resources should be reallocated to other uses. For example, does expanding prenatal care reduce total healthcare costs? The cost is the monetary expense of expanding prenatal services, while the benefits are fewer premature births, lower use of neonatal intensive care units (NICUs), and lower inpatient costs. Research indicates prenatal care lowers subsequent healthcare expenditures by an amount greater than their cost and thus reduces total healthcare spending. When multiple means are available to achieve an objective, CBA can identify the method that creates the largest monetary benefit per dollar expended.

Cost-effectiveness analysis (CEA) quantifies the outcome (benefit) of an activity costs in nonmonetary units and compares the cost measured in dollars of alternative means of achieving an end. In CEA, an explicit or implicit understanding has been reached that the end is worthwhile, and the question is, what is the most efficient means to reach the end? CEA would be used to determine the best way to reduce neonatal deaths. The benefit of a human life does not need to be quantified in dollars; the only thing that must be determined is the cost per life saved. CEA could compare the cost per life saved from expanding prenatal care against expanded NICU funding and possibly increases in nutrition, housing, and education programs to determine which alternative has the lowest cost per life saved.

The analysis of preventive care can be either CBA or CEA; decision theory illuminates the choice between prevention, screening, and early, low-cost treatment and no screening and later, higher-cost treatment. The key factors in CBA examining whether prevention is cheaper than cure are prevalence, screening and prevention costs, early treatment costs, and later treatment costs. The benefit of screening, prevention, and early treatment is avoided healthcare cost, that is, the difference between the cost of early and late treatment. The cost of screening and prevention is the cost per recipient. **TABLE 14.1** describes the screening and prevention decision: if a person does not have a disease, the only cost is screening; if a person is ill, screening and/or prevention may accelerate treatment and lower costs. When no screening or prevention is undertaken and a patient does not contract the disease, no cost is incurred. If a person gets sick and treatment is delayed, resulting in higher costs, avoidable costs are incurred. The fourth factor is **prevalence**, the proportion of a population with a disease at a point in time.

The breakeven point between screening, prevention, and early treatment and curative care, that is, the prevalence of the out-of-control state, $P_{\text{O-O-C}}{}^*$ is calculated as follows:

TABLE 14.1 Decision Theory and Early versus Late Treatment

	In Control (No Disease)	Out of Control (Disease)
Screening and prevention	Total screening cost, $5 * n$	Early treatment, $10,000
Curative care	$0	Late treatment, $20,000

$$P_{\text{O-O-C}} = \frac{\text{Total screening cost}}{(\text{Late treatment cost} - \text{Early treatment cost})} \quad (14.1)$$

If 1000 people are screened, $n = 1000$ and $P_{\text{O-O-C}}* = (\$5.00 * 1,000)/(\$20,000 - 10,000)$, or 0.5. That is, if exactly 0.5 people per 1000 contract the disease, there is no difference in the total medical cost between early and later treatment. Screening costs $5000 ($5 * 1000). If 0.5 cases produce $5000 in treatment cost (0.5 * $10,000), the total cost is $10,000. If screening is not undertaken and cases are treated as they are identified, $10,000 in curative costs will be incurred (0.5 * $20,000). If $p > 0.5/1000$, screening is cheaper than curative care. For example, if $P_{\text{O-O-C}} = 1.0/1000$, screening costs $5000 plus $10,000 (1 * $10,000), or $15,000, versus $20,000 to delinquently treat one patient. If $P_{\text{O-O-C}} = 0.25$, screening is costlier ($5,000 + [0.25 * \$10,000] = \$7,500$) than delayed treatment (0.25 * $20,000 = $5,000). Screening and prevention become more economical as prevalence and late treatment costs increase and screening and early treatment costs decrease. One means to increase the desirability of screening and prevention is to target high-risk groups rather than the general population and increase the rate of prevalence.

Program evaluation provides a third methodology for assessing the merits of an activity or department. Program evaluation is used extensively in medicine, education, and the social sciences to assess new technologies, initiatives, and interventions and can be productively applied to any field to collect information, assess performance, and identify opportunities for improvement. Unlike CBA and CEA, program evaluation takes a retrospective view and focuses on what was achieved rather than what is planned.

There are many ways to achieve an end, and unfortunately, people often become set in their ways and fail to consider other possibilities; incremental budgets provide a prime example of a system that actively discourages change. For most objectives, there are high- and low-cost alternatives with varying degrees of effectiveness. When possible, the lowest-cost and most effective methods should be employed. When the lowest-cost method is not the most effective, decisions should weigh costs and effectiveness. CBA, CEA, and program evaluation are tools that should be regularly employed to examine what we do and how we do it in order to ensure the right ends are pursued by the right means.

▶ Cost–Benefit Analysis

CBA is a tool that on first appearance appears simple: Add up the benefits and costs of an activity in dollars; if benefits equal or exceed costs, undertake the activity, and if costs exceed benefits, do not undertake the activity. When costs exceed benefits, undertaking the activity reduces well-being, and a search for other opportunities that can provide a greater return on resources should occur. Complications, however, immediately arise in determining "what is a benefit?" and "what is a cost?" and setting monetary values for nonpecuniary benefits and costs. If costs and benefits are paid and received in different years, future benefits and costs must be discounted to compare monetary magnitudes across years because of the declining purchasing power of money.

CBA and capital budgeting follow the same general steps, but capital budgeting generally focuses on a single alternative: is investing in X worthwhile? CBA begins more broadly: what is the goal, and in how many ways can it be reached? The first step in CBA (**BOX 14.1**) is to identify whether the goal should be pursued and, if pursued, the optimal alternative to employ. The "if it should be done" and "how it should be done" questions are often one and the same in capital budgeting. In contrast, Carande-Kulis, Stevens, Florence, Beattie, and Arias (2015) wanted to reduce falls in older adults and began by identifying three potential interventions to prevent falls and injury. Each intervention was determined to create value; the expected benefits (i.e., avoided medical costs) were greater than prevention costs, and later steps identified the alternative that provided the greatest financial return, that is, the highest avoided cost per dollar of intervention.

Step 2 details the resources needed to run each program and the expected outcomes. Resources are specified as the number of workers, units of supply, square footage, etc., and outcomes may be quantified as units of output, reduction in errors, etc. Step 3 monetizes inputs: What is the total compensation per worker and the total labor cost, what is the input price for each unit of supply and the total supply expense, and what is the cost of buying or leasing space and equipment? When outcome is specified as higher output, the benefit is the change in output multiplied by output price, that is, revenue. When outcome is specified as a reduction in error, the benefit may be calculated as avoided cost: what is the cost of reworking or discarding defective outputs, and how many units will no longer need remediation?

A major issue in quantifying costs and benefits is determining which costs and benefits to count: are only the costs incurred and benefits received by a department or organization to be considered or the total societal costs? Healthcare organizations are likely to include only their own costs and benefits and ignore social costs like medical expenses incurred outside their organizations, lost output due to absence from work, or the benefits of successful treatment that increase productivity and wages. CEA is employed when benefits cannot be easily monetized, for example, what is the value of a human life or pain and suffering?

CBA, like capital budgeting, often entails aggregating costs and benefits spanning multiple years, requiring later benefits to be discounted to their present value (PV) to achieve equivalent purchasing power comparisons. For example, should a person be vaccinated in his or her teens or twenties for human papillomavirus (HPV), when HPV-caused cancer may take decades to develop? This is a time-value-of-money problem, where an immediate cash outlay is made to obtain future benefits. In the case of HPV, the cost per dose is approximately $135, and three doses are required for a total outlay of $405. The question is, what is the future value of $405 compounded over 40 years, or what is the discounted value of treatment received in 40 years? The point emphasized in the chapter "Capital Budgeting" is that when costs and benefits are received at different points in time, the time value of money should be recognized to ensure that real, as opposed to nominal, benefits exceed real costs.

BOX 14.1 The Cost–Benefit Analysis Process

1. Identify objectives and alternatives.
2. Identify the inputs and outcomes of each alternative.
3. Monetize inputs (costs) and outcomes (benefits).
4. Discount costs and benefits.
5. Summarize, compare, and evaluate alternatives.
6. Perform sensitivity analysis.

Step 5 defines how alternatives will be compared: will alternatives be evaluated on the basis of which alternatives generate the highest net present value (NPV) or which provide the highest return, depending on resources employed, the internal rate of return (IRR) or the benefit–cost ratio (BCR)?

-Stand-alone decision rule: benefit ≥ cost (NPV ≥ 0.00, IRR ≥ discount rate, or BCR ≥ 1.00)

-One of multiple alternatives decision rules: max. NPV, IRR, or BCR

Step 6, sensitivity analysis, asks how the desirability of an investment changes when key variables change. How will marginal benefit change, given changes in output, output prices, and expenses? Sensitivity analysis calculates how much output or revenue projections can be overstated or expenses understated before other investments become more desirable. Managers should consider how much variation in expected values is needed to change program rankings and assess how likely that amount of change will occur. The more insulated a project's net benefit is to fluctuations in output, output prices, and expenses, the less risky the investment. Microsoft Excel's sensitivity analysis function, **Goal Seek** under **Data** and **What-If Analysis**, was discussed in the chapter "Capital Budgeting."

Example of a Cost–Benefit Analysis

In the chapter "Capital Budgeting," an investment choice was presented as go/no-go: should a plant be built to produce 1,250,000 units of output over its useful life? Determining whether the investment should be made requires summarizing the expected cost and revenues. The investment in plant and equipment is expected to run $4,000,000, and the variable cost per unit of output is $2.00. Each unit of output is expected to sell for $7.5172. The NPV is $2,897,000 ($9,387,000 − $4,000,000

− $2,500,000), and the BCR is 1.72 (($9,387,000 − $2,500,000)/$4,000,000). The investment should be undertaken since NPV > 0.00 and BCR > 1.00.

The problem is only one option is presented and it meets the financial criteria for acceptance under stand-alone decision rules, but no other alternatives are considered. The question should be, is this option the best use of limited investment dollars? Should a plant be built to produce more or less than 1,250,000 units? Consider the discounted benefits and costs in **TABLE 14.2**. It would be tempting to invest in a plant that could produce 1,450,000 units as costs and benefits are equal, BCR = 1.00, and NPV = 0.00. In a capital-rationing situation, where the best of multiple alternatives is selected, the NPV is maximized with a plant that produces 950,000 units and the BCR is maximized with a capacity of 550,000.

Browning and Browning (1994) emphasize that investment decisions should not necessarily be undertaken as long as the benefits equal or exceed costs, nor should the choice be based on maximizing the NPV. **TABLE 14.3** shows that if a plant with a capacity of 1,450,000 units is built, expected benefits and cost are $10,900,000 and the investment should be undertaken. However, it is clear that building a plant to this scale is undesirable; expanding capacity from 1,250,000 to 1,450,000 units increases the fixed cost by $4,000,000 and the total variable cost by $400,000 and increases revenue only by $1,503,000. The marginal benefit is $0.3416 for every dollar expended ($1,503,000/$4,400,000) to expand capacity, or 34.16¢ is earned (or 65.84¢ are lost) per dollar expended.

Similarly, building a capacity of 1,250,000 units is financially undesirable despite the fact that NPV ≥ 0.00 and BCR ≥ 1.00. The marginal benefit of a plant this size is less than 1.00 again, indicating the additional costs required for expansion are not met by additional revenues. Cost increases by $2,600,000 over a plant with a capacity of 950,000 units, while revenue

TABLE 14.2 Determining the Efficient Plant Size

Q (000)	TFC	TVC	Total Cost	Total Revenue	Profit	BCR	MB
0	0	0	0	0	0	0.00	0.00
250	$500	$500	$1,000	$1,879	$879	2.76	1.88
550	$1,000	$1,100	$2,100	$4,134	$2,034	3.03	2.05
950	$2,000	$1,900	$3,900	$7,141	$3,241	2.62	1.67
1250	$4,000	$2,500	$6,500	$9,397	$2,897	1.72	0.87
1450	$8,000	$2,900	$10,900	$10,900	$0.00	1.00	0.34

TFC, total fixed cost; TVC, total variable cost; MB, marginal benefit.

TABLE 14.3 CBA of Fall Prevention Programs

Program	Outcome: Fall Reduction (%)	Benefit ($)	Cost	Net Benefit	ROI (%)
Otago	35	$461.00	$339.15	$121.85	35.9
Tai Chi	55	$633.90	$104.02	$529.88	509.4
Stepping on	31	$345.75	$211.38	$134.37	63.6

only increases by $2,256,000. The size of the plant that maximized the NPV was 950,000 units, and its marginal benefit was 1.67 (each dollar of cost generated $1.67 in revenue); the size of the plant that maximized the BCR was 550,000 units (each dollar of investment, each dollar of fixed cost, generated $3.03 of profit). Marginal benefit analysis by explicitly recognizing the change in revenue and expenses clarifies the decision between plant sizes; select the plant that maximizes the marginal benefit. If additional money is available, investment should be expanded until the marginal benefit equals 1.00.

Investments should not be made when marginal benefit < 1.00; investing in a plant to produce 950,000 units is appropriate if no other investments are available that can produce a marginal benefit greater than 1.67. Expanding beyond 550,000 units increased costs by $1,800,000 and revenue by $3,007,000; if the next-best alternative offers a marginal benefit of 1.66 or less, for example, 1.50, it is clear that expanding capacity from 550,000 to 950,000 will create more value ($3,007,000 ($1,800,000 * 1.67)) than investing the $1,800,000 elsewhere ($2,700,000). If another opportunity

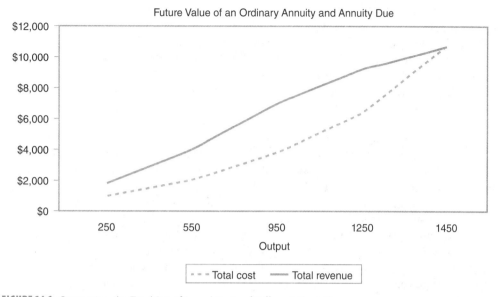

FIGURE 14.1 Comparing the Total Benefits and Costs of Different Plant Sizes

could provide a marginal benefit of 1.80, the 550,000-unit plant should be built and the $1,800,000 saved should be invested in the other opportunity; total return would be $2,034,000 plus $3,240,000 ($1,800,000 * 1.80).

FIGURE 14.1 illustrates the investment choice for program size but fails to highlight opportunity costs, that is, if the investment is not undertaken or its size is reduced, what other options are available for the funds and what benefit will they provide? **FIGURE 14.2** provides the answer: projects and their sizes should be ranked according to the marginal benefit they generate.

Figure 14.2 demonstrates that if the return on the smallest plant is acceptable, then the next-largest plant should be built as its marginal benefit exceeds that of the smallest plant (2.05 versus 1.88). This outcome is the result of economies of scale: the average total cost falls as capacity increases. Beyond 550,000 units, diseconomies of scale arise, reducing the marginal benefit to 1.67. The decision on whether to expand plant size to 950,000 units should be based on opportunity costs: if another project offers a return greater than 1.67, funds should be invested there; if the next-best alternative is less than 1.67, the current project should be expanded. Plants with

capacities of 1,250,000 or 1,450,000 units should not be built as they fail to generate benefits equal to the resources expended, that is, they have a marginal benefit less than 1.00.

Cost–Benefit Analysis Cases

The preceding example provided a standard business approach to CBA; the cases of Carande-Kulis et al. (2015) and McKinnell, Bartsch, Lee, Huang, and Miller (2015) demonstrate how CBA has been applied in health care.

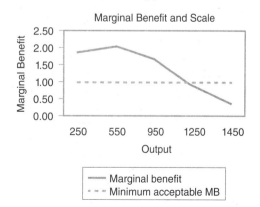

FIGURE 14.2 Comparing the Marginal Benefits and Costs of Different Plant Sizes

Carande-Kulis et al. (2015) used CBA to examine three fall prevention programs: *Otago* an individually designed, muscle-strengthening and balance training delivered by a physical therapist; *Tai Chi*, emphasizing weight-shifting, postural alignment, and coordinated movement demonstrated by Tai Chi instructors; and *Stepping on*, group exercises and fall discussions led by an occupational therapist. Carande-Kulis et al.'s goal was to determine whether fall preventions should be undertaken and, if so, which method to pursue. Steps 2 and 3 identified the inputs and outcomes of each alternative and their costs and benefits. The cost per participant was $339.15 for Otago, $104.20 for Tai Chi, and $211.38 for Stepping on. If these programs were equally effective in reducing falls, Tai Chi would be the optimal choice, given its lower cost.

Effectiveness, however, was not equal; the authors reported that falls were reduced by 35% by Otago, 55% by Tai Chi, and 31% by Stepping on, which amounted to monetary benefits (avoided medical costs per participant) of $461.00, $633.90, and $345.75, respectively. Tai Chi not only costs less per participant than Otago and Stepping on but also provides the largest reduction in falls.

Step 4, discounting of costs and benefits, was not performed as cost and benefits were assumed to be incurred and received in the same period, so step 5 simply involved subtracting costs from benefits to determine the net benefit and dividing the net benefit by cost to calculate the return on investment (ROI). Table 14.3 summarizes.

On the basis of the accounting of costs and benefits, all three fall prevention programs are financially viable: avoided medical costs exceed program costs, and fall prevention should be undertaken. In comparing the effectiveness of each program, it appears Tai Chi should be the first choice, given it reduces falls the most and has the lowest cost per participant. Tai Chi's ROI of 509.4% reflects the fact that more people could be served and a greater reduction in falls can be achieved; for every Otago participant, 3.26 ($339.15/$104.20) people could be instructed in Tai Chi. For every 1 fall prevented by Otago (2.85 * 35%), 5.12 (3.26 people * 2.85 * 55%) falls may be prevented by Tai Chi.

Tai Chi should be funded first if funds are limited; sensitivity analysis shows that even if the effectiveness of Tai Chi is overstated by 20%, it is still as good as Otago. Likewise, the cost per Tai Chi participant could increase by 226.04% and still be comparable to Otago. Given the positive ROI on the other two programs, they may also be considered, especially as the effectiveness decreases and the cost of Tai Chi increases as the program expands. A second consideration is the receptivity of the target population: are there individuals who may refuse to participate in or be incapable of practicing Tai Chi who could benefit from the other two programs?

McKinnell et al. (2015) studied the economic impact on hospitals of universal screening for Methicillin-resistant *Staphylococcus aureus* (MRSA). The research was motivated by prior research that concluded that universal MRSA screening generated a net social benefit, and highlights a key issue in CBA: whose costs and whose benefits are included in the analysis? In the McKinnell et al. study, only hospital costs to run the screening program and avoided medical costs (benefit) were included. Their cost benefit measure was as follows:

$$\left(\begin{array}{c} \text{No. of infections averted} * \\ \text{MRSA LOS} * \text{Cost/day} \end{array} \right) -$$

Cost of screening plus contact precautions,

where LOS is the length of stay.

The low-cost alternative was chromogenic agar screening (nares) and had an intervention cost of $252,234 (range: $209,295–$299,142) for swabs, testing, gloves, gowns, and nursing time (largest cost component) per 1000 tests. The intervention identified 2.7 (2.1−3.4) MRSA cases per 1000 and averted $24,740 in medical cost, or costs exceeded benefit by −$227,494 (−$189,867 to −$273,610). The high-cost alternative was polymerase chain reaction screening (nares) with an intervention cost of $669,420 ($608,348–$732,835) for swabs, testing (increase of 5.88x over the cost of chromogenic agar screening [nares] and the largest cost component), gloves, gowns, and nursing time. Polymerase chain reaction screening (nares) identified more MRSA cases per 1000 tests, that is, 4.2 (3.4–5.1), and averted $37,630 in medical costs, but costs exceeded benefit by −$631,790 (−$577,609 to −$689,002).

McKinnell et al. (2015) concluded that regardless of the intervention used and assumptions made concerning costs and benefits, universal MRSA screening increases total hospital costs. Unlike other studies that concluded universal screening is beneficial from a societal perspective, McKinnell et al. raise the question of who should pay the additional costs and whether reimbursement to hospitals should be increased. A second point is, what method should be used? It appears that the low-cost alternative of chromogenic agar screening (nares) should be used over the high-cost polymerase chain reaction screening (nares) as the 55.6% increase in MSRA case identification (4.2 versus 2.7) does not seem to warrant the 165.4% increase in screening and prevention costs ($669,420 versus $252,234). Of course, there is more to life than the weighing of monetary benefits and costs, so the next section examines the cost of reaching nonmonetary objectives.

CBA requires clear thinking: what is the desired goal? The goal must be specific and concrete, identifying exactly how benefit will be measured. Once the goal is clear, CBA facilitates a focused search for alternatives to reach the goal. A common failure is to suspend the search for alternatives after one viable method is identified; in most cases, multiple alternatives exist with different degrees of effectiveness and costs that also provide different incentives and disincentives on affected parties. It is vital that CBA recognizes to the extent possible how the different alternatives affect all parties and any potential unintended consequences. Finally, the acceptability of any program will be affected by who gains (benefits) and loses (pays) from the program. While

we would like to believe that any program that generates net benefits would be pursued, we must recognize that garnering support for the expenditure of resources will be easier when more people gain than lose. Value-creating programs that serve a small constituency may need to restructure their output and costs to gain widespread support from affected parties. All managers should be skilled in CBA to determine when goals are worth pursuing, what the best means to achieve a goal are, and how to gain public support.

▶ Cost-Effectiveness Analysis

CEA is used to assess alternative means to achieve an objective after its desirability has been established. Unlike CBA, CEA does not have to justify whether an end is worth pursuing; it begins with the assumption that increasing life expectancy, knowledge, etc., is worthwhile, and seeks the most efficient means to reach the end. CEA avoids endless debate on what the value of human life is and how much should be spent to prolong life. Many believe life is priceless, but day-to-day living does not allow us to allocate resources on this idea. If life were indeed priceless, society would be willing to spend whatever was necessary to save a life, for example, $1 million or $10 million on an experimental treatment with a low probability of success. Knowledge of opportunity costs, however, makes us allocate our limited resources to their best ends, eliminating low-return expenditures.

Doubilet, Weinstein, and McNeil (1986) note that the term "cost effective" has been used in medicine with four distinct meanings. The first equates it to cost savings, similar to CBA, and the second to achieving a desired goal at any cost. Neither definition is appropriate, as cost-effectiveness deals with cost and outcomes. A third definition holds that "cost effective" is cost savings with equal or better outcome. While most people would agree this combination is cost-effective, it excludes any intervention that increases cost regardless of whether people are willing to pay more for a better outcome. The final definition of "cost effective" is a change that produces a marginal benefit that exceeds its marginal cost; this definition embraces interventions that produce better health outcomes at higher cost—the critical factors are how much are health outcomes improved and how much do costs increase?

Typically, CEA compares the cost per outcome for different treatments for a single condition to determine which treatment is more desirable and treatments across conditions to determine which conditions should be given priority. Priority setting was the objective of zero-base budgeting (ZBB) and program budgeting, and the chapters "Zero-Base Budgeting" and "Program Budgeting" presented cases of how to maximize health services and outcomes to a population. When comparisons are made across conditions, the results are presented in **league tables**. Simple league tables list interventions on the basis of the lowest to the highest cost per outcome; detailed league tables list interventions from the lowest to the highest cost per outcome and provide the expected changes in cost and outcomes (**TABLE 14.4**).

Cost-effectiveness logic is illustrated by a case from 1993 where conjoined twins were born in Chicago and the probability of successfully separating them was reported to be 1.0%. The cost of separating the twins was estimated to be $1 million, and at best, only one baby would survive. Undertaking surgery in this case places an implicit value of $100,000,000 ($1,000,000/0.01) on life. Obviously, no society could commit $100 million to saving the lives of all their citizens as none has sufficient wealth for this level of investment. A Chicago hospital declined the surgery because of the low probability of success, and the twins were flown to Philadelphia, where they underwent surgery; both died.

The case highlights an important point about life-saving efforts: not all lives are equal, and in the case of infants, many of us agree that more money should be spent on the young. When medical resources are used, we should strive to obtain the maximum-possible benefit, and that benefit is directly proportional to remaining life expectancy. A newborn female in the United States can be expected to live to 81.2 years, while a 65-year-old women can expect to live another 20.5 years (Centers for Disease Control and Prevention [CDC], 2015). If each needs $100,000 in healthcare services, the expected cost per life year added is $1232 for the infant versus $4878 for the 65-year-old. A 95-year-old woman would be expected to survive only 3.3 years, and the cost per life year added is $30,303. Decisions should be made recognizing where finite resources will produce the greatest benefit, and if resources must be rationed, we should want to fund infant care before care for 65-year-olds (4.0 times greater benefit) or 95-year-olds (24.6 times greater benefit), assuming treatments have the same probability of success and do not produce undesirable side effects.

The value of life is not based solely on the quantity of life, and we should recognize that the value of one more year of life is not homogenous. The quality of life matters as much as or more than the quantity of life. For example, Beresniak et al. (2015) sought to determine peoples' preferences between living without a physical disability, walking with a limp, walking with a rollator, and being confinement to a wheelchair. Most people expressed that they prefer shorter lives without a disability or with a minor disability to longer but more restricted lives. Beresniak et al. found among the people they surveyed, 10 years of living with a limp or walking with a rollator would be "worth" 7.8 and 6.9 years, respectively, without a disability, that is, the average person is indifferent to 10 years of limping and 7.8 years with full function. If an intervention increases life expectancy by more than 2.2 years, from 7.8 to 10 years, and produces limping, the average

TABLE 14.4   Detailed League Table

Intervention	Change in Cost (2010 Dollars)	Change in QALY	Cost-Effectiveness Ratio	Source
Early surgery compared to prolonged conservative care to treat patients with sciatica from lumbar disc herniation	−$10	0.02–0.04	Saves money and improves health	van den Hout et al. (2008)
Coumadin (warfarin) compared to aspirin for 70-year-olds with atrial fibrillation	$3,000	0.81	$3,704	O'Brien and Gage (2005)
Daily dialysis compared to dialysis every other day for 60-year-old critically ill men with kidney injury	$13,000	2.14	$6,075	Desai et al. (2008)
ICD compared to current standard of care to prevent sudden cardiac death for patients at risk for sudden death due to left ventricular systolic dysfunction	$113,000	3.00	$37,667	Sanders, Hlatky, and Owens (2005)
Spine surgery compared to nonoperative treatment for adult patients with confirmed spinal stenosis and spinal nerve-based (radicular) leg pain	$15,000	0.17	$88,235	Tosteson et al. (2008)
Annual CT screening compared to no screening for 60-year-old heavy smokers who are eligible for lung reduction surgery	$6,000	0.04	$150,000	Mahadevia et al. (2003)
Heparin sodium and alteplase compared to heparin sodium for hemodynamically stable patients with submassive pulmonary embolism and right ventricular dysfunction	$700	−0.05	Increases cost and worsens health	Perlroth, Sanders, and Gould (2007)

QALY, quality-adjusted life year; ICD, implantable cardioverter defibrillator; CT, computed tomography.

person would see this as a desirable healthcare choice. If the intervention expands life expectancy by less than 2.2 years and is accompanied by limping, the average person would theoretically forego treatment.

Quality-adjusted life years (QALYs) recognize that every year of life is not created equal in order to rationalize resource allocation by directing resources to interventions on the basis of the increased life expectancy and value of the years gained. QALYs ascribe a value of 1.00 (100%) to 1 year of perfect health and 0.00 to death. Between these two poles lie many alternatives; years with reduced mobility, confined to home or hospital, with depression, etc. Sackett and Torrance (1978) reported the value of hospital confinement due to contagious diseases decreased with the length of confinement; confinement for 3 months was worth 1.7 months (56%) of perfect health, and confinement for 8 years was seen as equivalent to 2.6 years (33%) of perfect health. Torrance (1987) reported how the severity of disease influenced people's evaluation of various health states; mild angina was evaluated at 90%, while severe angina and the loss of sight, hearing, or speech were evaluated at 50% and 39%, respectively, of perfect health. Torrance's paper was noteworthy in that he reported that people evaluate certain health states as less desirable than death (0.00); these included quadriplegic, blind, and depressed patients, those confined to bed with severe pain, and unconscious people (<0.00).

There are three primary methods of determining the quality of life or preferences between health states: rating scale, standard gamble, and time trade-off. The use of a rating scale simply asks people to rank the values of different health states on a scale from 0.00 to 1.00. If people rank condition X as 0.50, then the average person would be willing to accept 2 years with X or 1 year of perfect health, that is, the value of life with X is one-half the value of life without the medical condition.

The **standard gamble** offers people the choice between a less than perfect health state and a treatment that will return them to perfect health but carries a risk of immediate death. The value placed on the health state is the highest probability of death the individual is willing to accept for a chance to return to perfect health. For example, if hospital confinement due to a contagious disease is worth 0.16, an individual should be willing to accept a treatment with a 16% chance of restoring him or her to perfect health and an 84% likelihood of killing him or her. When calculating these odds, the probability of success is increased and the probability of death lowered until people accept the gamble. The value of the health state is thus the highest probability of death (or 1.00 minus the lowest probability of success) people are willing to assume.

The third method is the **time trade-off**, which again provides respondents with choices. Assume you could live 10 years with a disease or disability or 9 years in perfect health; which would you choose? If the respondent selects perfect health, the number of years of perfect health is reduced (to 8 years...) until the respondent selects life with the disease or disability. The value of the health state is the lowest number of years a person is willing to accept to move from his or her health state to perfect health.

QALYs are simply the change in life expectancy expected from treatment multiplied by the value of the added years (Equation 14.2).

$$\text{QALYs} = \text{Number of life years} \\ * \text{Quality of life (0.00 – 1.00)} \quad (14.2)$$

QALYs allow disparate interventions to be compared. For example, Torrance (1987) reported life with the side effects of hypertension treatment was worth 0.97 (0.95–0.99) and with a kidney transplant was worth 0.84. Both treatments can be compared since we have a common metric of outcome: an additional 10 years of life from these interventions would be worth 9.7 and 8.4 years, respectively, and the only remaining question is, what is the cost of treatment? **TABLE 14.5** highlights time-trade-off utilities

TABLE 14.5 Quality-of-Life Adjustment Factors Across Countries

	Anchor, Skin and Joints	Mild, Skin and Joints	Moderate, Skin, Joints, Hematology, and Heart or Lungs	Severe, Skin, Joints, Hematology, and Heart or Lungs	Severe, Skin, Joints, and Central Nervous System	Severe, Skin, Joints, and Renal
Australia	0.75	0.60	0.41	0.23	0.30	0.35
Canada	0.76	0.65	0.42	0.28	0.35	0.37
Spain	0.80	0.71	0.53	0.33	0.45	0.43
France	0.80	0.64	0.46	0.26	0.34	0.33
Japan	0.66	0.55	0.38	0.19	0.33	0.36
United Kingdom	0.82	0.71	0.48	0.29	0.36	0.45
Average	0.77	0.64	0.45	0.26	0.35	0.38

for varying degrees of lupus on the basis of a study by Pollard et al. (2015).

Table 14.5 shows remarkable consistency in the evaluation of health states across six countries. Spaniards generally evaluate each health state the highest and the Japanese the lowest. As expected, the time-trade-off utilities decline as lupus becomes more severe; when lupus is limited to skin and joint involvement (the anchor state), 1 year is valued at 0.77 years of perfect health. As organ involvement increases, the reported quality of life declines, with a year of severe lupus involving skin, joints, hematology, and heart or lungs, valued at 0.26.

The value of health states in QALYs is influenced by how choice is structured and produces inconsistencies when choices are presented as the probability of success or failure. People consistently place a higher value on alternatives with an 80% chance of

success versus a 20% chance of failure, despite the fact that both probabilities describe the same underlying risk. A second source of bias arises from the number of health states compared. Context bias depresses the value of health states when they are compared with better health states and increases valuations when they are compared with worse states. A third factor that affects valuation is who is evaluating the health state; those without the condition tend to place a lower value on each health state than those currently with the condition, that is, the fear of living with cancer (or another disease) is worse than actually living with cancer.

Despite the limitations of QALYs, it is imperative that consideration be given to the quality of life. If the quality of life is not considered, interventions that extend life would always be favored over those that improve life. For example, a pill that costs $50,000 and extends life by 1 month for cancer patients would be favored over treatments that restore sight, hearing, and/or mobility for the duration of one's life but do not extend life. If the quality of life is not considered, a treatment that extends life by 1 month but makes one blind, deaf, and immobile would be favored over treatments that improve sight, hearing, and mobility. CEA using QALYs is also called cost utility analysis.

The cost-effectiveness ratio (CER) is Δcost/Δoutcome. **TABLE 14.6** highlights the choices individuals and society face in making medical decisions when interventions have different degrees of effectiveness and cost. The change in outcomes are categorized as high, increasing QALYs by 1 or more years; low 0 to 0.99 years; and negative, reducing life expectancy. Cost is categorized as cost saving, that is, reducing health expenditures; low cost, that is, less than $10,000 per QALY; and high cost, that is, $10,000 or more per QALY.

Any interventions that increase QALYs and reduce medical spending should be funded. While interventions falling into cell I are preferred, it behooves society to pursue interventions that may only marginally increase QALYs but reduce costs (cell IV). Cell II interventions in a health system that rations resources are clearly superior to interventions

in cells III and V. CER_{II} is $10,000 or less (<$10,000/>1.0) per life year. Cells III and V highlight the need for CEA as people and society should balance costs and outcomes to determine which interventions are more desirable.

Assume intervention A (cell III) increases QALYs by 2.0 years and costs $5000 and intervention B (cell V) increases QALYs by 0.5 and costs $1250—the CER for both is $2500 (A: $5000/2; B: $1250/0.5). An increase in the effectiveness of A or B or a reduction in their costs, however, would create a clear preference for one intervention over the other. Interventions in cell VI would fall into the "nice to have if you can afford it" category. Assume intervention C increases QALYs by 0.5 and costs $15,000; its CER is $30,000 (12 times the cost of interventions A and B). Those afflicted with the condition that C treats may believe this is a good use of resources, but society should recognize that every half year gained using C consumes the same level of resources that would increase life by 6 years using A or B. As a rule, interventions that reduce the quantity and/or quality of life (interventions VII–IX) should not be utilized. A case can be made that cell VII interventions should be used in countries where healthcare expenditures must be cut. If an intervention can substantially reduce costs with only

TABLE 14.6 Decision-Making and Cost-Effectiveness

Effectiveness (ΔQALY)	ΔCost		
	Cost Saving	**Low Cost** ($\leq$$10,000)	**High Cost** (>$10,000)
High ($x \geq 1.0$)	I	II	III
Low ($0.0 \leq x < 1.0$)	IV	V	VI
Negative ($x < 0.0$)	VII	VIII	IX

marginal reductions in health, for example, generic drugs versus reformulated, marginally better, and substantially higher-priced patent drugs, they should be considered.

The Cost-Effectiveness Analysis Process

CEA is used to select an intervention from mutually exclusive alternatives to meet a need and select the needs to be met. The first step in the CEA process identifies the research question, what is the goal or outcome sought? When choosing among competing alternatives, the question may be, what is the best way to treat heart disease? Zierler and Gray (2003) rightly argue that framing the research question as "Is intervention$_1$ better than intervention$_2$ for heart disease?" is incomplete. Better framing defines the perspective (society, patient), specifies the type of heart disease and target population to be treated, and defines what a better outcome is. Does "better" indicate an improvement in survival rates,

decrease in morbidity or cost, or a combination of factors?

When CEA is used to decide which needs should be met, that is, allocate resources, a common metric is needed. The research question would be, what interventions produce the largest improvement in health at the lowest cost? This is where QALYs become imperative; selecting the conditions to fund requires a common measure to account for increases in life years and the value of the years added.

Step 2, data collection, is simpler than CBA. In CEA, we do not have to assign a monetary value to the outcome (how much should we pay for one additional year of life or to avoid an infection, etc.), so data collection can be limited to the change in outcomes and relevant medical costs, including intervention costs and the cost of adverse outcomes (see **BOX 14.2** for the steps in CEA).

Skipping ahead to step 5 facilitates understanding. Muennig (2002) provides the following formulas for CERs and ICERs:

$$CER = \frac{(\text{Cost of intervention} - \text{Costs averted by intervention})}{\text{QALYs gained}} \quad (14.3)$$

$$ICER = \frac{(\text{Total cost intervention}_1 - \text{Total cost intervention}_2)}{(\text{QALYs intervention}_1 - \text{QALYs intervention}_2)} \quad (14.4)$$

The formulas break neatly into costs and benefits, steps 3 and 4. The numerator is the direct and indirect costs associated with an intervention. Direct costs are treatment costs, including the labor, supplies, equipment, and utilities required to deliver care. The author favors an activity-based costing approach that tracks the amount of resources consumed to provide an intervention and their input prices to determine costs but recognizes that cost is often determined using the output prices of services and a cost-to-charge ratio. The pitfall

---

BOX 14.2 The Cost-Effectiveness Analysis Process

1. Develop a research question.
2. Collect and organize data.
3. Calculate the change in costs.
4. Calculate the change in outcome.
5. Calculate CERs or incremental cost-effectiveness ratios (ICERs).
6. Perform sensitivity analysis.
7. Recommend and conclude.

of a charge-based cost estimate is that prices are set to maximize revenue without regard to cost and thus may not reflect actual cost. Indirect costs include the time a patient spends in treatment and the costs of getting to and from treatment.

Offsetting the cost of an intervention are costs averted by intervention: does a new therapy offset current costs? The best-case scenario would be a treatment that is more effective (increases QALYs) and replaces current therapies at a lower cost. When outcomes improve and costs decrease, the CER is negative: the intervention saves money and improves health. This situation could also be analyzed as CBA. In most cases, the cost of new interventions will (and should) exceed current treatment costs: a treatment increasing life expectancy and/or improving quality of life should be expected to be costlier than existing therapies.

The denominator, QALYs gained, is the expected change in the quantity or quality of life expected. Muennig (2002) notes the denominator is the repository for intangible costs—those hard-to-quantify factors that are reflected in the change in QALYs, such as pain and suffering. The denominator thus attempts to capture the impact of the disease and/or intervention on labor productivity or enjoyment of leisure.

Step 6, sensitivity analysis, examines how much the CER or ICER will change on the basis of changes in model variables and identifies when other alternatives become more desirable. How much can the chosen intervention's effectiveness decrease or its cost increase before another intervention becomes more desirable? Actual outcomes and costs often vary from expectations, so sensitivity analysis quantifies how far off the estimates of effectiveness or cost can be and whether this amount of variation is likely to arise before another alternative becomes viable.

Step 7, recommendation and conclusion, returns to the research question formulated in step 1. What intervention is being recommended for what condition and target group and on what grounds (ability to produce the best outcome, lowest cost, or lowest cost per outcome)? Does the data provide a clear case, does one intervention dominate others, or are differences in outcomes across interventions so marginal that treatment choices should be left to the preferences of patients and their physicians?

An Example of a Cost-Effectiveness Analysis

Step 1: Develop a research question.

Assess whether robotic gastrectomy is superior to open gastrectomy on the basis of a study of 200 stomach cancer patients between the ages of 55 and 65. Of these, 100 patients underwent each treatment, and costs were estimated on the basis of total charges multiplied by the cost-to-charges ratio for the hospital. No significant difference in mortality or complications was noted, so the outcome will be measured as the change in inpatient length of stay (LOS). Robotic gastrectomy was costlier because of equipment, maintenance, and licensing costs but reduced the LOS because of smaller and more precise incisions.

Step 2: Collect the outcome, cost, and demographic data.

Are experimental (robotic surgery) and control (open gastrectomy) groups comparable? Randomization of groups should result in each group having similar patients on the basis of age, gender, and medical condition.

Step 3: Calculate the difference in costs.

Robotic =	$24,522.27
Open =	21,615.92
	$2,906.35

Step 4: Calculate the difference in outcome.

Inpatient LOS:

Robotic =	10.98 days
Open =	12.96 days
	−1.98 days

Step 5: Calculate the ICER.

($24,522.27 − 21,615.92)/(10.98 − 12.96 days) =

$2,906.35/−1.98 days = −$1,468.47 per day

Robotic surgery reduces the LOS at a cost of $1468.47 per day.

Step 6: Perform sensitivity analysis.

If the cost of robotic gastrectomy falls by 11.9% or more or the cost of open gastrectomy increases by 13.4% or more, robotic gastrectomy would dominate open gastrectomy—a lower LOS at the same cost. Similarly, if the LOS for robotic gastrectomy increases by 18.0% or the LOS for open gastrectomy falls by 15.3%, open gastrectomy would dominate robotic gastrectomy.

Step 7: Make recommendations.

Given the shortcomings of charge-based cost determination, changes of 11.9% or 13.4% in cost can be expected, but given a sample of 200 patients, it is clear that robotic surgery reduces the length of inpatient hospitalizations by almost 2 days and increases total inpatient costs. The estimate of an increase in cost of $2906 creates a quandary for healthcare providers: are healthcare purchasers willing to pay $1468.47 per day for quicker discharge from the hospital? While patients may find it desirable to be discharged faster and return to work quicker, widespread adoption of robotic gastrectomy may be hampered if the additional costs are not covered by higher reimbursement.

Cost-Effectiveness Analysis Cases

Hopkins et al. (2011) examined the use of nurse-/nephrologist-supported care for patients with stage 3 to 4 chronic kidney disease versus standard care. The nurse-/nephrologist-supported care was directed at assisting patients in managing current health factors such as blood pressure and cholesterol levels that could lead to chronic kidney disease. Data was collected from 238 patients in the nurse-/nephrologist-supported (intervention) group and 236 patients in the standard care (control) group. Cost and outcome data are shown as follows:

	Cost	QALYs	CER
Intervention	$4,631	1.502	$3,083/QALY
Control	$5,741	1.456	$3,943/QALY
	−$1,109	0.046	
ICER	−$1,109/0.046 = −$24,109		

Hopkins et al. provide a clear case for the use of nurse-/nephrologist-supported care over standard care for chronic kidney disease. The CERs indicate both interventions increase QALYs at a relatively low cost; however, the ICER shows that nurse-/nephrologist-supported care dominates standard care in that it produces increases QALYs at a lower cost.

Pataky et al. (2013), assessed whether the use of magnetic resonance imaging (MRI), in addition to mammography, was cost-effective for breast cancer screening in *BRCA1* or *BRCA2* mutation carriers versus only mammography. Data was generated using a Markov model with sensitivity values of 89%–100% for MRI with mammography and 33%–50% for mammography alone. Specificity values accounting for more false positives and higher costs were 73%–80% for MRI and mammography and 91%–99% for mammography alone. Cost and outcome data are shown as follows:

	Cost	QALYs	CER
MRI + mammog-raphy	$9,893	22.66	$437/ QALY
Mammog-raphy	$5,201	22.57	$231/ QALY
	$4,692	0.092	
ICER	$4,692/0.092 = $50,911		

Pataky et al. provide a more interesting case as both options have a low cost and increase life expectancy substantially. The CER for MRI with mammography is $437 per QALY produced; if the choice were MRI with mammography but do nothing, the decision would clearly favor the use of MRI. The comparison, however, must be made against the next-best alternative, mammography only; the use of MRI increases QALYs by an additional 0.092 years and cost by $4692. Whether MRI should be used in conjunction with mammography comes down to what the value of an additional life year is. Is 1 year of life worth $50,911 ($4,692/0.092)? If you agree a life year is worth $50,911, there remains the larger societal or opportunity cost question of, could $50,911 employed in other areas increase life expectancy by more than 1 year? If maximization of health is the goal, it behooves society to allocate resources to interventions that extend life at a lower cost, and fund high-cost interventions as budgets allow.

CEA, by explicitly quantifying the cost per outcome, can be seen (or feared) as the first step toward healthcare rationing. Many of us do not like assigning any value to human life, yet in our daily lives, we make decisions and undertake activities that demonstrate we do not think our lives our priceless. We make trade-offs between safety and cost when we purchase cars; we undertake risky behavior, jaywalking rather than walking to a crosswalk and waiting for the WALK signal; and we smoke, drink, overeat, and fail to exercise. All of these choices can shorten our lives, but we do these things believing the benefits of these choices and behaviors exceed the potential shortening of our lives.

While we are comfortable with our own choices, concerns arise when healthcare choices (i.e., access) are dictated by third-party payers or the government. Beresniak et al. (2015) note the Patient Protection and Affordable Care Act (PPACA) does not recommend the use of cost-per-QALY estimates for healthcare decisions. CEA, despite starting with the assumption that life years should be prolonged, cannot help highlighting the different costs of life-prolonging treatments. It is only a matter of time before treatments are ranked from least expensive to most expensive and someone draws a line between an acceptable cost per QALY and unacceptable, that is, unreimbursed, treatments (see the Oregon Health Plan in the chapter "Program Budgeting"). It behooves all of us to understand how CEA defines the end pursued (value of added life years) and costs. Muennig believes that "cost-effectiveness analysis has become the standard (over CBA) for evaluating interventions in the health care field."

▶ Program Evaluation

CBA and CEA provide unique perspectives on whether future activities should be undertaken, but neither involves a comprehensive assessment of operations. CBA seeks to determine whether the benefits of an activity will exceed its expected cost, and CEA attempts to identify the best method of pursuing an objective. Both are forward-looking and rely on idealized operations, assuming things operate as planned. Program evaluation, on the other hand, is a wide-ranging and loosely defined methodology for assessing the actual performance of organizations. Program evaluation is concerned with what programs are supposed to do and what they actually achieve, similar to the relationship between prospective budget building and retrospective variance analysis.

Public dissatisfaction with government services, health care, education, and other professions is rising and highlights a clear disconnect between what the public wants and what it receives. Gallup reports 65% of Americans were dissatisfied with government in 2014 versus 30% in 2001 (McCarthy, January 22, 2014). The lack of comprehensiveness and other shortcomings of CBA and CEA provide opportunities for managers to present information in the most flattering light. Managers highlight successes and ignore everything else—no questions please. The counter to strategic behavior is comprehensive program evaluation specifying what will be examined and how it will be assessed. Life is more than "do benefits exceed cost?" or "what is the cost per outcome?"; managers should understand all aspects of their operations. The goal of program evaluation is not simply to document what is accomplished but also to assess how things are accomplished.

Program evaluation means different things to different people and disciplines. People trained in medicine, finance, and education have different ideas of what is valuable and how it should be measured. This text emphasizes financial analysis: costs and benefits are measured in dollars, but everyone recognizes there are other factors that outweigh monetary calculation. The balanced scorecard, Chapter 1, set the financial perspective and profit maximization as the primary goal of organizations but recognized that selling goods and services for more than their cost of production requires giving customers what they want, employing effective and efficient processes, and motivating and developing employees. Balanced scorecards offer one framework for developing a comprehensive program evaluation framework spanning multiple perspectives and potentially thwarting partial and self-serving analyses.

Rossi, Lipsey, and Freeman (2004, p. 18) provide five areas program evaluation should assess: (1) what need does the program fulfill, (2) how were processes designed, (3) how was the program implemented and how is it managed, (4) what outcomes are produced, and (5) are resources used efficiently? CBA and CEA, like budget building, focus on need and design, including expected costs and benefits; program evaluation, like variance analysis, adds actual output, expenses, and benefits. Program evaluation emphasizes what is achieved, more than what is produced, and how systems are implemented and managed. The five areas assessed connect why the program exists, how it should operate, how it operates, and what it produces.

The starting point for program evaluation identifies the need the program seeks to fulfill. What is the problem, how large is it, when and where does it arise, is it changing, and, if so, how is it changing? Answering these questions facilitates identifying the target population and the desired outcome. Identifying who (age, gender, race, ethnicity, income, etc.) and what change is sought sets the stage for identifying alternatives and determining which interventions may be more effective for a given group and outcome (**FIGURE 14.3**).

The second step assesses the evidence between the desired goal and possible interventions. Program design should specify the inputs needed, the processes expected to be

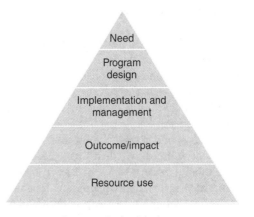

FIGURE 14.3 Program Evaluation Areas

used, the outputs expected to be produced, and the outcomes the outputs will advance. Program designers are building systems, and there should be clear links between the ends sought, the needs to be fulfilled, and the means selected to achieve the ends. Rossi et al. (2004, pp. 157–158) recommend the following questions when assessing program design:

- Are objectives well defined and feasible?
- Can the target population be identified and services maintained until the objectives are reached?
- Are processes defined and capable of promoting the desired objectives?
- Does the program have sufficient resources?

Broad objectives such as improving health (or increasing quality or reducing costs) are not helpful; specificity is essential, and cascade metrics are needed to identify where, when, how, and by whom objectives will be reached. Cascade metrics provide a roadmap from the big picture (organizational objectives such as reducing the cost per patient day or reducing adverse events) to specific actions to be taken at the department level (Nelson, Batalden, Godfrey, & Lazar, 2011). Specificity allows employees tasked with achieving the goals and evaluators to determine whether the end sought is consistent with existing research and/or practice or, when previously untried methods are considered, whether preliminary observation suggests an innovation can produce the desired goals.

For previously untested methods, plan-do-check-act (PDCA) cycles are a means to test-drive innovations before wide-scale implementation. In the PDCA cycle, **planning** identifies a need and means to achieve the goal, **do** is a small-scale test of the innovation, and **check** summarizes the results of the test. If the results are positive, then full-scale implementation is undertaken, that is, **act**; if outcomes are less than desired, program designers return to planning to develop and test other alternatives.

Identifying a need and an intervention capable of meeting the need is the easy part; the challenging part is putting a program into action and fulfilling the objectives at a reasonable cost. The third level assesses whether the program was implemented as planned and operated as expected. Assessing implementation and management is inextricably tied to impact and cost, the last two areas that should be reviewed. Well-managed programs efficiently achieve their goals; poorly run programs do not accomplish goals and/or consume excessive resources.

Assessing program management explores the target users of goods and services, the goods and services they actually receive, the adequacy and organization of human and physical resources, compliance with directives and legal and regulatory requirements, and consumer satisfaction. Implementation and management are concerned with how processes are organized, completed, and utilized; whether the desired outcome is realized at a reasonable cost is addressed in the fourth and fifth areas.

Rossi et al. (2004, pp. 172–173) provide a series of questions to assess utilization, organization and management, and consumer satisfaction. The first question is, how many people are receiving goods and services? Is the volume greater than, equal to, or less than expected? The second question is, are the intended targets receiving goods and services? Even if the expected number of people is receiving the goods and services, the objective may not be reached if the intended targets are not reached. One of the goals of *Sesame Street* was to narrow educational performance between children from high- and low-income families by creating programs for children from low-income families. The fact that the program reached beyond its intended audience (children from high-income families also watched *Sesame Street*) may have undermined the goal of narrowing the performance gap but increased the number of children benefitting from the program. When intended and actual consumers differ, managers should address why intended targets are not receiving services: is the target population unaware of or unable to access services? When unintended groups are being served, is this a good thing, or should the program be restructured to reach only the intended groups?

The third question is, are the goods and services produced capable of and meeting the desired goal? Are outputs of the correct type, produced in the appropriate quantity, and meeting generally accepted standards? Providing the wrong types of goods and services, in too high or low quantities, and/or low-quality output may inhibit reaching the desired outcome and efficient resource use. How outputs are produced may be as important as the output produced. Do processes follow generally accepted ways, and is performance adequate? Is the number and skills of the staff sufficient to meet program and consumer demands? Are physical resources such as facilities, equipment, and information systems sufficient to meet program and consumer demands? Are processes well organized, and does the staff work together? Does the staff work effectively with other programs that are required to achieve goals? If services are provided at multiple sites, is performance consistent across sites? When performance is inconsistent across sites, low-performing sites should be able to emulate the activities of higher-performing sites and improve their outcomes. The questions above are designed to determine whether managers can identify the appropriate outputs to realize the program's goals, assemble the necessary resources to complete work, and organize systems.

Does the program comply with the governing board's directives? The need was identified in step 1: are managers pursuing the goals specified by their governing bodies? Principal–agent theory holds that managers (agents) work for compensation to fulfill the interests of owners (principals). Principal–agent problems arise when principals delegate decision-making authority to others, that is, managers and managers forsake the principals' interests to pursue their own desires. The principal–agent problem is inherent in any organization where ownership and management are separated. In addition to board directives, programs must also satisfy federal, state, and local laws and regulations and professional standards.

Of course, it is possible to correctly identify need, produce a technically correct product, and follow all governing directives, laws, and regulations but still fail to satisfy consumers. The fourth area is concerned with consumer satisfaction with the goods and services received and their satisfaction with staff and procedures. Does a gap exist between what program designers and employees think consumers want or should have and what consumers actually want? Assuming what the program provides is what consumers want; there remains the issue of how it is provided. For example, a business, a healthcare provider, or a government agency may provide what consumers want but may force consumers to endure long wait times and/or tolerate poor customer service. Consumer satisfaction may be completely undermined despite the fact that the consumers received the product and outcome they wanted. Another metric of consumer satisfaction is the rate at which recommended follow-up visits or activities are completed. High rates of follow-up visits and activities not only validate management competency but also increase the probability that programs will meet their objectives.

The above questions are geared toward evaluating processes in place, but when objectives are not met, evaluators should determine whether this failure is due to current management or implementation. Implementation failures may prevent senior managers from reaching desired goals or efficient use of resources. Implementation failures (Rossi et al., 2004, pp. 191–194) include nonprograms, incomplete interventions, minimal delivery, "ritual compliance," wrong intervention, and unstandardized interventions.

Evaluation of management should be based on whether the need the program was created for was met and what amount of resources were consumed. Outcome assessment directly measures the results identified in needs assessment: who is the target population, what change is sought, what are the outcomes, and how should they be measured? Outcome assessment determines whether the expected results were obtained.

Measuring outcomes is often difficult and attributing outcomes to programs even more so. **FIGURE 14.4** demonstrates part of the problem: the desired outcome was increasing over time, and the program may have accelerated the increase. The challenge for evaluators is to identify how much of the change is due to the program and how much is due to chance or other factors. Statistical tests provide a clear rule; there must be less than a 5.0% probability that the change observed is due to chance before a researcher concludes the effectiveness of an intervention is supported. Figure 14.4 highlights the challenge of evaluating outcome: the desired outcome was improving before the program and should continue to improve; therefore, any change should be decomposed into trend improvements and program impact.

When outcomes are more than expected, it behooves managers and evaluators to determine why better-than-expected results arose and whether they can continue. When results are less than expected, their causes should be identified and remedies enacted, including considering whether different methods should be used. When funding is greater than or less than expected, actual and expected results should vary accordingly; however, differences in outcomes may or may not be related to funding. The value of a program is predominantly determined by whether it produces the intended effect.

The final issue deals with resources consumed: is value created and/or are outcomes efficiently produced? Even if the intended impact is produced, there remains the question of how much it cost to achieve and how much it should have cost. CBA or CEA should be used to compare expected and actual costs to determine whether a program is operating as expected and how it compares to relevant benchmarks. When actual costs are significantly higher than expected or the costs of similar programs per outcome produced, then the evaluation should return to implementation and management to determine where resources can be saved. A primary goal of program evaluation is to establish accountability and improve outcomes.

Shadish (2006) noted that the common threads of program evaluation are (1) a concern for constructing valid knowledge, including what can be known, and methodology, including defining measurement and analytical techniques; (2) recognizing what value is; (3) knowing how programs change and making improvement; (4) communicating results; and (5) developing a framework for conducting

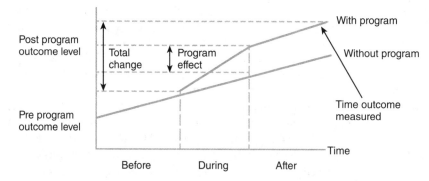

FIGURE 14.4 Outcome Assessment

evaluations. At the conclusion of a program evaluation, the answers to the following questions should be clear: Why is the program needed, and what does it hope to achieve? How was the program implemented, and how is it run? What has it achieved? Shadish recognizes that the primary focus of an evaluation should change with the age of a program. New programs should focus on need and implementation, while evaluation of mature programs should emphasize management and outcomes (2006, p. 3).

Rossi et al. (2004) provided the framework for "what should be assessed and how it should be assessed," which is invaluable in designing a program. However, most managers and evaluators will not be involved in program design but will, rather, be brought in after implementation to manage and/or assess performance. The Centers for Disease Control and Prevention (CDC) (1999) provides a six-step framework for conducting program reviews, beginning with stakeholder engagement and ending with dissemination of findings (**BOX 14.3**). The first step is to engage stakeholders, including those served by the program (patients, customers, etc.), those operating the program (employees, suppliers, etc.), and the users of the evaluation (senior managers, public officials, regulators, etc.). It is vital that all stakeholders be involved in the evaluation process; evaluations should be tailored to the needs of those expected to use the information so that their questions and concerns are addressed. Questions about

effectiveness and outcomes cannot be assessed without talking to the consumers of services, and questions of efficiency require understanding how work is performed, which can only be gained by talking to workers.

Step 2, describing the program, follows the framework suggested by Rossi et al. (2004), beginning with the need: what is the problem, including its extent, who is affected, is the need changing, and, if so, how is it changing? The discussion of need should conclude with a statement of intended outcomes and how they will be measured. Program design is next: how is the system supposed to operate, are expected processes mapped out, and are they conceptually sound? The next step determines whether actual operations conform to design: was the program implemented effectively, and is it well managed? The description of actual operation should draw a flowchart of or map program activities and identify resources (labor, supplies, equipment, buildings, etc.) consumed.

The primary reason for the existence of a program is to produce an outcome: what outcomes are produced and how do they compare with the outcomes described in the need statement? The CDC notes that outcomes evolve over time, so program administrators and evaluators should distinguish short- and long-term outcomes and report unintended consequences. When outcomes are less than expected, is it due to a changing need, poor program design, implementation, management, or deficiency of resources? While recognizing a need and fulfilling the need are the sine qua non for a program, the ability to produce an outcome or impact at a reasonable cost may determine its continuation. Program evaluators should be able to compare actual costs to expected costs and similar programs to determine whether more or less resources should be consumed.

Step 3, designing and focusing the evaluation plan, requires identifying the purpose of the program evaluation. The purpose may be one or all of the following: improvement, accountability, knowledge generation, and

---

BOX 14.3 CDC Program Evaluation Process

1. Engage stakeholders and define goals and measures.
2. Describe the program.
3. Focus the evaluation design.
4. Collect data.
5. Justify conclusions.
6. Disseminating findings.

public relations. The purpose of the evaluation should have been determined in step 1: what do stakeholders want? After the purpose is identified, how outcomes will be measured must be determined. Outcome methods include experimental (random assignment to intervention and control groups), quasi-experimental (potentially nonequivalent groups based on location), and observational (case studies) methods. The evaluation method defines the next step, data collection, and affects the validity, reliability, and generalizability of the results.

Step 4 collects data on the measures defined in step 1; measures should be relevant, credible, and comprehensive, that is, provide a comprehensive picture of program operation. Sources of reliable and valid information should be identified, and data collection should be delegated to parties who do not have an interest in over- or understating outcomes. The quantity of data collected should balance the need for accurate information against the cost of collecting large amounts of data.

Step 5, justifying conclusions, should tie data collected to standards: Are the desired results being achieved at the expected costs, and are stakeholders satisfied? What are the programs strengths and weaknesses, and where should resources be increased to expand or improve activities? Should activities be contracted? What does the evidence demonstrate about the performance of the program, and what value judgments are incorporated into decisions regarding the expansion, contraction, or continuation of activities? Finally, recommendations are made setting forth the actions that should be taken by decision-makers.

Disseminating findings is the final step. Findings and lessons learned should be shared with stakeholders, who should be given an opportunity to comment, and ultimately, the evaluation's findings should be put to use. The goal of program evaluation to facilitate informed decision-making and positive action can only be achieved if results are communicated to and accepted by stakeholders.

Program Evaluation Cases

Kleinsorge, Roberts, Roy, and Rapoff (2010) performed a program evaluation for a pediatric primary care training clinic to determine whether it met the standards of primary care and medical homes and satisfied the parents of the children treated. Kleinsorge et al. defined six relevant medical home dimensions: accessibility, continuity, coordination, comprehensiveness, communication and compassion, and cultural competency. Accessibility was measured as driving distance, scheduling and wait times, and insurance and payment options. Continuity was measured by the rate at which a patient was seen by the same healthcare professional. Coordination of care examined whether healthcare providers collaborated with other healthcare workers in developing and carrying out care plans, including sharing of information and referral rates. Comprehensive care assessed whether prevention and treatment covered all of a patient's physical and mental health needs. Interpersonal communication and compassion encompassed listening, explaining, spending time with patients, and incorporating family input into treatment decisions. Cultural competency was defined as recognizing and incorporating the family's cultural beliefs into treatment plans.

The study was notable for the incorporation of existing measurement instruments to assess the clinic's performance. The Client Satisfaction Questionnaire-8 (CSQ-8) was used for parent satisfaction, the Parent's Perception of Primary Care (P3C) was used to assess quality of care, communication and compassion were assessed using the Consumer Assessment of Health Plan Study (CAHPS) 2.0 Child Core Questionnaire, and additional questions were written to assess cultural competency. While parents and their children were one group of stakeholders, Kleinsorge et al. recognized the program evaluation would be incomplete if attitudes of employees were not assessed. The Job Satisfaction Questionnaire developed by

Byers, Mays, and Mark (1999) was used to obtain worker feedback.

Parents indicated they were happy with accessibility (appointment scheduling and ease of travel) and conformance with primary care and medical home standards. Unsurprisingly, Kleinsorge et al. found parents were dissatisfied with waiting times, continuity (40.2% could not name a specific provider as their child's regular provider), and cultural competency (nearly half indicated their cultural beliefs were not elicited).

Employees indicated they were most satisfied with the care they were delivering (self-evaluation of performance) and expressed the least satisfaction with the support services they received and the benefits of employment. In both cases, the input of parents and employees identified opportunities for the clinic to improve its operation.

Kleinsorge et al. concludes, "The results of the present study indicate this clinic could improve services and satisfaction ratings by decreasing the time families spend waiting and by emphasizing continuity, coordination, and comprehensiveness of care." The value of this program evaluation was its clear enunciation of what would be measured and the conformance of performance data to primary care and medical home standards—it provided clear direction on how performance should change. The weakness of the study was its disregard for resource use: it did not determine whether the clinic had the necessary resources to reduce waiting times or whether current resources were used efficiently.

Riley et al. (2015) sought to determine the effect of remote monitoring on heart failure patients, given the number of heart failure admissions each year and their impact on patient life expectancy and quality of life. The primary stakeholders were heart failure patients and their healthcare providers as well as employees of the Internet service provider and physiologic monitoring equipment company. The program was designed to measure the weight, blood pressure, heart rate, and pulse oximetry of rural heart failure patients at their residences and relay this information over the Internet to healthcare workers with the goals of improving transitional care by earlier detection of deterioration in health status and initiation of care.

The evaluation design centered on three groups of patients: those agreeing to participate, those refusing to participate, and a matched cohort paralleling participants—a quasi-experimental design. The outcome measures were the number of emergency room (ER) and inpatient admissions, the number of ER and inpatient days, and total charges prior to and after program initiation. Data was collected for 45 participants, 45 matched cohorts, and 57 nonparticipants. **TABLE 14.7** reports the findings after 182 days.

Table 14.7 documents a reduction in admissions, inpatient days, and charges for all groups. The largest reduction in admissions occurred in the matched cohort, while the largest reduction in charges occurred in the monitored participant group. The reduction in inpatient days was highest in the monitored group, but the decline was closely matched by nonparticipants. Although the evaluation design attempted to match participants by age, gender, and ethnicity, Table 14.7 demonstrates that pre-intervention utilization of healthcare services was 49.1% higher in the monitored group than the matched cohort and 83.5% higher than nonparticipants. The authors note (2015, p. 161) they were unable to match patients on the basis of type and severity of conditions, comorbidities, and the home environment, which could explain the different utilization of healthcare services. The authors also note that several heart failure management programs were introduced concurrently with remote monitoring, which may explain the across-the-board declines and the small differences observed between patient groups.

Riley et al. concluded that the observed reductions in healthcare utilization cannot

TABLE 14.7 Impact of Remote Monitoring on Heart Failure Outcomes									
	Admissions			**Inpatient Days**			**Charges**		
	Pre-	**Post-**	**Change (%)**	**Pre-**	**Post-**	**Change (%)**	**Pre-**	**Post-**	**Change (%)**
Participants	3.31	1.87	−43.5	14.22	5.24	−63.2	$138,600	$44,674	−67.8
Matched Cohort	2.42	1.22	−49.6	8.11	7.05	−13.1	$92,930	$39,732	−57.2
Non-participants	1.86	1.49	−19.9	8.36	4.60	−45.0	$75,549	$73,593	−2.6

be attributed to remote monitoring, given the other interventions concurrently introduced, but caution readers that the ability of remote monitoring to improve outcomes cannot be ruled out. The authors encourage others interested in the impact of remote monitoring to learn more about the technology, expand the outcome measures assessed to include mortality and quality-of-life measures, and utilize a random control trial design to create equal intervention and control groups. The limitation of the study was its failure to incorporate the costs of remote monitoring so that cost–benefit ratios (CBRs) or CERs could be calculated.

As noted earlier, managers have a vested interest in presenting their departments in the best light, and it is probably impossible that program evaluation can be separated from program administration. The remedy is the development of comprehensive and generally accepted program evaluation standards where the absence of major factors will be tantamount to acknowledging program deficiency. One of the primary purposes of program evaluation is improvement, and improvement can only occur when the right things are measured in the right way and effective action is taken when inadequacies are identified.

Summary

CBA and CEA are means of organizing information for assessing current operations and structuring future operations. In CBA, benefits and costs are denominated in dollars and the following questions are answered: should an activity be undertaken, are benefits greater than cost, and in the presence of more than one alternative where not all activities can be undertaken, which projects should be tackled?

CEA begins with the assumption that a particular end should be pursued, and is used to identify the alternative that best balances outcome and cost. In CEA, costs continue to be denominated in dollars but outcomes are measured in natural units such as lives saved, additional life years, and infections prevented. CEA does not require a monetary value to be placed on life, a year of life, or an avoided infection. The goal is simply to identify the means that produces the lowest cost per desired outcome and direct resources to more effective activities. CBA can be used to determine the level of activity, alternatives, and size of the budget; CEA is more appropriate for identifying alternatives and allocating resources within a budget.

Program evaluation differs from CBA and CEA as it is often retrospective rather than prospective, practical versus theoretical, and concerned with effectiveness rather than efficacy. Program evaluation requires understanding the original need and the alternative programs available to satisfy the need, assessing the performance of the implemented program, including its expected outcomes and costs, and assessing whether needs have changed. Program evaluation focuses on a wider range of questions than CBA or CEA: has the need changed, have new and superior alternatives been developed, was the program implemented properly and does it continue to function properly, are expected outcomes being achieved, and have costs been minimized? Program evaluation, by focusing on the totality of operations, is better designed to facilitate improvement and establish accountability than CBA or CEA; program evaluation should be used to determine whether the promised benefits and costs projected by CBA or CEA were realized.

Key Terms and Concepts

Cost–benefit analysis (CBA)
Cost-effectiveness analysis (CEA)
League tables

Prevalence
Program evaluation
Quality-adjusted life years (QALYs)

Standard gamble
Time trade-off

Discussion Questions

1. Explain the factors that should be considered when evaluating the cost-effectiveness of preventive care.
2. Explain the major differences between CBA and CEA.
3. Briefly explain the main steps in CBA or CEA and the purpose of each step.
4. Define cost-effectiveness.
5. What is the purpose of a QALY, and how does it fulfill this role?
6. Discuss how quality of life or preferences between health states are measured.
7. According to Rossi et al. (2004), what are the five domains or dimensions a program evaluation should assess. Provide at least one question that focuses on a critical element of each domain.
8. Describe the difficulties that arise in measuring program outcomes.

Problems

1. (A) Calculate the $P_{\text{O-O-C}}$ for the fecal occult blood test (FOBT) for colon cancer, given the prevalence of 45 per 100,000 population. (i) What are the total medical costs with and without screening (assume $n = 1000$)? (ii) Should the FOBT be performed? (iii) Colonoscopy costs \$1127. (B) What is the $P_{\text{O-O-C}}$ for colonoscopy? (i) What are the total medical costs with and without screening ($n = 1000$)? (ii) Should colonoscopy be performed? (C) How can the cost-effectiveness of the FOBT and colonoscopy be improved?

	No Disease	Disease
Screening	$99	$30,000
No screening	$0	$120,000

2. A hospital is considering building a freestanding physician practice, and the key decision is how many physicians it should accommodate. The table given shows the number of employees needed to staff the operation, an average salary of $100,000, the total number of supplies needed, the average number of supply units used per patient of four at a cost of $2.50, and the building size at a cost of $240 per square foot per year. Expected revenue is $120 per patient. Calculate the total cost, total revenue, profit, and marginal benefit. What size facility (the number physicians to be accommodated) should be built?

# of Physicians	Patients (Q)	# of Staff	# of Supplies	Building Size (sq. ft.)	Total Cost	Total Revenue	Profit	Marginal Benefit
0	0	0	0	0				
1	5,000	3	20,000	500				
2	10,000	5	40,000	800				
3	15,000	8	60,000	1,100				
4	20,000	12	80,000	1,400				

3. It is estimated that 25% of persons over the age of 65 fall every year and 10% of those that fall require hospitalization costing $10,000. In a group of 1,000 people, 250 will fall and 50 will require hospitalization. Three fall prevention programs are being considered. Use CBA and $n = 1000$ to (A) complete the table given, (B) determine whether only one program can be funded (which one should it be on the basis of the return on investment [or ROI] or CBR), and (C) assuming unlimited funding is available which programs should be funded?

Program	Cost per Participant	Reduction in Falls Requiring Hospitalization (%)	# of Falls Reduced	Avoided Hospital Costs	CBR or ROI
Exercise	$200	50			
Home modification	$1000	45			
Clinical (vitamin D)	$300	30			

4. Three alternatives are being considered to reduce childhood obesity: improving school lunches, mandatory exercise programs, and year-round health classes. The table given provides expected reduction in the body mass index (BMI) and the annual cost per participant. (A) Calculate the CER for each program. Which program should be funded first? (B) Assuming a budget of $56B is established to fight childhood obesity and there are 70,000,000 children in the United States between the ages of 4 and 18, which programs should be funded? (C) Assume the total, discounted lifetime cost of childhood obesity per excess BMI point is $10,000, would it be cost-beneficial to expand the budget? Explain your answer.

Program	Reduction in BMI	Cost per Participant	CER
School lunches	0.50	$300	
Exercise programs	1.00	$500	
Health classes	0.75	$700	

5. Calculate the CER and ICER for interventions X and Y. X increases QALYs by 5 years and costs $40,000; Y increases QALYs by 6.0 years and costs $60,000. Only one intervention can be funded; what is your recommendation? If widespread adoption of intervention Y reduces its cost to $55,000, will your recommendation change?

References

Beresniak, A., Medina-Lara, A., Auray, J. P., De Wever, A., Praet, J. C., Tarricone, R., ... Duru G. (2015). Validation of the underlying assumptions of the quality-adjusted life-years outcome: Results from the ECHOUTCOME European project. *Pharmacoeconomics, 33*(1), 61–69.

Browning, E. K., & Browning, J. M. (1994). *Public finance and the price system* (4th ed.). Englewood Cliffs, NJ: Prentice Hall.

Byers, V. L., Mays, M. Z., & Mark, D. D. (1999). Provider satisfaction in army primary care clinics. *Military Medicine, 164*(2), 132–135.

Carande-Kulis, V., Stevens, J. A., Florence, C. S., Beattie, B. L., & Arias, I. (2015). A cost-benefit analysis of three older adult fall prevention interventions. *Journal of Safety Research, 52*, 65–70.

Centers for Disease Control and Prevention. (1999). Framework for program evaluation in public health. *MMWR Recommendations and Reports, 48*(RR-11), 1–40.

Centers for Disease Control and Prevention. (2015). *Health, United States, 2015. With special feature on racial and ethnic health disparities.* Retrieved December 2, 2016, from www.cdc.gov/nchs/data/hus /hus15.pdf#14

Desai, A. A., Baras, J., Berk, B. B., Nakajima, A., Garber, A. M., Owens, D., & Chertow, G. M. (2008). Management of acute kidney injury in the intensive care unit: A cost-effectiveness analysis of daily vs alternate-day hemodialysis. *Archives of Internal Medicine, 168*(16), 1761–1767.

Doubilet, P., Weinstein, M. C., & McNeil, B. J. (1986). Use and misuse of the term "cost effective" in medicine. *New England Journal of Medicine, 314*(4), 253–255.

Hopkins, R. B., Garg, A. X., Levin, A., Molzahn, A., Rigatto, C., Singer, J., ... Goeree, R. (2011). Cost-effectiveness analysis of a randomized trial comparing care models for chronic kidney disease. *Clinical Journal of the American Society of Nephrology, 6*(6), 1248–1257.

Kleinsorge, C. A., Roberts, M. C., Roy, K. M., & Rapoff, M. A. (2010). The program evaluation of services in a primary care clinic: Attaining a medical home. *Clinical Pediatrics (Phila), 49*(6), 548–559.

Mahadevia, P. J., Fleisher, L. A., Frick, K. D., Eng, J., Goodman, S. N., & Powe, N. R. (2003). Lung cancer screening with helical computed tomography in older adult smokers: A decision and cost-effectiveness analysis. *JAMA, 289*(3), 313–322.

McCarthy, J. (2014). In U.S., 65% dissatisfied with how gov't system works. Retrieved from http://news .gallup.com/poll/166985/dissatisfied-gov-system-works.aspx

McKinnell, J. A., Bartsch, S. M., Lee, B. Y., Huang, S. S., & Miller, L. G. (2015). Cost-benefit analysis from a hospital perspective of universal active screening followed by contact precautions for methicillin-resistant *Staphylococcus aureus* carriers. *Infection Control and Hospital Epidemiology, 36*(1), 2–11.

Muennig, P. (2002). *Designing and conducting cost-effectiveness analyses in medicine and health care.* San Francisco, CA: Jossey-Bass.

Nelson, E. C., Batalden, P. B., Godfrey, M. M., & Lazar, J. S. (2011). *Value by design.* San Francisco, CA: Jossey-Bass.

O'Brien, C. L., & Gage, B. F. (2005). Costs and effectiveness of ximelagatran for stroke prophylaxis in chronic atrial fibrillation. *JAMA, 293*(6), 699–706.

Pataky, R., Armstrong, L., Chia, S., Coldman, A. J., Kim-Sing, C., McGillivray, B., ... Peacock, S. (2013). Cost-effectiveness of MRI for breast cancer screening in BRCA1/2 mutation carriers. *BMC Cancer, 13*, 339.

Perlroth, D. J., Sanders, G. D., & Gould, M. K. (2007). Effectiveness and cost-effectiveness of thrombolysis in submassive pulmonary embolism. *Archives of Internal Medicine, 167*(1), 74–80.

Pollard, C., Hartz, S., Liu Leage, S., Paget, M. A., Cook, J., & Enstone, A. (2015). Elicitation of health state utilities associated with varying severities of flares in systemic lupus erythematosus. *Health and Quality of Life Outcomes, 13*(66), 10.

Riley, W. T., Keberlein, P., Sorenson, G., Mohler, S., Tye, B., Ramirez, A. S., & Carroll, M., (2015). Program evaluation of remote heart failure monitoring: Healthcare utilization analysis in a rural regional medical center. *Telemedicine Journal and E-Health, 21*(3), 157–162.

Rossi, P. H., Lipsey, M. W., & Freeman, H. E. (2004). *Evaluation: A systematic approach* (7th ed.). Thousand Oaks, CA: Sage.

Sackett, D. L., & Torrance, G. W. (1978). The utility of different health states as perceived by the general public. *Journal of Chronic Diseases, 31*(11), 697–704.

Sanders, G. D., Hlatky, M. A., & Owens, D. K. (2005). Cost-effectiveness of implantable cardioverter-defibrillators. *New England Journal of Medicine, 353*(14), 1471–1480.

Shadish, W. R., (2006). The common threads in program evaluation. *Preventing Chronic Disease, 3(1), A03.*

Torrance, G. W. (1987). Utility approach to measuring health-related quality of life. *Journal of Chronic Diseases, 40*(6), 593–600.

Tosteson, A. N., Lurie, J. D., Tosteson, T. D., Skinner, J. S., Herkowitz, H., Albert, T., ... Weinstein, J. N. (2008). Surgical treatment of spinal stenosis with and without degenerative spondylolisthesis: Cost-effectiveness after 2 years. *Annals of Internal Medicine, 149*(12), 845–853.

van den Hout, W. B., Peul, W. C., Koes, B. W., Brand, R., Kievit, J., & Thomeer, R. T. (2008). Prolonged conservative care versus early surgery in patients with sciatica from lumbar disc herniation: Cost utility analysis alongside a randomised controlled trial. *British Medical Journal, 336*(7657), 1351–1354.

Zierler, B. K., & Gray, D. T. (2003). The principles of cost-effectiveness analysis and their application. *Journal of Vascular Surgery, 37*(1), 226–234.

PART 4

Financial Functions for Finance and Planners

Part 4, "Financial Functions for Finance and Planners," shifts from departmental financial management issues to issues that affect the entire organization. If a manager was successful in leading a department, he or she may be promoted to oversee multiple departments and with continued success may become the chief executive officer (CEO). Prior chapters largely focused on how to manage the financial affairs of a department, although zero-base and program budgeting cater more to the planning than line item budgeting. The next two chapters focus on financial functions performed in finance and in support of planning.

The chapter "Financial Functions in Finance" explores financial activities performed by finance professionals. Financial reporting concerns the information provided to the public and affects what the public thinks about organizations. A major decision that affects the cost of acquiring assets is the mix of debt and equity in an organization's capital structure. The use of debt should not be the balancing factor between desired investment and equity but rather a conscious decision by senior managers and the board to balance minimizing financing costs and taking financial risk. Similarly, finance must ensure the organization has sufficient funds to pay obligations as they come due, through accurate cash budgets, given the time between when healthcare providers deliver care and when payments are received. Finally, the proliferation of non-charge-based reimbursement has exposed healthcare providers to new risks that must be understood, managed, and communicated to employees to ensure financial success.

"Strategic Financial Planning" charts a multiyear financial plan detailing where the organization expects to be in the future, that is, an investment plan and how the assets will be financed. The idea of sustainable growth is a key element in the strategic financial plan, as assets cannot grow faster than equity without increasing the organization's reliance on debt. The strategic financial plan establishes multiyear net income projections and a system to monitor organizational performance. The chapter also discusses the role of finance in the larger strategic management process in setting achievable long-term goals, strategy selection, and strategy implementation.

It is only fitting that the text conclude with an eye toward the future. Healthcare costs have soared in the past 50 years in absolute dollars and as a share of the gross domestic product (GDP). The chapter "Financial Management and Health Care" recaps budget systems, summarizes the role of managers vis-à-vis their departments' budgets, and speculates on the role budgeting may play in the evolving healthcare economic environment. If cost increases in health care are going to be controlled, managers are first going to have to understand budgeting systems and their incentives and use budgets that focus on effectiveness and efficiency. Second, managers are going to have to understand costs better; activity-based budgets and variance analysis that recognize the impact of changes in efficiency and intensity on costs must become common tools in managers' work. Third, value, as defined as output divided by cost, must be internalized by all employees. When employees work every day to increase output or, better yet, improve outcomes, while maintaining or reducing costs, we will take the first steps away from an unsustainable *status quo* to a better health system for patients, healthcare workers, and healthcare payers.

CHAPTER 15

Financial Functions in Finance

CHAPTER OBJECTIVES

1. Explain the purpose of financial reporting.
2. Calculate the cost of capital and demonstrate the impact of financial leverage on the return on equity.
3. Explain the timing difference between cash outflows and inflows.
4. Calculate a cash budget.
5. Explain the different types of risk and how they are distributed between healthcare providers and insurers.

▶ Introduction

The topics covered in this chapter deal with matters that are primarily the responsibility of the finance department, that is, finance professionals determine what should be done and are tasked with executing their decisions. Operating managers should understand these issues and how they affect the organization and their departments, even though they may not be responsible for setting direction or executing action. The first topic, financial reporting, determines how external parties think about the organization. Organizations that provide transparent financial information generally garner greater public support; organizations that withhold or manipulate information are responsible for increasing calls for government oversight.

Decisions on capital structure, the mix of debt and equity used to finance assets, has a direct impact on investment decisions. The higher the cost of acquiring funds, the lower the number of desirable investments. Operating managers should understand why desired investments are financially unacceptable, given the organization's cost of acquiring funds. The cost of acquiring funds can be reduced through the judicious use of debt, but everyone should understand the risks of overreliance on debt.

The goal of working capital management is to ensure cash is available to pay bills as they come due and to reduce cash outflows by avoiding excessive investment in low-performing current assets. There is a profound difference between earning profits and having money in the bank to pay wages, bills, and taxes. While ensuring cash is available to pay bills is the responsibility of finance, the amount of money flowing into and out of an organization is determined by all managers. Department managers can minimize cash outflows by prudent use of labor and assets such as inventories, and revenue-producing departments can facilitate cash inflows by prompt and accurate charge capture.

The primary cash inflows come from third-party payers, and negotiating contracts and payments rates in hospitals is a finance function. However, the impact on the organization is determined by how well front-line departments structure their processes. In physician practices, negotiation and managing contracts may fall on a physician or practice manager, so understanding financial risk is vital. Financial risk management requires that employees recognize what is required for success under the terms of contracts and work toward maximizing the returns to the organizations. These topics must be understood, and budgeting and employee evaluation systems should ensure employees work toward the organization's goals by synchronizing employees' and employers' interests.

▶ Financial Reporting

A key point in prior chapters was that managers often present data to maximize their interests, and systems are needed to ensure that self-interest, organizational goals, and public interest coincide. Financial reporting standards are designed to ensure that external parties receive valid and relevant information, or "financial statements should be designed and prepared to reasonably assure complete and understandable reporting of all significant information relating to the economic affairs of the accounting entity" (Welsch, Zlatkovich, & White, 1976, p. 26). High-profile organization failures ranging from Enron and nonprofit hospitals to the city of Detroit indicate the financial reports and management of for-profit, nonprofit, and public organizations are

deficient—reasonable people have been misled and injured by deceptive financial reports.

External financial statements, including income statements, balance sheets, and cash flow statements, should be constructed according to generally accepted accounting principles (GAAP), but recent failures have led the accounting profession to reassess the role of and establish consistent principles for financial reporting. The Sarbanes–Oxley Act of 2002 (SOX Act) was the result of the large-scale failures of publicly held organizations in 2001. These failures demonstrated the inadequacy of financial reports and highlighted managerial and audit–consultant conflicts of interests.

Major provisions of the act included requiring chief executive officers (CEOs) and chief financial officers (CFOs) to certify that financial and other information in their companies' quarterly and annual reports do not contain untrue statements or material omissions. A major change was requiring organizations to disclosure all material off balance sheet transactions, such as those used by Enron to conceal the extent of its liabilities. Although the disclosure provision was adopted in 2003, the issue arose again with the collapse of Lehman Brothers in 2007. The SOX Act also requires organizations to establish and report on internal controls aimed at ensuring the validity of financial statements and increased penalties on individuals for violations.

Although the SOX Act does not apply to nonprofits, public demand for greater accountability suggests that nonprofits should increase the quantity and quality of financial information available to the public. One of the primary roles of financial reporting is to ensure external parties who may invest money in or make loans to organizations that their investment is safe. Nonprofit organizations should adopt similar disclosure policies to ensure their access to capital (debt and philanthropic) and enhance their public image. Another key issue is tax-exempt status; nonprofit hospitals are increasingly scrutinized by the Internal Revenue Service (IRS) to determine whether they perform sufficient public service via charity care in order to warrant tax exemption.

Valletta (2005) catalogs the type of information being requested from nonprofits, including charity care and bad debt, joint venture and cost-sharing arrangements, and expense allocations. Beyond these issues, he suggests organizations should inform their publics of their growth strategies, people issues, market share, and supply chain performance using nonfinancial quantitative measures (p. 60). While healthcare providers routinely report admissions, patient days, and reimbursement, Valletta suggests managers should understand and communicate more information on the cost of charity care, compliance costs, capital needs and capital-raising strategies, cost of recruiting personnel, malpractice costs, and the cost associated with quality improvement and consumerism (pp. 60–61).

A key provision of the SOX Act was CEO and CFO attestation to the accuracy of financial statements, and Valletta suggests nonprofits should voluntarily follow suit and develop systems for officers to certify and disseminate operating results on a quarterly basis (p. 62). The idea of **stewardship**, managers should not only safeguard the resources of others but also ensure assets are used in the most effective and efficient ways possible, has been a main theme of this book. Financial reports should be the means by which external parties can determine whether resources are effectively and efficiently used.

Given the IRS's focus on the tax-exempt status of nonprofits and the amount of charity care provided, Valletta explores the vagaries surrounding how charity care is reported. Hospitals report that 5.0% of net operating income is committed to providing charity care, but how hospitals account for this service is problematic. Some hospitals report charges that vastly overstate costs, others fail to differentiate charity cases from bad debt, and still others include contractual discounts. The differences have led to calls to standardize charity care reporting by excluding contractual discounts from Medicare and Medicaid,

excluding any patients who were subject to bill collection efforts, and requiring charity care to be reported at cost rather than charges or other statistical measures (p. 64). Providing clear financial information on charity care should not only improve a hospital's image in its community but also avert challenges to the organization's tax-exempt status.

The three main financial reports are income statements, balance sheets, and cash flow statements. Income statements report financial performance over time, the relationship between revenues and expenses. Balance sheets provide a snapshot of assets and liabilities at a point in time. Income statements and balance sheets provide insight into an organization's viability and solvency: will it be able to maintain itself and meet its obligations? Cash flow statements report the change in an organization's cash balance over time and its sources and uses of cash.

Recent financial machinations have increased skepticism over income statements and balance sheets, and more people today recognize that income, assets, and liabilities can be and have been manipulated by opportunistic managers. This skepticism has increased the attention given to the cash flow statement as cash is easy to count and hard to manipulate—an organization either has or does not have cash in the bank. The cash flow statement contains four sections. The first section reports cash flows emanating from operations primarily net income, changes in current assets, and noncash expenses. The bottom line should be positive; operations should generate cash for the organization. The second section recounts changes in cash arising from investment activities. Healthy organizations should be investing in their future, purchasing property and equipment to maintain competitiveness and facilitate future production. Investment activities also report the purchase (outflow) or sale of securities (inflow). Investment activities should record the use or outflow of funds and hence be negative.

The third section, financing activities, reports the acquiring (inflow) or discharging (outflow) of debt. While we would like to think healthy organizations would be repaying previously borrowed funds, an outflow or use of cash, section 3, may show an organization is taking on additional debt (an inflow) to lower its cost of financing assets and/or purchase more assets to maximize net income. The last section recounts how operations, investments, and financing explain the change in cash available from one fiscal period to the next.

TABLE 15.1 shows the statement of cash flows for Oyam Hospital. The sources of cash are indicated as (s) and the uses as (u). Oyam's income statement and balance sheet were reported in Tables 2.2 and 2.3. Operating activities generated $154,902,000 of cash, primarily due to net income, but cash also increased due to depreciation, $32,247,000 (a noncash expense); a decrease in accounts receivable, $19,926,000 (a noninterest-bearing asset); and an increase in accounts payable, $3,706,000 (a non-interest-bearing liability). Cash was reduced because of the increased investment in inventories, −$5,462,000 (a non-interest-bearing asset).

Section 2, investment activity, shows that the organization aggressively reinvested money into its operations and related organizations. Oyam purchased $199,891,000 in plant and equipment, a use of funds, and partially financed this investment by reducing its security holdings, a source of funds.

Section 3, financing activity, demonstrates that besides devoting all the cash generated from operations into property and equipment investment, an additional $20,350,000 of long-term debt was contracted. The impact of operating, investment, and financing activities was a negligible reduction in cash on hand. The overall evaluation of management on the basis of the cash flow statement is positive. Management generated high profits, reinvested in operations, and partially financed this investment by improved management of short-term assets and liabilities—only 12.0% of reinvestment ($21,050,000 of $176,117,000) was funded by debt.

The goal of financial reporting is to provide useful information to external parties to assess the operations of an organization. The primary sources of information are income statements, balance sheets, and cash flow statements. While accounting information is subject to variation due to how financial variables are measured, it should never mislead the public. Past financial malfeasance has resulted in increased government scrutiny of financial reports and increased emphasis on the statement of cash flows due to its lower susceptibility to accrual accounting measurement issues.

▶ Capital Structure and Financial Leverage

Capital structure is the mix of equity and debt used to finance assets. For-profits can sell ownership (equity) interests in the organization and make conscious decisions on how much debt and equity they use. Nonprofits have less access to equity since they cannot sell equity interests, but they can utilize retained earnings, the net income from operations, or philanthropy, and they should also be making a conscious decision on how much debt is used to acquire assets. The use of debt should *not* be the go-to or default option when net income or charitable giving is inadequate. Overreliance on debt increases the cost of debt and reduces the access to debt. Organizations with excessive debt often find that lenders who once were willing to give high-interest loans are unwilling to provide additional funds at any interest rate.

Prudence requires an explicit debt policy built on understanding the cost of acquiring funds to run an organization. The cost of acquiring funds is determined by the risk the organization faces. Organizations face two types of risk, business risk and financial risk. **Business risk** is the risk inherent in an organization's operations that may reduce profit, including changing consumer tastes leading to a loss of customers, increased competition,

TABLE 15.1 Cash Flow Statement	
Operating Activities	
Net income (s)	$104,485,000
Adjustments:	
Depreciation (s)	$32,247,000
Accounts receivable (u)	$19,926,000
Inventory (u)	−$5,462,000
Accounts payable (s)	$3,706,000
Total	$154,902,000
Investment Activities	
Property and equipment (u)	−$199,891,000
Securities (s)	$23,774,000
Total	−$176,117,000
Financing Activities	
Long-term debt (s)	$20,350,000
Short-term debt (s)	$700,000
Total	$21,050,000
Change in cash (u)	−$165,000
Beginning balance	$25,435,000
Ending balance	$25,270,000

increased input prices, changes in technology, and/or changes in laws and regulations. **Financial risk** is the risk associated with meeting contracted interest and principal payments on debt. The **risk/return trade-off**, the idea that higher financial returns can only be earned if investors accept higher risk, requires investors seeking higher returns to accept higher risk.

For-profit operations can be funded by issuing debt or equity instruments; debt is less expensive than equity for the simple fact that in the event of failure, that is, bankruptcy, debt holders are paid *prior* to equity holders. The fact that debt obligations must be met before any resources are distributed to equity holders reduces the risk to creditors and thus the cost of debt. Beyond liquidation issues, debt often specifies a fixed interest rate and defined payment dates guaranteeing creditors an income stream.

Equity holders have the residual claim on both income and assets. In the event of liquidation, equity holders are only paid if assets remain after all prior claimants are satisfied. In bankruptcy, equity holders may receive a fraction or none of their investment; following GM's 2009 bankruptcy, existing equity shares were cancelled and stockholders received no shares in the reorganized company. In regard to income, equity holders "own" any residual income, but distribution as dividends is determined by management. Management may elect to retain part of or all after-tax earnings.

The cost of acquiring funds can be minimized by using a mix of debt and equity financing. Given that debt is less expensive than equity, managers seeking to minimize the cost of funds want to increase the organization's debt financing, that is, **financial leverage**. Financial leverage is measured as the ratio of debt to total assets and is used to increase returns to equity holders by lowering financing costs.

Managers may be tempted to fund the majority of assets, if not all, by debt, given its cost is lower than equity; however, as the ratio of debt to assets increases, debt holders become de facto equity holders. If an organization's assets were funded completely by debt, creditors would have no cushion in liquidation and losses would come directly from their accounts. Creditors realize their risk increases as the use of debt increases and thus require higher-interest payments. If 100% of assets were financed by debt, debt holders should demand the same return as equity holders. **TABLE 15.2** and **FIGURE 15.1** demonstrate how increasing debt affects an organization's **cost of capital**, the overall cost of

TABLE 15.2 Cost of Capital

Debt in Capital Structure (%)	Debt (R_d) (%)	Equity (R_e) (%)	WACC (%)
0	4.5	10.0	10.0
20	5.0	10.0	9.0
40	5.5	10.0	8.2
50	6.0	10.0	8.0
60	7.0	10.0	8.2
80	8.5	10.0	8.8
100	10.0	10.0	10.0

WACC, weighted average cost of capital.

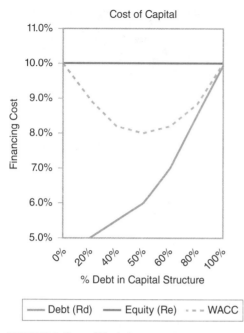

Cost of Capital

— Debt (Rd) — Equity (Re) · · · WACC

FIGURE 15.1 Cost of Capital

acquiring funds based on its mix of debt and equity financing.

$$\text{Cost of capital} = \left(\% \text{ Debt} * R_d * (1-t)\right) \\ + \left(1 - \% \text{ debt}\right) * R_e, \quad (15.1)$$

where % debt is debt/total assets; R_d is the cost of debt, that is, the interest rate; t is the tax rate; and R_e is the cost of equity, that is, dividend and growth.

Figure 15.1 shows that the minimum cost of capital is achieved when debt provides 50% of total financing. Under 50%, the organization is using too little debt (or financial leverage); every additional dollar of assets can be financed under the return on equity (ROE) of 10%. Over 50%, the organization is too highly financially leveraged; the increasing risk of principal loss to creditors drives up the interest rate on the entire debt. At 40%, while the average cost of debt is 5.5%, the marginal cost of debt is 6.0%: 5.0% on the first 20% financing and 6.0% on the additional 20%. The higher marginal rate of 6.0% pulls the average cost of debt up to 5.5%,

but the 6.0% debt is still cheaper than the 10% cost of equity. At 50% debt, the marginal rate of debt financing is 8.0%, but at 60% debt financing, the cost of additional debt leaps to 12% above the cost of equity.

A major factor influencing capital structure decisions is the availability and cost of equity funds, including ownership interest such as stock, retained earnings, and philanthropy, and debt, including bonds, fixed- or variable-rate mortgages, and private debt placement with banks or insurance companies. Other factors influencing the choice between equity and debt include the expected growth rate and stability of future revenues, the competition, the type of assets employed, and the attitudes of owners, managers, and lenders. Organizations that use more debt typically enjoy high growth and stable revenues, have less competition, purchase nonspecialized assets, and have owners and managers willing to cede control to lenders (Weston & Brigham, 1978, pp. 684–685).

Recognizing increased reliance on debt increases interest rates, it is important to understand how higher use of debt can increase returns to equity holders. The key point is as long as the cost of debt is lower than the cost of equity, increasing debt reduces the cost of acquiring assets and increases the ROE. The ability to enhance profit is even greater in for-profit organizations, where corporate profits are taxed; hence, as long as the after-tax cost of debt is lower than equity, it is advantageous to replace equity with debt. **TABLE 15.3** demonstrates that while debt reduces taxable income, before-tax profit, it increases the ROE for non-profits and for-profits.

Funding 40% of assets with debt carrying an interest rate of 7.0% reduced taxable income and increased the ROE. This counterintuitive outcome is the result of reduced earnings before interest and taxes (EBIT), $12.20 versus $15.00, but a higher rate of earning on a smaller investment, $12.20 on $60.00 versus $15.00 on $100; earnings on equity declined by 18.7%, but equity financing decreased by 40%.

TABLE 15.3 Impact of Debt on the ROE

Balance Sheet	No Debt	40% Debt
Total assets	$100.00	$100.00
Total debt	$0.0	$40.00
Total Equity	$100.00	$60.00
Income Statement		
Total revenue	$100.00	$100.00
Operating expenses	$85.00	$85.00
EBIT	$15.00	$15.00
Interest expense (7%)	$0.0	$2.80
Taxable income	$15.00	$12.20
Tax (40%)	$6.00	$4.90
After-tax profit	$9.00	$7.30
ROE	15.0%	20.3%
ROE after tax	9.0%	12.2%

EBIT, earnings before interest and tax.

As discussed in the chapter "Cost–Benefit Analysis, Cost-Effectiveness Analysis, and Program Evaluation," the financial question of whether to increase debt revolves around the return the $40 in equity freed up by increased debt can bring. If the $40 can be reinvested at a rate that returns more than $2.80 (7%), then the use of debt is warranted. If the $40 can be reinvested at 15%, producing $6, the total return will be $18.20 ($12.20 on $60 + $6 on $40), superior to the $15 and 15% earned when the $100 is invested in a single venture. If the $40 investment cannot generate 7.0%, it is better to use 100% equity financing. If only 6.0% can be earned on the freed-up $40, then the total return would be $14.60 ($12.20 on $60 + $2.40 on $40).

The higher ROE from financial leverage does not come without cost; using debt requires ceding control to external creditors and increasing overall risk. When assets were 100% equity-financed, revenues could fall by 15% and the total expense could be covered. Using 40% debt financing increases the total expense by $2.80, and thus if revenue falls by more than 12.2%, the organization may be unable to meet its obligations.

Working Capital Management

The goal of working capital management is to ensure an organization has enough cash to continue operations, that is, to purchase resources as needed and pay bills as they come due. **Net working capital** is the difference between current assets and current liabilities, that is, does the organization have sufficient readily converted assets available to pay short-term obligations? Organizations typically purchase variable and fixed inputs to produce goods and services in advance of when they are produced, sold, and paid for. The difference between when inputs are purchased and consumed and when payments for goods and services sold are received varies greatly across industries.

If you are reading this text as part of a college degree program, your university demanded you pay your tuition prior to the start of the semester. Your university then pays its variable expenses, such as salaries, supplies, and utilities, across the semester. The CFO of the university does not have to worry about where money will come from to pay salaries and bills, since it was collected prior to the start of classes. The challenge for a CFO of a university or an insurance company is to invest tuition dollars or insurance premiums until they are needed to pay professors' salaries or claims.

Healthcare organizations purchase inputs well in advance of receiving payment for services. Wages paid to labor to produce exams or treatments today may not yield cash for 60–90 days in the future. The **revenue cycle** begins when patients are scheduled for services and ends when no further payment is expected for the goods or services delivered. Healthcare providers must pay staff to set up appointments, deliver care, bill for services delivered, and collect the appropriate reimbursement on the basis of each patient's insurance status and the contractual arrangement with third-party payers. Ratio analysis, discussed in Chapter 12, uses days in accounts receivable to assess an organization's ability to collect cash for the services it produces. The 2015 hospital benchmark for days in accounts receivable was 47.3 days. An average hospital, therefore, pays its employees at least 33 days (47.3 days − 14 days, assuming biweekly pay periods) for their labors *prior* to obtaining payment from patients or third-party payers for exams and treatments. Likewise, supplies may be purchased in advance of use (cash on delivery) or paid 30 days after delivery. Utilities typically billed on actual usage depart from the paid-before-revenue-is-received model, as utility customers may have 30 days after the close of the billing period to pay their utility bills.

The challenge facing healthcare providers is they must pay most of their expenses prior to receiving payment for the services they provide. Assume a hospital has $500,000 in cash expenses daily and 47.3 days in accounts receivable. The hospital would need to pay out up to $23,650,000 in salaries, supplies, and other expenses before any money is received. The problem is, does the organization have the ability to front this money and wait for payment? Insolvency was previously defined in the chapter "Accounting and Economics" as having more liabilities than assets. In actuality, there are two types of insolvency: **balance sheet insolvency**, which arises when liabilities exceed assets, and **cash flow insolvency**, which arises when an organization does not have sufficient liquid assets to pay bills as they come due. Both types of insolvency can lead to bankruptcy, although in cash flow insolvency, creditors may be willing to wait until less liquid assets are converted to cash rather than force the organization into bankruptcy. Prudent working capital management (securing financing, accelerating cash inflows, and/or delaying outflows) should avoid cash flow insolvency rather than rely on the benevolence of creditors.

Working capital is not a problem most department managers must worry about; it is the job of finance to ensure the organization has sufficient funds to meet payroll and pay suppliers, but all departments affect the inflow and outflow of cash. The flow of funds in an organization (**FIGURE 15.2**) parallels the system model (Chapter 1). The first component is inputs, which sometimes must be paid for before the organization obtains the benefit of the inputs (prepaid insurance) or promptly after receiving or using them. Biweekly payroll requires that employees be paid for their services within 14 days of performance and payments for supplies often requires payment in 30 days regardless of whether the resource is used or placed into inventory.

The second phase, producing goods and services, is throughput; in most cases, consumers do not pay for goods and services until after they are completed and delivered. The length of the throughput process thus increases the difference between when inputs are consumed or paid for and when payment for outputs can be received.

The third phase, the billing process or charging consumers for what they received, generally begins when an output is produced, but inefficiency in billing may increase the time needed to obtain payment. In hospitals, if the average length of stay (LOS) is 5 days (the production process) and it takes an additional 4 days to bill a patient and/or his or her

third-party payer (the billing process), this adds 9 days between when resources were expended and when cash could be collected. The last phase, collection, is responsible for the biggest gap between when the input costs are paid and when the revenue they generate is received. Third-party payers must receive the bill, adjudicate it, pay the claim, and distribute payment. On the basis of an average of 47.3 days to payment, this suggests that the claims review and payment processes of third-party payers may add 38 (47.3 – 9.0) days to the cash collection process. The challenge for hospitals and other healthcare providers is to pay their expenses prior to receiving revenue.

Although the vast majority of the cash collection process is the purview of finance, all departments can facilitate working capital management by judicious purchase of inputs, foregoing unnecessary expenditures and acquiring resources when they are needed (rather than in advance) to reduce and/or delay cash outflows. Revenue-producing departments can accelerate billing and cash inflows by submitting accurate charges when activities are completed. While billing and collection are primarily the responsibility of finance, all managers should understand the organization's need to balance cash outflows and inflows and how they and their employees can improve the cash collection process. All employees should understand the revenue and expense cycles, that is, healthcare workers should understand the medical revenue cycle and improve the scheduling, registration, production and charge capture, coding, billing, and collection processes to reduce the time between cash outflows and inflows.

The Cash Budget

When revenue budgets are created, they typically reflect accrual accounting: revenues are recognized when an obligation to pay is created. The obligation to pay is often different from the actual inflow or outflow of cash. The statement of cash flows plows the same territory by recognizing the difference between net

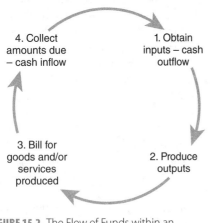

FIGURE 15.2 The Flow of Funds within an Organization

income, earning money, and changes in cash balances—having money to spend. Creditors do not want obligations to pay; they want cash, and the job of the cash budget is to ensure funds are available to pay bills promptly and excess cash is productively invested. Organizations cannot spend profit; they can only spend cash.

The cash budget recognizes when revenue is actually collected and bills are paid. The largest difference between income statements and budgets and the cash budget is the lag between when goods and services are billed to customers and when payments are received. The cash budget in **TABLE 15.4** assumes payments for services billed in 1 month will be received over 3 months. For example, payment for 35% of services rendered in January is expected to be collected in January, 50% in February, and 15% in March. Table 15.4 also shows the difference between gross and net revenues, which should be monitored to ensure that neither contractual discounts nor bad debt is excessive.

TABLE 15.4 A Cash Budget for a Going Concern

Inflows	March	April	May	June
Gross revenue	$587.00	$572.00	$528.00	$520.00
Net revenue	$293.50	$286.00	$264.00	$260.00
0–30 days	$102.70	$100.10	$92.40	$91.00
31–60 days	$138.00	$146.80	$143.00	$132.00
61–90 days	$41.30	$41.40	$44.00	$42.90
Total collections	$282.00	$288.30	$279.40	$265.90
Outflows				
Wages paid	$146.80	$143.00	$132.00	$130.00
Supplies	$58.70	$57.20	$52.80	$52.00
Utilities	$29.40	$28.60	$26.40	$26.00
Other	$47.00	$45.80	$42.20	$41.60
Capital expenditures	——	$50.00	——	——
Total payments	$281.80	$324.60	$253.40	$249.60
Net cash from operations	$0.20	−$36.30	$26.00	$16.30
Beginning cash balance	$22.00	$22.20	−$14.10	$11.90
Net cash from operations	$0.20	−$36.30	$26.00	$16.30
Ending cash balance	$22.20	−$14.10	$11.90	$28.20

Cash budgeting is often less important to going concerns that have previous revenues and substantial cash balances but is often critical for start-ups. Let us return to the start-up physician practice introduced in the chapter "Scratch Budgeting." The budget indicated expenses have to be cut by $65,284 to break even, which will be taken out of the physician's income, reducing the physician's first-year income to $114,000. The pro forma income statement indicates revenue and expenses will be equal, but the cash budget examines whether the practice will have sufficient funds to pay wages and other expenses as they come due. **FIGURE 15.3** presents the expected cash inflows and outflows over the first 9 months of the budget year.

The challenge presented by the lag between billing and collection is that expenses are primarily incurred and paid in the month services are billed. Figure 15.3 shows that net cash from operations is negative for the first 2 months of the year despite net revenue exceeding expenses; it also shows that the $22,000 cash balance to get the operation started will be insufficient to fund operations. Cash outflows exceed cash inflows by $25,515 in the first 2 months of operation, exhausting the physician's cash reserves. The ending cash balance only maintains a positive balance starting in the seventh month of the budget year. The physician may be surprised that even if the budget projections are correct he or she will be unable to pay himself or herself the expected salary of $9,500 ($114,000/12) per month.

The cash budgets for the going concern and start-up highlight the two roles of cash budgeting. The going concern is generating excess cash, which should be invested in interest, or income-generating assets (the $50 expenditure in April), to improve financial performance. The start-up has more money going out than coming in and needs to locate low-cost, short-term financing. Short-term financing is available through trade credit, that is, accounts payable, credit lines, and/or short-term notes. The working capital manager in

Days in month	21	20	22	17	20	22	18	21	22
Visits	378	360	396	306	360	396	324	378	396
Inflows	Jan	Feb	Mar	Apr	May	Jun	Jul	Aug	Sep
Gross revenue	$54,872	$52,259	$57,485	$44,420	$52,259	$57,485	$47,033	$54,872	$57,485
Net revenue	$32,923	$31,356	$34,491	$26,652	$31,356	$34,491	$28,220	$32,923	$34,491
0-30 days	11,523	10,974	12,072	9,328	10,974	12,072	9,877	11,523	12,072
31-60 days		16,462	15,678	17,246	13,326	15,678	17,246	14,110	16,462
61-90 days			4,939	4,703	5,174	3,998	4,703	5,174	4,233
Total collections	$11,523	$27,436	$32,688	$31,277	$29,474	$31,748	$31,826	$30,807	$32,767
Outflows									
Wages paid	$21,338	$21,338	$21,338	$21,338	$21,338	$21,338	$21,338	$21,338	$21,338
Supplies	2,835	2,700	2,970	2,295	2,700	2,970	2,430	2,835	2,970
Utilities	3,269	3,113	3,425	2,646	3,113	3,425	2,802	3,269	3,425
Other	4,037	3,844	4,229	3,268	3,844	4,229	3,460	4,037	4,229
Total payments	$31,478	$30,996	$31,961	$29,547	$30,996	$31,961	$30,030	$31,478	$31,961
Net cash from operations	-$19,955	-$3,559	$727	$1,730	-$1,521	-$214	$1,796	-$672	$805
Beginning cash balance	$22,000	$2,045	-$1,515	-$788	$943	-$579	-$792	$1,004	$332
Net cash from operations	-19,955	-3,559	727	1,730	-1,521	-214	1,796	-672	805
Ending cash balance	$2,045	-$1,515	-$788	$943	-$579	-$792	$1,004	$332	$1,138

FIGURE 15.3 Screenshot of Cash Budgeting for a Start-Up

the going concern looking to balance the rate of return and liquidity must choose between short-term, lower interest rates and long-term securities offering higher interest rates. Projecting cash balance is essential for both organizations to determine how much financing is needed for how long or how much can be invested in long-term securities.

Management requires metrics, and managing the revenue cycle requires understanding and controlling multiple departments. **BOX 15.1** highlights some of the measures managers should monitor to ensure departments from registration to revenue generation to patient accounting are doing their job.

Understanding cash and working capital management is essential to understand why an organization may be earning profit yet have no funds to invest in operations. Managers should recognize the difference between revenue and cash in the bank, understand the timing of cash outflows and inflows, and take action to improve financial performance, especially when cash shortages are predicted. Working capital management may appear to be a purely financial function, but this view ignores the impact all areas have on cash inflows and outflows.

BOX 15.1 Revenue Cycle Metrics

Scheduling/Pre-registration/Registration

Percentage of pre-registered accounts
Percentage of insurance cards copied
Turnaround time on precertifications
Registration error rates
Percentage of copayments collected
Cash receipts as a percentage of net revenue

Charge capture

Delay between delivery and charge
Error rate

Coding

Percentage of correct procedure codes
Percentage of correct diagnostic codes
Discharged but not final-billed due to coding, sign-off, etc.
Percentage of present on admission complications recorded
Percentage of correct diagnosis-relation group (DRG) assignment

Billing

Days between discharge and bill
Percentage of clean claims
Percentage of rejected claims

Payment

Average days in accounts receivable
Receivables as a percentage of revenue
Bad debt as a percentage of gross/net revenue

▶ Contract and Financial Risk Management

A theme of this text is that achieving superior performance requires understanding what needs to done and how it should be done, exemplified in the ability to create and operate under a budget that provides only enough resources to satisfy customers and equity suppliers. Meeting the budget requires knowing what is being done and improving processes when they are less than optimal. Healthcare providers long ago moved away from charge-based reimbursement, where they totally controlled their revenues. The shift to fixed reimbursement subjected healthcare providers to various risks that can reduce revenues and profits and in the extremis lead to the failure of the organization.

The problem in many healthcare organizations is too many managers and employees are unaware of the financial constraints and operations are carried on without regard to financial considerations. The idea that health care is a right and therefore funding will be provided and medical personnel can utilize all the resources they think appropriate is unsustainable. Healthcare purchasers are putting greater pressure on providers to use resources wisely, and superior performance cannot be achieved when personnel silo themselves and act in a parochial manner without concern for organization goals or the work of others. Negotiating reimbursement contracts may be the responsibility of finance personnel, but finance has a duty to ensure other employees understand financial constraints and how operations should be carried on to succeed under the negotiated rates.

Managing contract and financial risk requires understanding the risks faced by the organization. The three types of financial risk faced by healthcare providers are cost, utilization, and actuarial. Cost, or input price, risk arises when increases in input costs cannot be passed on to patients and third-party payers. Utilization risk prevents providers from recouping the costs of providing more or higher-cost services. Actuarial risk prevents providers from increasing revenues when more care is needed by patients.

Under charge-based reimbursement, there is no cost risk as providers can simply increase prices to pass on increases in wages, supplies prices, utility rates, and insurance premiums to patients and third-party payers. While charge-based reimbursement provides a small incentive to keep costs down (to increase profits by increasing the spread between revenue and costs), under cost reimbursement, there is no incentive to control input prices since increases in cost automatically produce higher revenue. The expected gain to payers from using cost reimbursement was the elimination of profit; however, the incentive problem under cost reimbursement led to the rapid escalation of healthcare costs from 1966 to 1981. The rapid escalation of costs led to the implementation of fixed reimbursement systems to shift financial risk to providers to restrain healthcare spending.

Utilization risk focuses on the use of inputs and/or number of services delivered rather than prices or input costs. Is a provider using more resources than necessary to produce services? Greater than necessary costs can arise from producing and providing more services than a patient needs (unnecessary, too much care) or using too many inputs to produce necessary care (inefficiency, too many inputs for care delivered). Per procedure or per diem reimbursement increases revenue with the number of medically necessary services delivered or medically necessary days a patient is hospitalized. If sicker patients are seen or admitted and more services, tests, procedures, patient days, etc., are needed, per procedure or per diem reimbursement compensates providers for necessary expenses. Both reimbursement systems, however, force providers to shoulder costs arising from inefficiency. Per procedure or per diem reimbursement sets a fixed rate per procedure or inpatient day, and revenue will not increase if a provider consumes more labor, supplies, or other inputs to produce an output. The incentive is to ensure care, a procedure or patient day, can be produced at a lower cost than the contracted payment; providers have incentives to increase their efficiency by reducing either the cost of inputs or the number of inputs consumed per output.

Under per procedure or per diem reimbursement, providers continue to have an incentive to increase the number of services for which they are paid, so per case reimbursement (a single payment received for an episode of care) was instituted. Per case reimbursement is independent of the number of tests, procedures, or patient days a provider delivers, and thus an incentive is created to provide the correct amount of intermediate services to treat a patient: are too many tests or procedures being produced, or is the LOS too long? Per case reimbursement supplies an incentive to encourage providers to be circumspect in their use of tests, procedures, and days.

Actuarial, or occurrence, risk arises from patients' need for care. All previous reimbursement systems operated on increasing provider revenue when a patient presented for care—the number of visits or admissions. Capitation supplies a fixed payment for every covered member for a period and encourages reduced use of health care. No additional payment is received when a patient presents for care, nor are payments reduced if patient utilization of care is lower than expected. Providers have an incentive to keep patients healthy, provide preventive care, and avoid unnecessary patient encounters that will consume resources and increase costs but bring no additional revenues. Preventing unnecessary patient encounters has been a vexing problem for health care, resulting in the use of deductibles and copayments to force patients to shoulder some of the cost of seeking care and question whether care is really needed to physician gatekeepers and second opinion requirements to limit patient access to specialists and procedures.

TABLE 15.5 shows how financial risks are distributed between healthcare providers and payers under five reimbursement systems. Charge and cost reimbursement place all risks on the payer. Increases in input prices (when output prices are raised), the number of resources consumed to produce a service, the number of services provided, and the number of times care is sought increase payment to providers. In the per diem or per procedure system, payers continue to pay providers for increases in the number of services provided and the number of patient care episodes, but capping payment by procedure or day forces providers to absorb increases in cost due to higher input costs or higher use of resources.

Per case reimbursement completes the shift of utilization risk from payer to provider; under per case reimbursement, providers only see higher revenues when patients need additional episodes of care, that is, medically necessary hospitalization. Providers can increase their own revenues under per case reimbursement by admitting higher numbers of patients.

All the reimbursement systems discussed to this point were based on paying providers for delivering curative care, leading some to conclude that the U.S. healthcare system should be called a sickness system—the provider incentive is to wait until people get ill and then treat them.

Capitation was designed to encourage healthcare providers to keep patients healthy though preventive care and screening to detect illness in its early stage and initiate potentially lower-cost treatment. In capitation, all risk is shifted to providers. Healthcare providers under capitation essentially function as insurance companies; they must assess the need for care (number of occurrences), the extent of care that

TABLE 15.5 Financial Risk and Reimbursement

Reimbursement System	Cost	Utilization	Actuarial
Charge/% of charge	Payer	Payer	Payer
Cost	Payer	Payer	Payer
Per diem/procedure	Provider	Payer, intensity Provider, efficiency	Payer
Per case	Provider	Provider	Payer
Capitation	Provider	Provider	Provider

will be needed (types of service and their cost), and obtain payments (premiums) that cover the expected medical outlays and administrative costs. Failure to accurately assess the need for care, manage the health delivery process and the cost of care provided, or obtain sufficient capitation payments results in operating losses.

The degree of contract risk a provider faces is inversely proportional to the provider's ability to manage the need for care (actuarial risk), the use of services (utilization risk), and the cost of services. That is, providers that can reduce patients' need for care through prevention or compliance to treatment protocols, minimize waste (including errors and idleness in their production processes), and not overpay for resources should succeed under a capitated rate. While Table 15.5 provides an esoteric view of financial risk, **TABLE 15.6** provides a more useful look at the actions providers can implement to increase their net revenue under each reimbursement system.

The ability of a provider to manage financial or contract risk is based on the provider's ability to control (reduce) the use of care (prevention and control over physician-admitting habits), the delivery of care (LOS and use of medical services while hospitalized), and input costs. Under charge-based reimbursement, all risk is held by payers and hospitals largely exercise complete control over their revenues. Hospitals could increase output prices at their discretion to obtain higher revenues and profits and would automatically benefit from increases in the quantity of care provided (number of patient care episodes), the LOS of each episode, or the number of services provided per day. Providers had explicit financial incentives to increase output prices, the number of patient care episodes provided, and the number of services provided in each episode and reduce costs. Cost reduction, however, was not a high priority given providers' ability to increase revenue.

The change between charge and cost reimbursement is that prices become irrelevant since payment is based on the cost of care delivered rather than the price of care. Under cost reimbursement, cost is typically determined using cost-to-charge ratios, so astute charge setting can change calculated costs and subsequent payments—this nuance, however, will be ignored. The big change between cost and charge reimbursement is the elimination of the ability to earn profit (total revenue > total cost), which essentially precludes using prices, quantity, the LOS, or the number of services provided to increase net income. However, most managers want to grow their organizations (and increase the size of their budgets), so increasing the quantity of patients treated, the LOS, and/or the number of services can be used to increase revenues. It is natural for people to want to control more resources, and cost reimbursement encourages providers to increase cost rather than reduce cost in charge-based reimbursement. The incentive to increase cost manifests itself as paying more for inputs, that is, salaries can be increased for employees and higher-priced supplies, equipment, and buildings can be purchased. In addition to paying more than necessary for resources, cost reimbursement also encourages overstaffing and less expectation from deployed resources, that is, employees are allowed to take more time per test or procedure than necessary and high error rates are tolerated. Overinvestment in equipment and buildings also arises when duplicate resources are purchased for patient or employee convenience and are underutilized.

The shift between cost and per diem reimbursement includes restoring the incentive to reduce the cost of tests and procedures and establishing an incentive to reduce the number of tests and procedures. Since a fixed amount is paid per day of hospitalization, providers have an incentive to be circumspect in their use of tests and procedures. The desirability of per diem reimbursement increases with a provider's ability to change the ordering habits of its physicians, that is, reduce the number of unnecessary tests and procedures (because of defective performance, inability to recognize a service has already been performed, or

TABLE 15.6 Incentives in Each Reimbursement System

	Price	Q (admits)	LOS	Tests and Procedures per Day	Cost of Tests and Procedures
Charge/% of charge	↑	↑	↑	↑	↓
Cost	Does not affect	↑ (Does not affect net income)	↑ (Does not affect net income)	↑ (Does not affect net income)	↑ (Does not affect net income)
Per diem/per procedure	Does not affect	↑ if medically necessary	↑ if medically necessary	↓	↓
Per case	Does not affect	↑ if medically necessary	↓	↓	↓
Capitation	Does not affect	↓ (Does not affect revenue but reduces net income)	↓	↓	↓

inability to recognize a service that provides no benefit), and lower the cost of tests and procedures (better processes and/or lower input costs). Providers under per diem reimbursement can improve their financial performance by increasing the number of medically necessary admissions or the LOS and reducing the number or cost of services provided.

The major change between per diem and per case reimbursement is the elimination of the incentive to increase the LOS. Under per case reimbursement, providers receive the same payment, whether a patient stays for 4 or 5 days, so quicker discharge should reduce costs and increase net income. The desirability of per case reimbursement is contingent upon a provider's ability to create a care process that allows faster discharge and change physician discharge practices. Financial performance under per case payment can be improved by increasing the number of medically necessary admissions and reducing the LOS, the number of services provided, and the cost of services.

Capitated reimbursement presents the greatest risk to providers as they are paid a flat rate to provide all necessary medical services for a defined group of people for a unit of time, i.e., a month or year. The flat rate does not change on the basis of whether individuals seek care or the level of care provided when people seek care. Financial success hinges on the ability to keep patients out of the hospital, that is, can hospitals enact effective prevention programs and change physician treatment patterns? The previous incentives to reduce the LOS, the number of services provided, and the cost of services continue.

Success under fixed reimbursement systems requires hospital managers to have productive partnerships with their medical staff and employees to ensure effective and efficient delivery of care. This partnership should be built on every employee understanding the financial risks each reimbursement system imposes on the provider, knowing how financial performance can be improved, and accepting that the financial performance of the organization is not only everyone's responsibility but also in their best interest. Information systems that can track and report what has been done to avoid needless duplication of tests and/ or procedures and what needs to be done to eliminate unneeded services is essential to provide frontline employees with the information necessary to function effectively and efficiently.

The three main ways to handle risk are risk avoidance, transfer, and retention. **Risk avoidance** occurs when providers recognize an attempt to shift cost, utilization, or actuarial risk through a managed care contract and do not accept it. Maintaining charge or cost reimbursement avoids risk, but this option may not be viable if other providers accept the proposed reimbursement methods. A second means of risk avoidance is to carve out high-risk services or those that fall outside the organization's expertise. **Risk transfer** accepts the risk but attempts to shift its impact; stop-loss and re-insurance arrangements for low-probability, high-cost medical expenses are two methods of transferring risk. Care that falls outside an organization's expertise can be accepted but subcontracted to other providers as a second means to transfer risk. The third option is **risk retention**, where a provider

understands the monetary risk assumed and can negotiate a reimbursement rate to cover the potential cost. The ability of a provider to successfully manage risk unfortunately may depend upon the willingness of its competitors to accept unfavorable contract terms or reimbursement rates. Organizations operating in highly competitive markets may have to accept risk to be included within a payer's preferred provider network.

Pumpian (2012) discussed how Sharp HealthCare approaches risk management primarily through patient steering. Effectively using preventive care and steering patients to the most appropriate provider for their condition, including primary care over emergency rooms, skilled nursing facility versus acute care, and transfer to hospice, not only improve treatment but also lower costs. A second aspect utilizes team-based negotiation with payers recognizing hospitals control inpatient costs and medical groups control office visits and success requires effective coordination of both. Sharp's approach also recognizes the inherent risks associated with medical services that are not provided by either the provider or the payer, such as ambulance, skilled nursing facilities, and home health care. These services require actuarial analysis of the potential patient population, age, sex, and payer (benefit plan), to assess financial exposure. Other programs Sharp has initiated include 24-7 nursing hotlines, disease management programs, out-of-network follow-up and transfer, and hospitalist care. Finance plays a large role in contract management, including analyzing cost by population, contracting with payers and out-of-network providers, estimating reserve models, providing authorizations for services, identifying capital needs, verifying eligibility for services, billing, and collecting for services delivered.

Organizations that struggle with contract management often lack effective management systems. Abernathy (2000) cites three common problems. The first is inadequate information technology systems for contract provisions, that is, information systems either do not track risk exposures or cannot provide timely information to mitigate loss. Second, contract targets are not based on historical experience, that is, providers accept contract terms without understanding what the financial impact would be on prior financial performance. A third problem is unclear contract terms; each party needs to understand who is responsible for what, and any ambiguity will result in a shift of costs to the provider. Tiscornia, Wilson, Orlikoff, and Totten (2009) propose five indicators of higher financial risk: (1) declining patient volume, (2) declining efficiency (costs increasing faster than patient volume), (3) lower profits or cash flow, (4) declining liquidity, and, finally, (5) a highly leveraged financial structure. They also present five actions to improve financial performance: (1) revenue cycle enhancement; (2) targeted price increases (versus across-the-board increases); (3) improved contract negotiations with payers; (4) nonlabor cost savings via renegotiation of service contracts, outsourcing, and standardization; (5) and reduction of labor costs by comparing current performance with industry standards.

Summary

This chapter began by reviewing the obligation of healthcare organizations to supply valid and reliable financial information to outside parties; it ended with noting the responsibility of employees to ensure the efficient functioning of the revenue cycle and adapting healthcare delivery processes to minimize financial risk. While decisions on what financial information is reported, the mix of equity and debt in the capital structure, the level of cash to hold, and which contracts should be entered into are primarily the responsibility of finance, every manager and employee should understand how the choices made affect what ends the organization can pursue and how goals are pursued.

The use of debt in financing assets is a double-edged sword. When debt is less expensive than equity financing, increasing debt lowers costs and expands the number of profitable investment opportunities. On the other hand, increasing use of debt increases the power of creditors over the organization and increases cash outflows, that is, mandatory interest payments. Working capital management recognizes the time lag between when resources are purchased and when payment is received for goods and services produced. Effective working capital management requires that finance hold the appropriate amount of cash to pay bills, minimize cash outflows, and maximize cash inflows by making all employees aware of their roles in the revenue cycle. Similarly, contract management touches on all aspects of an operation by setting the terms under which the organization receives reimbursement and the extent of the payment.

The financial performance of an organization is determined by how well managers and employees understand their roles in maximizing outcomes under the incentives and constraints established by the capital structure and third-party payer contracts. The job of finance is to ensure managers understand these incentives and constraints; the job of managers is to ensure all employees work to improve organizational performance. The chapter "Strategic Financial Planning" takes the information of prior chapters and develops a multiyear plan to determine where an organization will go and how it can get there.

Key Terms and Concepts

Business risk	Financial risk	Risk transfer
Cash flow statement	Risk avoidance	Stewardship
Cost of capital	Risk retention	Working capital
Financial leverage	Risk/return trade-off	

Discussion Questions

1. What is the role of financial reporting?
2. What impact did the SOX Act have on financial reporting?
3. What should we observe on the cash flow statement in the operations, investment, and financing sections for a financially strong organization?
4. Explain why higher use of debt can lower the cost of capital and why beyond a certain point the cost of capital increases with the amount of debt.
5. What types of organizations or what characteristics are common among organizations that use high levels of debt?
6. Explain the timing difference between cash outflows and inflows and how employees can narrow the time between resource payments and receipt of payment for goods and services sold.
7. Explain the different types of risk and how they are distributed between healthcare providers and insurers under charge, cost, per diem, per case, and capitation reimbursement systems.
8. Explain how risk is managed using risk avoidance, risk transfer, and risk retention.

Problems

1. Interpret the given cash flow statement. Discuss operating, investment, and financing activities. What were the primary sources of cash each year? Comment on management performance.

Operating Activities	2017	2018
Net income	−$238,454	$278,650
Adjustments		
Depreciation	$87,215	$73,635
Accounts receivable	−$85,830	−$83,759
Inventory	−$11,652	−$1,612
Accounts payable	$15,128	$15,294
Retirement plan	$188,442	−$49,240
Other	$55,079	−$83,695
Total	$9,928	$149,273
Investment Activities		
Property and equipment	−$284,697	−$216,404
Securities	$206,313	−$114,537
Total	−$78,384	−$330,941

Financing Activities		
Long-term debt	$107,057	$51,467
Short-term debt	−150,915	31,200
Total	−$43,858	$82,667
Change in cash	−$112,314	−$99,001
Beginning balance	$153,388	$252,389
Ending balance	$41,074	$153,388

2. Calculate the WACC for each level of debt in the table given. Produce a line graph with the cost of debt, equity, and WACC. What level of debt produces the lowest cost of capital?

Debt in Capital Structure (%)	Debt (%)	Equity (%)	WACC
0	5	10	_____
20	6	10	_____
40	7	10	_____
60	9	11	_____
80	11	12	_____
100	14	14	_____

	No Debt	50% Debt
Total assets	$400.00	$400.00
Total debt	$0.0	_____
Total equity	_____	_____
Total revenue	$200.00	$200.00
Operating expense	$170.00	$170.00
EBIT	_____	_____
Interest expense	_____	_____
Net income	_____	_____
ROE	_____	_____

3. Calculate the impact of debt on the ROE for the organization in the table given, assuming the interest rate is 5.0% and 50% of assets are financed by debt. What is the ROE with and without debt financing? Assume the organization is taxed at 40%; what is the after-tax ROE with and without debt?

4. Calculate the cash budget for the organization. Net collections average 50% of gross revenue, and 20% of payments are received within 30 days of billing, 50% in 31–60 days, and 30% between 61 and 90 days. The physicians are planning to purchase $50,000 in equipment in the second quarter; will a bridge loan be necessary? What is the expected cash balance at the end of the fourth quarter?

Dollars in 000				
Inflows	**1st Quarter**	**2nd Quarter**	**3rd Quarter**	**4th Quarter**
Gross revenue	$1000.00	$1010.00	$1020.00	$1030.00
Net revenue	_____	_____	_____	_____
0–30 days	_____	_____	_____	_____
31–60 days	$249.00	_____	_____	_____
61–90 days	$148.00	$149.00	_____	_____
Total collections	_____	_____	_____	_____
Outflows				
Wages paid	$325.00	$328.00	$332.00	$335.00
Supplies	$50.00	$51.00	$51.00	$52.00
Utilities	$40.00	$40.00	$41.00	$41.00
Other	$75.00	$76.00	$89.00	$77.00
Capital expenditures		$50.00		
Total payments	_____	_____	_____	_____
Net cash from operations	_____	_____	_____	_____
Beginning cash balance	$65.00	_____	_____	_____
Net cash from operations	_____	_____	_____	_____
Ending cash balance	_____	_____	_____	_____

References

Abernathy, M. (2000). Avoid common problems in risk sharing contracts. *Managed Care, 9*(4), 29–30, 32.

Pumpian, A. (2012). Sharp healthcare's risk-sharing strategy. *Healthcare Financial Management, 66*(11), 32–34.

Tiscornia, J. R., Wilson, R. E., Orlikoff, J. E., & Totten, M. K. (2009). Strategies to reduce financial risk in a perilous economy. *Trustee, 62*(7), 13–16.

Valletta, R. M. (2005, August). Clear as glass, transparent financial reporting. *Healthcare Financial Management, 59*(8), 58–66.

Welsch, G. A., Zlatkovich, C. T., & White, J. A. (1976) *Intermediate accounting* (4th ed.). Homewood, IL: Richard D. Irwin, Inc.

Weston, J. F., & Brigham, E. F. (1978). *Managerial finance* (6th ed.). Hinsdale, IL: Dryden Press.

CHAPTER 16

Strategic Financial Planning

CHAPTER OBJECTIVES

1. Explain the role and phases of strategic management.
2. Explain the role of finance in formulating and implementing strategic plans.
3. Develop a multiyear financial plan.
4. Compare actual financial performance with the multiyear targets.
5. Explain sustainable growth.

▶ Introduction

As you climb the ladder in your organization, your focus shifts; initially, you are concerned with day-to-day operations, that is, managing defined processes and meeting your budget. Managers at the top of the organization focus on where the organization should go, in addition to directing day-to-day operations. Senior managers are tasked with decisions regarding what customers want in the future and the evolution of technology and how both may affect products, production processes, and organizational goals. Whether Henry Ford ever said, "If I had asked people what they wanted, they would have said faster horses," is unclear; his point, however, is obvious. The task he set for himself was to show the public the superiority of a new method of transportation. Senior managers work with uncertainty: consumers may not accept

new products, technology may not work as expected, input prices increase or fall, etc. Strategic management is a means to assess an organization's situation and potential strategies and select and pursue an optimal course of action.

Financial information documents the health of the organization and is a key component in strategic management. Is the organization achieving its potential, and is financial performance improving or declining? Financial management should move the organization to higher performance, and the strategic financial plan is the vehicle to set long-term goals and assess management's ability to achieve strategic goals. Not every plan can be met, so the strategic plan should be altered as events expand or reduce what is achievable. When financial performance exceeds expectations, hard work and good fortune should be built upon and operations and investments should be expanded. When financial results are less than expected, the strategic plan should be reassessed. Planned investments should be reconsidered and possibly delayed or cancelled, given the lower-than-expected net income, and actions should be taken to improve net income.

The primary difference between operating budgets and strategic planning is the number of years covered and the detail. Operating budgets are a detailed plan of how goals will be accomplished in a year, whereas strategic plans set broader goals over a multiyear horizon at a lower level of detail. In some cases, strategic plans are little more than wishful thinking. Strategic plans should define where the organization wants to be in the future, but this vision should be accompanied by a financial plan that covers the same period to be credible. If a 5-year strategic plan is constructed, it should contain a 5-year financial plan defining the goods and services to be sold or provided; market forecasts; expected revenues, expenses, and net income; a set of investment priorities (to support the output forecasts with expected financial performance); and sources of financing.

The strategic plan, in addition to presenting a financial plan, should specify the organization's mission, vision, and values; its strengths, weaknesses, opportunities, and threats (SWOT); and its competitive advantage, objectives, strategies, action plans, and mechanisms for assessing performance. Strategic planning is often criticized for producing little tangible results; this happens when form supersedes substance. It is possible to produce a strategic plan with all the required components that totally fails to meet the goals of strategic planning. Strategic planning fails when critical data is not collected, undesired information is minimized or ignored, goals and/or strategies are determined before data is collected, and/or the plan is poorly implemented. Common implementation problems include lack of employee commitment and no mechanism to connect the plan to budgets or performance evaluation.

Multiyear financial planning is one way to avoid a common pitfall of strategic planning—the lack of feasible goals. Ensuring ambitious goals are realizable requires rigorous data collection and analysis. Can the vision be achieved under existing practices? Finance should not shy away from judgment when resources are inadequate to fund operations. Financial planners should specify the degree of improvement required to achieve the vision when funds are inadequate. Is the organization capable of or prepared to improve existing practices to achieve the vision? If not, how should the vision be altered, which goals should be pursued, and which should be discarded?

Financial planning is a tool to assess the vision, that is, budgeting and finance do not set the vision; they supply input, assess the feasibility of the plan, and provide feedback on performance. There are two primary financial relationships, between revenue and expenses (net income) and between assets and liabilities (equity). The relationship between revenue and expenses determines viability—the ability of the organization to continue operations. When organizations generate net income, that is, create value, they can continue operating. When expenses exceed revenues, value is destroyed, and managers must secure other sources of support or go out of business.

The relationship between assets and liabilities determines solvency—the ability to pay creditors. As discussed in the chapter "Financial Functions in Finance," creditors want a cushion of equity to fall back on if operating losses occur. In for-profits, net income from the income statement can be either distributed to owners or reinvested in the organization to increase equity on the balance sheet. In nonprofit organizations, net income and retained earnings largely determine the growth in equity and the extent of investment.

The climate for hospitals has been hostile since 1990; there are 1085 fewer hospitals in 2015 than there were in 1990, a reduction

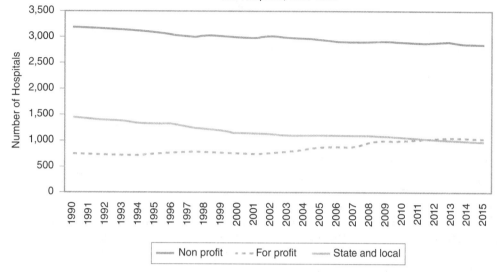

FIGURE 16.1 U.S. Hospitals, 1990–2015

of 16.3%. **FIGURE 16.1** shows how the number of hospitals in the United States has changed since 1990 by ownership: there are 461, or 31.9%, fewer public hospitals, while for-profit hospitals have increased by 285, or 38.1%. The results speak for themselves: better managed organizations thrive, while poorly managed organizations cease to exist. For-profit managers planned to grow their organizations and did so despite the general contraction in the industry, while managers of public hospitals did little planning and left their patients and employees to fate. In 2000, there were 695 more public hospitals than for-profits; in 2015, there were 51 more for-profit than public hospitals.

Leaving the well-being of patients, the livelihoods of employees, and millions of dollars of plant and equipment to fate is neither sensitive nor wise. Besides the negative impact on patient health, when a hospital shuts down, that is, a major employer leaves town, there is also severe economic dislocation. This chapter describes the roles of strategic management and how strategic financial planning should assist in realizing strategic goals. Previous

chapters emphasized planning was essential for the efficient allocation of resources; this chapter expands beyond a 1-year operating budget or a single-investment capital budget to focus on the entire organization and its performance over a multiyear horizon.

▶ Strategic Management

Successful individuals, organizations, and countries focus on what they do best, improve their strengths, and correct, minimize, or avoid their weaknesses. David Ricardo described the law of comparative advantage almost 2 centuries ago, where two countries enjoy more goods if each specializes on what it does best. Ricardo's insight was that it does not matter if one country can produce goods at a lower absolute cost; gains from trade occur if the higher-cost country specializes in what it does best and trades with a lower-cost country. Similarly, managers should identify and focus on their organization's strengths: is its strength in capital resources, human resources, or the ability to organize resources that provide an advantage in the marketplace?

A successful strategy is built on exploiting advantage, but what is strategy? According to Webster's dictionary, strategy is the science and art of employing political, economic, psychological, and military forces of a nation . . . to afford the maximum support to adopted policies in peace or war. Hellriegel, Jackson, and Slocum (2005) define strategy as the major course of action an organization takes to achieve its goals. Both definitions emphasize goals, but Webster's definition makes clear that strategy-making is not mechanistic or programmatic—it is art as well as science and alerts the reader that one should assess all critical elements before a course of action is selected. Tactics are often confused with strategy; tactics are the science and art of maneuvering forces in combat (Webster's) or detailed decisions about what to do, when to do it, how to do it, and who should do it (Hellriegel et al., 2005). Hellriegel et al. provide the superior definition by alerting the reader to the information needed (the what, when, how, and who) to undertake action.

Strategic management is the process of setting organizational goals and instituting systems capable of reaching the goals set. The strategic decisions managers must make include defining the organization's future mission, goals, customer mix, service area, and competitive strategies (Swayne, Duncan, & Ginter, 2008). These decisions should be guided, but not straightjacketed, by the organization's current mission, vision, and values; its strengths and weaknesses; and the opportunities and threats posed by its current environment. The acronym **MOST**, **m**ission, **o**bjectives, **s**trategy, and **t**actics, encapsulates the role of strategic planning, starting with why the organization exists and ending with what specific actions it expects to take. The mission defines why an organization exists and specifies its customers, services, geographic area, values, and philosophy (Swayne et al., 2008, p. 169). **BOX 16.1** provides examples of mission statements that

BOX 16.1 Examples of Mission Statements

Nike:	"Crush Reebok"
Walmart:	"To give ordinary folk the chance to buy the same things as rich people"
Walt Disney:	"To make people happy"

clearly define the organizations' goals, are readily understandable, are direct, and motivate employees in their work.

After the mission is defined, what objectives or goals will the organization's employees pursue? Objectives should be related to mission-critical activities and be specific, easily understood, and limited in number. Objectives should be developed in concert with major constituencies and be widely accepted, motivating, and inspiring (for stakeholders). Objectives are measureable outcomes such as expanding sales or market share, improving quality, or innovating.

Third, what strategy do senior managers believe will allow the objectives to be reached? What major factors will the organization capitalized on to achieve its objectives? Organizations typically pursue strategies based on providing high-quality or lower-cost products or specializing in niche markets. Implementing these strategies may require expanding, contracting, altering, or maintaining current operations. When expansion or contraction is required, managers must determine the best method. Expansion can be accomplished by building, buying, or partnering, while contraction requires reducing the scale or scope of activity through retrenchment, divestiture, or liquidation. Each method has advantages and disadvantages, and the choice should be based on the organization's SWOT analysis.

Finally, what actions are expected from managers and employees to make the chosen strategies work? Implementation of strategy should not be left undefined; every manager should know what is expected of him or her and the employees. New and existing activities critical to achieving strategy should be explicitly defined: what is required, how will it be measured, and when is it expected to be completed? Managers and employees should not only understand what is expected but also believe it is achievable.

While MOST encapsulates the main decisions that must be made and clarifies the goal of strategic management, selecting the best or superior alternatives and effectively implementing choices requires a process. The four distinct and interdependent steps in the strategic management process are data collection, analysis, strategy formulation and selection, and implementation (Swayne et al., 2008, p. 33). Data collection is the identification of critical factors and gathering of data. Data collectors should be intimately familiar with the organization, industry, and environment to gather pertinent and accurate data. In organizations with multiple products, processes, and/or markets, the breadth of information needed and the validity of data collected often require input from multiple stakeholders, customers, equity providers, employees, regulators, etc. (**FIGURE 16.2**).

Analysis separates the "wheat from the chaff": data must be organized into information after it is collected. Analysis should identify what matters and which internal and external factors present a competitive advantage to capitalize on or a competitive disadvantage to overcome. After completing this step, planners and managers should have a clear understanding of the demands of their environment (opportunities and threats) and their ability to meet those demands (strengths and weaknesses).

The third step, strategy formulation and selection, requires planners and managers to determine what the organization wants to do (on the basis of its mission), what it can do (its strengths and weaknesses) to meet the needs and challenges of its operating environment (opportunities and threats),

and which strategy offers the greatest probability of success. Strategy setters must understand the linkage between the organization's strengths and weaknesses and the advantages and disadvantages of potential strategies to ensure the strategy pursued makes the best use of the skills and resources the organization possesses. The third step converts information into knowledge—knowing what to do in a particular situation.

The final step, implementation, carries the plan into action and hopefully to completion; this is where the "rubber meets the road." Successful implementation requires explicit goals and expectations, a clear means to achieve goals, including who is responsible for what actions and what resources they will have at their disposal, and monitoring of activity and outcomes with correction taken when plans are not realized. Poor performance at any point—failure to collect data, transform the data into information, select an achievable plan, or act on one's knowledge—increases the probability of failure, given the interdependency of steps.

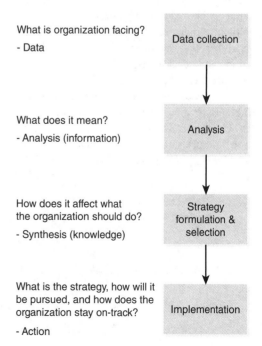

What is organization facing?
- Data

Data collection

What does it mean?
- Analysis (information)

Analysis

How does it affect what the organization should do?
- Synthesis (knowledge)

Strategy formulation & selection

What is the strategy, how will it be pursued, and how does the organization stay on-track?
- Action

Implementation

FIGURE 16.2 The Four Steps of Strategic Management

Objective and strategy setting is always subservient to the organization's mission, vision, and values; where the organization goes should be determined by what equity suppliers and customers want rather than what the current SWOT analysis says. Neither current capabilities nor environmental demands should dictate goals, but each should be understood to inform knowledgeable decision-making and action. Understanding the internal and external environments informs what can be and should be done, but ultimately, owners and senior managers will determine what will be pursued by focusing on the strengths or opportunities that support the desired goals or addressing the remediable weaknesses or threats to move them into line with goals.

The goal of **internal analysis** is to identify and evaluate an organization's key strengths and weaknesses to improve management and planning. Swayne et al. (2008) structure internal analysis around the **value chain** that divides organizational functions into service and support functions (**FIGURE 16.3**). Service functions encompass all activities (preservice, service, and postservice) of an organization that interact with customers. Assessing preservice functions examines the organization's ability to design goods and services desired by customers and produce them at prices they are willing to pay.

The **four Ps of marketing**, that is, the marketing mix, examine an organization's choices for products, prices, physical distribution, and promotion and provide a framework for assessing the preservice capabilities of the organization. The product or mix of products sold should be determined by what patients want. The design of products should meet the tangible and intangible desires of patients and specify the necessary functional, psychological, and social attributes. Product design should encompass the good or service (what is delivered), the service experience (how the good or service is delivered), the environment (where customer transactions occur, including climate and location), choice (depth and width of the product mix), timeliness, and price.

The goal of pricing is to clear the market, equate supply with demand, and fulfill the organization's objective. The objective could be to maximize the return on equity (ROE) (for-profits), maximize services to the community and generate an adequate ROE to support growth (nonprofits), or achieve optimal use of services, while equitably spreading costs among clients and taxpayers (public organizations). The pricing of services in public healthcare organizations should ensure that needed services are obtained via subsidies but that services are not consumed to the point where marginal cost exceeds marginal benefits, that is, minimize moral hazard. Many organizations view market share as an indicator of success, that is, increasing market share indicates superior performance to competitors and vice versa. Intelligent price setting requires understanding production costs, customer price sensitivity (i.e., price elasticity), and competitor prices.

Physical distribution (i.e., place) decisions determine where products will be sold.

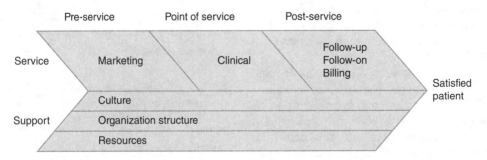

FIGURE 16.3 The Healthcare Value Chain

Intensive distribution is used for convenience products where consumers want to minimize search and travel costs. Multiple outlets are required to maximize sales as consumers will not bypass one seller for another. Selective distribution is used for high-price products where consumers routinely shop around and expect higher service. Sellers do not have to have to provide multiple outlets if they can attract customers through superior service. Exclusive distribution is used for specialty or unique products; in this case, customers may have no choice but to travel extensive distances to obtain the product. Physical distribution determines time and place—where and when customers want the product. In health care, multiple examples of all three exist: routine care is available through physician offices and urgent care facilities, hospitals provide selective services, and tertiary care and level I trauma centers may be the only source for some services across wide geographic areas.

The last **P** is promotion. The goal of promotion is to create product awareness. There are divergent beliefs on promotion, especially in medicine: does advertising fill in the gaps in patient knowledge of needed goods and services, or does it create artificial demand? In health care, the question is, does advertising prevent underuse of medical care or encourage overuse?

The second element in the service value chain is the actual delivery of goods and services to customer, that is, point-of-service (POS) activity. Important attributes include the technical and interpersonal skills of the staff; the age of, cleanliness, and ease of movement around a facility; time to complete transactions; and fulfillment of customer needs or desires. Product delivery goals are often stated as better, cheaper, and faster. In hospitals, the question, who is the customer? is not trivial; product design depends on whether the primary customer is the patient, admitting physicians, or third-party payers. When hospital customers are defined as physicians, the hospital may promote better outcomes and state-of-the-art medical technology. If customers are defined as patients, emphasis may be placed on better outcomes, amenities, and short waiting times. When third-party payers are targeted, the hospital may want to promote lower-cost and better outcomes.

The final link in the service value chain is postservice activity, that is, the events arising after a good or service has been delivered to the customer. Postservice activities include billing, follow-up, and follow-on. Bills for products should be prompt, accurate, and understandable, and customer inquiries should be quickly and courteously handled. Follow-up seeks to determine customer satisfaction with the product and, in health care, deals with the patient's response to care and early detection of complications. Follow-on activities seek to identify additional needs or wants the organization could fulfill, for example, what additional procedures, tests, and/or therapies could a patient benefit from? Follow-up and follow-on activities demonstrate the organization is committed to building a long-term relationship with its customers rather than viewing sales as one-time transactions.

Preservice, POS, and postservice activities must be performed well to ensure a positive customer experience. Providing exceptional POS and postservice work cannot salvage poorly designed goods and services. Similarly, organizations can design perfect products and deliver them without error, but lack of follow-up or errors in billing may convince customers the organization is indifferent or incompetent.

Just as all service functions must be performed competently, all service personnel, whether engaged in preservice, POS, or postservice activities, must be provided with the resources they need to do their jobs. Support functions define the culture and decision-making structure of an organization and assess the resources supplied to frontline employees. The ability of service personnel to complete their jobs effectively, efficiently, and promptly depends on the support they receive from management, finance, information technology (IT), human resources, facilities, and other areas of the organization. Customers value demand-centered cultures, where their needs and desires are placed above employee desires, versus supply-centered organizations, where processes are designed for the convenience of employees. Effective cultures are also team- and goal-oriented. How much authority frontline personnel are given will determine how fast decisions are made and customer-pleasing actions taken.

Organizational architecture examines the symmetry of decision-making rights, incentive systems, and performance evaluation systems. Decision-making rights focus on who makes decisions, incentive systems examine whether decision makers have explicit encouragements to maximize the value of the organization, and performance evaluation systems examine whether employee actions are monitored, that is, whether controls are in place to ensure decision makers are taking actions that increase the value of the organization. When any component is absent, it is unlikely the organizational value will be maximized. If employees have decision-making rights and incentives but no monitoring is in place, the desired action may not occur. If incentives and monitoring systems are in place but employees are not allowed to make decisions, improvements cannot be introduced. The extent of decision-making authority granted must be proportional to the incentives given to undertake organizational value–increasing actions and the ability to monitor actions.

Efficient production requires resources be in place, maintained, and integrated into workflows. Does finance provide the monetary resources to purchase up-to-date equipment and facilities, does the human resources department identify and recruit the best staff, does IT provide timely and relevant information, and does the facility services department optimize workspaces and maintain plant and equipment? The question addressed by examining support functions is, are service personnel operating in an environment that places customers first; expects, monitors, and rewards performance; and supplies employees with the resources they need to complete their jobs?

The desired outcome of internal analysis is the identification of a **competitive advantage**—the things the organization does better than its rivals that are valued by current or potential customers and that should be incorporated into strategic plans and pursued to improve performance. Typical competitive advantages include an organization's ability to provide products at lower cost, higher quality, provide products faster, and/or provide products adapted to the specific need or desire of the customer. Equally important is the recognition of competitive disadvantages (or the competitive advantages of rivals). Recognizing competitive disadvantages allows organizations to focus on correcting remediable shortcomings or crafting strategies that avoid disadvantages such as discontinuing a product or exiting a market.

FIGURE 16.4 presents a hypothetical internal analysis with an organization having a clear POS competitive advantage from providing superior outcomes and eliciting higher-than-average patient satisfaction plus above-average management and financial performance. On the negative side of the ledger, the organization has older facilities than its rivals and poorer information systems. Assessing the overall capability of the organization, it can be concluded that strengths exceed weaknesses as the number of unweighted strengths exceeds weakness, 3S > 2T, net +1. A more sophisticated analysis could attempt to assess the magnitude of each strength or weakness on a five-point scale to incorporate the intensity of each strength and weakness, 9S (4 + 3 + 2) > 6T (−4 − 2), net +3.

The assessment of the overall strength or weakness of an organization provides some indication of what the organization can do—the greater the overall strength, the more aggressive the goals and vice versa. The identification of

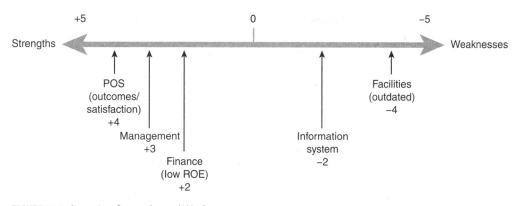

FIGURE 16.4 Assessing Strengths and Weaknesses

individual strengths and weaknesses provides insight into what the organization should do. In the example above, managers may want to market the superior outcomes to third-party payers and physicians, as well as marketing higher satisfaction scores to patients. The intensity of the facility weakness (−4) suggests that if patients are selecting providers on the basis of facility age and appearance, the strategic plan should include significant capital upgrades.

Internal analysis assesses what an organization can and should do (capitalize on strengths and/or correct weaknesses); the strategic plan (including what to produce, where, etc.) should also consider the needs of customers and the strengths and weaknesses of competitors. **External analysis** is the process of identifying and evaluating the opportunities and threats in an organization's operating environment to recognize issues the strategic plan should address. External issues are typically divided into the general environment, the industry (health care), the organization, and specific products and services. The external issues are analyzed from the most far-reaching ones, those affecting all organizations, to those that only affect the products of the particular organization. At each level, issues can be categorized as political/regulatory, economic, social/demographic, technology, and competition (PEST-C) to aid data collection and analysis.

General environmental issues include which political party holds power and its orientation toward taxing, spending, and regulation. Economic issues include the overall state of the economy: is the per capita gross domestic product (GDP) expanding or contracting? The level of changes in per capita income affects the revenues of all industries as well as the government. High and increasing per capita income spurs higher consumer spending and tax revenues. Increasing per capita income also increases the demand for the products of most industries and funding for government agencies.

Social issues include population growth, average age of the population, and educational achievement. The overall demand for goods and services should increase proportionately with an increase in the population, and changes in the average age or educational levels can increase or decrease the demand for particular goods and services. Technologies that affect all industries include computer, the Internet, and communication; the impact of these forces varies by industry. General competitive issues include the impact of global competition on the national economy; in the United States, the increase in global competition has exerted pressure on low-technology goods but stimulated high-tech exports. The goal of examining and projecting changes in the general environment is to determine the favorableness of the overall business climate, that is, how industries will be affected.

The shift to industry issues identifies factors that will have a disproportionate impact on the industry the organization inhabits. For example, the Affordable Care Act had some impact on nonhealthcare industries but a profound impact on health insurance, hospitals, pharmaceuticals, and medical supply organizations. Similarly, the impact of changes in per capita income will have differential effects on organizations that produce durable goods, nondurable goods, and services. During economic expansion, the demand for durable goods increases faster than the overall economy, and during recession, it falls more. Industries supplying services may see little change in the demand during expansion or recession. In health care, an aging population, a social or demographic factor, should produce a higher demand for care and revenues. On the other hand, an aging population may produce lower revenues for the entertainment industry. Changes in technology and competition in an industry may have a profound impact on cost, prices, and demand. The goal of industry analysis is to determine how an organization operating in an industry may be affected by industry-wide trends.

The next step, from the most far-reaching to a specific impact, studies factors in the market where an organization operates. Per capita income and population growth are examined at the national level, but the specific markets in which an organization functions, its city, county, or state, may see opposite movements. For example, the U.S. population may be growing roughly by 1.0% per year, but the population in Colorado is growing at a significantly faster rate and West Virginia has been contracting. Demand projections for either Colorado or West Virginia providers should be based on state or local growth rates rather than national trends. Similarly, local economic and competitive factors are far more important than national trends. The goal of organizational analysis is to determine how the

organization should perform on the basis of market-specific factors—will the organization see a higher or lower demand for its products than its industry? See **FIGURE 16.5**.

The most important analysis takes places at the product and service levels. Rational planning requires specific planning for each product or product line; just as an organization should not blindly expect to see the same change in demand for its services as the industry, each product line should not expect to see the same change as the overall organization. The question that should be addressed is in light of general and industry changes: how will a change in the operating environment of organization X affect the demand for service Y? The goal is to develop specific expectations for the goods and/or services produced by the organization to facilitate rational resource planning: will this service grow faster or slower than the overall organization, industry, and economy, and what resources should be committed to it?

FIGURE 16.6 demonstrates a hypothetical analysis of an organization with two general opportunities, population growth and economic growth, and one specific threat, an increase in competition in its market. An unweighted analysis concludes that opportunities exceed threats, $2O > 1T$, net $+1$, but a weighted analysis concludes the opposite, $+3O$ $(+2 + 1) < -5T$, net -2. The weighted analysis concern for local competition outweighs the advantages of positive but low population and economic growth.

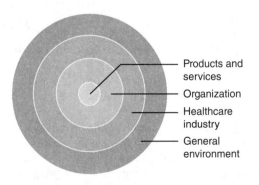

FIGURE 16.5 External Analysis

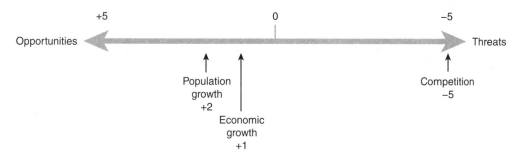

FIGURE 16.6 Assessing Opportunities and Threats

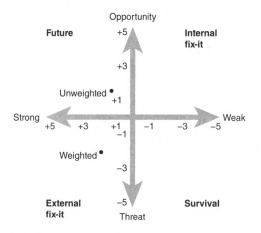

FIGURE 16.7 Assessing the Competitive Position

SWOT diagrams plot an organization's strengths, weaknesses, opportunities, and threats in a four-quadrant space to assist planners in identifying the competitive position of the organization and optimal strategies. **FIGURE 16.7** identifies the four quadrants as future, internal fix-it, external fix-it, and survival. The best position for an organization is the future—a strong organization operating in a hospitable environment. The stronger and more opportunistic the environment, the better for the organization; as the assessment shifts to the upper-left corner of the future quadrant, the possibilities of the organization expand and it could pursue more aggressive strategies. An organization with small strengths and opportunities, operating near the intersection of the *x* and *y* axes of Figure 16.7, should be more conservative.

An organization with more weaknesses than strengths, operating in an opportunistic environment, would reside in the internal fix-it quadrant. An appropriate strategy would focus on correcting weaknesses to shift the organization from the internal fix-it to the future quadrant.

A strong organization operating in a threatening environment resides in the external fix-it quadrant. An appropriate strategy involves improving the environment, perhaps changing it, lobbying policy makers, or taking a wait-and-see approach with the goal of changing threats to opportunities and shifting the organization into the future quadrant.

The worst position is survival—a weak organization in a threatening environment. Improving self and the environment is needed. Managers operating in the survival quadrant should pursue defensive strategies. The SWOT diagram allows planners and managers to visualize the competitive position of the organization and whether an aggressive, passive, or defensive strategy is appropriate.

The shift from data collection and analysis to strategy formulation begins by recognizing where an organization exists on the SWOT diagram. In the example above, the internal analysis yielded unweighted +1 and weighted +3, and the unweighted external analysis yielded +1 and weighted −2. Combining the analyses concludes that the organization is either slightly in the future quadrant (unweighted, +1S, +1O) or moderately strong but facing moderate external threats (weighted, +3S, −2T).

Strong organizations operating in opportunistic environments (upper-left corner of the SWOT diagram) should pursue aggressive strategies. Weak organizations in threatening environments (lower-right corner) should pursue conservative strategies. **FIGURE 16.8** lists the strategies available to an organization and their relationship to the competitive position of the organization. The strategy chosen by managers should be based on the capabilities of the organization and the structure of its operating environment.

The easiest-to-see relationship between organizational strengths and weaknesses and environmental opportunities and threats and a desirable strategy is seen in the survival quadrant. Organizations with modest weaknesses in a mildly threatening environment may simply want to address their weaknesses or insulate themselves against the threats, that is, pursue an enhancement strategy. Managers should take more evasive or defensive actions as organizational weaknesses grow or external threats increase. Action that is more drastic would move the organization away from its traditional products to a more favorable product mix through unrelated diversification. The final four strategies require more and more movement away from the organization's *status quo;* harvesting signifies maintaining operations but restricting or ending new investment. Retrenchment is a conscious attempt to

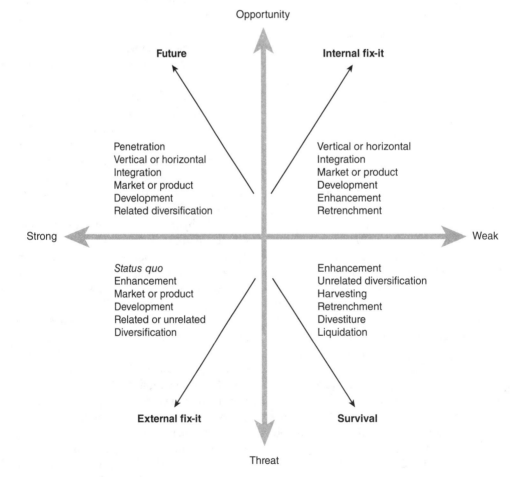

FIGURE 16.8 Competitive Position and Potential Strategies

scale back operations and conserve resources. Divestiture and liquidation involve disinvesting (selling assets) and recognizing that the organization cannot and should not continue at the present size and/or scope of operations.

In the future quadrant, strong organizations can do more of the same, that is, possess good management, deep resources, and low-cost processes that produce high-quality products; these organizations can go head-to-head with competitors to seize the market share, that is, pursue a penetration strategy. As strengths or opportunities diminish, managers may pursue less aggressive strategies such as vertical or horizontal integration or market or product development. These strategies seek growth opportunities along the distribution chain by acquiring competitors, customers, and/or suppliers entering new markets, and/or introducing new products (**BOX 16.2**).

The final and most challenging step is implementing the selected strategy. In implementing a strategy, employees should be clear on what actions are needed, who will undertake the actions, when the actions should occur, and what resources will be provided. It is at this point where financial planning increases its profile from defining what is possible to providing active support. Finance must first provide the necessary monetary resources to carry out the strategy, and second, it must provide the information to determine whether the organization is on track.

▶ Strategic Financial Planning

Finance plays a critical role in the strategic management process; it introduces realism and limits to a process that often leans toward excessive ambition. Strategic planning often trumpets that it will "remake" an organization into an industry leader or some other grandiose goal without supplying a plan, leadership, or resources. Building castles in the air is only

---

BOX 16.2 Strategy Definitions

Penetration: Pushing more products into existing markets

Vertical integration: Acquiring suppliers (backward integration) or customers (forward integration)

Horizontal integration: Acquiring competitors

Market development: Entering new geographic markets with current products

Product development: Introducing new products into current markets

Diversification: Expanding into goods or services that overlap current products to take advantage of the customer base, distribution channels, or technological expertise (concentric/related diversification) or moving into goods and services with no connection to existing products (conglomerate/unrelated diversification)

Status quo: Continuing current operations

Enhancement: Doing current things better

Harvesting: Continuing current operations and minimizing investment

Retrenchment: Reducing the scope or scale of operations

Divestiture: Selling viable operations and exiting markets

Liquidation: Selling nonviable operations and exiting markets

---

worthwhile if a foundation can be built under them; finance's role is to determine whether the organization has the resources for the castle *and* the foundation. Successful strategic management relies on finance to determine resource needs and the availability of funds to meet those needs across a multiyear horizon. Like in operational budgeting, the question is, is the plan feasible?

Beyond assessing the feasibility of the initial strategic plan, finance should monitor actual performance: were resource needs accurately estimated, and did the expected financial performance occur? Underestimation of funding needs, due to poor planning or unforeseeable inflation, and/or overstatement of output and revenue will create a funding gap that should be addressed. At what point does a funding gap become unsustainable and planned investments should be pulled back or other sources of funding explored? In the event that financial performance is better than expected, how should the additional funds be used?

Lastly, finance plays a direct role in implementing strategy: whether the organization pursues expansion, enhancement, or contraction. Finance has a duty to monitor financial performance to ensure the organization receives the maximum benefit from the resources it employs and meet its targets when possible. When actual performance does not meet expected performance, finance should identify where deviations occur and provide timely information to managers so they can take prompt, corrective action. Finance also plays a key role in obtaining financial resources, assessing acquisitions or divestitures, and targeting improvement efforts.

The need to move from 1-year operating budgets to multiyear financial plans is clear; resource needs, whether for new construction or replacement, span multiple years, and organizations must be able to fund these needs across time. For example, building a nuclear power plant takes 6–7 years from the start of construction; obtaining the permits to start construction may take as long or longer. Neither equity nor debt funding will be forthcoming if managers cannot demonstrate long-term viability.

Long (1976) demonstrated that a positive return must be earned on employed assets as breakeven financial performance is unsustainable in the long run, even for nonprofit organizations. A primary role of finance is to ensure suppliers of funds receive adequate and predictable returns on their investments. Long noted that the required return on assets (ROA) was 10.8%, but more important than this rate of return is understanding the factors it was designed to cover. First, input prices are increasing, so the ROA must supply enough

funds to replace existing assets in the future at higher prices. The increase in consumer prices from January 1, 2000, through January 1, 2016 (Table 13.1) was 39.4%, meaning an input originally purchased in 2000 would cost 39.4% more in 2016. A facility that cost $50,000,000 in 2000 would require $69,683,500 to replace; if the organization had fully depreciated the asset and saved the funds for replacement, it would only have enough funds to purchase 71.7% ($50.0 million/$69.7 million) of the resource.

Other factors that must be accounted for in the return needed over time include the cost of improved technology. Healthcare equipment, buildings, and supplies are increasing in price because of inflation and innovation. Advances in imaging equipment, robotic surgery, and designer pharmaceuticals provide a small sample of new high-cost innovations; some believe that advancing technology accounts for 40%–60% of the annual increase in healthcare costs. Health care, unlike most industries, adopts cost-increasing technologies, and organizations must invest in these technologies if they are going to stay competitive. The third factor is expanding capacity; the U.S. population is growing, and organizations that do not grow lose their market share to competitors. Healthcare resources should be expected to grow at least as fast as the population, and as the population ages, the need for care and investment may exceed the growth rate in the population.

The fourth factor is the cost of altering operations. Health care, like many industries, is introducing cost-increasing amenities to retain and attract customers. Upgrading patient rooms and furniture, expanding dining options, and providing concierge and valet parking services, as well as altering facilities to accommodate the shift from inpatient to outpatient care, have added and continue to add to hospital costs. The fifth factor identified by Long is uncertainty; organizations need a reserve for unforeseen and unforeseeable economic and political events. Long recognized that his estimates for inflation, technology and other factors were likely to variability, so he added a 10% hedge. So if inflation is underestimated by 10%, an adequate return would still be earned. **TABLE 16.1** provides Long's original required return calculation and an update to 2016.

Updating Long's work to 2016 suggests that healthcare managers need to produce a 6.0% ROA simply to maintain their position. The role of finance is to ensure organizations survive and grow by continuously raising, allocating, and managing funds.

Sustainable Growth

Finance holds that over the long run, the change in assets must equal the change in equity, that is, organizations cannot indefinitely rely on debt to acquire assets. The two limitations on the use of debt are (i) as the amount of debt increases, lenders face more risk and charge a higher interest rate and (ii) excessive debt may make lenders unwilling to provide funds at any interest rate. Given the costs of excessive reliance on debt, the change in equity often determines how much debt can be obtained and the maximum amount of investment that can be undertaken.

TABLE 16.1 Required Return on Assets		
	1976 (%)	**2016 (%)**
Inflation	5.5	1.3
Technology	2.0	2.0
Expansion	1.0	1.0
Alteration	0.5	0.5
Uncertainty	0.5	0.5
Hedge	0.9	0.7
Required return	10.8	6.0

The starting point for determining sustainable investment is assessing the historical change in revenue and expenses (see growth rates in the chapter "Output Forecasts and Revenue Budgets"). Are historical patterns likely to continue? What factors are likely to change, and what effects will they have? Assuming the historical growth rates of revenues and expenses is 10%, **TABLE 16.2** demonstrates the impact on net income of changes in revenue growth rates.

The table illustrates when that revenues and expenses are growing at the same rate, the operating margin and ROA are constant, that is, the organization will be able to replace, expand, and alter operations. Scenario 2 shows an organization that will have difficulty in replacing assets in the future because expenses are growing faster than revenues and operating margin and ROA are declining. This organization will have to increase its use of debt to replace assets. Scenario 3 shows an organization creating value; the value of its output exceeds its cost, net income is growing, and it should have more than sufficient funds to pursue aggressive growth strategies.

The second major accounting relationship is the change in assets, liabilities, and equity. The accounting identity $A = L + E$ demonstrates that all assets are owned by equity holders or creditors. The left side of the equality represents the total assets in use, and the right side divides these assets into who owns them. Organizations must maintain a balance between assets, debt, and equity. The "acceptable" amount of debt in an organization's capital structure will be determined by organizational and industry characteristics. Weston and Brigham (1978, pp. 684–685) identify the growth rate and stability of future sales, the competitive structure of the industry, lender attitudes toward the organization and industry, the asset structure of the organization, and the attitudes of owners and managers toward risk as the key factors determining the extent of debt in the capital structure. Low-risk industries such as health care, utilities, and

TABLE 16.2 Impact of Changes in Revenue Growth Rates on Net Income				
	Baseline	**Scenario 1**	**Scenario 2**	**Scenario 3**
Revenue growth	–	10%	5%	15%
Revenue	$1000.00	$1100.00	$1050.00	$1150.00
Expense (growth = 10%)	$935.00	$1028.50	$1029.50	$1029.50
Net income	$65.00	$71.50	$21.50	$121.50
Operating margin	6.5%	6.5% (n/c)	2.0% (↓)	10.6% (↑)
Assets (growth = revenue growth)	$833.00	$916.30	$874.70	$958.00
ROA	7.8%	7.8% (n/c)	2.5% (↓)	12.7% (↑)

consumer products typically use more debt than other industries. **TABLE 16.3** explores how changes in revenue growth and net income, from Table 16.2, impact the need for debt, assuming assets grow by 10%.

The key variable in Table 16.3 is debt; the goal of management should be to reduce reliance on debt and the financial risk of the organization. Table 16.3 highlights the concept of **sustainable growth**—the maximum rate of growth in assets an organization can maintain without increasing financial leverage, that is, the debt-to-equity ratio. Scenario 1, column 3, demonstrates that when revenue, expenses, net income, and assets are increasing at 10%, equity is built and the debt-to-equity ratio is reduced. Total debt is increasing, but its share in the capital structure is lower, and the ability of the organization to carry debt (in the absence of an interest rate increase) is improved; this is sustainable growth. Sustainable growth also includes financial results that leave the equity financing or debt-to-equity ratios unchanged. That is, if net income had been $41.7, equity growth would have been 10.0% and the capital structure ratios would not change.

Scenario 2, column 4, shows a reduction in the equity financing ratio and an increase in the debt-to-equity ratio, signifying a deterioration in the capital structure of the organization. Assets are increasing at 10.0% ($83.30), but equity is only growing by 5.2% ($21.50); therefore, debt must be used to fund the majority of asset growth ($61.80). External parties would own a larger proportion of the assets, and the organization would be weaker and more reliant on external parties to finance their assets. This trend is unsustainable over the long run. The problem is that if this performance continues, the board of directors may refuse to approve an increase in self-imposed debt limits or creditors may refuse to extend additional funds.

Scenario 3, column 5, demonstrates the advantage of increasing net income; the organization could pay down the debt and own a larger proportion of its assets. Paying down debt reduces financial risk and strengthens the organization. On the other hand, if desirable investment opportunities are available, managers could increase the rate of investment to 29.2% (the same as the growth in equity),

TABLE 16.3 Impact of Changes in Net Income on the Capital Structure				
	Baseline	**Scenario 1**	**Scenario 2**	**Scenario 3**
Net income	$65.00	$71.50	$21.50	$121.50
Equity growth	–	17.2%	5.2%	29.2%
Total equity	$416.50	$488.00	$438.00	$538.00
Assets (growth = 10%)	$833.00	$916.30	$916.30	$916.30
Debt	$416.50	$428.30	$478.30	$378.30
Equity financing ratio	0.50	0.53 (↑)	0.48 (↓)	0.59 (↑)
Debt-to-equity ratio	1.00	0.88 (↓)	1.09 (↑)	0.70 (↓)

while maintaining the current equity financing and debt-to-equity ratios. In summary, when the increase in equity equals the increase in assets, the capital structure is constant; when the increase in equity is lower than the change in assets, the capital structure deteriorates and financial risk increases; and when the increase in equity exceeds the increase in assets, the capital structure improves and financial risk decreases.

Tables 16.2 and 16.3 demonstrate the simple idea that sustainable organizational growth rates can be no more than the rate of growth in equity. If managers want assets to grow faster than the equity growth rate, they should recognize the necessity of higher debt and higher financial risk. If owners and/or managers do not want to increase the proportion of debt in the capital structure, then investment must be reduced, profitability must be improved by increasing revenues and/or reducing expenses, and/or equity must be increased through non operating means, that is, seeking donations for nonprofits or selling stock in for-profits.

Multiyear Financial Planning

One-year operating budgets are insufficient for strategic management; funds must be committed for multiple years, and shortfalls in financial performance may cause significant problems in out years if improvements are not made. A 5-year financial plan provides the means to evaluate the ends sought in the strategic plan: is the organization on track, and if not, where should action be taken to move it toward its target?

The fundamentals of a multiyear financial plan were introduced in previous chapters: First, it is a **budget** specifying expected performance during the life of the strategic plan. Second, it sets the standard against which actual performance will be evaluated—**variance analysis**. Third, it relies on the use of **financial ratios** to evaluate performance (this chapter uses DuPont analysis to pinpoint where performance can be improved). Fourth and fifth, a multiyear financial plan proposes a set of investments, **capital budgeting**, and specifies how they will be financed, **capital structure**.

Building a 5-Year Financial Plan

A master budget is the consolidation of all department budgets and provides a basis for building a multiyear financial plan. While past and current operating results and the master budget are the foundation for a multiyear financial plan, the plan should *not* be a simple extrapolation of historical trends and the current budget. Senior management should set definitive expectations on output, investment, and debt in light of what is achievable, given external factors that may make the future easier or tougher than the past. The position of the organization at the end of the strategic plan should not be the result of carrying on current operations but rather improving internal processes and guiding the organization to a more favorable position.

Unlike operating budgets, a multiyear financial plan is less concerned with line item detail at the department level and more concerned with overall financial performance. Ratio analysis in general and DuPont analysis in particular (Chapter 12) provide critical insight into the key elements determining financial performance and how it can be improved by altering current processes to lower expenses or increase prices, investing in programs and assets that yield more revenue, and altering the capital structure to reduce financing costs. DuPont analysis highlights that the ROE is the product of the total margin, total asset turnover, and equity multiplier:

$$\text{ROE} = \text{Total margin} * \text{Total asset turnover} \\ * \text{Equity multiplier} \qquad 16.1$$

$$\text{ROE} = \frac{\text{Net income}}{\text{Total revenue}} * \frac{\text{Total revenue}}{\text{Total assets}} \\ * \frac{\text{Total assets}}{\text{Total equity}}$$

The total margin specifies the expected relationship between revenue and expenses:

how much net income is generated from one dollar of revenue? The total margin assesses management's ability to control costs; the net income increases when costs are reduced and revenue is comstant. The total asset turnover documents the productivity of assets and investment in assets: how many dollars of revenue are generated from $1 of assets. Are managers obtaining the maximum revenue from employed assets, and should assets be increased or decreased? The equity multiplier defines the current capital structure: should the organization have more assets for the equity employed, or are financing costs too high due to overreliance on equity? These three ratios define how management expects the organization to operate in terms of efficiency, productivity, and asset financing.

Let us build a 5-year financial plan for the start-up physician practice introduced in the chapter "Scratch Budgeting" and revisited in the chapter "Financial Functions in Finance," since the physician's first-year salary was less than hoped. **TABLE 16.4** omits the physician's salary from wages, and thus, the practice's profit is the physician's income. The physician wants to know how much could be earned in 5 years. The budget created in the chapter "Scratch Budgeting" assumed that 90 patients per week would be seen, the practice would operate 48 weeks per year, and the average revenue per visit would be $87.10. The first-year net revenue is expected to be $376,267, and all expenses other than the physician's wages would be $261,946. The net income for the practice (or the maximum salary the physician could take without reducing equity) is $114,321.

As seen in capital budgeting, Chapter 13, the key variables in creating a multiyear financial plan are output, output price, and expenses and their expected rates of growth. Unlike capital budgeting, the financial plan adds assets and equity and tracks the total margin, total asset turnover, and equity multiplier. The current-year performance and future projections are built on a 30.4% total margin

TABLE 16.4 Building a 5-Year Financial Plan for a New Physician Practice

	Current year	Year + 1	Year + 2	Year + 3	Year + 4	Year + 5
Visits/week	90.0	94.5	99.2	104.2	109.4	114.9
Price	$87.10	$89.71	$92.40	$95.18	$98.03	$100.97
Net revenue	$376,267	$406,933	$440,098	$475,966	$514,757	$556,710
Staff wages	$142,053	$145,605	$149,245	$152,976	$156,800	$160,720
Supplies	$32,400	$34,830	$37,402	$40,123	$43,001	$46,045
Rent/utilities/ housekeeping	$49,360	$50,594	$51,859	$53,155	$54,484	$55,846
Other	$38,133	$39,086	$40,063	$41,065	$42,091	$43,144
Total expenses	$261,946	$270,115	$278,569	$287,319	$296,377	$305,756
Practice/physician income	$114,321	$136,818	$161,529	$188,647	$218,380	$250,954
Cash flow	$118,321	$140,818	$155,529	$192,647	$222,380	$244,954

(continues)

TABLE 16.4 Building a 5-Year Financial Plan for a New Physician Practice *(continued)*

Investment	$80,000		$20,000		$20,000
Assets		$76,000	$92,000	$88,000	$84,000	$100,000
Equity	$40,000	$40,000	$50,000	$50,000	$50,000	$60,000
Total margin	30.4%	33.6%	36.7%	39.6%	42.4%	45.1%
Total asset turnover	4.70	5.35	4.78	5.41	6.13	5.57
Equity multiplier	2.00	1.90	1.84	1.76	1.68	1.67
Q	5%					
Anticipated output price increase	3.0%					
Anticipated input price increase	2.50%					

(30.4 cents of every dollar of net revenue can be retained in the practice or taken as physician income), a total asset turnover of 4.70 (each dollar of assets produces $4.70 of net revenue), and an equity multiplier of 2.00 (each dollar of equity supports $2.00 of assets).

The financial plan assumes that output (patient visits) will increase by 5.0% per year over the next 5 years and the net revenue (reimbursement) per case and expenses will increase by 3.0% and 2.5%, respectively. The plan projects $20,000 in additional assets will be required in years + 2 and years + 5 and these expenditures will be 50% equity (retained earnings) and 50% debt-financed, maintaining an equity multiplier of 2.00 or lower. If these assumptions are realized, the physician will see practice income increase to $250,954 in year + 5 (see Chapter16.xlsx, Table 16.4 tab).

DuPont analysis demonstrates that the improvement in practice/physician income is due to increasing total margin and total asset turnover. The total margin is increasing because of widening the spread between per visit reimbursement and expense—primarily the result of better utilization of fixed staffing resources (more visits per staff member) rather than reimbursement increases. Similarly, the total asset turnover is improving because of the growing number of patient visits for every dollar of investment. Of course, predictions are simply predictions, and factors ranging from almost completely uncontrollable (per visit reimbursement) to highly controllable (expense per case) will determine actual performance.

Assessing Performance

Growth rates for output, prices, and expenses cannot be accurately predicted; a year ahead, forecasts are challenging, and multiyear forecasts are subject to countless events that were not and could not be foreseen when projections were made. The goal of financial planning is not to obtain perfection in forecasting but rather to quickly and effectively respond to internal or external factors that affect financial performance. Minor changes made early are easier than major changes made late. Assume Medicare freezes reimbursement (50% of patients), so per visit reimbursement increases at a lower rate (1.5%) than the expected increase in expenses (2.5%). The impact of this change is substantial; the first-year net income falls by $5926, and the reduction increases to $39,374 in year 5. The first-year shortfall is only 1.5% of net revenue; if changes are not undertaken until year 5, the shortfall may grow to 7.6% (**FIGURE 16.9**).

The reduction in expected income over 5 years is $107,855 if no effective action is taken; for an individual, an income loss of this size may have a substantial impact on lifestyle choices. The goal of assessing performance is to ensure operating results are as expected and, if not, to take action to move them toward the plan or, when results are less than expected and improvement cannot be made, to assess the strategic plan and retrench, if necessary. The physician can accept the lower income for the next 5 years or seek ways to increase the number of patients seen, increase the revenue generated from each patient, or reduce operating expenses.

Pinpointing Product Lines for Improvement

While pinpointing differences between actual and budgeted revenues and expenses is the purpose of variance analysis, assessing the accumulative impact of these differences and determining whether operational changes are needed or plans should be altered must be done at the product level. The financial plan for a physician producing a single output was straightforward; the situation facing a hospital with multiple medical lines is more complex. Senior managers of large organizations need to build and assess performance by product line, similar to zero-base or program budgeting. Product line costs cross multiple department, so traditional department accounting provides

Visits/week	90.0	94.5	99.2	104.2	109.4	114.9
Price	$87.10	$88.41	$89.73	$91.08	$92.44	$93.83
	Current year	+1	+2	+3	+4	+5
Net revenue	$376,267	$401,007	$427,373	$455,473	$485,420	$517,336
Staff wages	$142,053	$145,605	$149,245	$152,976	$156,800	$160,720
Supplies	32,400	34,830	37,402	40,123	43,001	46,045
Rent/utilities/housekeeping	49,360	50,594	51,859	53,155	54,484	55,846
Other	38,133	39,086	40,063	41,065	42,091	43,144
	$261,946	$270,115	$278,569	$287,319	$296,377	$305,756
Practice/physician income	$114,321	$130,892	$148,804	$168,154	$189,043	$211,581
Cash flow	$118,321	$134,892	$142,804	$172,154	$193,043	$205,581
Investment			$20,000			$20,000
Assets	$80,000	$76,000	$92,000	$88,000	$84,000	$100,000
Equity	$40,000	$40,000	$50,000	$50,000	$50,000	$60,000
Total margin	30.4%	32.6%	34.8%	36.9%	38.9%	40.9%
Total asset turnover	4.70	5.28	4.65	5.18	5.78	5.17
Equity multiplier	2.00	1.90	1.84	1.76	1.68	1.67
Q	5.0%	vs.	5.0%			
Anticipated output price increase	1.5%		3.0%			
Anticipated input price increase	2.5%		2.5%			
Baseline, output price = 3.0%	$114,321	$136,818	$161,529	$188,647	$218,380	$250,954
Actual output price = 1.5%	$114,321	$130,892	$148,804	$168,154	$189,043	$211,581
Difference	$0	-$5,926	-$12,725	-$20,493	-$29,337	-$39,374
Difference as % net revenue		-1.48%				-7.61%

FIGURE 16.9 Screenshot of Assessing First-Year Performance under the 5-Year Plan

an inadequate foundation for decision-making and improvement. The first step is to build an accounting system that supports product line decision-making. The accounting system should provide an aggregate patient accounting perspective, where the costs of treating a patient in a product line, whether it is cardiology, maternity, or oncology, are based on the services they consume from each department.

The 5-year financial plan in **TABLE 16.5**, for the sake of brevity, only reports net revenue, expenses, and investment by product line. Currently, the organization earns 7.2% on invested equity on the basis of a 4.0% total margin, a 1.20 total asset turnover, and a 1.50 equity multiplier. The ROE for product lines varies from 2.62% to 10.69%, given differences

in their total margin and total asset turnover. No difference in ROE is ascribed to the use of debt, since all product line assets are assumed to be financed at the organization equity multiplier.

The financial plan anticipates improvement in the total margin as revenues grow faster than expenses—5.5% revenue versus 5.0% expenses. Planned investment is expected to outpace the growth in revenue and reduce the total asset turnover. Finally, the promulgated debt policy calls for maintaining the current equity multiplier. If things go as planned, the net income will more than double to $169.9 from $83 and the ROE will increase to 9.4% in year 5. Table 16.5 demonstrates the performance expected from each product

TABLE 16.5 A 5-Year Financial Plan for a Hospital by Product Line

Net Revenue	Previous Year	Net Revenue (%)	Budget Year + 1	Net Revenue (%)	Year + 2	Year + 3	Year + 4	Year + 5
Product line 1	$101.00	4.8	$106.60	4.8	$112.40	$118.60	$125.10	$132.00
Product line 2	$201.00	9.6	$212.10	9.6	$223.70	$236.00	$249.00	$262.70
Product line 3	$302.00	14.5	$318.60	14.4	$336.10	$354.60	$374.10	$394.70
Product line 4	$392.00	18.8	$413.60	18.7	$436.30	$460.30	$485.60	$512.30
Product line 5	$496.00	23.8	$523.30	23.6	$552.10	$582.40	$614.50	$648.30
Product line 6	$593.00	28.4	$625.60	28.2	$660.00	$696.30	$734.60	$775.00
Net revenue	$2085.00	100.00	$2199.70	100.0	$2320.70	$2448.30	$2582.90	$2725.00
Expenses								
Product line 1	$95.00	4.7	$99.80	4.5	$104.70	$110.00	$115.50	$121.20
Product line 2	$198.00	9.9	$207.90	9.4	$218.30	$229.20	$240.70	$252.70
Product line 3	$292.00	14.6	$306.60	13.8	$321.90	$338.00	$354.90	$372.70
Product line 4	$382.00	19.1	$401.10	18.1	$421.20	$442.20	$464.30	$487.50

(continues)

TABLE 16.5 A 5-Year Financial Plan for a Hospital by Product Line *(continued)*

Net Revenue	Previous Year	Net Revenue (%)	Budget Year + 1	Net Revenue (%)	Year + 2	Year + 3	Year + 4	Year + 5
Product line 5	$466.00	23.3	$489.30	22.1	$513.80	$539.50	$566.40	$594.70
Product line 6	$569.00	28.4	$597.50	27.0	$627.30	$658.70	$691.60	$726.20
Total Expense	$2002.00	100.00	$2102.10	94.88	$2207.20	$2317.60	$2433.40	$2555.10
Profit	$83.00	4.0	$97.60	4.4	$113.50	$130.70	$149.50	$169.90
					$113.50	$130.70	$149.50	$169.90
Assets								
Product line 1	$98.00		$106.30		$115.90	$127.00	$139.20	$152.50
Product line 2	$172.00		$186.50		$203.40	$222.90	$244.20	$267.60
Product line 3	$224.00		$242.90		$264.90	$290.30	$318.10	$348.50
Product line 4	$312.00		$338.40		$369.00	$404.30	$443.00	$485.40
Product line 5	$421.00		$456.60		$497.90	$545.60	$597.80	$655.00
Product line 6	$506.00		$548.70		$598.40	$655.70	$718.50	$787.20
Total Assets	$1733.00		$1879.40		$2049.60	$2245.80	$2460.70	$2696.20

Equity	$1155.00	$1252.60		$1366.00	$1496.80	$1646.30	$1816.20
Organization	7.2%	7.8%		8.3%	8.7%	9.1%	9.4%
Total margin	4.0%	4.4%		4.9%	5.3%	5.8%	6.2%
Total asset turnover	1.20	1.17		1.13	1.09	1.05	1.01
Equity multiplier	1.50	1.50		1.50	1.50	1.49	1.48
Product line 1	9.19%	9.61%		9.94%	10.19%	10.40%	10.59%
Total margin	5.94%	6.39%		6.83%	7.27%	7.71%	8.15%
Total asset turnover	1.03	1.00		0.97	0.93	0.90	0.87
Product line 2	2.62%	3.34%		4.00%	4.59%	5.12%	5.60%
Total margin	1.49%	1.96%		2.42%	2.89%	3.35%	3.80%
Total asset turnover	1.17	1.14		1.10	1.06	1.02	0.98

line, its total margin and asset productivity, to achieve the organization's long-run goals.

FIGURE 16.10 assesses first-year performance against the multiyear financial plan targets; it allows managers to see which product lines are outperforming expectations—those with a higher-than-expected total margins and total asset turnovers. The assessment starts by examining total profit and profit by product line. The organization has fallen short of its first-year goals, actual ROE was only 5.7% versus a budget of 7.8% or 26.9% lower than expected, and profit is down $27.57 or 28.3%. Deviations of this magnitude in the first year will make it extremely difficult to realize the 5-year goals unless rapid and effective action is undertaken. The DuPont formula shows that the primary reason for the shortfall was the reduction in the total margin for the

organization, 3.2% actual versus 4.4% projection. Revenues were less than planned, $25.68 (1.2%), and expenses were modestly higher, $1.90 (0.1%), but before action can be taken, these changes must to be traced back to each product line.

Examining performance by product line (see Chapter16.xlsx, Figure 16.10 tab) reveals all product lines except product line 4 missed their targets. Product line 4 produced a higher margin (3.8% versus 3.01%) and ROE (6.74% versus 5.53%) than expected. The product line falling furthest from its projections was line 2; the actual ROE of −2.38% versus a budget of 3.34%. Product lines 2, 3, and 6 accounted for 77.4% of the missed profit projection, but although product line 2 missed its budgeted profit by $7.15 versus $7.16 for product line 6: it missed its forecast by −172.2%, that is, it lost

Profit	Budget +1	Actual +1	Variance	%Variance
Product line 1	6.80	3.00	-$3.80	-55.9%
Product line 2	4.15	-3.00	-$7.15	-172.2%
Product line 3	12.01	5.00	-$7.01	-58.4%
Product line 4	12.46	16.00	$3.54	28.4%
Product line 5	33.98	28.00	-$5.98	-17.6%
Product line 6	28.17	21.00	-$7.16	-25.4%
Total Profit	97.57	70.00	-$27.57	-28.3%

Organization	Budget +1	Actual +1	Variance	%Variance
ROE	7.79%	5.71%	-2.08%	-26.6%
Total margin	4.44%	3.22%	-1.22%	-27.4%
Total asset turnover	1.17	1.15	-2.20%	-1.9%
Equity multiplier	1.50	1.48	-1.59%	-1.1%

Product line 2	Budget +1	Actual +1	Variance	%Variance
ROE	3.34%	-2.45%	-5.80%	-173.4%
Total margin	1.96%	-1.49%	-3.44%	-175.8%
Total asset turnover	1.14	1.07	-6.81%	-6.0%

Product line 3	Budget +1	Actual +1	Variance	%Variance
ROE	7.42%	3.21%	-4.21%	-56.8%
Total margin	3.77%	1.66%	-2.11%	-56.1%
Total asset turnover	1.31	1.25	-5.85%	-4.5%

Product line 4	Budget +1	Actual +1	Variance	%Variance
ROE	5.53%	6.95%	1.42%	25.7%
Total margin	3.01%	3.80%	0.79%	26.1%
Total asset turnover	1.22	1.18	-3.97%	-3.2%

FIGURE 16.10 Screenshot Assessing First-Year Performance by Product Line

rather than made money. The main problem was that the total margin was budgeted at 1.96 and the line lost 1.49 cents per dollar of revenue, that is, expenses exceeded revenues. Asset productivity was 6.0% lower than the expected $1.14: $1.07 in revenue was earned for every $1.00 of assets.

Product line 3 was the second-worst performer: its profit was 58.4% below expectations, with an actual ROE of 3.11% versus a forecast of 7.42%. The drop was primarily due to lower-than-expected revenues and higher cost, reducing the total margin to 1.66 versus the forecast of 3.77, 56.1% below expected. Asset productivity was 4.5% lower than expected: each dollar of assets produced 1.25 in revenue versus a forecast of 1.31.

Putting the organization back on track with its financial targets will require senior and mid-level managers to determine why product lines 2 and 3 are not meeting targets; product line 6 contributed 26.0% of the missed profit, but this was largely driven by the size of the program, and it accounts for roughly 28% of net revenue. Once the causes of the higher costs and lower revenues in product lines 2 and 3 are identified, the next step is to determine whether the causes can be remediated. Managers will have to examine (i) the number of patients seen and the payer mix composition to determine why net revenue is behind targets and/or (ii) the composition of expenses to determine what type of expenses are leading to higher-than-expected costs. Action plans should be implemented if revenue deficiencies and/or expenses overages are remediable and the financial plan reassessed to determine whether revision is needed. Product line 4 indicates the problem in total margin is remediable, that is, not an uncontrollable, organization-wide phenomena, as product line 4 increased its margin by 26.1% through a combination of increasing revenues or decreasing costs. If the problems in product lines 2 and 3 cannot be controlled, the strategic financial plan should be revised. After product lines 2 and 3 are reviewed, management

should also examine product lines 5 and 6 for improvement.

Supporting the Selected Strategy

Strategy involves expansion, reprioritization and reallocation of assets, maintenance of the *status quo*, or contraction. Finance plays a major role in realizing goals besides assessing the feasibility of strategic plans and assessing performance. When expansion is pursued through building or purchase, finance should identify where funds will come from to complete these transactions. The strategic financial plan should identify whether funds are expected from net income, cash or investment holdings, and/or debt. Owners (or nonprofit board members) and senior managers should approve the financing method. When funds are targeted from operations (net income and cash flow), there should be a detailed plan identifying what each department or product line is expected to contribute. If borrowing is a primary source of funds, then finance should identify debt instruments with the lowest interest rates.

When expansion is pursued by purchasing rivals, mergers, partnerships, or alliances, finance should assess the financial strength of the potential partners. The goal is to ensure the organization does not pay more than necessary for an acquisition or be saddled with weak partners. Finance should determine whether the financial statements accurately represent the potential partner's financial position, that is, the nature of their assets and liabilities, as well as identify trends: how has the quantity of service produced changed, is market share increasing or decreasing, and have expenses increased faster than revenues?

When strategy calls for maintaining the size of the organization, that is, the same total assets but reallocated to maximize organizational value, finance should identify underperforming areas to subtract resources from and identify higher-performing areas to add resources to. In Figure 16.10, product line 4 has the highest ROE and is outperforming expectations, while product line 2 has a negative ROE. Should product line 2 be reduced in scale or closed to increase resources for product line 4?

A *status quo* strategy suggests operations will continue as in the past, that is, the same level of resources allocated to each area. Even when the *status quo* is pursued, it behooves managers to identify areas for improvement. A *status quo* strategy, that is, making absolutely no changes to operations, is not viable, because competitors are constantly seeking improvement, so managers should pursue enhancement, doing the same things but doing them better. Enhancement strategies require that finance identify areas where financial performance can be improved by identifying areas with underutilized resources, i.e., low asset turnover ratios and/or excessive costs, i.e., low margins.

When contraction is pursued, finance should identify areas where new investment will be minimized, reduced, or eliminated.

When operations are sold off, finance should evaluate their worth to ensure assets are sold at the highest-possible price, hopefully by identifying purchasers who could profitably add the service to their existing operations. Liquidation is the last resort, but finance can again play a role in identifying when the operation should be sold, that is, balancing the capital loss on the sale of assets against continuing operating losses.

▶ Long Range Forecasting: Medicare 2090

Previous chapters highlighted the higher growth occurring in Medicare compared to the GDP. This trend is unsustainable in the long run. Medicare prepares 75-year estimates to project outlays and financing, that is, taxes. In the current year, 2015, Medicare is 3.61% of the GDP. Medicare is funded by payroll taxes of 2.90%, so tax revenues were below expenditures. Equalizing inflows and outflows would

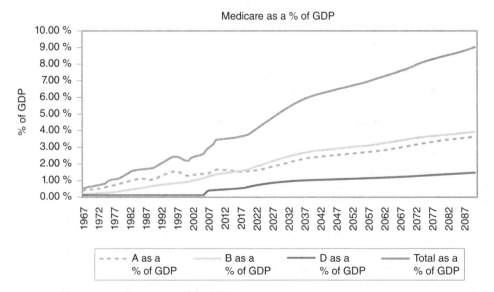

FIGURE 16.11 Medicare as a Percentage of the GDP

require an immediate tax increase of 25% or a 16% reduction in outlays (Centers for Medicare & Medicaid Services, 2016).

Beyond the current revenue shortfall, there is the larger question of how much of the GDP will Medicare outlays consume in the future. **FIGURE 16.11** shows one set of assumptions; the key variable is growth in Medicare expenditures, Parts A, B, and D; economic variables include growth in the GDP, wage, productivity, and consumer price index (CPI); and demographic variables include fertility rates and reduction in death rates. Ten-year intermediate growth estimates for Parts A, B, and D are 6.01%, 7.39%, and 9.18%, respectively. The estimates for GDP growth range from 2.7% (worst case) to 5.0% (best case) with an intermediate estimate of 3.9%. From 2000 through 2016, the GDP increases from $11,226B to $18,569B, a compound growth rate of 3.2%. The fertility estimates, that is, how many people will pay tax in the future, range from 1.80 (worst case) to 2.20 (best case) with an intermediate estimate of 2.00. The current U.S. fertility rate is 1.87 and falling (Central Intelligence Agency, 2017). To meet the intermediate projection, substantial increases must occur in GDP growth and fertility rates.

On the positive side, Part A payroll taxes are not indexed to inflation and workers (but not employers) are taxed 0.9% over $200,000. By 2090, it is estimated that inflation will result in 79% of the workers earning over $200,000 and hence taxed.

Between 1967, the first year of Medicare, and 2015, expenditures have grown from 0.55% of the GDP to 3.61%. In the next 25 years (by 2040), when my current students will be halfway through their careers, Medicare outlays may consume 6.20% of the GDP, and by 2090, the end-year projection, 9.06%. There are three alarming aspects of this analysis: first, these projections may understate Medicare outlay growth; second, they may overestimate income growth and the number of people in the workforce;

and third, even if the projections are accurate, they ignore other government spending. On top of 6.20% or 9.06% of the GDP required to fund Medicare, taxpayers will have to fund other federal expenditures, including Medicaid and defense and local and state expenditures. Assuming other government spending does not increase, an unlikely assumption, future taxpayers may be facing tax rates over 44%. The problem we face is far from a simple budgeting problem, yet because so few people are aware of the magnitude of the threat, we are placing a huge and unjust burden on future generations. Our unwillingness to face the current Medicare deficit (2015) does not bode well.

Summary

Strategic management defines the vision and objectives of an organization; it requires understanding what the organization wants to do (mission, vision, and values), what it can do (its strengths and weaknesses), and what it should do (the needs of its markets and capabilities of competitors). The outputs of strategic planning are a set of goals and strategies and should include detailed activities defining how the goals will be met. Included in the strategic plan should be a long-range financial plan that specifies what is expected, establishes benchmarks for performance, and identifies where resources will come from to support the plan.

Strategic financial planning touches upon each of the major financial functions, including budgeting, variance analysis, ratio analysis, capital budgeting, and capital structure. Strategic financial planning should play a major role in strategic management, including determining whether the organization has sufficient resources to meet the plan, assessing overall performance toward meeting the plan, and contributing to performance by increasing financial resources, assessing potential partners, and identifying specific areas for improvement or reduction.

The first step in the strategic financial planning process is building a multiyear plan. DuPont analysis provides an easy-to-conceptualize framework for the plan: what net income is expected from each dollar of revenue (total margin), how many dollars of revenue are expected from every dollar of assets (total asset turnover), and how many dollars of assets are supported by every dollar of equity (equity financing ratio)? DuPont analysis specifies how the ROE is earned or how the strategic financial plan expects future ROE to be earned. The second step is to assess whether operations are meeting the plan: are costs being controlled, is the productivity of assets meeting expectations, and is more or less equity employed to support invested assets? Finally, when operations diverge from expectations, managers should take action to ensure the organization obtains the maximum benefit from its assets. When operations fall short of expectations, early and minor corrective action is necessary to avoid the need for later and larger corrections.

Determining the strategic plan and strategic financial plan is the duty of the highest-ranking members of an organization, but the financial plan and performance must be effectively communicated to all employees to ensure it is more than a plan. Employees should know their role in achieving the plan and when performance must be improved; a plan is only a plan unless it is effectively used. Financial management must ensure that operating budgets and strategic plans are used to improve the performance of organizations; plans must become tools to justify their creation.

Key Terms and Concepts

Competitive advantage	Internal analysis	Strategic management
External analysis	Mission, objectives, strategy,	Sustainable growth
Four Ps of marketing (or	and tactics (MOST)	SWOT diagram
marketing mix)	Organizational architecture	Value chain

Discussion Questions

1. Explain the role and phases of strategic management.
2. What is the purpose of internal analysis, and how does the value chain provide a structure to internal analysis?
3. Discuss the four areas that should be assessed in external analysis. What is the purpose of each assessment?
4. Discuss why breakeven is an unsustainable situation for any organization. What factors should be considered in setting a target for an ROA?
5. Explain the role of finance in formulating and implementing strategic plans.
6. Explain the concept of sustainable growth.

Problems

The next four problems use the table given (amounts in millions).

Income Statement	2014	2015	2016	2017	1018	2019	2020	2021	2022	2023
Revenues	100	106	112	119	127	____	____	____	____	____
Expenses	97	103	111	117	125	____	____	____	____	____
Profit	3	3	1	2	2	____	____	____	____	____
Balance sheet										
Assets	80	82	85	86	90	99	109	120	132	145
Liabilities	50	50	52	53	54	____	____	____	____	____
Equity	30	33	34	36	38	____	____	____	____	____

1. The chief executive officer (CEO) of a hospital has announced an ambitious building and renovation project that will increase total assets by $55 million over the next 5 years, ending in 2023. You are the chief financial officer (CFO). Determine whether the plan is feasible. Calculate the compound growth rates for revenue, expenses, profit, and equity from 2014 through 2018.

   Compound growth rate, revenues: _____
   Compound growth rate, expenses: _____
   Compound growth rate, profit: _____
   Compound growth rate, equity: _____

2. Forecast the revenue and expenses for 2019 through 2023. Calculate the profit, equity (prior year equity + profit), and liabilities (assets – equity) for the plan.

3. Calculate the ROE, total margin, total asset turnover, and equity multiplier for all years (2014 through 2023). Comment on the changes in financial performance.

4. Assume the board of directors will not approve a plan if the equity multiplier exceeds 3.00. Is the plan feasible? If not, what actions should be taken?

	2014	2015	2016	2017	1018	2019	2020	2021	2022	2023
ROE	___	___	___	___	___	___	___	___	___	___
Total margin	___	___	___	___	___	___	___	___	___	___
Total asset turnover	___	___	___	___	___	___	___	___	___	___
Equity multiplier	___	___	___	___	___	___	___	___	___	___

References

Centers for Medicare & Medicaid Services. (2016). *2016 Annual report of the boards of trustees the Federal Hospital Insurance and Federal Supplementary Medical Insurance Trust Funds*. Retrieved from https://www.cms.gov/research-statistics-data-and-systems/statistics-trends-and-reports/reportstrustfunds/downloads/tr2016.pdf

Central Intelligence Agency. (2017). *The world factbook*. Retrieved from https://www.cia.gov/library/publications/the-world-factbook/rankorder/2127rank.html

Hellriegel, D., Jackson, S. E., & Slocum, J. W. (2005). *Management: A competency based approach* (10th ed.). Cincinnati, OH: South-Western College.

Long, H. W. (1976). Valuation as a criterion in not-for-profit decision-making. *Health Care Management Review*, *1*(3), 361–381.

Swayne, L. E., Duncan, W. J., & Ginter, P. M. (2008). *Strategic management of health care organizations* (6th ed.). San Francisco, CA: Jossey-Bass.

Weston, J. F., & Brigham, E. F. (1978). *Managerial finance* (6th ed.). Hinsdale, IL: Dryden Press.

CHAPTER 17

Financial Management and Care

▶ Introduction

Managers are responsible for means and ends, and their primary focus changes as they climb the organization; entry-level managers are responsible for how things are done, while senior managers are responsible for what is done. Activity-based, flexible, and incremental budgets address how things are done—the steps and processes taken to produce an output. It is only by knowing how things should be done that entry-level managers identify excessive costs and where improvements can be made. Zero-base and outcome budgets address the questions of what outputs should be produced and what outcomes should be pursued. Answering these questions is essential for structuring the decision-making processes of senior managers.

Managers oversee multiple aspects of a business, including operations, finance, human resources, and information management. In many cases, managers are promoted from within on the basis of their expertise in a job—they know and have excelled in one part of the production process and are promoted to oversee an entire department. With the promotion, they are expected to perform in the areas of finance, human resources, and information technology (IT) and may be called upon to market products, lobby politicians and regulators, and develop organizational strategy. The challenge is that their training often lies in a single area, and neither on-the-job training nor college classes fully prepare them to excel in all their areas of responsibility.

Learning how to interact with employees requires more than reading a human resource textbook. Building effective interpersonal skills requires repeated experience dealing with different personalities to learn communication skills and acquire the knowledge to implement different approaches in different situations. Similarly, financial management, although less ambiguous than managing human beings, requires broad knowledge before a manager can achieve a high level of competency. The role of financial management in some textbooks is defined as assessing the financial condition, determining the asset structure, and determining the capital structure. In the real world, entry-level managers are rarely called upon to perform these tasks, and most organizations settle for managers who can continue business as usual; senior managers are content with people who can maintain production, retain employees, and submit budgets similar to those prepared in the past.

A simple replication of past performance should neither be encouraged nor be tolerated, but where can managers learn better financial, or other, skills? Organizations need managers who understand what is and what could be. University courses in finance focus on finance for finance professionals, that is, financial reporting, capital structure etc.—issues entry-level managers are rarely involved in but are of greater importance to senior managers. The topics that are lightly covered, budgeting and variance analysis, are issues all managers are involved with on a monthly basis. Budgeting and variance analysis provide the critical elements needed for line managers to understand what an organization does. Budgeting and variance analysis for senior managers provide information to set and monitor organizational strategy.

Budgets are an organization's operating plans specified in monetary terms; they identify goals, the expected cost of meeting those goals, and where the organization will be if the goals are reached. While ratio analysis was introduced as a tool to assess an organization's financial condition, the analysis is performed at the organizational level and does not illuminate departmental performance and is therefore less relevant to operating managers. According to the chapter "Ratio Analysis and Operating Indicators," ratio analysis should be the starting point to examine opportunities for improvement, while specific action requires operating indicators to document performance at the organizational and departmental levels. Operating indicators, when used as benchmarks for specific departmental processes and outputs, can illuminate what performance could be. Operating indicators can identify departments consuming too many resources and propel improvement in departmental processes and organizational outcomes. Financial acumen is a necessary precondition for understanding how departments operate, including what is produced, what outputs cost, and what actions can lead to improvement.

This text has turned the typical financial perspective on its head; it has not been a top-down, 40,000-foot perspective of financial management but a bottom-up approach illuminating the financial functions frontline managers perform. The text was designed to provide nonfinancial managers with the tools to get greater value out of the budgeting process and understand why actual operating results differ from budgets. The first step toward developing financial acumen is developing the skill to construct a realistic budget that supplies the appropriate level of resources for the expected output. The second required skill is the ability to analyze and explain actual operating results. A manager's ability to explain and respond to budget variances may be the difference between a rewarding and successful career and a dead-end job. For variances beyond managerial control, the ability to demonstrate that overruns were due to factors other than poor management may be crucial.

The purpose of management is to obtain the maximum value possible from the resources it oversees. Maximizing value requires much more than managing crises and writing or forwarding emails; it requires understanding how work is done, and one test of this understanding is whether a manager can assemble a budget. Can a manager identify needed resources and what they should cost to produce the expected quantity of goods or services? The first step toward ensuring the best resources are assigned to each task is knowing what needs to be done and what are the minimum resources necessary to complete work. Henry Ford perfectly understood his role; in his autobiography, he noted that building a car required 7882 activities (1923, p. 108). More importantly, he understood the capabilities each activity required: 4034 did not require full physical capability, 670 could be completed without legs, 2637 required only one leg, 2 could be performed without arms, 715 required one arm, and 10 did not require sight. Ford did not pay employees with disabilities less than other workers but rather assigned them to jobs where they could be most productive and demanded high performance. Beyond understanding what was, Ford had the vision to see what the production process could be. He understood his role was to facilitate work by bringing the product to the worker rather than having the worker move to the product. The assembly line, a change in production technology, reduced the time to assemble a car chassis by 87.5% (pp. 81–82). The gains from this innovation were shared with consumers through lower car prices and workers who received higher wages. Ford's innovations and success were the result of achieving a thorough understanding of the production process, capitalizing on improvement opportunities, and demanding high and consistent performance.

▶ Bringing It All Together

Budgeting and finance, relying heavily on accounting and economics, is the means to define performance standards and institute operational control. Accounting supplies the basic framework to evaluate financial performance; the two accounting identities (profit = total revenue − total cost; equity = assets − liabilities) are the barometers of success. Accounting generally records past performance, whereas finance involves planning future performance and initiating action to improve financial results. Profit measures viability: can the organization be sustained over the long run? Equity measures solvency: do assets exceed liabilities? Accounting documents how much wealth is created by an organization and supplies the framework for annual budgets and multiyear financial planning. The beauty of accounting is the elegance of its system: accounting is an information system that summarizes voluminous and complex financial transactions to succinctly define performance.

Economics introduces the concepts of marginalism, opportunity costs, and efficient markets (Case & Fair, 1989, pp. 4–7). Marginalism recognizes that expanding activity leads to diminishing returns or eventually fewer outcomes should be expected from increasing output. Managers contemplating expanding output need to understand that eventually prices decline, unit costs increase and profits will fall. Opportunity costs recognize that undertaking one activity necessitates forgoing other alternatives and raises the question of what the best uses for limited resources are and which markets and investments maximize value. Efficient markets recognize that people look for and act on opportunities to maximize their well-being; profit opportunities are not left unexploited. Efficient markets drive inefficient producers out of business. If an organization's prices are too high because its costs are too high, more efficient producers will enter the market, offer customers lower prices, and give inefficient producers two choices: reduce costs to current market prices or go out of business.

Financial management should use accounting information and economic concepts to improve performance. Typical financing decisions include how money should be raised to minimize the cost of capital and where the raised funds should be invested to maximize net income. Beyond these infrequent decisions, financial education should build skills that can be used to improve day-to-day choices and actions. While the majority of nonfinancial managers see finance as a bookkeeping task occasionally concerned with raising capital and periodic investing in high-cost assets, all managers should see it as essential to the day-to-day operation of their departments. Finance can achieve no greater impact than by improving the performance of individual departments. The first step toward capturing the benefits that finance can provide is to stop seeing budgets as attempts to foresee the future and view them as the financial specification of an operating plan to be followed or refined as conditions dictate.

The financial operating plan should communicate to all employees what is expected and coordinate the disparate operations of an organization. Planning is undertaken to identify challenges and avoid problems. Planning defines expected output, and the first, prospective part of the budgeting process estimates revenues and expenses on the basis of the type and quantity of anticipated output. Issues of output, output and input prices, and productivity that were not or could not be foreseen must be dealt with in the second, concurrent phase of budgeting. Facilitation and control of the plan attempt to recognize deviations from expected performance as soon as practical, typically on a monthly basis, so that action can be taken as quickly to minimize adverse effects. The role of budgeting in phase 2 is to recognize what could and should be controlled.

The final stage of budgeting, retrospective evaluation, determines how effective managers were in operating according to the plan. Did a manager produce the expected outcomes, satisfy customers, and meet his or her budget? How did managers perform when reality did not meet budget assumptions because of higher or lower output or changes in input or output prices, production technology, or competition? Retrospective evaluation should also assess the accuracy of planning (what was the difference between predicted and actual output?) and budgeting (did estimates identify the maximum achievable revenue and minimum achievable costs?). Budgets should provide appropriate performance targets and incentives so that managers and employees pursue activities that maximize organizational value.

Financial management is about planning and performance, *not* data collection. Accounting provides the tools to analyze performance; finance takes this information and improves performance. A budget is the output of planning and finance that charts the direction the organization wants to go, monitors performance along the route, and assesses whether the goals were achieved and whether opportunities were maximized. The first step required to fulfill these roles is to create a realistic and challenging budget.

The chapter "Financial Planning and Management" discussed how budgeting is reviled as a tool to indiscriminately cut costs whether the expense is or is not necessary and micromanage operations. We have seen that budgeting is an attempt to understand where an organization wants to go and how it expects to get there, and this requires knowing what resources are necessary to achieve goals. The idealistic goal of budgeting is to derive the maximum output from a set of resources using foresight rather than relying on history or spur-of-the-moment action. The goal of managers and budgets should be to maximize value rather than cut costs; budgets should indicate where costs should be increased when outcomes are less than what they could be and additional resources would create value. To obtain additional resources, managers must make a compelling case for the need, the solution, and the value that additional resources will create. When costs should be reduced, budgets should identify where efficiency can be increased.

For-profit and nonprofit organizations operating in competitive markets will be driven toward efficiency by cost-cutting competitors and consumers seeking maximum benefit from their purchasing dollar. Enterprises shielded from competition, public organizations and monopolies, tend to drift to higher levels of inefficiency—it is these organizations that are most in need of effective budgeting practices.

The budgeting systems reviewed sought to not only guide but also improve the allocation of scarce resources in organizations. Few should object to this goal, but in practice, budgeting often misallocates resources, producing fewer than possible highly valued goods and overproducing less desired outputs at too high a cost. It is important to understand that this failure does not lie with budgeting theory and techniques but rather with the budgeting system employed and the way it is used. Common budget strategies employed by managers to unnecessarily increase the size of their budgets were reviewed in the chapter "Budget Incentives and Strategies"; whether a budget actually increases or reduces value will be determined by how people harness its positive aspects and prevent budget gaming. The goal of this book was to increase the reader's understanding of budgeting and ability to improve budgeting practices. Whether budgeting practices and operations improve is up to the reader; in the division of labor between knowledge and application, I have the easier task.

Budgets should specify decisions in concrete terms. Budgets are not straightjackets requiring managers to meet their budgets at all costs but rather a means to assess when ignoring the budget is prudent. When do the benefits, additional revenues or avoided costs, that could be obtained by disregarding budget limits exceed the cost of going overbudget? When should customer-pleasing demands be met, damn the cost? Any evaluation of manager competence must balance the desire to encourage creativity and innovation against innovation excess that could bring dire financial consequences. Budgets are perfect vehicles to identify and assess assumptions and risks built into organizational plans.

▶ Building a Budget

Building a budget involves seven steps, beginning with deciding on the type of budget to construct and ending with the implementation of a budget (**FIGURE 17.1**). The first step in building a budget is to determine the aim: what are the organization's goals, and what type of budget provides the greatest support for the desired ends? Unfortunately, most managers skip the first step and/or fail to understand that a choice can be made. Budgets are created as they were in the past—typically, an incremental budget with its well-known flaws. Building an incremental budget does not demand skill or provide direction—little is asked and little is received. Does an incremental budget create value? Probably not.

Selecting the best budgeting system cannot occur if alternatives and their strengths and weaknesses are unknown. There are five types of budgets with different foci and strengths and weaknesses: incremental, flexible, zerobase, program, and activity-based budgets. As demonstrated in previous chapters, different budgeting systems are more appropriate to fulfill the duties of managers at different levels of the organization.

After a budgeting system has been selected, the data required to run it must be collected, step 2. Incremental budgets require the least data; managers need to know only the amount spent in each object code in the base period (year-to-date [YTD] spending, current budget, or prior-year spending) and expected price increases for outputs and inputs to produce a budget. Expense estimates should be increased or decreased when substantial changes in output are expected. Data requirements increase exponentially as more advanced budgeting

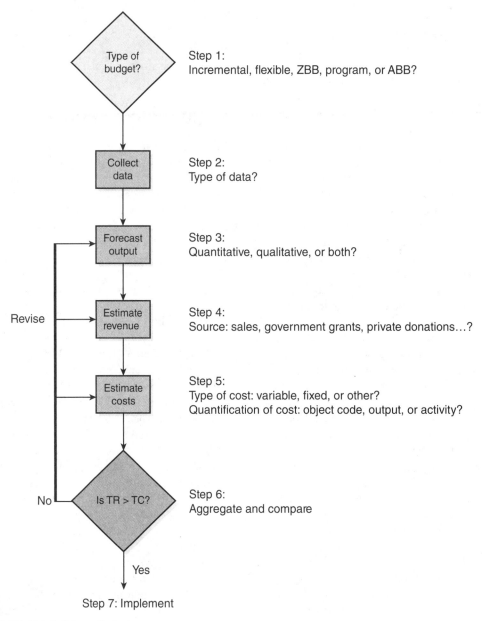

Step 1:
Incremental, flexible, ZBB, program, or ABB?

Step 2:
Type of data?

Step 3:
Quantitative, qualitative, or both?

Step 4:
Source: sales, government grants, private donations…?

Step 5:
Type of cost: variable, fixed, or other?
Quantification of cost: object code, output, or activity?

Step 6:
Aggregate and compare

Step 7: Implement

FIGURE 17.1 Building a Budget

systems are employed; flexible and zero-base budgets require quantifying output. Program budgets need desired outcomes, which may reside outside the organization, to be defined and quantified. Activity-based budgets require the number of tasks per output and the resources needed per task. Ford (1923) noted that 7882 activities were required to produce a car; healthcare outputs like an admission or a patient visit require dozens, if not, hundreds, of tasks to be identified along with the resources needed to complete each task to create an activity-based budget.

Once the necessary data has been collected, step 3 quantifies expected output in the budget year. The starting point for output forecasts is historical output and how it has changed over time. In large organizations, department managers may or may not be involved in generating output forecasts; in most cases, senior management or finance develops forecasts, and expense, cost, and revenue center managers are responsible only for determining the expenses and/or revenues arising from the projected output. Managers of profit and investment centers in large organizations or owners/managers of small organizations are responsible for developing their own output forecasts.

Output forecasts are developed using quantitative and/or qualitative methods. Quantitative methods assume the future can be determined by the past, that is, past changes in output can predict future changes. The chief drawback of quantitative methods is change; consumer needs and preferences change, increasing or decreasing demand for goods and services; technological improvement introduces new products and production technologies that may destroy existing needs, preferences, and/or production methods; and competition can increase or decline affecting the particular demand for an output. Recognizing the unpredictable nature of demand and technological change opens the door for qualitative methods that rely on the judgment of senior managers or outside futurists to assess the potential impact of non-quantifiable factors.

Revenue estimates, step 4, are frequently handed down by senior management or finance in large organizations, and again profit and investment center managers and owners/managers of small organizations often develop their own revenue forecasts. After forecasted output is determined, the next step is to estimate prices for the forecasted outputs. Managers responsible for setting prices should consider the impact of price elasticity; the law of demand states that quantity sold moves inversely with prices, so any planned price increases (or decreases) should consider how much output sold will decrease (or increase).

Steps 3 and 4 provide the foundation for creating expense budgets; forecasted output should have a direct impact on production costs, and the product of expected quantities and prices ($P * Q$) may place an upper limit on sustainable costs. Estimating expenses is the primary responsibility of department managers. Managers should be capable of identifying costs that increase and decrease with output and determine how much they will change, that is, what is the average variable cost (AVC)? Fixed costs do not change with output, but that does not mean fixed costs are constant from year to year as price changes and resources may be added or subtracted.

Step 6 aggregates variable and fixed costs within a department and the organization to determine whether the financial plan is viable (total revenue > total cost). If total revenue exceeds total cost by the desired margin or more (provides an adequate return to owners), the budget can be implemented, step 7. If the budget does not produce an adequate return or total revenue is less than total cost, the budget must be reworked, and the process returns to steps 3 through 5 to determine whether output, revenue, and/or expenses can be raised or lowered to produce the desired margin.

While budgeting steps are straightforward, the relationships between variables are not. As seen in the chapter "Output Forecasts and Revenue Budgets," the selection of a forecasting method and expenditure base produces output forecasts that widely vary. Expected output (Q) has a direct impact on revenue ($P * Q$), total variable cost (TVC = AVC $*$ Q), and average fixed cost (total fixed cost [TFC]/Q); in the presence of economies of scale, higher output reduces the average total cost (ATC) as fixed costs are spread over additional units. If costs can be lowered by increasing output, can prices be reduced to increase demand? On the other hand, will higher output produce diseconomies of scale, increase the ATC, and can this cost be paid? Revenue shortfalls cannot be eliminated by simply increasing prices; managers should understand the impact price increases may have on demand (i.e., how much will sales decrease?) and ATC (i.e., if sales decline, will the ATC increase or decrease?). The interrelationships between output and revenue, revenue and cost, and cost and output are complex and should be understood and addressed.

Incorporating these interactions into the budget may not be the responsibility of operating managers, who do not estimate output or set prices, but understanding these relationships is important to understand the constraints on the organization and the impact they place on department budgets. Managers that internalize the goals of the organization, understand their departments' operations and the larger operations of the organization, and strive to improve will be more effective and valued than those content to maintain the *status quo* and cash a paycheck.

Choice is always constrained by knowledge, and it is improbable that managers who are unfamiliar with the different types of budgets will select the right tool for the right job. In fact, the choice of a budgeting system is frequently left to finance, not operating managers, who use it on a regular basis, or senior managers, who set strategy. The choice, therefore, often begins and ends with incremental budgeting as it most readily supports the accounting view: expenses are categorized by object code and can be rolled into financial statements.

The problem is that the accounting view does not provide optimal support for either day-to-day or strategic management. Managers need more than simply knowing expenses are above or below the budget; they need to know why expected expenses were not realized. Are budget overruns due to changes in the quantity of output, type of output produced, changes in production technology, prices of inputs, or management of resources? Likewise, strategic planners need to understand how customer demands and production processes are changing in order to set direction.

Choosing the right tool, that is, a budgeting system, for the right job demands ends and means thinking: what is the goal, how much authority do managers have, how predictable are revenues, and how stable is the operating environment? Incremental, flexible, and activity-based budgets should be relied on when the primary goal is to estimate expenses. When the goal is to define organizational direction, zero-base and program budgeting provide the means to assess what outputs should be produced and what outcomes should be pursued.

FIGURE 17.2 demonstrates that different budgeting systems target different parts of a production system and that the goal should dictate the budgeting system used. If the organization is concerned about ensuring no more resources are used than budgeted, an incremental budget suffices. Activity-based budgets, built on activities and their expected quantities, are optimal if the goal is to monitor work and ensure the necessary tasks are performed in the proper quantity.

If activities, that is, the tasks performed, are not as important as producing output, flexible budgets are appropriate. Flexible budgets increase and decrease with output and allow managers to determine how productivity and cost standards will be met. Zero-base and program budgets take a more top-down approach: while expenses are estimated by department managers, senior managers determine what should be produced. Zero-base and program budgets are driven by the idea of opportunity

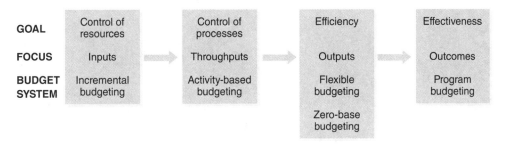

FIGURE 17.2 Budgeting Systems

cost: what are the costs of outputs and outcomes, and should funds be shifted from one purpose to others to maximize value?

The authority of a manager over the mix of inputs used, the quantity of output, pricing, product mix, and capital expenditures should factor into the decisions of what budgeting system should be employed and how managers are evaluated. Managers should not be evaluated on factors beyond their control. When a cost center manager decides the mix of inputs and cost of output, he or she should be evaluated on efficiency, and a flexible budget produces the optimal metric. Profit and investment center managers who establish input mixes, product mixes, and prices should be evaluated on what they achieve, that is, profit, where a program budget may best assess the quality of their decisions and actions.

The last two conditions, predictability of revenues and environmental stability, should be assessed to identify the proper budget for the operating conditions the organization faces. If revenues change proportionately with output, expense allocations should rise and fall with output, and flexible and activity-based budgets provide this feature. If an organization receives fixed funding divorced from output, increasing output will not generate additional funds and expense should not be allowed to rise to exceed expected revenue. Incremental budgets provide managers with a fixed and known budget constraint. Budgeting system choices should be contingent on whether output increases

generate sufficient funds to cover additional expenses to expand output (sales-based) or whether revenue is fixed (government grants, fund-raising, etc.).

Environmental stability asks how quickly the operating environment is changing and whether rapid managerial decision-making and action are needed. In static environments with slow change in consumer demand, production technology, and resource prices, slow-moving, if not static, budgeting systems can be employed. Incremental budgets are appropriate in stable environments, where what was done last year may be appropriate to continue. Zero-base and program budgets that elevate the decisions on trade-offs to senior managers and remove budget choices from frontline managers are slow to respond to changes. In a rapidly evolving environment, where managers need to make rapid product choice and production method decisions, flexible and activity-based budgets provide the greatest support and proper incentives for rapid decision-making. Different budgeting systems are more appropriate for cost, expense, revenue, profit, and investment centers and the goal of the budget. Once a budget is constructed, the hardest tasks remain: the budget must be used to facilitate and control operations and evaluate managers.

TABLE 17.1 highlights the primary differences in budgeting systems; managers should understand their assumptions, structures, strengths, and weaknesses and pick the system that is most likely to provide the maximum support for organizational objectives.

TABLE 17.1 Overview of Budgeting Systems

Budgeting System	Assumptions	Structure and Design	Strengths	Weaknesses
Incremental	- No change in total expense with output or constant output - Effective and efficient production methods - Goods and services needed or desired	- Internal and operational focus - 1-year horizon - Input-driven - Metric: total cost, actual ≤ budget	- Easy to construct - Focus on change - Fixed spending target provided	- Lack of focus on efficiency or effectiveness - Budget not tied to actual output - Institutionalization of past practices - Dependence on accuracy of output forecast - Adverse incentives
Flexible	- Change in total expense directly with output - Fluctuation in output precluding precise forecasts - Variable (marginal) cost identifiable	- Internal and operational focus - 1-year horizon - Output-driven - Metric: actual cost per unit ≤ budgeted cost per unit (↓ ATC)	- Deeper understanding of operations required - Increase and decrease of budget with actual output - Decentralized decision-making - Simplified review and evaluation - Efficiency emphasized	- More time to prepare and restate budget required - Increase and decrease of budget with actual output - Unstable budget target - Decoupled revenue and expense
Zero-base	- Need for every dollar spent to be justified every year - Current output probably unnecessary and unmet needs probably arising - Alternative production methods and sizes to be explored - Competition to created between alternative outputs	- Internal and planning focus - 1-year horizon - Throughput-, output-, and outcome-driven - Metric: marginal cost/output ≤ other decision packages	- Explicit priorities - Bottom-up construction - Understanding of expenses, output, and value - Creates choice - Creates competition across departments - Identifies redundancies - Emphasizes efficiency	- More time required to construct multiple budgets - Difficulty in reducing existing programs - Data-gaming

	Description	Focus	Advantages	Disadvantages
Program	- Budgets based on results, that is, outcomes - Goals set by senior managers - Outcomes requiring input across departments and costs to reflect *all* costs regardless of origin - Competition to be created between alternative methods to reach goals	- External and planning focus - Multiyear horizon - Outcome-driven - Metric: cost/outcome ≤ other programs	- Focus on goals - Pursues lowest cost means to an end - Creates competition across goals and methods - Identifies redundancies - Emphasizes effectiveness	- Difficulty in defining and measuring outcomes - Administrative problems for programs spanning multiple departments - Allocating costs for programs that produce more outcome - Allocation of overhead
Activity-based	- Existing budgets designed for accounting rather than management, that is, lack of useful cost information - Resources often misdirected - Output prices probably not reflecting costs	- Internal and operational focus - 1-year horizon - Throughput-driven - Metric: cost per cost object, including cost/activity ≤ budgeted cost/activity; and number of activities ≤ budgeted activity	- Process view of work provided - Responsibility and accountability placed on employees - Cause of budget variances identified - Accuracy of product costing improved - Visibility of capacity issues elevated - Improved ability to control and manage work: what should occur versus what is occurring	- Complexity, requiring manager training and understanding - Time to prepare and maintain

▸ The Financial Role of a Manager

Managers are expected to be competent in a broad range of fields; at a minimum, managers should be expected to be proficient in the field of activity they are managing, such as medicine, nursing, dietary, etc., summarized as operations management, in **FIGURE 17.3**, and in the supporting fields of finance, human resources, and information management. Figure 17.3 recognizes the multidiscipline responsibilities of managers and highlights the role of budget construction and variance analysis in the pantheon of finance. All managers are responsible for financial performance, whether they create a budget or they don't, as they are entrusted with the use of resources, and no organization can provide unlimited resources to complete tasks. Human resources and IT skills are needed as managers select, train, motivate, and/or supervise subordinates and produce and use information on a daily basis. The primary

financial roles of a department manager are building and using budgets.

Managers should be coaches and facilitators for their employees. They should monitor employee performance, identify opportunities for improvement, demonstrate improved methods, and provide necessary resources. Managers should also be expected to ensure the quality of work performed in their departments and steward nonhuman resources. The budget should provide standards to monitor employees, output (defects, etc.), outcomes (customer satisfaction, etc.), and assets. Budgets should encourage managers to expand their roles from safeguarding resources to improving and optimizing. As seen in the life and work of Henry Ford, astute managers can produce a profound change beyond their industry and benefit the lives of their customers and workers and all humankind.

Fulfilling these roles does not require the vision of Ford, but it can be driven by effective financial tools that focus managers' attention on how operations can be improved. These tools include budgeting, variance analysis, and

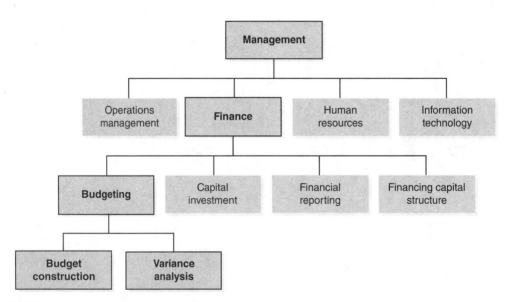

FIGURE 17.3 Management Functions and Primary Financial Responsibilities

ratio analysis. Budgeting is a financial plan of where an organization wants to go and how it expects to get there, and provides a simplified model of the interrelationships between output, revenue, and costs. The first task of a manager is to understand how work is performed and how costs are incurred in his or her department on the basis of what it produces and achieves.

Once the budget is constructed, it must be used to justify its creation. Managers should be capable of using variance analysis to explain deviations between actual and expected performance. Why are expenses greater or less than the budget? Is it because of price, efficiency, intensity, and/or volume variances, and are these factors within the control of the manager? If an expense is controllable, is the manager using variance information to control operations? Variance analysis supplies the answers to "what is occurring" questions; why it is occurring and how performance can be improved is up to the manager.

The third essential financial tool to improve operations is ratio analysis, including operating indicators and benchmarking. Ratio analysis and operating indicators address "what is" questions and are used in conjunction with industry averages and more so with best-in-class benchmarks to provide insight into what could be. How does the organization perform relative to the industry average or industry leader, what aspects of the organization could be improved, and how can these opportunities be tracked to the performance of individual departments? Managers who understand the information that accounting supplies and are given appropriate incentives will distinguish themselves in the organization.

As managers with financial acumen advance within the organization, achieving greater decision-making authority, they require competency in higher-level financial functions such as capital budgeting (Chapter 13); cost–benefit and cost-effectiveness analyses (Chapter 14); financing, working capital management, and financial risk management (Chapter 15); and strategic financial planning (Chapter 16).

▶ Financial Management and the Future of Health Care

It is unlikely that financial management will do anything other than increase in importance and prominence in health care. Recent demographic and economic changes in society and the healthcare industry point toward

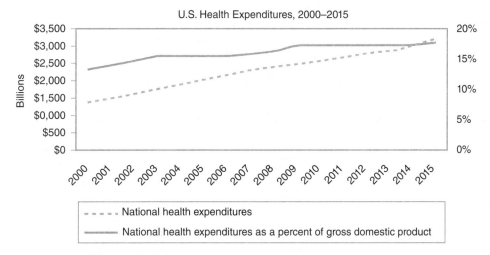

FIGURE 17.4 Growth in Health Expenditures

continuing growth in healthcare expenditures, and questions of whether citizens and patients are receiving appropriate value for their healthcare dollars will grow with expenditures. **FIGURE 17.4** shows the growth in healthcare expenditures in the United States; total expenditures show constant growth, but the acceleration of growth in the percentage of the gross domestic product (GDP) spent on health care is alarming. The growth in the percentage of economic output devoted to health care starkly demonstrates the concept of opportunity costs; the 17.8% of U.S. GDP spent on health care cannot be used for education, nutrition, housing, or any other goods. Contrasts of U.S. spending with other countries (U.K. 8.8%, Canada 10.7%) are regularly reported to suggest U.S. healthcare spending is excessive and wasteful.

Before delivering any judgment on the appropriateness of healthcare spending (which is not coming from this author), it is important to understand why healthcare costs continue to increase. First, the U.S. population is growing by appropriately 1.0% per year, and the population is aging as baby boomers enter retirement. The shift to an older population will accelerate spending as people over the age of 65 consume roughly three times the amount of healthcare services as those under 65. Second, labor-intensive industries, like health care, have severe limits on productivity growth. Capital-intensive industries and agriculture continue to demonstrate astounding ways to increase output and lower costs. Health care, on the other hand, is limited by how fast and long humans can work, and thus the share of our economy or any other economy consumed by labor-intensive industries must increase as capital-intensive industries become more productive. A third factor is that the technology introduced in health care generally increases cost rather than lowering costs. Two recent innovations provide stark examples: electronic medical record systems and robotic surgery impose millions of dollars of cost, while benefits so far appear limited.

While the appropriateness of total spending will not be judged, there is evidence the money is not being used in the most efficacious manner. **FIGURE 17.5** provides an example. In community hospitals, the average cost of an admission is significantly higher in nonprofit and public hospitals than in for-profit hospitals. The cost per admission in for-profit hospitals averages 88.7% of the cost of an admission in a public hospital, while costs in nonprofits are 2.2% higher than public hospitals and 15.2% higher than for-profit hospitals. This difference, evident in operating ratios and indicators, should be investigated. How do for-profit hospitals control costs, and can nonprofit and public hospitals create higher value from their resources? Researchers and writers who cite that the lower costs in other countries have to date failed to identify any concrete lessons that the U.S. public is willing to accept to reduce spending and/or improve health outcomes.

There is an obvious need for better financial management in the U.S. healthcare system. Industry and policy leaders need to understand how the industry functions (positive analysis—what is) before pursuing what should be (normative solutions). The U.S. healthcare system has not benefited from medical personnel and patients seeking to maximize the amount of services delivered and received, lawyers writing legislation, or financial personnel working to maximize profits. The incomplete and parochial views of each guarantee nonoptimal solutions.

What is needed is an improved understanding of the demand for health care, including the uncertainties surrounding government regulation and patient tastes and preferences as well as the impact of income and price elasticities. In conjunction with demand, costs should be better understood; rather than blindly inflating expenses from 1 year to the next, budgets should be created that evaluate the cost of inputs, labor, supplies, machinery, buildings, etc., and assess what they produce. Are outputs effective, and do patients benefits from all the tests and treatments

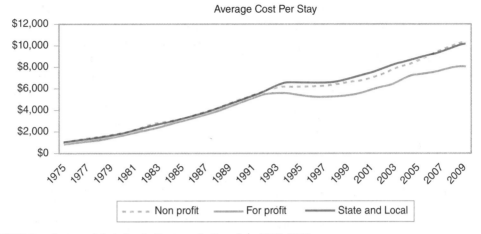

FIGURE 17.5 Cost per Admission in Community Hospitals, 1975–2009

ordered? The blind arms race in medical technology should also be examined: when should a lower-cost X-ray replace a computed tomography (CT) scan or a generic drug be used in place of a name-brand pharmaceutical? Is technology being fully utilized? Similarly, the distribution of health resources should be examined: are there too many providers in urban areas, reducing value by duplicating resources and providing marginal care, while necessary care in rural areas is not delivered?

While these larger issues cannot be addressed in individual organizations, all organizations can benefit from better planning and oversight (what services they provide and how work is performed) and a continual focus on how things can be improved. Improvement at the organizational and department levels is where financial management and budgeting can provide immense benefits. The challenge for physicians, nurses, and other healthcare workers is that if they do not develop financial skills, they will have to rely on nonmedical staff. Rather than being dependent on, if not at the mercy of, financial staff, it is imperative that healthcare professionals recognize the role finance plays in their organizations and take the necessary steps to develop financial competence. Financial competency starts with budgeting and variance analysis.

What individual employees can do to improve health care is clear when value is defined as follows:

$$\text{Value} = \frac{\text{Output}}{\text{Cost}} \qquad (17.1)$$

Value will increase if current output can be produced at lower cost ($\uparrow$value = output/ $\downarrow$cost) or if superior outputs and outcomes are produced from existing resources ($\uparrow$value = $\uparrow$output/cost). Both goals require knowing the desired output, the goal it is designed to fulfill, and the resources currently being consumed. The eight Lean wastes highlight what everyone can do to increase value by reducing overproduction, overprocessing, excessive motion, excessive transport, excess inventory, defects, and idleness and ensuring resources are employed in their best use. The majority of these wastes speak directly to reducing costs (the denominator), but three deal with improving/increasing output (the numerator), that is, lowering defects and idleness, and using resources to the extent of their capabilities. While overproduction, overprocessing, excessive motion, excessive transport, and excess inventory speak to reducing unnecessary output and improving systems and processes to use less resources, lowering defects and idleness and directing resources to their best uses are means to increase the desirability and functionality of the outputs produced.

Equation 17.1 also presents two other possibilities to increase value:

- Value will be greater if an increase in cost produces proportionately larger increases in output ($\uparrow$ value $= \uparrow\uparrow$ output/$\uparrow$ cost). If more output is desired by consumers and a 10% increase in cost produces a greater than 10% increase in output, value increases. This possibility is realizable if current resources are idle or underemployed and only need complimentary inputs to produce more output.

- The second option is interesting as it recommends counterintuitive action: value can be increased when output is lowered if costs fall by a greater percentage ($\uparrow$ value $= \downarrow$ output/$\downarrow\downarrow$ cost). In health care this could be accomplished by reducing overproduction, that is, is the number of tests and procedures critical to patient care? Do tests that reveal the absence of disease add value? The answer is yes; there is a benefit to knowing what you do not have, but is the value of peace of mind worth the cost of the test? Many studies indicate that hundreds of billions of dollars are spent annually for tests and procedures that may have minimal impact on patient health. In 1999, the Institute of Medicine (IOM) reported in *To Err is Human* that medical errors cost the United States between $17 and $29 billion (in 1997 dollars), half of which was attributed to additional medical spending and the other half to lost wages. In 2013, the IOM released *Best Care at Lower Cost*, which concluded that $750 billion (25% of all healthcare spending) was lost to medical error. Given the difference in these two estimates, it is clear that healthcare professionals first need the skills to identify low-value services and second need the courage to reduce these services.

Equation 17.1 highlights what all employees should understand: value is determined by what is produced and how it is produced. The net value of output is determined by the worth consumers place on the quantity and quality of the product produced (the consumption side) less the value of resources consumed (the production side). We should never lose sight of the fact that the goal of health care is not to produce goods and services but rather to improve the health of patients, so outcomes as well as outputs must be considered when allocating resources. *A Comprehensive Guide to Budgeting for Health Care Managers* encourages readers to see and use budgets as a tool to illuminate how operations function and the trade-offs managers face every day—will increasing or decreasing the use of an input increase or decrease the worth of goods and services produced to consumers and the value of the organization? The simple calculus between inputs consumed and the value of outputs must be understood by managers to ensure operations are effective and efficient.

Summary

Every system is perfectly designed to produce the results it achieves. If a budget produces dysfunctional behavior (shoddy high-cost goods and services), it is due to the fact that it was *designed* to do so and no one wishes it to produce a better result. On the other hand, a budget that encourages employees to do their best—produce the best product for the customer at the lowest-possible price—is a result of conscious design. Incremental budgets are designed to ensure employees spend every dollar allocated, and we can hardly criticize people for responding to the primary incentive incremental budgeting offers.

Use of other budgeting systems encourages different behavior; if we want budgets that encourage efficiency or maximize outcomes, we must implement new tools and incentives. Once new budget tools and incentives are in place, they must be used rather than placed on a shelf to be referenced when the next budget is constructed. Improvement cannot be achieved by doing the same things in the same way as they were in the past, yet administrative practices are often set in the past. The usefulness of budgeting, an administrative practice, will increase when it is viewed as a help rather than a hindrance to managers. Budgeting should be viewed as a way to simplify and understand what a department and the larger organization do and judge performance. Activity-based budgeting offers the best guide to operational improvement by focusing on what products are produced, specifying what activities should be performed, and defining the cost per activity. Activity-based budgeting provides the elements to identify the eight Lean wastes: overproduction, overprocessing, excessive motion, excessive transport, excess inventory, disproportionate defects, underutilized resources, and idleness.

A budget is only the first step toward effective financial management; managers should be guided by the budget, and this requires identifying variances and taking action to minimize unnecessary expenditures. Managers should be able to compare their operations to similar organizations and identify where they can do a better job. Financial ratios and operating indicators provide the information to identify improvement opportunities and drill down into operations to determine which factors can be improved. More challenging is the ability to recognize and act on future prospects; cost–benefit analysis, cost-effectiveness analysis, and capital budgeting provide the framework to assess future investments.

Skills in budgeting, variance analysis, ratio analysis, and capital budgeting must be supplemented as a person moves up the management ladder; senior managers must ensure departments work together, sufficient resources are available to meet short- and long-term obligations, cost of capital and risks are minimized, and a feasible strategic financial plan is in place. These higher-level responsibilities are predicated on budgets; estimates

of cash reserves and expansion plans should not exist independently of annual operating budgets. Senior managers, like department managers, must recognize when current operations are not advancing the organization's long-range plans and make appropriate adjustments whether this requires improving suboptimal performance, changing the mix of goods and services provided, or scaling back plans. Management is impossible without the understanding budgets and accounting provide—ensuring superiors and subordinates agree on what should be done and whether it is being accomplished. Budgets provide the assumptions, targets, and incentives detailing what constitutes superior performance and how it is rewarded.

In *The Art of War* (~400), Sun Tzu noted:

> The general who wins a battle makes many calculations in his temple, here the battle is fought. The general who loses a battle makes but few calculations beforehand. Thus do many calculations lead to victory and few calculations to defeat: how much more no calculation at all! It is by attention to this point that I can foresee who is likely to win or lose.

While a well-constructed budget cannot guarantee success, it is clear managers who understand the inflows and outflows of resources have a distinct advantage over rivals who do not know their products and costs or how costs should change with output. Budget-savvy managers know how much financial misfortune their organization can sustain and can see, when misfortune comes, how long it will take to return the organization to its desired financial position. While budgets will never allow managers to see the future, the skills gained from creating good budgets will make them more capable of dealing with unforeseeable changes and ensuring their own and their organization's success.

The central idea in finance is no margin, no mission; organizations that cannot cover their costs do not survive. *A Comprehensive Guide to Budgeting for Health Care Managers* was designed to demonstrate that producing a margin depends on accurately estimating revenues and costs and managing operations to the financial plan to the extent possible to ensure the highest-possible profit is earned so that the organization can continue to operate. No measurement → no management → no mission better emphasizes the desired role of managers; know the desired goals and how they are measured and take the necessary steps to achieve those goals. In the absence of unforeseen events, budget goals should be realized; when unforeseen events arise, the budget should specify the best-possible financial outcome and guide the steps necessary to achieve it. Budgeting is *the* tool that specifies organizational goals and allows managers to assess progress toward these goals. Managers, whether employed in for-profit, nonprofit, or public organizations, who do not master budgeting have their goals and destinies dictated by others.

If cost increases in health care are ever going to be controlled, healthcare managers must first understand budgeting systems and the incentives they establish. If effectiveness and efficiency are going to be improved, organizations must use budgets that focus managers' attention on these outcomes. Second, managers are going to have to understand costs better; activity-based budgets and variance analysis that recognize the impact of changes in efficiency and intensity on costs must become common tools in managers' work. Third, value, defined as output divided by cost, must be internalized by all employees. When employees come to work every day with the goal of maximizing value by increasing output or, better yet, improving outcomes, while maintaining or reducing costs, we will take the first steps away from the unsustainable *status quo* to a better health system for patients, healthcare workers, and healthcare payers.

References

Case, K. E., & Fair, R. C. (1989). *Principles of economics*. Englewood Cliffs, NJ: Prentice Hall.

Ford, H. (1923). *My life and work*. Garden City, NJ: Doubleday, Page.

Institute of Medicine. (1999). *To err is human*. Washington, DC: National Academies Press.

Institute of Medicine. (2013). *Best care at lower cost*. Washington, DC: National Academies Press.

Sun, T. (1910, original work published ~400). *The art of war* (G. Lionel, Trans.). Retrieved from http://classics.mit.edu/Tzu/artwar.html

Glossary

4 Ps of marketing product, price, physical distribution, and promotion.

5S a five-step process to organize work to optimize output.

A

Activity (in activity-based costing or budgeting) a step in a production process that generates expense.

Activity-based budgeting a budgeting system that bases resource allocations on the number of activities expected to be required to produce outputs.

Activity-based costing a cost accounting method that seeks to trace costs to output via activities performed to minimize reliance on cost allocation and produce more accurate product costs.

Activity cost assignment tracking of activities to cost drivers, recognizing that seemingly similar products or customers may consume different amounts of resources.

Adjusted R^2 (the coefficient of determination) the percentage of change in a dependent variable explained by changes in independent variables.

Allocative efficiency a situation in which a good or a service is produced up to the point where marginal benefit equals marginal cost.

Annualizing estimation of the expected total for an entire year, or 12 months, on the basis of partial-year or less than 12 months of data.

Annuities a series of equal payments.

Annuity due a series of equal cash flows paid or received at the start of a year.

B

Balanced scorecard an organizational assessment tool that evaluates financial performance, customer satisfaction, the effectiveness and efficiency of production processes, and learning and development activities.

Bankruptcy inability to satisfy creditor claims with existing assets.

Benchmarking comparison of an organization's processes and outcomes with those of other organizations.

Bounded rationality a constraint on reaching optimal decisions arising from the inherent limits of the human mind, incomplete information, and limited time to make decisions.

Budget the operating plan of a department or organization, expressed in monetary terms.

Budget standard budgeted input cost per output, cost standard plus expected price increase.

Business risk the risks inherent in an organization's operations that may reduce profit.

C

Capital structure the mix of equity and debt used to finance assets.

Capital structure ratios values that measure how assets are financed and the ability of the organization to meet all its financial obligations.

Cash flow statement a tool that reports a change in an organization's cash balance over time and its sources and uses of cash.

Chart of accounts an accounting system providing numeric codes for categorizing expenses, revenues, assets, and liability transactions.

Competitive advantage something an organization does better than its rivals that is valued by customers.

Compound growth rate the annual increase in a numeric series calculated using the formula $r = (Y / X)(1 / n) - 1$.

Consumer price index (CPI) the average price change seen for a market basket of goods and services purchased by an urban consumer.

Consumer sovereignty the assertion that consumer preferences determine the type and number of goods and services produced.

Contribution margin the difference between price and average variable cost or a change in profit from selling one additional unit.

Cost-benefit analysis (CBA) a tool that compares the benefits and costs of an activity measured in dollars to determine whether it creates value.

Cost-effectiveness analysis (CEA) a tool that quantifies the outcome (benefit) of an activity costs in nonmonetary units and compares the cost measured in dollars of an alternative means to achieve an end.

Cost driver an event that initiates activity and generates costs.

Cost object the final repository for cost collection, that is, the total cost of a product, customer, etc.

Cost of capital the amount an organization must pay to use money.

Cost standard input cost per output, the productivity standard multiplied by input price.

Cost variances differences between actual expenses and budgeted expenditures arising from the cost of inputs consumed, often inappropriately called price variance.

D

Decision package a description of an activity, its goals, how it is accomplished and how it could be accomplished, the resources consumed, and its benefits developed to allow comparison with other activities.

Delphi method a forecasting method that relies on anonymous input from two or more people who subsequently receive group feedback and can alter their forecast on the basis of the feedback they receive. The process of input, feedback, and revision continues until a consensus forecast is reached.

Depreciation the estimated cost of using buildings and equipment during an accounting period, a noncash expense.

Diminishing marginal returns the declining increase in output accompanying increases in variable costs when a fixed input is present.

Discount rate the interest rate used to determine the value of future cash flows.

Divisional organizational structures authority lines and operations organized around products or markets to concentrate knowledge of and ability to respond quickly to customer needs and desires.

Durable good a physical product that provides benefits to a consumer for a prolonged period, usually more than 3 years.

E

Economies of scale the reduction in cost per unit resulting from increasing the number of units produced or a situation in which the percentage increase in the average total cost is less than the percentage increase in output.

Effectiveness achieving a goal.

Efficiency minimizing the cost per output or maximizing output from a set of inputs.

Efficiency variances the difference between actual expenses and budgeted expenditures arising from over- or underconsumption of inputs.

Elastic a situation in which a percentage change in price results in a greater percentage change in the quantity sold in the opposite direction.

Element (in program budgeting) an alternative means to an end.

Equity the question of what is a "fair" distribution of a society's economic goods among its members.

Exponential smoothing a forecasting method that bases future estimates on a user-specified weighted average of actual results (α) and prior forecast ($1 - \alpha$).

External analysis the process of identifying and evaluating the opportunities and threats in an organization's operating environment.

External scan a study of changes in an organization's environment to identify opportunities and threats.

Externalities benefits received or costs imposed on nonparticipants to an economic transaction.

F

Featherbedding the employment of unnecessary resources.

Financial competence having the knowledge, skills, and ability to respond to issues and challenges to improve the economic performance of an organization.

Financial leverage the use of debt to increase returns to equity holders, measured as the ratio of debt to total assets.

Financial risk the risk associated with meeting contracted interest and principal payments on debt.

Fisher equation nominal interest rate (i), the expected inflation rate (π^e) + real interest rate (i_r).

Flexible budgeting a budgeting system that bases preliminary resource allocations on the expected output and retrospectively increases or decreases allocations on the basis of actual output.

Free riders individuals who do not contribute to the costs of goods but receive some benefit from the goods.

Full-cost pricing a process of establishing a minimum price for a good or service that covers its fixed and variable costs.

Full-time equivalents (FTE) the number of hours paid to a full-time employee, 2080 hours per year (40 hours/week × 52 weeks).

Functional organizational structures authority lines and operation organized around activities performed to maximize technical expertise.

H

Hawthorne effect the impact on a person's behavior resulting from being observed.

High/low method a method of estimating the fixed and variable components of a process by calculating the change in inputs used or costs incurred between the highest and lowest output periods.

I

Income redistribution the idea that income inequities should be remediated by government action, shifting resources from high-income groups to low-income groups.

Incremental budgeting a budgeting system that bases resource allocations on historical expenses adjusted for expected changes in input and output prices.

Inelastic a situation in which a percentage change in price results in a smaller percentage change in the quantity sold in the opposite direction.

Inflation a general increase in wages and prices.

Intensity variances differences between actual expenses and budgeted expenditures arising from changes in the output produced.

Internal analysis the process of identifying and evaluating an organization's key strengths and weaknesses.

Iron triangle the self-reinforcing relationship between interest groups, elected officials, and public employees supporting the continuation and expansion of public programs.

J

Job order costing a cost accounting method that determines the cost of a good or services on the basis of resources consumed.

L

Law of demand as prices increase, less product will be sold.

League tables a table ranking interventions by their cost-effectiveness ratio, typically from the lowest cost to the highest cost per outcome.

Liquidity a measure of how quickly an asset can be converted to cash at full value.

Liquidity ratios tools that measure the ability of an organization to meet its short-term financial obligations.

M

Marginal cost pricing the process of establishing a minimum price for a good or service that recoups the additional costs incurred to produce it (variable costs) and ignores the fixed cost that must be paid whether additional output is produced or isn't.

Marginal or incremental cost the change in total cost resulting from a one-unit increase or decrease in output.

Marginal product (MP) the change in output attributable to increasing an input by one unit while holding other inputs constant.

Marginal rate of technical substitution (MRTS) the rate at which one input must be increased while a second is decreased to maintain constant output.

Marginal revenue product (MRP) the change in total revenue attributable to increasing one input by one unit while holding all other inputs constant.

Marginalism the change in benefits and costs resulting from a decision or action.

Market failures the inability of economic markets to reach optimal resource allocations due to the existence of externalities, public goods, or monopolies.

Market organization a categorization system that classifies industries by the number of producers and extent of competition.

Master budget the compilation of departmental budgets into a single organizational budget to assess total inflows and outflows of funds.

Mission an organization's reason for existing.

Monopolistic competition a market with many producers who have limited control over price.

Monopoly a market where one firm produces a product that has no close substitutes and exercises complete control over price in the absence of price regulation.

Moral hazard the incentive created for an individual to consume larger quantities of a good or service when its price is partially or fully subsidized by others.

MOST mission, objectives, strategy, and tactics.

Moving average a forecasting method that calculates future estimates on an average of prior activity where the user determines the number of prior periods to use.

N

Net working capital current assets minus current liabilities.

Net worth the claim owners of an organization have on assets, that is, equity.

Nominal value the current price of a good or service.

Nondurable goods a physical product whose usefulness is exhausted in a short period, usually under 3 years.

O

Oligopoly a market with a small number of producers who consider the reactions of their rivals to their competitive actions and have extensive influence over price.

Operating indicators a method of measuring organizational performance by examining the relationship between financial measures and outputs and between outputs produced and inputs consumed.

Operating leverage the percentage of fixed costs to total cost in an organization's cost structure.

Opportunism the practice of exploiting situations for personal gain without regard for the impact on others.

Opportunity cost the alternative foregone.

Ordinary annuity a series of equal cash flows paid or received at the end of a year.

Organizational architecture a management system designed around decision rights, compensation structures, and performance reporting systems.

P

Pareto 80/20 rule 20% of causes (activities) account for 80% of effects (costs).

Pareto improvement reallocation of resources that makes one or more people better off without making anyone else worse off.

Pareto optimality a situation in which any reallocation of resources will have an adverse effect on one or more people.

Parkinson's law the idea that expense rises to meet revenues. Parkinson's corollary: financial success requires violating Parkinson's law, that is, keeping the increase in expenses under the increase in revenues.

Perfect competition a market with many producers where none can influence price.

Portfolio analysis a methodology for comparing alternatives on two criteria in a 2×2 matrix to illustrate choices (originally developed by the Boston Consulting Group on the basis of market share and growth).

Prevalence the proportion of a population with a disease at a point in time.

Price elasticity the ratio of the percentage change in demand for a product, given a percentage change in its price.

Price variances differences between actual expenses and budgeted expenditures arising from changes in input prices.

Pro forma financial statements what-if financial statements assuming future business transactions will be completed as contemplated.

Process (or absorption) costing a cost accounting method that estimates the cost of a good or service by dividing total cost equally over outputs.

Producer price index (PPI) the average price change seen by producers for the goods and services they purchase over time.

Product life cycle a model that predicts revenue on the basis of the age of a good or service.

Production function the relationship between the amount of inputs consumed and the amount of output produced.

Productivity output per worker.

Productivity standard input units per output.

Profitability ratios tools that measure the ability of management to generate more revenues than expenses, that is, create value.

Program (in program budgeting) the major goal of an organization and whom it will serve.

Program budgeting a budgeting system where resource allocations are based on the outcome produced.

Program evaluation a framework to evaluate the performance of systems that assesses goals, processes (what is done and how it is done), outcomes, and cost.

Public goods goods that can be consumed without reducing the benefit enjoyed by others (nonrival) and that cannot be withheld from individuals who do not contribute to their cost (nonexclusive).

p-Value the probability of obtaining a calculated coefficient when the independent variable is unrelated to the dependent variable.

Q

Quality-adjusted life year (QALY) a means to measure the effectiveness of healthcare treatment, given the change in life expectancy and the degree to which prefect health is achieved.

R

Ratio analysis a method of measuring and assessing financial performance by relating one financial variable to another.

Real value the price of a good or service based on the purchasing power of the dollar in a former time period.

Resource cost assignment input price divided by the expected number of activities the input will provide, that is, cost per activity.

Return on investment (ROI) the ratio of the net income generated from an expenditure of funds and its initial acquisition cost.

Revenue cycle the steps taken to obtain cash for goods and services produced.

Risk avoidance a situation that occurs when pro-viders recognize an attempt to shift cost, utilization, or actuarial risk through a managed care contract and do not accept it

Risk retention a situation that occurs when a pro-vider understands a monetary risk assumed and negotiates a reimbursement rate to cover its poten-tial cost

Risk transfer a situation where a provider accepts risk but shifts its impact to others through stop-loss or re-insurance arrangements.

Risk/return trade-off the idea that higher finan-cial returns can only be earned if investors accept higher risk.

S

Salvage value the expected resale price of an asset at the end of its useful life.

Services nonphysical products.

Silo thinking the unwillingness to share informa-tion or coordinate work between departments.

Social welfare the well-being of the entire society.

Solvency the condition of having more assets than liabilities.

Specialization limiting the number of tasks a worker performs to increase productivity; in some cases, maximum productivity is achieved when a worker performs a single task.

Standard gamble a means to determine the value of less-than-perfect health states by a person's will-ingness to accept a treatment that would cure his or her condition or end his or her life.

Stewardship the responsibility for safeguarding the resources of others.

Strategic decision-making selecting long-term goals and the means that will be used to achieve those goals.

Strategic management the process of setting organizational goals and instituting systems capable of reaching the goals set.

Structure-conduct-performance paradigm a framework that holds that the number of compet-itors in a market and the products sold determines competitive actions and financial performance.

Subprogram (in program budgeting) part of a program that satisfies one end of the major program goal.

Sunk costs costs of previously committed resources that cannot be controlled by current man-agers.

Sustainable growth the maximum rate of growth in assets an organization can maintain without increasing financial leverage, that is, debt-to-equity ratio.

SWOT diagram strengths, weaknesses, oppor-tunities, and threats diagrammatically shown in a four-quadrant space to assist planners in identifying the competitive position of their organization and optimal strategies.

System a set of inputs and procedures for accom-plishing a task or achieving a goal.

T

Tactical decision-making and action the day-to-day choices and alterations to resource use made to advance an organization's goals.

Target-base budgeting a zero-base budgeting (ZBB) process that requires review of only new and/or discretionary funds.

Technical efficiency a situation in which output cannot be increased by increasing the use of one input and decreasing the consumption of another.

Technology assessment the systematic evalu-ation of the effects of new technology on people, society, and the environment.

Time and motion studies a procedure for break-ing work into simple tasks and recording the time taken to complete each task.

Time-driven activity-based costing a method of determining the cost of an activity on the basis of how long a resource should be employed, depend-ing on direct observation and its acquisition cost.

Time trade-off a means to determine how many years a person would accept of perfect health in exchange for a higher number of years in dimin-ished health.

Total compensation the total cost of hiring an employee, including the salary and fringe benefits.

Turnover ratios tools that measure the productivity of assets

Two-part tariff expenses that include a fixed and per unit consumed charge.

U

Uncertainty the inability to know how a system operates, how it will evolve, and/or what impact actions will have on its performance.

Unitary elastic a situation in which a percentage change in price results in an equal percentage change in the quantity sold in the opposite direction.

Unity of command the principle that subordinates should report to a single superior.

V

Value chain the set of activities and resources an organization uses to deliver a product to customers.

Viability the condition of having higher revenues than expenses.

Voice of customer (VOC) a process for assessing the needs and requirements of customers before or after a product has been produced.

Volume variances differences between actual expenses and budgeted expenditures arising from producing more or less output.

W

Weighted cost of capital the average cost to an organization to acquire funds depending on its mix of debt and equity financing.

Z

Zero-base budgeting (ZBB) a budgeting system that assumes every dollar of expense should be justified and determines resource allocations by comparing different levels of expense and output.

Zero-base performance auditing an objective examination of operations focusing on whether the activities, costs, and benefits expected in the budget were realized.

Zero-base review a ZBB process that supplements annual budgeting processes where expenditures are examined annually every 5 years or so to determine whether reallocation is desirable.

Index

Page numbers followed by *b*, *f*, or *t* indicate material in boxes, figures, or tables, respectively.